Human reproductive behaviour

Human reproductive behaviour

a Darwinian

perspective

Edited by

Laura Betzig,
Monique Borgerhoff Mulder
and Paul Turke

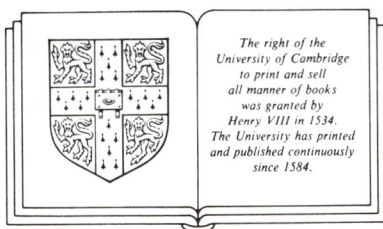

The right of the
University of Cambridge
to print and sell
all manner of books
was granted by
Henry VIII in 1534.
The University has printed
and published continuously
since 1584.

CAMBRIDGE UNIVERSITY PRESS

Cambridge

New York   New Rochelle

Melbourne   Sydney

Published by the Press Syndicate of the University of Cambridge
The Pitt Building, Trumpington Street, Cambridge CB2 1RP
32 East 57th Street, New York, NY 10022, USA
10 Stamford Road, Oakleigh, Melbourne 3166, Australia

First published 1988

Printed in Great Britain at The Bath Press, Avon

British Library cataloguing in publication data

Human reproductive behaviour: a Darwinian
perspective.—(Cambridge studies in
biological anthropology).
1. Sex (Psychology)   2. Reproduction
3. Evolution
I. Betzig, Laura   II. Mulder, Monique
Borgerhoff   III. Turke, Paul
155.3   BF692

Library of Congress cataloguing in publication data

Human reproductive behaviour.
1. Sex customs—Cross-cultural studies.   2. Marriage
customs and rites—Cross-cultural studies.   3. Child
rearing—Cross-cultural studies.   4. Human reproduction—
Cross-cultural studies.   I. Betzig, Laura L., 1953–
II. Mulder, Monique Borgerhoff.   III. Turke, Paul.
GN848.3.H85   1988   306.7   87–6629

ISBN 0 521 32738 5 hard covers
ISBN 0 521 33796 8 paperback

Contents

v

Contributors

Alexander, Richard D., Museum of Zoology, University of Michigan, Ann Arbor, MI 48109, USA

Berté, Nancy A., Department of Anthropology, Northwestern University, Evanston, IL 60201, USA

Betzig, Laura, Museum of Zoology, University of Michigan, Ann Arbor, MI 48109, USA

Boone, James L., III Department of Anthropology, University of New Mexico, Albuquerque, NM 87131, USA

Borgerhoff Mulder, Monique, Department of Zoology Large Animal Research Group, University of Cambridge, Cambridge, CB3 0DT, UK

Brown, Donald E., Department of Anthropology, University of California, Santa Barbara, CA 93106, USA

Chagnon, Napoleon A., Department of Anthropology, University of California, Santa Barbara, CA 93106, USA

Crook, John H., Department of Psychology, University of Bristol, Bristol, BS8 1HH, UK

Crook, Stamati J., St Catherine's College, Oxford University, Oxford, UK

Dunbar, Robin I. M., Department of Zoology, University of Liverpool, Brownlow Street, PO Box 147, Liverpool, L69 3BX, UK

Essock-Vitale, Susan M., Department of Psychiatry, School of Medicine, University of California at Los Angeles, Los Angeles, CA 90024, USA

Flinn, Mark V., Department of Anthropology, University of Missouri, Columbia, MO 65201, USA

Gaulin, Steven J. C., Department of Anthropology, University of Pittsburgh, Pittsburgh, PA 15260, USA

Hames, Raymond B., Anthropology Department, University of Nebraska, Lincoln, NE 68588, USA

Hewlett, Barry S., Department of Sociology and Anthropology, Southern Oregon State College, Ashland, OR 97520, USA

Hill, Kim, Department of Anthropology, Emory University, Atlanta, GA 30322, USA

Hoffman, Harol A., Department of Anthropology, University of North Carolina, Greensboro, NC 27401, USA

Hotra, Dana, Department of Anthropology, University of California, Santa Barbara, CA 93106, USA

Irons, William, Department of Anthropology, Northwestern University, Evanston, IL 60201, USA

Kaplan, Hillard, Department of Anthropology, University of New Mexico, Albuquerque, NM 87131, USA

Low, Bobbi S., Evolution and Human Behavior Program and School of Natural Resources, University of Michigan, Ann Arbor, MI 48109, USA

McGuire, Michael T., Psychiatry Service, Sepulveda Veterans Administration Medical Center, Sepulveda, CA 91343, USA

Turke, Paul W., Evolution and Human Behavior Program and Department of Anthropology, University of Michigan, Ann Arbor, MI 48109, USA

Voland, Ekhart, Institut für Anthropologie, Universität Göttingen, Göttingen D-3400, FRG

Preface

Right from the beginning we should stress that attempts to provide evolutionary explanations for the diversity of human social behaviour are just starting out. Empirical evidence is often limited; methods can often be improved; and many conclusions remain open to alternative explanations. Under such circumstances, two courses of action are open. One, by far the most often taken, is criticism. The other is an attempt to do better work. In this book, we have tried to put together some of the best studies to date that tackle the issue of the adaptive significance of human behaviour.

After arranging a series of symposia at the 1984 meetings of the American Anthropological Association in Denver, we invited anthropologists, biologists and psychologists interested in whether and how human action may have been shaped by natural selection to contribute chapters to a volume addressing two critical aspects of human reproductive behaviour – securing a mate and raising children. While each of the studies in this book leaves ends untied, and many raise more questions than they resolve, all provide novel insights into the adaptive significance of aspects of mating and parental behaviour, and all rely on quantitative data. This book is meant to remedy the fact that there has been so much rhetoric about evolution and human behaviour, and so little data. The work in it convinces us that there is plenty of promise in the Darwinian approach.

Five people whose names are not on the cover helped a great deal in editing. Martin Daly and Margo Wilson, both of the McMaster University Department of Psychology, Randy Thornhill of the University of New Mexico Department of Biology, Nancy Wilmsen Thornhill of the University of New Mexico Department of Anthropology, and Richard Alexander of the University of Michigan Museum of Zoology all made comments on several drafts that substantially improved the final results. Many others helped by reviewing individual chapters. Thanks to Steve Albon, David Buss, Tim Caro, Mildred Dickemann, Robin Dunbar, Mark Flinn, Steve Frank, Alan Grafen, Robert Hinde, Warren Holmes, William Irons, Phyllis Lee, Beverly Strassmann and Donald Symons. The book has benefited greatly from such a collaborative effort.

During the period of editing, we have received financial support from a number of sources. LB thanks the University of Michigan Museum of Zoology for a fellowship during 1985–86, and the University of Michigan Department of Social Psychology for an NIMH fellowship during 1986–87, as well as Billy E. Frye and Gene Burnstein for making these fellowships possible. MBM thanks Northwestern University Department of Anthropology for fellowships during 1985–86 and 1986–87. PT thanks the Population Council for a fellowship during 1986–87. MBM is especially grateful to Tim Clutton-Brock and all the members of the Large Animal Research Group at the Department of Zoology, University of Cambridge, for providing space, facilities, and stimulating ideas; and LB and PT are grateful to Richard Alexander and all the friendly inhabitants of the University of Michigan Museum of Zoology for affording a perfect atmosphere in which both to work at evolutionary biology and raise a family.

Laura Betzig
Monique Borgerhoff Mulder
Paul Turke

Introduction

Laura Betzig[1]

Mating and parenting in Darwinian perspective

In the beginning, there were no females, and there were no males. Like dandelions, successfully established strawberries, and Portuguese man-of-war polyps, the first parents might have made nearly identical offspring, without help or interference from a mate. Barring mutation and other forms of recombination, the first parents and offspring could have shared a perfect identity of genetic interest, and lived and died without conflict (e.g. Alexander 1987).

But females and males evolved. As a result, mothers and fathers had to contend with genetically dissimilar daughters and sons, and with a continuum of increasingly dissimilar kin. And they had, first, to contend with genetically dissimilar mates, before they could even produce them!

For the sake of sex, men and women, like the vast majority of organisms, incur both the costs of mating (e.g. Daly 1978) and of parenting genetically dissimilar children, grandchildren, and non-descendent kin (e.g. Williams 1975, theories of sex include Parker *et al.* 1972, Williams 1975, Maynard Smith 1978, Hamilton 1980). For the sake of sex, human reproductive effort, like the *reproductive effort* (Fisher 1958) of any sexual species, involves both *mating effort*, including effort spent competing for, attracting, and provisioning a mate, and *parental effort* (Low 1978), including effort spent to raise both

[1] Museum of Zoology, University of Michigan, Ann Arbor, MI 48109, USA

3

daughters and sons and those of close kin (cf. Alexander and Borgia 1979).

What follows in this chapter reviews the theory and evidence to date on human mating and parenting from a Darwinian perspective. Theory on the allocation of reproductive effort is interspersed with a review of evidence that people mate and parent in adaptive ways. The chapter concludes with arguments as to why they might not, and implications for further research.

What follows in the rest of the book builds on these theoretical and empirical foundations. These chapters make up the latest attempt to find out whether or not human reproductive behavior is adaptive in a variety of places and times, ranging from contemporary Paraguayan hunters and gatherers to 15th century élite Portuguese.

Mating

As Darwin pointed out, 'It is certain that amongst all animals there is a struggle between the males for possession of the female. This fact is so notorious that it would be superfluous to give instances. Hence, the females have the option of selecting one out of several males' (1871:571). He went so far as to trace sex roles, the 'great eagerness' of males, and relative caution of females, to the fact that 'the female has to spend much organic matter in the formation of her ova, whereas the male expends much force in fierce contests with his rivals' (p. 581).

The reproductive effort of any individual is finite: in theory, effort spent in any one activity precludes spending effort in another (see Fisher 1958, Gadgil and Bossert 1970, Hirschfield and Tinkle 1975, Stearns 1976, 1977). Low (1978) distinguished between two kinds of reproductive effort, mating and parental effort, the last including effort spent raising both offspring and other kin. For any individual female or male, reproductive effort is devoted to parenting at the expense of mating (e.g. Trivers 1972); and effort devoted to mating is made at the expense of parenting (e.g. Wade 1979).

How much reproductive effort should be spent on mating or parenting depends on how much effort is devoted to each by the opposite sex (see e.g. Darwin 1871). Where the amount of parental effort offspring need stays the same,

one sex may benefit by devoting more effort to mating to the extent that the other devotes more effort to parenting. This argument has been used to explain why females and males evolved: as eggs devoted more effort to nurturing offspring, sperm devoted more effort to seeking out eggs (Parker et al. 1972). In almost every case, males can benefit reproductively by mating with more than one female, while females cannot benefit by mating with more than one male (Bateman 1948). More females than males will, then, contribute to the next generation: the effect will be a polygynous breeding system (see Daly and Wilson 1980:80; discussion in Wade and Arnold 1980 and Clutton-Brock 1983; reviews in Partridge and Halliday 1984 and Vehrencamp and Bradbury 1984).

Generally, the sex allocating a smaller proportion of reproductive effort as parental effort benefits most, then, from competing for mate quantity (Bateman 1948, Trivers 1972, Wade 1979). Both sexes, though, may benefit from choosing high quality mates and from excluding others from mates of their choice (see Darwin 1871, Trivers 1972).

Mate competition

In raising children, women are physiologically committed to spending nine months gestating and up to nine years lactating (Howell 1979) although 2–3-years lactating is usual in traditional cultures (Bongaarts and Potter 1983). Men need only to spend as much time as it takes to make enough viable sperm. On the other hand, children are sufficiently altricial (e.g. Lovejoy 1981) that their ability to survive and reproduce may be substantially enhanced by resources provided by a father (e.g. Lancaster and Lancaster 1983; see too Alexander and Noonan 1979, Strassmann 1981, Turke 1984, 1987); and a discriminating mother may demand enough reproductive effort from a mate to help raise not only his daughters and sons, but generations of descendants as well.

Though the reproductive effort of any individual is finite, it can be increased by exploiting others' labors. By doing so, human males can win as many mates as they can impregnate, offering each of them resources with which to raise children. Although members of communally breeding species (see Emlen 1984) may use help from both related and unrelated individuals to their reproductive advantage, the potential for appropriating the fruits of others' labors is particularly marked in the human case. Historically, the heads of most states have managed to take enough tribute and labor from subjects to attract, and help rear children by, hundreds of women (Betzig 1986a).

As men have the potential to father many more children than women can mother, they should have been selected to compete for both the number and quality of their mates. An important part of this mate competition will involve contests over resources their wives will need to raise children. To the extent that male mate quality varies, women, and the kin who share their interests, should also be expected to compete for men. Mate quality will vary among men, in part, to the extent that some do successfully exclude others from resources required to raise children.

A number of studies have worked from the proposition that competition among men has evolved as a means to reproduction. For example, Wilson and Daly (1985), in a study of 512 closed cases of homicide in Detroit, found that murder was much more often a crime by and against men, rather than women (see too Daly and Wilson 1987c). In a large number of cases, the explicit motive was sexual jealousy (see too Daly et al. 1982). Both victims and offenders tended to have less to lose, and more, reproductively, to gain, than others: they tended to be unmarried and unemployed, compared to the population at large. Along similar lines, Boone (1986; see also Boone this volume (Chapter 12)), in a study of 15th and 16th century Portuguese élites, showed that the less his inheritance, due either to birth order or rank, the more likely a young man was to undertake risk, presumably in order to raise his reproductive prospects. Lower status and later-born sons were more likely to campaign in expansionist wars, to die as a result, and to die farther from home. These two and other studies (e.g. Alexander 1979: 240–8, Shields and Shields 1983, Thornhill and Thornhill 1983, 1986) suggest that men with fewer resources may be more likely to undertake risk, in order to increase their access to resources, or, more directly, to women.

A critical question has been whether winners of competition among men have higher mating and reproductive success. Evidence from a large

and growing number of studies suggests that they do, at least in traditional groups. Dominance, or the ability to win conflicts of interest (see e.g. Dewsbury 1982, Fedigan 1983, Gray 1985), and the spoils of dominance, especially status and wealth, have been shown to predict a number of measures of reproductive success.

The first formal test was done in the book *Evolutionary Biology and Human Social Behavior: An Anthropological Perspective* (Chagnon and Irons 1979). In it, Irons (1979; see too Irons 1980) found that men in the richer half of a group of Persian Yomut Turkmen had significantly higher age-specific fertility than did poorer men. Other studies since have shown relationships between measures of success in male–male competition, including dominance, status, and wealth, and (1) fertility to date, (2) age-specific or completed fertility, and (3) mechanisms promoting fertility.

Correlations of the first sort, between status or wealth and fertility to date, have been found for both the Venezuelan Yąnomamö (Chagnon et al. 1979:318 and Chagnon 1979a, 1980) and rural Trinidadians (Flinn 1986). Stronger evidence of an association between means and reproductive ends controls, however, for age. Among Paraguayan Ache foragers, better hunters matched for age with poorer hunters have been found to have more surviving children (Kaplan and Hill 1985a); and age-specific fertility has been found to vary with both status and wealth among men on Ifaluk, a Micronesian atoll (Turke and Betzig 1985, Betzig, this volume (Chapter 2)). Completed fertility has been predicted by both rank and wealth in a 19th century cohort of Utah Mormons (Mealey 1985), by rank within 15th and 16th century Portuguese élites (Boone 1986, Boone, this volume), and by wealth, in number of cows or acres of land, in three cohorts of 20th century Kenyan Kipsigis men (Borgerhoff Mulder 1988).

Finally, dominance, status, and wealth have all been positively associated with a variety of mechanisms promoting men's reproductive success, including number of serial or simultaneous conjugal unions, number of reported extramarital liaisons, age at first marriage or reproduction, spouse's age at first reproduction, interbirth intervals, longevity, offspring survival, and probability of cuckoldry. This is, of course, not an exhaustive list of mechanisms; nor does each measure contribute equally to reproductive variance; nor are the measurements made with equal precision.

The correlation most often demonstrated has been between measures of success in male–male competition and number of conjugal unions. The latter has been positively associated with status or wealth among the Yąnomamö (Chagnon *et al.* 1979:318 and Chagnon 1980), polygynous Mormons (Faux and Miller 1984, Mealey 1985), rural Trinidadians (Flinn 1986), élite Portuguese (Boone 1986, Boone this volume), and Kipsigis (Borgerhoff Mulder 1987a, 1987b). And, in a cross-cultural study, dominance, or ability to win conflicts of interest, was found a powerful predictor of harem size in 104 politically autonomous societies (Betzig 1986a).

'Illegitimate' unions have been reported to be more frequent among Ache who were above the median in calories brought home per time spent hunting (Kaplan and Hill 1985a, Hill and Kaplan, this volume (Chapters 17 and 18)), and among high-ranking élite Portuguese (Boone 1986, Boone, this volume). Salaried men on Ifaluk were found to have started reproducing younger, had wives who started reproducing younger, and to produce children at shorter interbirth intervals (Turke and Betzig 1985, Betzig this volume); and both longevity and earlier age at marriage were found to contribute to higher completed fertility among Mormon men (Mealey 1985). Offspring survival has been positively associated with Ache hunting success (Kaplan and Hill 1985a, Hill and Kaplan, this volume (Chapters 17 and 18)), élite Portuguese rank (Boone 1986, Boone this volume), and wealth among some US (Essock-Vitale 1984) and Kipsigis women (Borgerhoff Mulder 1987a). And, rich Trinidadians have been putatively cuckolded less often (Flinn 1987).

Correlations between products of dominance, usually wealth and status, and various measures of reproductive success, have also been found among modern Iranians (Miller and Windel 1960) and Nigerians (Sween and Clignet 1974, Grossbard 1976), the African Ife (Driesen 1972), in the New Guinea highlands (Wood *et al.* 1985) and in rural Bangladesh (Shaikh and Becker 1985). Qualitative evidence of such associations has been presented by Dickemann (1979a), van den Berghe (1979), and Hill (1984).

Evidence from a broad range of social and eco-logical contexts, then, shows measures of success in male–male competition to vary with measures of differential reproduction. Further work can, though, make improvements in three areas common to studies of adaptation. First, better measurements might be made. In the studies above, there is relatively little difficulty operationalizing access to resources. It is more difficult to measure reproductive success. One long-term consequence of interest in any study of adaptation is always the effect of the trait in question on fitness. But fitness is not easy to measure (e.g. Dunbar 1982). The approximations used so far vary, as noted above, in precision; and better approximations, involving counts of collateral and direct descendants over more than one generation, and electrophoretic analyses, have yet to be made (e.g. Gray 1985).

Second, where other theories fit the facts, they must be tested against. In the studies above, measures of resource access may predict men's reproductive success *both* because men compete for resources, and because women choose for them. Few studies have determined whether these associations result from competition among males, or female choice, or both. Effects of mate competition and mate choice are exceedingly hard to factor out. In social species, for example, even dominance, or success in male–male competition, can be effected in part by support from others, including females who have chosen to back them (e.g. DeWaal 1982).

Finally, variation in behavior across cultures needs to be explained. Though the proper study, taking into account such important ends of the reproductive spectrum as reproductive failures and serial monogamists, has yet to be done, the associations between status or resource access and reproductive success do not seem to hold up in modern contexts (see Freedman and Thornton 1982, Mueller and Short 1983, Betzig 1986a). The apparent dislocation between the means and ends of reproductive success in modern cultures constitutes what I consider a major challenge to a Darwinian view of human behavior (see Betzig 1986a, Alexander, this volume (Chapter 20)).

In stark contrast to the volume of evidence devoted to male–male competition, virtually nothing quantitative has been done to date to address the question of whether women raise their reproductive success through competition for men. The importance and pervasiveness of dowry competition in societies with great differentials in wealth has, though, been interpreted in this light (Dickemann 1979a, 1979b, 1981, Irons 1983), and seems an especially worthwhile topic for further work.

Mate choice

Generally, where one sex competes for mates, mate choice is expected among the other. Women should have been selected to choose carefully for a mate's willingness and ability to expend effort which will help raise children. They should also choose against men who have, or are likely to have, attracted so many women that the resources allotted to each falls below what they might get from a less polygynous mate (Orians 1969, Borgerhoff Mulder and Caro 1983).

Where they attract more women than they can mate, men may also be expected to choose among women. Women with the most to offer in this respect will be capable of bearing and rearing many children; they should be young and healthy (Fisher 1958, Williams 1975, Symons 1979), and able to provide child-rearing resources themselves. Men should also be expected to choose against women who have children by other men, to whom their resources may be diverted, and against those who are pregnant by other men, or who are likely to *become* pregnant by other men, that is, promiscuous women (e.g. Trivers 1972).

Finally, though both theory and evidence on this subject remain open to considerable argument, both women and men might choose mates for their supposed ability to transmit fit traits, genetically, to their progeny. That is, besides choosing for reproductive effort, they may choose for 'good genes' (e.g. Hamilton and Zuk 1982, contrast Taylor and Williams 1982).

As suggested above, all of the associations between men's status or wealth and reproductive success may reflect choice on the part of women and their kin for husband's ability to provide parental effort, as much as mate competition among men. Very indirect evidence that this might be the case is that ornamentation is more common in groups with greater differences in wealth (Low 1979), which suggests that men

might ornament themselves, and even their wives, in part to signal ability to spend reproductive effort on women and children. Another indirect suggestion that women and their families are choosing well-off men is that bride price, also a possible signal of investment potential, is much more commonly found in societies with inherited wealth and status differentials (Hartung 1976, 1982, Flinn and Low 1986). More directly, Buss (1986), in a review of seven earlier studies, found that American women consistently valued ambition, industry, and 'good earning capacity' above all in prospective mates.

Other research has addressed the problem of whether or not becoming a new addition to a harem will allow a woman to raise as many children, grandchildren, and other kin, as would becoming an addition to a less abundantly provisioned, but smaller, harem. Early evidence (e.g. Dorjahn 1958), and many more recent studies (e.g. Smith and Kunz 1976, Mealey 1985), suggested that, at least in the first generation, perhaps it would not. Borgerhoff Mulder (1987a), on the other hand, found that though reproductive success among women was affected by the amount of wealth available per wife, monogamously and polygynously married Kipsigis women of the same cohort differed neither in the amount of wealth available per wife, nor in number of children raised. Furthermore, polygynously married women experienced more available caretakers for their infants than did monogamously married women (Borgerhoff Mulder and Milton 1985).

There is, then, some evidence that women choose men for the provisions they offer, but a lot of work remains to be done. Future comparative studies might try to explain cross-cultural variation in female choice. They might, for example, explore whether women's preferences for well-provisioned men are more marked in societies where resource differentials among husbands have the greatest effects on reproductive differentials. This might be effected by the extent of stratification among men, the ability of women to get support from kin, and sex restrictions in the division of labor (see Borgerhoff Mulder 1987c). Conversely, where provisioning by men is less important, a woman might be expected to value other attributes, possibly strength, health, and willingness to spend time with children, in so far as these might enhance

7

both her own reproductive success and, where they are heritable, that of her children. Last, there is no evidence yet that women actually promote their reproductive success by choosing particular kinds of mates.

That men also choose among mates has been borne out in several studies. Using census data from greater Seattle in 1976, Lockhard and Adams (1981) showed that, in most age groups, older men tended to marry younger women. They also found, using observational data from shopping centers in the census area, that older-looking men were seen with younger-looking women much more often than older-looking women were seen with younger-looking men. This is consistent with qualitative evidence from a number of societies, which suggests that dominant men successfully sequester the youngest, and 'prettiest', women themselves (see Dickemann 1979a, Betzig 1986a). It is consistent, too, with Buss' (1986, 1987) finding that American men have been repeatedly reported to place strongest emphasis on physical atrractiveness in prospective mates. Buss argued, following Williams (1975) and Symons (1979), that attractiveness in women might signal youth, health, and other important components of reproductive potential.

Other studies have addressed the question of whether a man chooses a woman who is likely to allot effort to his, rather than someone else's, children. Dickemann (1981) has suggested that sexual modesty among women, including such strict institutions as veiling, footbinding, and claustration, might function to raise the paternity confidence of their consorts. Similarly, Daly et al. (1982), following Symons (1979), have suggested that male sexual jealousy might diminish the probability of cuckoldry. Consistent evidence is that sexual jealousy is an often cited motive for homicide (Darwin 1871:871, Daly et al. 1982, Wilson and Daly 1985, Betzig 1986a). Flinn (1987) has presented further, quantitative evidence that men are concerned with their mates' fidelity. He used behavioral observations from instantaneous scans made in rural Trinidad to show that men interested in the same woman were overtly competing 30% of the time they were seen together. Men were seen much more often with co-resident mates who Flinn suggested were more likely to be fertile; and men with such mates were significantly more often

seen behaving agonistically (see too Flinn this volume (Chapter 11)).

Other evidence that men choose faithful mates comes from studies of divorce. Daly et al. (1982) found that, cross-culturally, though women were less likely to have reported that they committed adultery, men were more likely to cite their spouse's adultery as a cause for divorce. Essock-Vitale and McGuire (1985a, Essock-Vitale and McGuire this volume (Chapter 13)) found that, among 300 Los Angeles women, those who reported having had extramarital affairs were divorced on average about twice as often as those who did not. And Betzig (1986a:83) found a wife's infidelity listed as a cause for conjugal dissolution in 48 of a sample of 104 societies, while, in others, more severe measures were taken to end the union. In none of these groups was adultery by a husband a cause for conjugal dissolution where adultery by a wife did not result in her divorce or death.

Finally, in making a choice, Darwinian theory suggests that both women and men should be concerned about their mate's fertility. Among the most direct evidence that they are is the finding that infertile spouses are often divorced. Essock-Vitale and McGuire (1985a, Essock-Vitale and McGuire this volume), in their Los Angeles study, found that marriages were significantly more likely to end in divorce if no children had been produced. Over three-quarters of first marriages which had produced no children ended in divorce, compared to only 30% of those to which a child had been born. Strong evidence that infertility causes divorce must, however, control for marital duration (e.g. Thornton 1977). Last, Betzig (1986a:83) found ethnographic statements that sterility was a cause for divorce for 37 of a sample of 104 societies; including related factors, such as impotence, sexual neglect, the death of children, too few children, and the wife's being too old to produce children, infertility has been noted as a cause for divorce in accounts of at least 53 of those groups.

There is, then, more substantial evidence that men with a lot to offer choose wives for various indices of reproductive potential, especially, youth and lack of children by another spouse. As already noted, however, for studies of female choice, the effect of male choice on reproductive success remains to be shown, and effects of each of different attributes of mate quality on mate choice must be separated out. It is often not clear, for example, to what extent men are choosing wives for their attractiveness or nulliparity, in so far as older women are more likely than younger women to have produced children and to have had extramarital affairs. Finally, future comparative studies might try to quantify the extent to which choice for female attributes, including fidelity and youth, increases with variation in male attributes, including status and wealth.

Parenting

The object of mating – competing for mates with reproductive effort to spend, and choosing among the competitors – must of course be parenting. But parenting – raising the number and kind of kin most likely to be successful themselves at reproducing – is no simpler than mating.

On the face of it, for instance, it would seem the best way to get genes into later generations would be by producing the most young. Not so: as Lack (1954) cleverly showed, a parent who produces more young than it can raise is likely to end up with fewer of them surviving, compared to one who has fewer in the first place, but raises every one. The number of young which can be raised successfully to maturity will, though, vary. Parents should be selected to determine both the amount of reproductive effort they will have at their disposal, and when, and to produce offspring accordingly. Important determinants of parents' reproductive potential will include available resources, spouse's resources, and age (e.g. Fisher 1958).

Besides producing an optimum number of offspring, at optimum times, parents should have been selected to raise them according to the number of surviving young they, in turn, are likely to reproduce. In other words, they should have evolved to expend parental effort according to the reproductive potential of their offspring (Fisher 1958). Two primary factors will contribute to a child's reproductive potential: first, his or her ability to survive, and, later, his or her ability to reproduce. As Hamilton (1966) argued, parents may have been selected to stop caring for young unlikely to live to maturity,

and to replace them as soon, i.e. with as little wasted reproductive effort, as possible. By the same logic, older offspring should, other things being equal, be favored over their younger sisters and brothers, at least until their reproductive values are reversed (Fisher 1958, Schulman and Chapais 1980, Charlesworth and Charnov 1981, but see Horrocks and Hunte 1983). One important thing which will not, in this case, be equal, is need: younger offspring in many cases will benefit more than older sibs from an equal expenditure of effort.

Having assessed the survivability of offspring, parents may be expected to try to determine how reproductive each is likely to become. Trivers and Willard (1973) have suggested that sex should be an important predictor. Given that females are usually the reproductively limiting sex, successful males will outreproduce their sisters. At the same time, where females and males exist in about equal numbers (see Fisher 1958), the least reproductively successful females will generally outreproduce their brothers. Assuming that parental resources will affect the reproductive success of their offspring, parents with lots of resources at their disposal may benefit most by producing sons, while those with relatively few resources may do best by producing daughters (see too Charnov 1982, Clutton-Brock and Albon 1982, Hrdy 1987).

Finally, besides assessing, first, their ability to expend reproductive effort, i.e. their own reproductive potential, and, second, the recipients' ability to use those resources to survive and reproduce, i.e. recipients' reproductive potential, parents must also determine each recipient's relatedness to them. Again, sex assures that any mother or father shares half its genes by descent with daughters and sons, half, as well, with full sisters and brothers, a quarter with nieces and nephews, and so on. Hamilton (1963, 1964) has made the essential point that where the ratio of reproductive benefit to cost will be higher, parents will do well to invest in, for example, a brother rather than a son; where the pay-off will be more than twice as great, they should do better to invest in, for example, a niece rather than a daughter. In short, wherever $k > 1/r$, where k is the ratio of benefit to cost, and r is the proportion of genes identical by descent, individuals should be selected to help their kin reproduce.

Reproductive potential

Since so much parental effort must be expended to bring up children, human parents should have been selected to be careful about how they spend it. They should be good at assessing their own reproductive potential, and that of their children. Some evidence suggests they might be, and that they use their own and their mate's parental resources, and recipients' survivability, age, and sex, as cues.

Blurton-Jones and Sibley (1978) and Blurton-Jones (1986) have looked at birth spacing among the Kalahari !Kung. On the basis of both empirical evidence and assumptions about the costs and benefits involved in a number of expenditures of parental effort, they have argued that !Kung women adaptively space their children, at an average interbirth interval of between 4 and 5 years.

In addition, several recent studies have shown that reports of abortion, infanticide, and child abuse are more likely when mothers are uncertain of whether parental effort will be forthcoming from fathers. Bugos and McCarthy (1984) collected 54 accounts of infanticide among the Ayoreo of Bolivia and Paraguay (38% of all livebirths to sampled women), and found that firstborn children were significantly more often victims, and that lack of parental investment was a commonly cited cause. Daly and Wilson (1984) found that, cross-culturally, lack of a father's support was frequently cited as a cause for infanticide ethnographically. Essock-Vitale and McGuire (1985a, Essock-Vitale and McGuire this volume (Chapter 13)), in their study of Los Angeles women, found only a small proportion, 7%, of pregnancies reported to have ended by voluntary abortion. In stark contrast, women without husbands ended 64% of reported pregnancies voluntarily, as did 57% of those who were married but unsure who had fathered the child. And, in their recent Hamilton, Ontario, study, Daly and Wilson (1985) found that reported child abuse is more common when mothers are single, and when they are young.

Evidence that parents invest according to a child's survivability and age also comes from child abuse studies. Lenington (1981) and Daly and Wilson (1981a) cited previously published data suggesting that abuse risk is substantially higher among children with congenital physical problems. And Lightcap et al. (1982), using observational data from rural Pennsylvania, found that children with such abnormalities were more likely to suffer abuse than those without. Younger children have been found to be severely abused more often (e.g. Lenington 1981, Daly and Wilson 1985, but see Lightcap et al. 1982).

Last, several studies have shown that parents appear to evaluate reproductive potential by sex, and accordingly invest. The first such study was Dickemann's (1979b). She looked at demographic records from British colonial India, traditional China, and early modern Europe, and found that, in each case, parents of the highest caste or class produced dramatically fewer reproductive daughters than sons. Dickemann reported childhood sex ratios, based on census figures, for India at around two to one, and for China as high as four to one; in both cases, female infanticide was reported to have been extremely common. For Europe, Dickemann reported sex ratios often greater than one to one, and evidence that aristocratic women were routinely kept from reproducing in nunneries.

Voland (1984), using historical data from German Schleswig-Holstein for 1720 to 1869, found evidence that infant mortality in prosperous families was dramatically female-biased compared to the male-biased mortality in less prosperous families. He pinpointed the period of differential survival as the first 120 days of life, and suggested that differences in infant death by sex were affected largely by child abuse and neglect. Boone (1986, Boone this volume (Chapter 12)), in his Portuguese study, found the marriage probability of élite women decreased with parents' status. And Betzig and Turke (1986a) found that, on Ifaluk, parents of traditional and salaried status spent about twice as much time with sons as with daughters, while among parents without such status the pattern was reversed. If association frequency reflects parental investment, these results also indicate favoring of sons among high status parents.

These studies, again, provide some support for evolutionary predictions; they also raise some interesting questions. The first is, again, how much do these actions, as opposed to alternatives, raise parental fitness? Infanticide, for example, should be adaptive only where a child presents a greater cost to parental fitness than an asset. Whether the children of unmated women, the children of young women able to find better mates, low status sons or high status daughters constitute such costs is hard to find out (see too Kitcher 1985). Second, which factors contribute most? We should know, for example, whether child abuse is more common among single mothers because they are single or because they are young (see Daly and Wilson 1985). And third, what accounts for cross-cultural variation? Where a behavior, like female infanticide, is supposed or shown to be adaptive in one context, what accounts for its absence in another? Variables must be sought which explain why, for example, colonial Indian élites practiced female infanticide, early modern European élites cloistered their daughters, and Yąnomamö parents of high status failed to adjust sex ratio in either way (Chagnon et al. 1979).

Relatedness

As humans have for a long time lived socially, with number of kin of varying degrees of relatedness available as recipients of their reproductive efforts (e.g. Lee and DeVore 1968), women and men should be good at discriminating among others according to relatedness, and at caring for them accordingly. Human mothers and fathers seem able to discriminate relatedness both by protracted and more immediate cues. The finding that Israeli children brought up together in kibbutzim refused to marry one another, even against their parents' wishes (Spiro 1958, Shepher 1971), has been cited in support of Westermarck's (1891) early hypothesis that people learn incest avoidance by close childhood association. Presumably, if children learn, by being brought up with them, not to interbreed with close kin, they might also, by that mechanism, learn to help kin when they can. Evidence that humans can discriminate kin on the basis of less experience is accumulating as well; parents and children have been shown to use voice (DeCasper and Fifer 1980), smell (e.g. Russell et al. 1983), and facial features (Daly and Wilson 1982a) to recognize one another (review in Porter 1986).

More has been written about whether or not people take kinship into account when they expend reproductive effort than about any other problem in the study of human reproductive

behavior. People have been shown (1) to prefer proximity to kin (presumably, the better to help them), (2) to actually help their kin (presumably, in ways likely to enhance their reproductive success), and (3) to produce more children and grandchildren when they live close to and/or are helped by kin.

In one of the first explicit applications of Darwinian theory to human behavior, Chagnon (1979b, 1981; see too Chagnon 1975) used extensive demographic data on the Venezuelan Yąnomamö to show that, when villages fission, people take their kin along with them. Specifically, the average coefficient of genealogical relatedness among village members is higher after than before a fission. In another Yąnomamö study, Chagnon and Bugos (1979) showed that men stay in proximity to kin in a crucial context – during an ax fight. Using notes taken at the time of one fight, still photographs, and a 16-mm film, they determined that people in each of the two groups involved were more closely related among themselves than they were, on average, to members of the other group. Other studies showing that proximity varies with genealogical kinship include Hames' (1979) of Venezuelan Ye'kwana association patterns, and Hurd's (1983, 1985) of Pennsylvania Amish church group fissions.

Evidence that kin actually help kin includes Silk's (1980) reanalysis of adoption in Oceania. She showed that adoption in the 11 societies for which she found data was most common when adoptors and adoptees shared a 0.25 genealogical tie, and that in 76.5% of all reported cases the relationship was closer than or equal to that of first cousins. Though 'adoption' does not, in most of these groups, entail the expenditure of parental effort it does in Western cultures, it probably does in every case entail some, and in many cases a major, expenditure (e.g. Carroll 1970, Brady 1976). In this study, Silk looked at costs and benefits, that is, at reproductive potential, as well as relatedness. She found that household heads with fewer young children of their own (i.e. with a lower cost to incur) were more likely to adopt those of their kin.

Other evidence of actual helping according to kinship includes results of six studies. Daly and Wilson (1982b) found that co-resident Detroiters were less likely to murder kin than non-kin. Hawkes (1983; cf. Hawkes 1977, Dow

1984) showed that more closely related New Guinea Binumarien helped one another garden more often. Fredlund (1985) reported that four Yanomamö informants were more likely to classify marriages made by distant kin as 'incestuous,' or against the rules. Kaplan and Hill (1985b, Kaplan *et al*. 1984) found that food brought home by Ache women, though not Ache men, most often went to nuclear family members. Essock-Vitale and McGuire (1985b) reported that, for their Los Angeles women, help was more likely to be reciprocated among non-kin than among kin, that large amounts of aid were allocated according to closeness of relationship, and that the generational age of related recipients was significantly lower (i.e. they were better able to benefit) than that of givers of help (cf. Essock-Vitale and McGuire 1980). And Betzig and Turke (1986b) found that closely related households on Ifaluk shared food more often, that among food sharers relatedness increased with distance, and that the consumer to producer ratio in recipient households was higher than it was among donors.

In addition, a number of studies have addressed the more specific proposition that men should invest in children according to their confidence that they fathered them. An association between a high overall incidence of female adultery within a society and a tendency on the part of men to care for their sisters' sons, rather than their own, has been noted for over a century in anthropology (review in Hartung 1985). Following arguments by Alexander (1974, 1977), Greene (1978), and Kurland (1979), Gaulin and Schlagel (1980), Flinn (1981), and Hartung (1985) found cross-cultural correlations between matrilineal inheritance and the incidence of infidelity by women.

Another line of evidence that parents prefer to invest in genetic rather than putative children comes from studies of step-parenting. In a number of papers, Daly and Wilson (1980, 1981a, 1981b, 1984, 1985, 1987a, 1987b, Wilson and Daly 1987, Wilson *et al*. 1980, 1983) have used data from different cultures to show that child abuse and neglect occur more often in households with single or substitute parents than in households with both genetic parents. In their latest study (Daly and Wilson 1985), of families in Hamilton, Ontario, they found that both child abuse and police apprehension are significantly more likely in step-parent and in single-parent homes. They found, too, that while low income is associated with abuse, income varies little between 'natural' and step-families in the study, that is, that income alone could not predict child abuse. Similarly, Lightcap *et al*. (1982), in a study of 24 rural Pennsylvania households with two parents and at least one victim of child abuse, found that while abuse occurred in only 17 of 157 (putative) genetic parent–child dyads, it occurred in 13 of 27 step-parent–child pairs, and that, when they lived with both, parents abused step-children significantly more often than genetic children (see too Lenington 1981).

Finally, evidence that kin may actually help other kin have children comes from studies in four societies. Chagnon (1982) showed that, among the Yanomanö, married men, both monogamous (with one wife at once) and polygynous (with more than one wife at once), had more matrilineal relatives, ascending generation relatives, and own generation relatives co-resident in their villages than had single men. Faux and Miller (1984), in their study of Mormon polygyny, reported that the church founder, Joseph Smith, was able to appoint kinsmen to the hierarchy, and that, for all polygynous members of the hierarchy between 1830 and 1897, those related to Smith had significantly more wives than his non-relatives had (see too Mealey 1985). Turke and Betzig (1985) found that, controlling for age, both men and women on Ifaluk produced significantly more children as the number of parents they had living on the island went up. And Flinn (1986) found that Trinidadian men with fathers presently co-resident in their village had had significantly more children.

The literature on whether or not kinship affects expenditures of reproductive effort is, like the literature on topics already reviewed, both persuasive and provocative. Calculating coefficients of relatedness from genealogical data can be difficult; both ethnographers and fathers, for a number of reasons, may be misled (e.g. Gray 1985). Corroborations by independent interviews, and especially with electrophoretic data (as, e.g. by Smouse *et al*. 1981), will increase the accuracy of genealogies. Better behavioral and demographic measures will help in the difficult task of demonstrating inclusive fitness effects (e.g. Grafen 1982, 1984).

The prediction that kin prefer to help kin will be made more precise as more reproductive costs and benefits are factored in (Hamilton 1964); reproductive potential of parents and children are among the most important of these. Further studies should also look more closely at correlations between reproductive expenditures and relatedness in trying to sort out cause and effect. It is possible, for instance, that paternal effort varies inversely with women's adultery because men with few resources to offer their children are less able to demand fidelity in their wives, as much as because fathers uncertain of their paternity are less inclined to offer their children resources.

Finally, though reproductive potential on the part of parents and children, and relatedness between them, affect parental behavior in a number of cases, anomalies exist in several cultures. One of the most stubborn questions concerning kinship remains why the most powerful men in a number of societies transmit their status, resources, and even their harems to sisters' sons rather than to their own (cf. Betzig and Turke 1986a).

Problems with a Darwinian perspective

Most of the studies discussed above, and all of the work in this book, test the prediction that human behavior is adaptive in the place and time in which it is observed. They ask the question: Are men and women behaving in ways which should or do positively affect their reproductive success? For a couple of good reasons, they might not be.

First, the tacit or explicit assumption that natural selection has optimized the mechanisms responsible for the behaviors in question may not always be a valid one (e.g. Gould and Lewontin 1979). Other evolutionary forces, including random forces, may have fixed less than optimal traits; optimal variants may never have appeared by mutation; and phylogenetic constraints often make for jury-rigged rather than optimal adaptations (e.g. Gould 1980, Mayr 1983). To the most casual observer, however, it is clear that evolution has been shaped by more than random events: it is likely that enough heritable traits have had consistent effects on bearers' reproduction to produce adaptations. It should be reason-

able to assume that natural selection has produced mechanisms which underlie a broad range of actions (e.g. Wright 1983, Maynard Smith 1982). But it may not, in many cases, have produced an optimal result.

An example illustrates the point. Many studies summed up above test Hamilton's (1963, 1964) prediction that individuals have evolved to behave most altruistically toward closest kin. All of them use estimates of r, or proportion of genes identical by descent, to measure relatedness. But, as Hamilton (1964:23–8) himself has pointed out, kin recognition might have evolved by a number of mechanisms. Where individuals reliably encounter close relatives only, they might do well to behave altruistically according to proximity: 'A difference in the generosity of ... behavior according to whether the situations evoking it were encountered near to, or far from ... home might occasion an advantage' (p. 23). Where, on the other hand, kin are not always physically closest, we might expect greater discrimination: 'It seems a reasonable hypothesis that the ability to discriminate "own young" advances in step with the chance that without such discrimination ... parental care [would be] wasted on unrelated genes' (p. 26). Best of all, though, would be 'the discrimination of those individuals which do carry ... the behavior-causing genes from those which do not' (p. 27). By Hamilton's own admission, in this instance, 'At simplest we need to postulate something like a supergene affecting (a) some preceptible feature of the organism, (b) the perception of that feature, and (c) the social response consequent upon what was perceived' (Hamilton 1964:27). The extent to which altruism is allocated adaptively must, then, depend on the extent to which an accurate mechanism promoting kin recognition can evolve (see e.g. Holmes and Sherman 1983, Porter 1986, Fletcher and Mitchner 1987).

There is another important reason why people might not behave optimally. As a result of their own actions – and so presumably, at least at some point, in *some* of their interests – humans, like many other organisms, now live in environments in some ways very unlike those in which they are supposed to have evolved. Over the course of 99% of our evolutionary history as hominids, we are supposed to have lived in family-based hunting and gathering bands of 50 to 100 members (Lee and DeVore 1968). What does this mean? It means to some theorists (e.g. Symons 1979, 1986), who make the assumption that adaptive behaviors will be evoked only under circumstances very much like those under which we evolved, that people often will behave in not at all adaptive ways.

This point, too, can be illustrated with a kinship case. Suppose that we have evolved to recognize as closest kin those with whom we live during a critical period early in life. Suppose, too, that living arrangements are now importantly different from those which characterized our evolutionary history. In that case, we might find individuals behaving generously toward others distantly related genetically, and not very generously toward closer kin. This sort of maladaptive behavior would follow from an evolutionary prediction, based on an understanding of mechanisms supposed to have been shaped by evolution.

The study of contemporary societies

For this reason, a number of researchers have tried to make predictions about human behavior based on knowledge or, more often, assumptions about specific evolved mechanisms (see Tinbergen 1963). This approach is most common among researchers studying humans in the most modern contexts (e.g. Daly and Wilson 1986a).

Like any research, it is associated with some problems. Based on scenarios supposed to characterize evolutionary history, specific adaptations are argued to have evolved (e.g. Symons 1979, 1986). But such scenarios are often difficult to substantiate (see Caro and Borgerhoff Mulder 1987). Besides this, consistency between behavioral outcomes and postulated mechanisms is often accepted as evidence that such mechanisms exist (especially Symons 1979). But a single outcome might be the product of a number of possible mechanisms. Men able to win conflicts of interest might outreproduce losers because women choose winners, because women choose for resources winners control, or because men compete for women and the means to sustain them. It can be, as noted above, exceedingly difficult to determine which of these motivations contributes most. Nevertheless, an understanding of the mechanisms underlying behavior will lend precision to any Darwinian prediction. This

will be true whether the context in which the behavior takes place is, or is not, like the one in which the mechanism evolved.

Others (e.g. Alexander 1979, 1987) start out with the tacit or explicit assumption that *relevant* aspects of the environment (including, for instance, consumable resources, mates, and kin) are fairly invariant. This approach is common among researchers studying humans in more traditional contexts, from hunter–gatherer bands to horticultural tribes to historical states (e.g. Kaplan and Hill 1985a, 1985b, Chagnon 1982, Dickemann 1979a). It starts out with the more general prediction that behavior will promote reproductive success in the current context.

This approach, too, raises several problems. Besides problems with the measurement of behavioral cause and fitness effects, the attempt to distinguish among alternative predictions, and the explanation of behavioral variation, the constraints on behavior are often difficult to see or measure. Whether or not, under those constraints, an individual is behaving adaptively is often difficult to determine (cf. Hinde 1975). Whether, for example, a man who becomes a member of a harem is contributing to his fitness or not depends upon what other options are open (e.g. Crook and Crook, this volume (Chapter 5)). Along with an understanding of specific proximate mechanisms, an awareness of all of the relevant environmental determinants of an individual's actions will contribute to precise predictions and explanations (e.g. Betzig 1986b).

No doubt in part because the difference between evolutionary and present contexts is less stark, the last prediction, that behavior will be adaptive in current contexts, is very widely made in studies of the behavior of every other species (e.g. Alexander and Tinkle 1981, Rubenstein and Wrangham 1986, Clutton-Brock 1988). Again, most of the human work to date, and all of the work in this book, makes the same prediction.

The question, it seems to us, that should be asked at this point is not *whether* evolution has shaped behavior, but *how*. Present research should have a lot to say about each of the assumptions above. We should begin to determine, for example: are reproductive behaviors less than optimal because they have been drawn off track by novel environments, or because evolution did not produce an optimal mechanism, or both?

Last, it should again be pointed out that the discovery that behaviors are or are not adaptive says *nothing at all* about the possibility or desirability of changing them. The question of how easy or hard it may be to change a behavior can be an extremely important one, but it is independent of the question of whether or not that behavior is adaptive. And neither the prediction nor the finding that a behavior is adaptive amounts to a sanction. Natural laws often have little in common with the way we would have them. But our ability to understand them must often precede our ability to overcome them.

The plan of the book

Questions about whether or not men and women allocate their reproductive effort adaptively are asked, in the chapters that follow, of people in 13 different societies, and in two comparative studies. The book is split into two major sections, corresponding to each component of sexual reproduction: mating and parenting.

I should note at the outset that, in practice, it is often hard to determine whether a specific behavior amounts to mating or parental effort. For example, Aka men may spend time with children both to help raise them and in order to secure their mothers as mates (Chapter 16); Ache hunters may bring home extra game both to provision band members and because they are rewarded with sexual access to other men's wives (Chapter 17); and Ifaluk chiefs may procure more subsistence than they need themselves both to feed children and other kin and to attract women (Chapter 2).

At the same time, human mating is very rarely a two-party affair. Female choice, and probably male choice as well, can be compromised by the interests of families. Kipsigis bridewealth payments involve parental effort in sons' mating effort, as parents pay for their sons' first wives (Chapter 3); and K'ekchi' and Tibetan women and their families may choose husbands for their ability to get kin to help on the farm (Chapters 4 and 5).

Papers in the book's first section, on mating, look first at mate competition, through language (Chapter 1 [Chagnon]) and through resource acquisition (Chapter 2 [Betzig]) and allocation (Chapter 3 [Borgerhoff Mulder]). They then address the subject of mate choice, for available labor (Chapter 4 [Berté]), for wealth (Chapter 5 [Crook and Crook]), and for health (Chapter 6 [Low]). Last, they evaluate the effects of mate choice and mate competition on sex differences in psychology (Chapter 7 [Gaulin and Hoffman]) and in reproductive variance, in a 'monogamous' culture in this case (Chapter 8 [Brown and Hotra]). This part of the book is concluded with Dunbar's discussion (Chapter 9).

The second part of the book focuses on parenting, both of own and kin's children. Papers consider effects of many factors on expenditures of parental effort, including the availability of grandparents (Chapter 10 [Turke]), the fertility of daughters (Chapter 11 [Flinn]), as well as relatedness, resources, age, and sex (Chapters 12–16 [Boone, Essock-Vitale and McGuire, Hames, Voland, and Hewlett]). The last two papers in this section look at tradeoffs in the allocation of mating and parental effort (Chapters 17 and 18 [Hill and Kaplan]). The parenting section is concluded with Irons' discussion (Chapter 19). The book ends with Alexander's look at prospects for the study of human behavior from a Darwinian perspective (Chapter 20).

Acknowledgements

Thanks to Richard Alexander, Warren Holmes, and Don Symons for helpful discussions, and to Tim Caro, Monique Borgerhoff Mulder, and Paul Turke for copious criticisms. Support from the University of Michigan's Museum of Zoology and Department of Social Psychology are gratefully acknowledged.

References

Alexander, R. D. (1974) The evolution of social behavior. *Annual Review of Ecology and Systematics*, 5, 325–83.
Alexander, R. D. (1977) Natural selection and the analysis of human sociality. In *Changing Scenes in the Natural Sciences: 1776–1976*, ed. C. E. Goulden. Bicentennial symposium monograph, Philosophical Academy of Natural Science. Special Publication 12, 283–337.
Alexander, R. D. (1979) *Darwinism and Human Affairs*. Seattle: University of Washington Press.
Alexander, R. D. (1987) *The Biology of Moral Systems*. Hawthorne, NY: Aldine.

Alexander, R. D. and Borgia, G. (1979) On the origin and basis of the male–female phenomenon. In *Sexual Selection and Reproductive Competition in Insects*, ed. M. F. Blum and N. Blum. New York: Academic Press.

Alexander, R. D. and Noonan, K. M. (1979) Concealment of ovulation, parental care, and human social evolution. In *Evolutionary Biology and Human Social Behavior: An Anthropological Perspective*, ed. N. A. Chagnon and W. Irons. North Scituate, MA: Duxbury Press.

Alexander, R. D. and Tinkle, D. W. (1981) *Natural Selection and Social Behavior: Recent Research and New Theory*. New York: Chiron Press.

Bateman, A. J. (1948) Intrasexual selection in *Drosophila*. *Heredity*, 2, 349–68.

Betzig, L. L. (1986a) *Despotism and Differential Reproduction: A Darwinian View of History*. Hawthorne, NY: Aldine.

Betzig, L. L. (1986b) Vaulting, leaping, skipping, and trudging ambition. *Quarterly Review of Biology*, 61, 517–21.

Betzig, L. L. and Turke, P. W. (1986a) Parental investment by sex on Ifaluk. *Ethology and Sociobiology*, 7, 29–37.

Betzig, L. L. and Turke, P. W. (1986b) Food sharing on Ifaluk. *Current Anthropology*, 27, 397–400.

Blurton Jones, N. and Sibley, R. (1978) Testing the adaptiveness of culturally determined behavior: Do Bushman women maximize their reproductive success by spacing births widely and foraging seldom? In *Human Behavior and Adaptation*, ed. N. Blurton Jones and V. Reynolds. London: Taylor & Francis.

Blurton Jones, N. (1986) Bushman birth spacing: A test for optimal birth intervals. *Ethology and Sociobiology*, 7, 91–105.

Bongaarts, J. and Potter, R. C. (1983) *Fertility, Biology and Behavior: An Analysis of the Proximate Determinants*. New York: Academic Press.

Boone, J. L. (1986) Parental investment and elite family structure in preindustrial states: A case study of late Medieval–Early Modern Portuguese genealogies. *American Anthropologist*, 88, (4), 859–78.

Borgerhoff Mulder, M. (1985) Polygyny threshold: Application to a Kipsigis case study. *National Geographic Research Reports*, 21, 33–9.

Borgerhoff Mulder, M. (1987a) Cultural and reproductive success: Kipsigis evidence. *American Anthropologist* (in press).

Borgerhoff Mulder, M. (1987b) Resources and reproduction in women with an example from the Kipsigis. *Journal of Zoology* (in press).

Borgerhoff Mulder, M. (1987c) Is the polygyny threshold model relevant to humans? In *Human Mating Patterns*, ed. C. G. N. Mascie-Taylor and A. J. Boyce. Cambridge: Cambridge University Press (in press).

Borgerhoff Mulder, M. (1988) Reproductive success in three Kipsigis cohorts. In *Reproductive Success: Studies of Selection and Adaptation in Contrasting Breeding Systems*, ed. T. H. Clutton-Brock. Chicago: University of Chicago Press.

Borgerhoff Mulder, M. and Caro, T. M. (1983) Polygyny: Definition and application to human data. *Animal Behaviour*, 31, 609–10.

Borgerhoff Mulder, M. and Milton, M. (1985) Factors affecting infant care among the Kipsigis. *Journal of Anthropological Research*, 41, 231–62.

Brady, I. (1976) *Transactions in Kinship, Adoption, and Fosterage in Oceania*. Honolulu: University of Hawaii Press.

Bugos, P. and McCarthy, L. M. (1984) Ayoreo infanticide: A case study. In *Infanticide: Comparative and Evolutionary Perspectives*, ed. G. Hausfater and S. B. Hrdy. Hawthorne, NY: Aldine.

Buss, D. M. (1986) Sex differences in human mate selection criteria: An evolutionary perspective. In *Sociobiology and Psychology: Issues, Ideas, and Findings*, ed. C. Crawford, M. Smith and D. Krebs. Hillsdale, NJ: Erlbaum.

Buss, D. M. (1987) Human mate choice. *Journal of Personality and Social Psychology* (in press).

Caro, T. M. and Borgerhoff Mulder, M. (1987) The problem of adaptation in the study of human behavior. *Ethology and Sociobiology*, 7, (in press).

Carroll, V. (1970) *Adoption in Eastern Oceania*. Honolulu: University of Hawaii Press.

Chagnon, N. A. (1975) Genealogy, solidarity, and relatedness: Limits to local group size and patterns of fissioning in an expanding population. *Yearbook of Physical Anthropology*, 19, 95–110.

Chagnon, N. A. (1979a) Is reproductive success equal in egalitarian societies? In *Evolutionary Biology and Human Social Organization: An Anthropological Perspective*, ed. N. A. Chagnon and W. Irons. North Scituate, MA: Duxbury Press.

Chagnon, N. A. (1979b) Mate competition, favoring close kin, and village fissioning among the Yąnomamö Indians. In *Evolutionary Biology and Human Social Organization: An Anthropological Perspective*, ed. N. A. Chagnon and W. Irons. North Scituate, MA: Duxbury Press.

Chagnon, N. A. (1980) Kin selection theory, kinship, marriage and fitness among the Yąnomamö Indians. In *Sociobiology: Beyond Nature/Nurture?* ed. G. Barlow and J. Silverberg. Boulder, CO: Westview Press.

Chagnon, N. A. (1981) Terminological kinship, genealogical relatedness and village fissioning among the Yąnomamö Indians. In *Natural Selection and Social Behavior: Recent Research and New Theory*, ed. R. D. Alexander and D. W. Tinkle. New York: Chiron Press.

Chagnon, N. A. (1982) Sociodemographic attributes of nepotism in tribal populations: Man the rule breaker. In *Current Problems in Sociobiology*, ed. King's College Sociobiology Group. London: Cambridge University Press.

Chagnon, N. A. and Bugos, P. (1979) Kin selection and conflict: An analysis of a Yąnomamö ax fight.

In *Evolutionary Biology and Human Social Behavior: An Anthropological Perspective*, ed. N. A. Chagnon and W. Irons. North Scituate, MA: Duxbury Press.

Chagnon, N. A. and Irons, W. (1979) *Evolutionary Biology and Human Social Behavior: An Anthropological Perspective*. North Scituate, MA: Duxbury Press.

Chagnon, N. A., Flinn, M. V. and Melancon, T. F. (1979) Sex ratio variation among the Yąnomamö Indians. In *Evolutionary Biology and Human Social Behavior: An Anthropological Perspective*, ed. N. A. Chagnon and W. Irons. North Scituate, MA: Duxbury Press.

Charlesworth, B. and Charnov, E. (1981) Kin selection in age-structured populations. *Journal of Theoretical Biology*, **88**, 103–19.

Charlesworth, B. and Leon, S. A. (1976) The relation of reproductive effort to age. *American Naturalist*, **110**, 449–59.

Charnov, E. (1982) *The Theory of Sex Allocation*. Princeton: Princeton University Press.

Clutton-Brock, T. H. (1983) Selection in relation to sex. In *Evolution from Molecules to Men*, ed. D. S. Bendall. London: Cambridge University Press.

Clutton-Brock, T. H. (1988) Reproductive success. In *Reproductive Success: Studies of Selection and Adaptation in Contrasting Breeding Systems*, ed. T. H. Clutton-Brock. Chicago: University of Chicago Press.

Clutton-Brock, T. H. and Albon, S. D. (1982) Parental investment in male and female offspring in mammals. In *Current Problems in Sociobiology*, ed. King's College Sociobiology Group. London: Cambridge University Press.

Daly, M. (1978) The cost of mating. *American Naturalist*, **112**, 771–14.

Daly, M. and Wilson, M. (1980) Discriminative parental solicitude: A biological perspective. *Journal of Marriage and the Family*, **42**, 277–88.

Daly, M. and Wilson, M. (1981a) Abuse and neglect of children in evolutionary perspective. In *Natural Selection and Social Behavior: Recent Research and New Theory*, ed. R. D. Alexander and D. W. Tinkle. New York: Chiron Press.

Daly, M. and Wilson, M. (1981b) Child maltreatment from a sociobiological perspective. *New Directions for Child Development*, **11**, 93–112.

Daly, M. and Wilson, M. (1982a) Whom are newborn babies said to resemble? *Ethology and Sociobiology*, **3**, 69–78.

Daly, M. and Wilson, M. (1982b) Homicide and kinship. *American Anthropologist*, **84**, 372–8.

Daly, M. and Wilson, M. (1983) *Sex, Evolution, and Behavior*, 2nd edition. Boston: Willard Grant Press.

Daly, M. and Wilson, M. (1984) A sociobiological analysis of human infanticide. In *Infanticide: Comparative and Evolutionary Perspectives*, ed. G. Hausfater and S. B. Hrdy. Hawthorne, NY: Aldine Press.

Daly, M. and Wilson, M. (1985) Child abuse and other risks of not living with both parents. *Ethology and Sociobiology*, **6**, 197–210.

Daly, M. and Wilson, M. (1987a) Evolutionary psychology and family violence. In *Sociobiology and Psychology: Issues, Ideas, and Applications*, ed. C. Crawford, M. Smith and D. Krebs. Hillsdale, NJ: Erlbaum (in press).

Daly, M. and Wilson, M. (1987b) Children as homicide victims. In *Biosocial Perspectives on Child Abuse*, ed. R. Gelles and J. Lancaster. Hawthorne, NY: Aldine-de Gruyter (in press).

Daly, M. and Wilson, M. (1987c) *Homicide*. Hawthorne, NY: Aldine-de Gruyter (in press).

Daly, M., Wilson, M. and Weghorst, S. (1982) Male sexual jealousy. *Ethology and Sociobiology*, **3**, 11–27.

Darwin, C. R. (1859) *On the Origin of Species*. New York: Random House. (Modern Library edition published with *The Descent of Man and Selection in Relation to Sex*, pp. 1–386.)

Darwin, C. R. (1871) *The Descent of Man and Selection in Relation to Sex*. New York: Random House. (Modern Library edition published with *On The Origin of Species*, pp. 387–1000).

DeCasper, A. J. and Fifer, W. P. (1980) Of human bonding: Newborns prefer their mother's voices. *Science*, **208**, 1174–6

DeWaal, F. B. (1982) *Chimpanzee Politics: Power and Sex Among Apes*. New York: Harper and Row.

Dewsbury, D. A. (1982) Dominance rank, copulatory behavior, and differential reproduction. *Quarterly Review of Biology*, **57**, 135–59.

Dickemann, M. (1979a) Female infanticide and the reproductive strategies of stratified human societies: A preliminary model. In *Evolutionary Biology and Human Social Behavior: An Anthropological Perspective*, ed. N. A. Chagnon and W. Irons. North Scituate, MA: Duxbury Press.

Dickemann, M. (1979b) The ecology of mating systems in hypergynous dowry societies. *Social Science Information*, **18**, 163–95.

Dickemann, M. (1981) Paternal confidence and dowry competition: A biocultural analysis of purdah. In *Natural Selection and Social Behavior: Recent Research and New Theory*, ed. R. D. Alexander and D. W. Tinkle. New York: Chiron Press.

Dorjahn, V. R. (1958) Fertility, polygyny, and their interrelationships in Temne society. *American Anthropologist*, **60**, 838–60

Dow, J. (1984) The genetic basis for afinal cooperation. *American Ethnologist*, **11**, 380–3.

Driesen, I. (1972) Some observations on the family unit, relatedness, and the practice of polygyny in the Ife division of Western Nigeria. *Africa*, **47**, 44–56.

Dunbar, R. (1982) Adaptation, fitness, and the evolutionary tautology. In *Current Problems in Sociobiology*, ed. King's College Sociobiology Group. London: Cambridge University Press.

Emlen, S. T. (1984) Cooperative breeding in birds and mammals. In *Behavioral Ecology: An Evolutionary Approach*, ed. J. R. Krebs and N. B. Davies, 2nd edition. Sunderland, MA: Sinauer Associates.

Essock-Vitale, S. M. (1984) The reproductive success

of wealthy Americans. *Ethology and Sociobiology*, 5, 45–9.

Essock-Vitale, S. M. and McGuire, M. T. (1980) Predictions derived from the theories of kin selection and reciprocation assessed by anthropological data. *Ethology and Sociobiology*, 1, 233–43.

Essock-Vitale, S. M. and McGuire, M. T. (1985a) Women's lives viewed from an evolutionary perspective: I. Sexual histories, reproductive success, and demographic characteristics of a random subsample of American women. *Ethology and Sociobiology*, 6, 137–54.

Essock-Vitale, S. M. and McGuire, M. T. (1985b) Women's lives from an evolutionary perspective: II. Patterns of helping. *Ethology and Sociobiology*, 6, 155–73.

Faux, S. F. and Miller, H. L. (1984) Evolutionary speculations on the oligarchic development of Mormon polygyny. *Ethology and Sociobiology*, 5, 15–31.

Fedigan, L. M. (1983) Dominance and reproductive success in primates. *Yearbook of Physical Anthropology*, 14, 156–67.

Fisher, R. A. (1958) *The Genetical Theory of Natural Selection*, 2nd edition. New York: Dover Press.

Fletcher, D. and Mitchner, C. (1987) *Kin Recognition*. New York: Oxford University Press (in press).

Flinn, M. V. (1981) Uterine versus agnatic kinship variability and associated cousin marriage preferences: An evolutionary biological analysis. In *Natural Selection and Social Behaviour: Recent Research and New Theory*, ed. R. D. Alexander and D. W. Tinkle. New York: Chiron.

Flinn, M. V. (1986) Correlates or reproductive success in a Caribbean village. *Human Ecology*, 14, 225–43.

Flinn, M. V. (1987) Mate guarding in a Caribbean village. *Ethology and Sociobiology* (in press).

Flinn, M. V. and Low, B. S. (1986) Resource distribution, social competition, and mating patterns in human societies. In *Ecological Correlates of Social Behavior*, ed. D. Rubenstein and R. W. Wrangham. Princeton: Princeton University Press.

Fredlund, E. V. (1985) The use and abuse of kinship when classifying marriages: A Shitari Yąnomamö case study. *Ethology and Sociobiology*, 6, 17–25.

Freedman, D. S. and Thornton, A. (1982) Income and fertility: The elusive relationship. *Demography*, 19, 65–79.

Gadgil, M. (1982) Changes with age in the strategy of social behavior. *Perspectives in Ethology*, 5, 489–501.

Gadgil, M. and Bossert, W. H. (1970) Life historical consequences of natural selection. *American Naturalist*, 104, 1–24

Gaulin, S. and Schlagel, A. (1980) Paternal confidence and parental investment: A cross cultural test of a sociobiological hypothesis. *Ethology and Sociobiology*, 1, 301–9.

Gould, S. J. (1980) Sociobiology and the theory of natural selection. In *Sociobiology: Beyond Nature/Nurture?* ed. G. W. Barlow and J. Silverberg. Boulder, CO: Westview Press.

Gould, S. J. and Lewontin, R. C. (1979) The spandrels of San Marco and the Panglossian paradigm: A critique of the adaptationist programme. *Proceedings of the Royal Society of London, B*, 205, 581–98.

Grafen, A. (1982) How not to measure inclusive fitness. *Nature*, 298, 425–6.

Grafen, A. (1984) Natural selection, kin selection, and group selection. In *Behavioural Ecology: An Evolutionary Approach*, ed. J. R. Krebs and N. B. Davies, 2nd edition. Sunderland, MA: Sinauer Associates.

Gray, P. J. (1985) *Primate Sociobiology*. New Haven: HRAF Press.

Greene, P. (1978) Promiscuity, paternity, and culture. *American Ethnologist*, 5, 151–9.

Grossbard, A. (1976) An economic analysis of polygyny: The case of Maiduguri. *Current Anthropology*, 17, 701–7.

Hames, R. B. (1979) Relatedness and interaction among the Ye'kwana: A preliminary analysis. In *Evolutionary Biology and Human Social Behavior: An Anthropological Perspective*, ed. N. A. Chagnon and W. Irons. North Scituate, MA: Duxbury Press.

Hamilton, W. D. (1963) The evolution of altruistic behavior. *American Naturalist*, 97, 354–6.

Hamilton, W. D. (1964) The genetical evolution of social behavior, I. II. *Journal of Theoretical Biology*, 7, 1–52.

Hamilton, W. D. (1966) The moulding of senescence by natural selection. *Journal of Theoretical Biology*, 12, 12–45.

Hamilton, W. D. (1980) Sex versus non-sex versus parasite. *Oikos*, 35, 282–90.

Hamilton, W. D. and Zuk, M. (1982) Heritable true fitness and bright birds: A role for parasites? *Science*, 218, 384–7.

Hartung, J. (1976) On natural selection and the inheritance of wealth. *Current Anthropology*, 17, 607–22.

Hartung, J. (1982) Polygyny and the inheritance of wealth. *Current Anthropology*, 23, 1–12.

Hartung, J. (1985) Matrilineal inheritance: New theory and analysis. *The Behavioral and Brain Sciences*, 8, 661–88.

Hawkes, K. (1977) Cooperation in Binumarien: Evidence for Sahlins' model. *Man*, 17, 459–83.

Hawkes, K. (1983) Kin selection and culture. *American Ethnologist*, 10, 345–63.

Hill, J. (1984) Prestige and reproductive success in man. *Ethology and Sociobiology*, 5, 77–95.

Hinde, R. A. (1975) The concept of function. In *Function and Evolution in Behaviour*, ed. C. Beer and A. Manning. Oxford: Clarendon.

Hirschfield, M. F. and Tinkle, D. W. (1975) Natural selection and the evolution of reproductive effort. *Proceedings of the National Academy of Sciences, USA*, 72, 2227–31.

Holmes, W. G. and Sherman, P. W. (1983) Kin recognition mechanisms: A review. *American Scientist*.

Horrocks, J. and Hunte, W. (1983) Rank relations and vervet sisters: A critique of the role of reproductive value. *American Naturalist*, **122**, 417–21.

Howell, N. (1979) *Demography of the Dobe !Kung*. New York: Academic Press.

Hrdy, S. B. (1987) Sex-biased parental investment among primates and other mammals: A critical evaluation of the Trivers–Willard hypothesis. In *Biosocial Perspectives on Child Abuse*, ed. R. Gelles and J. Lancaster. Hawthorne, NY: Aldine-de Gruyter (in press).

Hurd, J. P. (1983) Kin relatedness and church fissioning among the 'Nebraska' Amish of Pennsylvania. *Social Biology*, **30**, 59–66.

Hurd, J. P. (1985) Sex differences in mate choice among the 'Nebraska' Amish of central Pennsylvania. *Ethology and Sociobiology*, **6**, 49–57.

Irons, W. (1979) Cultural and biological success. In *Evolutionary Biology and Human Social Behavior: An Anthropological Perspective*, ed. N. A. Chagnon and W. Irons. North Scituate, MA: Duxbury Press.

Irons, W. (1980) Is Yomut social behavior adaptive? In *Sociobiology: Beyond Nature/Nurture?* ed. G. Barlow and J. Silverberg. Boulder, CO: Westview Press.

Irons, W. (1983) Human female reproductive strategies. In *Social Behavior of Female Vertebrates*, ed. S. Wasser. New York: Academic Press.

Kaplan, H. and Hill, K. (1985a) Hunting ability and reproductive success among male Ache foragers. *Current Anthropology*, **26**, 131–3.

Kaplan, H. and Hill, K. (1985b) Food sharing among Ache foragers: Tests of explanatory hypotheses. *Current Anthropology*, **26**, 233–45.

Kaplan, H., Hill, K., Hawkes, H. and Hurtado, A. (1984) Food sharing among the Ache hunter-gatherers of eastern Paraguay. *Current Anthropology*, **25**, 113–15.

Kitcher, P. (1985) *Vaulting Ambition: Sociobiology and the Quest for Human Nature*. Cambridge, MA: MIT Press.

Kurland, J. A. (1979) Matrilines: The primate sisterhood and the human avunculate. In *Evolutionary Biology and Human Social Behavior: An Anthropological Perspective*, ed. N. A. Chagnon and W. Irons. North Scituate, MA: Duxbury Press.

Lack, D. (1954) *The Natural Regulation of Animal Numbers*. Oxford: Oxford University Press.

Lancaster, J. and Lancaster, C. (1983) Paternal investment: The hominid adaptation. In *How Humans Adapt: A Biocultural Odyssey*, ed. D. Ortner. Washington, DC: Smithsonian Institution Press.

Lee, R. B. and DeVore, I. (1968) *Man the Hunter*. Hawthorne, NY: Aldine Press.

Lenington, S. (1981) Child abuse: The limits of sociobiology. *Ethology and Sociobiology*, **2**, 17–29.

Lightcap, J. L., Kurland, J. A. and Burgess, R. L. (1982) Child abuse: A test of some predictions from evolutionary theory. *Ethology and Sociobiology*, **3**, 61–7.

Lockhard, J. and Adams, R. M. (1981) Human serial polygyny: Observational and demographic evidence? *Ethology and Sociobiology*, **2**, 177–86.

Lovejoy, C. O. (1981) The origin of man. *Science*, **211**, 341–50.

Low, B. S. (1978) Environmental uncertainty and the parental strategies of marsupials and placentals. *American Naturalist*, **112**, 197–213.

Low, B. S. (1979) Sexual selection and human ornamentation. In *Evolutionary Biology and Human Social Behavior: An Anthropological Perspective*, ed. N. A. Chagnon and W. Irons. North Scituate, MA: Duxbury Press.

Maynard Smith, J. (1978) *The Evolution of Sex*. London: Cambridge University Press.

Maynard Smith, J. (1982) The evolution of social behaviour – a classification of models. In *Current Problems in Sociobiology*, ed. King's College Sociobiology Group. London: Cambridge University Press.

Mayr, E. (1983) How to carry out the adaptationist program? *American Naturalist*, **121**, 324–34.

Mealey, L. (1985) The relationship between social status and biological success: A case study of the Mormon religious hierarchy. *Ethology and Sociobiology*, **6**, 249–57.

Miller, M. K. and Windle, C. (1960) Polygyny and social status in Iran. *Journal of Social Psychology*, **51**, 307–11.

Mueller, E. and Short, K. (1983) Effects of income and wealth on the demand for children. In *Determinants of Fertility in Developing Countries*. Volume 1, ed. R. A. Bulatao and R. A. Lee. New York: Academic Press.

Orians, G. H. (1969) On the evolution of mating systems in birds and mammals. *American Naturalist*, **103**, 589–603.

Parker, G. A., Baker, R. R. and Smith, V. (1972) The origin and evolution of gamete dimorphism and the male–female phenomenon. *Journal of Theoretical Biology*, **36**, 529–53.

Partridge, L. and Halliday, T. (1984) Mating patterns and mate choice. In *Behavioural Ecology: An Evolutionary Approach*, ed. J. R. Krebs and N. B. Davies, 2nd edition. Sunderland, MA: Sinauer Associates.

Porter, R. H. (1986) Kin recognition: Functions and mediating mechanisms. In *Sociobiology and Psychology*, ed. C. Crawford, D. Krebs and M. Smith. Hillsdale, NJ: Erlbaum Press.

Rubenstein, D. and Wrangham, R. W. (1986) *Ecological Correlates of Social Behavior*. Princeton: Princeton University Press.

Russell, M. J., Mendelson, T. and Peeke, H. (1983) Mothers' identification of their infants' odors. *Ethology and Sociobiology*, **4**, 29–31.

Schulman, S. R. and Chapais, B. (1980) Reproductive value and rank relations among macaque sisters. *American Naturalist*, **115**, 580–93.

Shaikh, K. and Becker, S. (1985) Socioeconomic status and fertility in rural Bangladesh. *Journal of Biosocial Science*, **17**, 81–9.

Shepher, J. (1971) Mate selection among second generation kibbutz adolescents: Incest avoidance and negative imprinting. *Archives of Sexual Behavior*, 1, 293–307.

Shields, W. M. and Shields, L. M. (1983) Forcible rape: An evolutionary perspective. *Ethology and Sociobiology*, 4, 115–36.

Silk, J. B. (1980) Adoption and kinship in Oceania. *American Anthropologist*, 82, 799–820.

Smith, J. E. and Kunz, P. R. (1976) Polygyny and fertility in America. *Population studies*, 30, 465–80.

Smouse, P. E., Vitzhum, V. and Neel, J. V. (1981) The impact of random and lineal fission on the genetic divergence of small human groups: A case study among the Yạnomamö. *Genetics*, 96, 179–97.

Spiro, M. E. (1958) *Children of the Kibbutz*. Cambridge, MA: Harvard University Press.

Stearns, S. C. (1976) Life-history tactics: A review of the ideas. *Quarterly Review of Biology*, 51, 3–47.

Stearns, S. C. (1977) The evolution of life-history traits: A critique of the theory and a review of the data. *Annual Review of Ecology and Systematics*, 8, 145–71.

Strassmann, B. I. (1981) Sexual selection, paternal care, and concealed ovulation in humans. *Ethology and Sociobiology*, 2, 31–40.

Sween, J. and Clignet, R. (1974) Type of marriage and residential choices in an African city. *Journal of Marriage and the Family*, 36, 780–93.

Symons, D. (1979) *The Evolution of Human Sexuality*. New York: Oxford University Press.

Symons, D. (1986) If we're all Darwinists, what's the fuss about? In *Sociobiology and Psychology: Issues, Ideas, Applications*, ed. C. Crawford, M. Smith and D. Krebs. Hillsdale, NJ: Erlbaum Press.

Taylor, P. D. and Williams, G. C. (1982) The 'lek paradox' is not resolved. *Theoretical Population Biology*, 22, 392–409.

Thornhill, R. (1980) Competitive, charming males and choosy females: Was Darwin correct? *Flavia Entomologica*, 63, 5–30.

Thornhill, R. and Thornhill, N. W. (1983) Human rape: An evolutionary analysis. *Ethology and Sociobiology*, 4, 137–73.

Thornhill, R. and Thornhill, N. W. (1986) On rape. In *Sociobiology and Psychology: Issues, Ideas, and Applications*, ed. C. Crawford, M. Smith and D. Krebs. Hillsdale, NJ: Erlbaum Press.

Thornton, A. (1977) Children and marital stability. *Journal of Marriage and the Family*, 39, 531–40.

Tinbergen, N. E. (1963) On aims and methods of ethology. *Zeitschrift fur Tierpsychologie*, 20, 410–33.

Trivers, R. L. (1972) Parental investment and sexual selection. In *Sexual Selection and the Descent of Man*, ed. B. Campbell. Hawthorne, NY: Aldine.

Trivers, R. L. (1985) *Social Evolution*. Menlo Park, CA: Benjamin/Cummings.

Trivers, R. L. and Willard, D. E. (1973) Natural selection of parental ability to vary the sex ratio of offspring. *Science*, 179, 90–2.

Turke, P. W. (1984) Effects of ovulatory concealment and synchrony on protohominid mating systems and parental roles. *Ethology and Sociobiology*, 5, 33–44.

Turke, P. W. (1987) Ovulatory concealment and menstrual synchrony. In *Biosocial Perspectives on the Family*, ed. E. Filsinger. New York: Sage Publications (in press).

Turke, P. W. and Betzig, L. L. (1985) Those who can do: Wealth, status, and reproductive success on Ifaluk. *Ethology and Sociobiology*, 6, 79–87.

van den Berghe, P. L. (1979) *Human Family Systems*. New York: Elsevier Press.

Vehrencamp, S. L. and Bradbury, J. W. (1984) Mating systems and ecology. In *Behavioural Ecology: An Evolutionary Approach*, ed. J. R. Krebs and N. B. Davies, pp. 251–78. Oxford: Blackwell Scientific Publications Ltd.

Voland, E. (1984) Human sex-ratio manipulation: historical data from a German parish. *Journal of Human Evolution*, 13, 99–107.

Wade, M. J. (1979) Sexual selection and variation in reproductive success. *American Naturalist*, 114, 742–7.

Wade, M. J. and Arnold, S. J. (1980) The intensity of sexual selection in relation to male sexual behavior, female choice, and sperm precedence. *Animal Behaviour*, 26, 446–61.

Westermarck, E. (1891) *The History of Human Marriage*. New York: Macmillan Press.

Williams, G. C. (1966) *Adaptation and Natural Selection: A Critique of Some Current Evolutionary Thought*. Princeton: Princeton University Press.

Williams, G. C. (1975) *Sex and Evolution*. Princeton: Princeton University Press.

Wilson, M. and Daly, M. (1985) Competitiveness, risk taking, and violence: The young male syndrome. *Ethology and Sociology*, 6, 59–73.

Wilson, M. and Daly, M. (1987) Risks to children in reconstituted families. In *Biosocial Perspectives on Child Abuse*, ed. R. Gelles and J. Lancaster. Hawthorne, NY: Aldine-de Gruyter (in press).

Wilson, M., Daly, M. and Weghorst, S. J. (1980) Household competition and the risk of child abuse and neglect. *Journal of Biosocial Science*, 12, 333–40.

Wilson, M., Daly, M. and Weghorst, S. (1983) Differential maltreatment of girls and boys. *Victimology*, 6, 249–61.

Wood, J. L., Johnson, P. L. and Cambell, K. L. (1985) Demographic and endocrinological aspects of low natural fertility in highland New Guinea. *Journal of Biosocial Science*, 17, 57–79.

Wright, S. (1983) Genic and organismic selection. *Evolution*, 34, 825–43.

Part I

Mating

Napoleon A. Chagnon[1]

Male Yąnomamö manipulations of kinship classifications of female kin for reproductive advantage

Introduction

Background to the data

This is a preliminary report on kinship knowledge and classification practices of the Yąnomamö Indians of southern Venezuela. Between January and March, 1985, I collected approximately 11 000 kinship responses from men and women in three Yąnomamö villages. These informants ranged in age from 5 years to approximately 75 years, the majority being between 15 and 30 years of age. Most of the residents were well known to me from previous visits to their villages between 1968 and 1975, during which period I collected detailed genealogical and demographic data on the population. The census and genealogical data were updated in 1985.

Theoretical dimensions of the study

The Yąnomamö kinship system

The Yąnomamö utilize a kinship classification system known as the Iroquois–Dravidian system (Chagnon 1966, 1968, 1983, Lizot 1971, Saffirio 1985). An important feature of that system is the classification of cross-cousins as the only legitimate marriage partners: both males and females must, according to the system's rules, select their marriage partners from the cross-

[1] Department of Anthropology, University of California, Santa Barbara, CA 93106, USA

cousin categories. Thus, a man must marry a woman who is classified into the categories Mother's Brother's Daughter (MBD) or Father's Sister's Daughter (FZD). These categories include cross-cousins of varying degrees of genealogical closeness or remoteness, i.e. first, second, third, etc. cross-cousins. Such women are called by the term *suaboyä* (or some equivalent, depending on the dialect area of the tribe) whether or not the man is married to them. It is considered incestuous to marry a woman of any other kinship category. The Yąnomamö kinship system thus operates as a component in what Levi-Strauss (1949 [1969]) has called a system of 'prescriptive marriage' (cf. Needham 1962).

It is important in such kinship classification systems that generational levels remain more or less in synchrony with relative ages of individuals: marriage with own-generation kin is, in effect, *prescribed* and marriage with any non-own-generation kin is proscribed. The demographic attributes of marriage among the Yąnomamö are such that males marry at about age 20 for the first time and females marry at about age 13. Thus, to marry according to the rules, a 20-year-old male not only must locate a cross-cousin, but one who should be about 13 years old.

For other matrimonial, social and economic reasons, it is likewise important to have a 'reasonable' relationship between generation level and ages of *all* kin, i.e. one's grandmothers should be older women, one's nieces should be younger girls, etc. Sisters and parallel cousins are classified as the same kind of relative and, since 'brother–sister' exchange (men giving their sisters in marriage to each other; see Figure 1.1) is an ideal and desirable practice, it is also important that a man's female 'siblings' (including his parallel cousins) be reasonably close to him in age.

Ideal models and socio-demographic reality

Most anthropological studies of primitive kinship systems focus primarily on the normative or 'ideal' rules of classification and attempt to view the specific taxonomic categories of such systems as 'roles' or 'statuses' with characteristic obligations, expectations, symbolic meanings, prescriptions, rules, etc. In such approaches, one can exemplify the ideal kinship relationships by giving cases of how two 'brothers' or 'cross-

cousins' should behave with respect to each other in particular circumstances. Most studies of primitive kinship invariably try to show how the kinship system articulates with other institutions in the society, such as the descent system, economic system, marriage system, etc. Such demonstrations usually take the form of diagrams or models, especially models that show the formal relationships between marriage rules, descent reckoning and kinship classification ... the 'structural' approach to social organization. (An 'ideal model' of Yąnomamö society is provided in Figure 1.1). However, these 'ideal' or 'formal' models can assume breathtaking complexity, as illustrated by Lane and Lane (1959), Eyde and Postal (1961) and Fox (1967).

These formal or structural approaches are used to characterize what the whole society is like as a *system* of social relationships that are defined in terms of ideal rules about kinship, marriage, or descent. Individuals within them, such as informants who provide the ethnologist with the rules, are occasionally 'used', along with other individuals, to provide examples of how the various rules operate – in a non-statistical sense. Neither the degree of deviation from the rules nor the degree of conformity to them by individuals is of concern in such approaches: it is immaterial what *all* or even the majority of individuals do in their actual marriages, exchanges, or classifications, since the formalist approaches are not concerned with explaining individuals as much as they are concerned about characterizing 'systems' (or models of systems) in some general sense.

Very few anthropological studies of kinship from any theoretical perspective provide much detail about the degree to which the kinship rules are followed by the people as they classify their kinsmen. I cannot think of any study where the actual kinship usage by a single individual for a large number of his/her co-residents was provided by the ethnographer, along with genealogical data that described how he/she was related to the individuals classified.

For reasons given above, the structuralist approach to kinship tends to view the system as an 'ideal' or 'perfect' system of classification and is not concerned with individual conformity or deviance. If we treat 'deviations' from the system as items that anthropologists 'sweep under the carpet,' the structuralist approach might be characterized as representing the kinship system as a perfectly flat carpet with nothing swept under it.

Most anthropologists are aware, however, that there are always some discrepancies between 'rules' and 'behavior' in all realms of culture. (See Fox (1982) for a superb illustration.) Manipulating or fudging of genealogies, for example, is commonly reported in the ethnographic literature, particularly for societies in which closeness to the chiefly line is advantageous (Polynesia, the Inca, etc.), or in agricultural areas where usufruct cultivation rights depends on genealogical connections (Melanesia, Micronesia). It is rare to find studies that focus on the discrepancies between kinship classification and the genealogical connections between individuals, i.e. that focus specifically on the statistical differences between what the people ought to be doing with their classifications and what they actually are doing. Most anthropologists would probably agree that deviations from the expected kin usage exist in all societies, but would probably regard them as more or less negligible and be willing to 'sweep them under the carpet' as a few small, discrete lumps.

For reasons given in more detail below, my own feeling is that in most primitive societies, especially in those where marriage possibilities are defined by kinship categories, there is more under the carpet (a larger lump) than we might like to admit, and what's under the carpet IS the system.

Kin classification discrepancies and demographic facts

In this analogy, there is a 'lump' under the carpet for very good reasons. Classification of kin and obtaining a satisfactory mate take place in a demographic milieu that demonstrably affects both. People cannot easily follow the 'rules' of either classification or marriage and the result is 'adjustments' or compromises in both realms. I want to explore just a few of the widely found demographic attributes of tribal populations in the context of some of the universal characteristics of male and female reproduction and show how the interaction of these must necessarily lead to manipulations of the kinship classification system in those societies where kinship classification defines marriageability. I have made

these arguments at greater length elsewhere (Chagnon 1982); I will simply summarize them now.

Before doing so, a note on my assumptions is in order. I assume at the outset that the facts of procreation in most societies are known to s members and that these serve in general as constraints on and guides for classification of kin (cf. Fortes 1969). Genealogy is a matrix used in most kinship classification systems in the tribal world, particularly for the closest kin of the individuals whose classifications are considered. I also assume that the degree to which classification reflects the genealogical relationships among individuals diminishes as the degree of kinship becomes increasingly remote. One is more likely to classify his genetrix by the term for mother than he is his mother's second matrilateral parallel cousin, even if the kinship rules indicate that both should be called by the term for mother.

Let me turn now to some of the more important demographic and physiological factors that impinge on the possible interplay of classification and genealogy. The major point is that *where kinship classification defines marriageability, individuals must necessarily manipulate kinship classification categories to keep generation level in synchrony with relative age.*

Age at reproduction and generation length

Because females are usually younger than males at the time of first marriage and because they have their first children at an earlier age, generation length through females will be shorter than it is through males (see Chagnon 1982). One major effect this short generation length through females has on kinship classification is that many individuals will have kin in the 'same' generation (traced back to the founder), but these kin will be of an absolute age that is inconsistent with their generational relationship. Five-year-old boys will have to classify 50-year-old women as 'sisters' or 'wives' in many cases. In a word, 'generation' gets out of 'synchrony' with absolute age and the two must be brought into some sort of harmony if the classification system is not to be used efficiently to designate marriageable individuals and assure that individuals of relatively comparable age are taxonomically eligible to get married. You can change taxonomy; you cannot change genealogy.

Reproductive lifespan of males and females

While females begin reproducing earlier in their lives than do males, men continue to reproduce longer than women (or are potentially able to do so). Many men in fact are producing children after 50 years of age in many tribal societies and, among the Yąnomamö, may have children by earlier wives who are 50 or more years older than their most recently born children. One of my best informants and dearest friends among the Yąnomamö is an elderly man who, in 1975 at approximately age 65, had a half-sister who was approximately 11 years old at that time. This has an effect similar to that described above: generation level and absolute age are incongruent with each other, and these incongruencies among siblings ramifies further when they marry and reproduce.

As is the case for age differences at first marriage and first reproduction by sex, the longer reproductive lifespan of males has an effect that necessitates chronic reclassification of some kin, probably by most individuals, to keep generation and age in relative harmony.

Inbreeding and how people are related genealogically

The necessity to chronically readjust classification takes place in a population where inbreeding levels are quite high and, therefore, people are related to each other in complex and multiple ways. Each of the genealogical connections between a pair of relatives is, or potentially is, associated with a specific kinship term or taxon, and therefore there is room for some ambiguity. This suggests that individuals have 'choices' regarding which genealogical connections to emphasize when they are related to a kinsman in multiple ways. Which ones they utilize can become the subject of great debate and conflict among their co-resident kin, since the act of classifying a kin can be a blatant attempt to gain advantage in the marriage competition. Examining the Yąnomamö marriage system as a set of ideal rules about marriage eligibility and reciprocal giving of females between descent groups will make clear how the multiplicity of genealogical links arise and how these lead to possible ambiguities and choices in kin classification.

The Yąnomamö marriage system entails reciprocal exchange over many generations between members of different (patrilineal) descent groups. This can be visualized as males exchanging sisters with each other within each generation, each marrying his bilateral cross-cousin as the 'ideal' diagram in Figure 1.1 suggests.

If everyone follows the rules, and each marriage produces one son and one daughter who survive to age of reproduction, then all men are married to women who are *simultaneously* their Father's Sister's Daughter (FZD) and their Mother's Brother's Daughter (MBD), i.e. their bilateral cross-cousins. Obviously these conditions cannot always obtain, but nevertheless a good deal of inbreeding does occur because groups of kin tend to exchange their marriageable daughters over several generations. The net result is that people are frequently related to their various kin in multiple ways, often in ways that are sometimes 'generation consistent' while simultaneously being 'generation inconsistent' (Figure 1.2)

One issue raised by this kind of example is the individual's 'choice' of which genealogical link to emphasize in classification when there are a number of choices possible. Some of the genealogical connections between the male and his spouse are consistent with the rule that he

Figure 1.1 Ideal model of the Yąnomamö social system showing how descent through the male line, brother–sister exchange, and prescriptive marriage by males with their bilateral cross-cousins articulate. Male members of two patrilineal descent groups (*x* and *y*) give females to each other in every generation. Each man is married to a woman who is simultaneously his Mother's Brother's Daughter (MBD) and Father's Sister's Daughter (FZD), i.e. his bilateral cross-cousin.

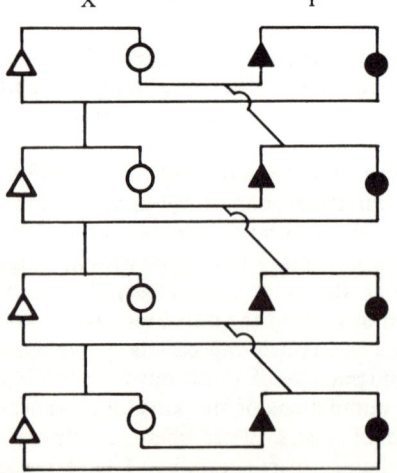

should marry a cross-cousin, but some are inconsistent with that rule, for the spouse is, genealogically, in a different generation than he is and therefore a prohibited mate.

Similar situations obtain between individuals and all other kinds of kin besides potential spouses and provide some 'choice' in so far as classification is concerned. There also appears to be a pattern to the choices people make as they go about adjusting the relationship between genealogical fact, rules of classification and competition for mates. The demographic necessity of reclassifying kin, in short, is also complicated by the fact that people are related to their kin in multiple ways. In general, the closest genealogical connections are the ones that should be used by the Yąnomamö, but that is not always the way individuals do it. I will return to this issue below.

Yąnomamö mortality and divorce rates and the 'decay' of the nuclear family
There are theoretical reasons to suspect that the use of kinship terms by male and female Yąnomamö is also affected by demographic attributes of the nuclear family, particularly high mortality rates in junior age categories and modestly high divorce rates. A critically important feature of

Figure 1.2 Pedigree of a typical Yąnomamö marriage showing the multiple relationships between a male and his spouse. Ego's wife is related to him as (a) MFSD, (b) FFSDD and (c) MFFSDDD where M = Mother, F = Father, S = Son, and D = Daughter. Only the first genealogical link conforms to the marriage rule since MFSD is Mother's (half)-Brother's Daughter. The two additional links are generation-aberrant and, by Yąnomamö definition, incestuous.

Yąnomamö marriage is that parents and elder kin, particularly kin on the father's side of the family, are very influential in arranging the marriages of their children and/or younger siblings. This is stated as a principle or belief by the Yąnomamö themselves, and numerous examples can be given to show that it indeed is the case for a large number of marriages. But the facts of demography as these relate to the duration of the nuclear family make it clear that it cannot always be the case. Indeed, the remarkable 'decay' rate of the Yąnomamö nuclear family raises a series of questions regarding kinship classification, and who actually arranges the marriages when genetic parents are dead or elsewhere, and how much 'choice' individuals have, particularly females, in obtaining a mate. Here, I will be concerned only with the issue of kinship classification and how the decay of the nuclear family in a society where parents are said to arrange marriages for their children possibly affects the way young individuals learn and utilize their genealogical and kinship skills.

The effects of mortality among young reproducing couples, combined with divorce frequency, leads to the dissolution of the nuclear family at a markedly high rate. As offspring go through infancy and childhood, the chances become increasingly remote that they will have genetic parents to look after their social and reproductive interests by the time they reach approximately age 20. While I have demonstrated this for the Yąnomamö (Chagnon 1982), I suspect that the pattern of nuclear family 'decay' is similar in all primitive populations where the 'demographic transition' has not yet

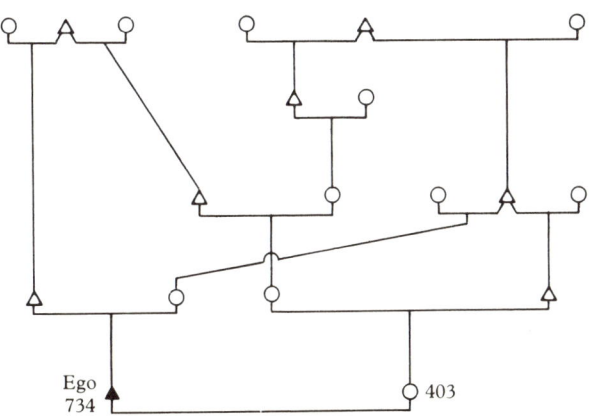

occurred, and where some divorce takes place. Let me explore this further.

Primitive populations are characterized by an age/sex distribution that reflects the relatively high birth rates coupled with relatively high death rates in younger age categories (Chagnon 1982). Moreover, marriage dissolution ('divorce') is fairly common in the primitive world, the median rate being approximately 30% of all marriages (Chagnon and Hames 1984).

While neither mortality rates nor divorce rates as such can be said to have a direct effect on how people classify their kin, they may have an important effect on who knows most about genealogy and kinship – males or females – and the rates at which both are acquired through enculturation where the following circumstances occur:

1. Marriageability is defined ('prescribed') by a kinship taxon, e.g. 'one should marry his matrilateral cross-cousin . . .'
2. One sex has more difficulty than the other in finding a suitable mate, e.g. male-biased sex ratio and/or polygyny leading to a 'wife shortage' for men.
3. Older kin have an important role in arranging the marriages of their sons and daughters, e.g. adult male agnates giving their sisters and daughters away in marriage in exchange for mates for their sons and brothers.

Many societies have all three features or a combination of some of these features (see also Murdock 1967 and Murdock and White 1969). Such situations exist (or have existed recently) in many tribal societies and the Yąnomamö are not an exception.

Before discussing how these factors are related to kinship and genealogy considerations, let me first put them into the context of the nuclear family.

If we define the nuclear family as consisting of a child, his or her monogamously married parents and at least one grandparent ('. . . an aged dependent . . .', Service 1971), approximately 25% of the individuals in the youngest age category (birth to age 5) live in that kind of nuclear family in my sample. This drops to just about 10% for children aged 6 to 10 years and is effectively zero thereafter (see Chagnon 1982:Fig.

14.6). After approximately age 15, almost no Yąnomamö would have a nuclear family defined as above.

If we consider a less 'stringent' definition of the nuclear family, such as both parents alive, monogamous and co-resident with the children, only about 18% of Yąnomamö have a 'nuclear family' by the end of their period of dependency on parents (age 16 to 20 years old). If we allow for the possibility that parents can have multiple spouses, only some 25% of the young people belong to nuclear families so defined.

Mortality among young parents and divorce therefore leads to a nuclear family arrangement such that most young individuals do not have both of their genetic parents co-resident and alive at the point they enter adulthood, at the point in their lives when they are looking for mates and, presumably, are most dependent on elder kin who arrange their marriages.

If young men have difficulty finding suitable mates in a milieu where male–male competition for mates is high, if their close kin in ascending generations are in any sense important in helping them find mates, and if there is a relatively low probability that their fathers, mothers and grandparents are around at this crucial time, then we have to examine more carefully the role of all individuals involved in marriage arranging. Empirically, we know that divorce usually separates the genetic father from his offspring, usually into different villages. The extent to which a non-co-resident father can aid his son in finding a suitable mate is probably extremely limited, and young males most probably have to develop their own strategies in circumstances where they cannot rely extensively on aid from older agnatic kin who have been compromised by subsequent marriages and the children they produce in them.

The above considerations raise important questions about fundamental anthropological theory, particularly the nature of lineal descent groups as marriage-arranging groups and the extent to which marriage is arranged by non-parental kin. For example, Leach (1961) argued that marriage-arranging groups in patrilineal societies like the Yąnomamö would consist of co-resident males representing, as a rule, three genealogical generations, namely: the old men or grandfathers, the normal adults or fathers, and the young adults or sons. While three generations of individuals who are co-resident might be involved in marriage arranging, it seems unlikely that they could be related genealogically in those societies where the mortality and divorce patterns are similar to those found among the Yąnomamö.

Important and new questions stem from the recent developments in theoretical biology with implications for kinship behavior and nepotism. We cannot continue to ignore the possibility that adult male (or female) marriage arrangers will 'favor' their own sons or grandsons over the less closely related offspring of deceased brothers in marriage arranging. Evidence is accumulating that closeness of kinship introduces a bias in the social interactions of members of many different species, including humans, and points more and more to the necessity of reconsidering some of our assumptions regarding indiscriminate nepotism (see Gray 1984). It is therefore quite possible that marriage arranging in primitive societies has nepotistic dimensions that we have consistently ignored.

Given the above data on nuclear family decay, it seems clear that few men will have their genetic fathers (or mothers) around to arrange their marriage, and fewer still will have their genetic grandfathers around. The problem will affect males far more than it does females, when females are in relatively short supply and some men are obliged to marry late, marry polyandrously, or not marry at all.

Reproductive striving and kinship knowledge by males

To the extent that Yąnomamö males are tracking their environment with their own fitness interests at stake, they should be aware that they will have to rely on a wider nexus of kin from whom aid and cooperation can be solicited in lieu of living, co-resident parents who would, if around, look after their marriage arrangements. Such a view makes kinship and genealogy a salient feature of the environment that the individual must manipulate and adapt to in striving for reproductive success and maximal inclusive fitness. Moreover, should we not also expect individuals to pay more attention to precisely those environmental features that most directly affect this pursuit and striving? I believe these are reasonable expectations and provide new ways to look at human kinship classifications and genealogical knowledge.

Kinship classification can thus be an intellectual tool that can be used to establish reproductively and socially useful relationships with one's neighbors. While genealogical connections that emanate from the facts of procreation impose constraints and limitations on classifications for close kin, kinship classification practices are seen here as highly flexible and situation-specific. It is predicted that individuals will manipulate kinship classifications and knowledge of genealogies to their own advantage, to advance their own survival possibilities and reproductive interests, as well as those of their closest kin. Individuals will, therefore, change their classifications of particular kin over a lifetime and probably nobody will consistently classify all their kin along the lines predicted by genealogy and the rules of their classification system.

Darwinian theory states that organisms strive to maximize inclusive fitness and adopt life strategies that, in general, lead to that end. Genealogical knowledge and kinship classification do not, at first blush, seem to be the kinds of topics where such arguments can be convincingly tested. In a society where mate competition is high among males, however, and where marriages are arranged by older kin for their younger siblings and children, it is possible to examine kinship usage from this perspective. Repeating some of the basic facts germane to the issue at hand, we have the following milieu:

1. Females are almost always married and have no difficulty finding suitable mates.
2. Males have difficulty finding mates.
3. Marriages are arranged by older kin, ideally by siblings, parents and siblings of parents.
4. The mortality patterns and divorce rates are such that neither males nor females have a high likelihood of having both natural parents alive and co-resident at the time they are most likely to obtain their first mate and must rely on more distant kin to help them in this regard.
5. The kinship system defines who is and who is not a legitimate mate.
6. People must manipulate kinship classification so that the relative ages of individuals is kept in synchrony with their generational relationships. This must be done for all kin.

29

Darwinian hypotheses derived from the sociodemographic attributes of Yąnomamö culture and population

A number of general hypotheses about kinship classification and genealogical knowledge suggested by the Darwinian approach follow from the above arguments. I will list a number of them, but explore only four of them in the next section of the paper.

1. Since age and generation become 'dysharmonic' because of the demographic factors described above, it is necessary to chronically 'adjust' kinship classifications to restore them to harmony. Thus, demographic factors allow us to predict only that reclassification of kin is necessary. Darwinian theory enables us to predict that individuals will move reclassified kin into categories that are socially and reproductively more useful to them rather than into categories that are less useful to them. For example, men should tend to move 'nieces' into 'wife' rather than 'sister' categories if they reclassify them into own generation and that they should call more women by 'wife' terms than are genealogically eligible to be called by wife terms.

2. If males have more difficulty finding mates than females do, and they are unlikely to have living parents and grandparents around when they most need them as 'marriage arrangers', men are more likely than women to make an effort to command knowledge of genealogy and kinship classification in order to better finesse a wider nexus of kin who would be potential wife-arrangers in lieu of actual parents and grandparents. These differences between Yąnomamö men and women should take several forms:

(a) First, males should have a more accurate knowledge of genealogies than females do, but will frequently conceal this knowledge when they classify kin. My past experience in collecting genealogies supports the first part of this claim (Chagnon 1974); projected analysis of male and female classification with respect to genealogical knowledge will be tested elsewhere.

(b) Second, males should know more about genealogies earlier in life than females do, i.e. learn genealogies and classifications sooner. Projected analyses of the differences in knowledge of young male and young female informants should reveal any existing differences.

(c) Third, males should 'manipulate' classifications more than females, i.e. *initiate* violations of the classificatory rules more often. This raises a difficult theoretical and practical problem. If men should know genealogies more accurately than females and simultaneously manipulate them more, how can you argue that the number of 'mistakes' they make represents 'greater knowledge'? Two kinds of 'solutions' might be explored. First, young males should be more accurate than young females, since the manipulations, as we shall presently see, usually do not begin until the males are at age of reproduction. Second, how males and females respond to questions of 'is this an incestuous marriage?' Males seem better able to explain why it is incestuous than females. They know how the classifications were modified in order to justify the illegitimate marriage. Although I do not plan to test greater male than female 'genealogical accuracy' in this paper, I am aware that this is a methodological problem at the outset. It is possible that self-deception is involved in the entire phenomenon of reclassification, an issue that lies beyond the scope of this paper.

(d) Fourth, males should have to ponder questions of genealogy and classification less than females do and respond more quickly and authoritatively to such questions.

3. Male siblings should tend to show a higher degree of conformity in the classification of their common relatives than either brother/sister dyads or sister/sister dyads. This is likely to be true for a number of reasons. The most important reason is that male siblings tend to cooperate in matters of politics and the politics of wife-giving more than either brother/sister or sister/sister dyads. I predict that they will show a greater tendency to contrive stories and classifications in cooperation with each other than they would with sisters.

4. Adult males should manipulate the classifications more frequently than juvenile males, since adults are already of reproductive age. Mistakes in classifying female kin by juveniles are probably more a reflection of ignorance and unfamiliarity with the genealogies and the rules

of classification and are likely to be more random than the 'mistakes' of their reproductively active older brothers.

I will focus on the following four arguments in the remainder of this paper:

1. Males will have kinship and genealogical information more immediately available, possibly reflecting a greater knowledge of both kinds of information compared to females.
2. When males reclassify female kin and move them from one category to another, there will be a bias toward creating more 'wives' than other categories of female kin.
3. Adult males will manipulate the classifications for their female relatives differently from juvenile males.
4. Adult males will show a tendency in reclassifying female kin to move females of higher reproductive value into the 'wife' category rather than women of lower-reproductive value.

Methods

Since the data in this paper are rather unusual,

Figure 1.3 Lineage composition of each of the three villages studied, and the three villages pooled. Note how predominant some lineages are in each village: 66% of the members of Village 93 belong to a single lineage, designated as Lineage 1222. Lineages are designated by the Identification Number of the founder.

I will take special pains to describe both the field and analytical methods. I do this not only in the spirit of clarity, but also to encourage others to collect similar data and provide comparative studies of other tribal populations. Moreover, I will describe the demographic attributes of the Yąnomamö population that are crucial for interpreting the results and deciding if the compared societies are indeed comparable. For example, a study of a population that was dwindling and had very few individuals in the junior age categories might not be as useful a comparison as one that, demographically, resembled the Yąnomamö population in age and sex distributions. Or, a study of a population most of whose members were unrelated to each other might not be useful for some comparisons, since the 'expected' classifications hinge on individuals being genealogically related to those they classify.

Most of the following analyses pool the data from the three villages that were studied. Subsequent analyses will focus on variations among the villages and among informants in the villages. It is important to point out, however, that the descent group characteristics of the villages vary somewhat, but it is not clear how, if at all, the data might be affected by the possibility that the informants' descent group membership biases the sample. Figure 1.3 summarizes the composition of all three villages by descent group representation. Several things should be pointed out here. First, the members of all three villages

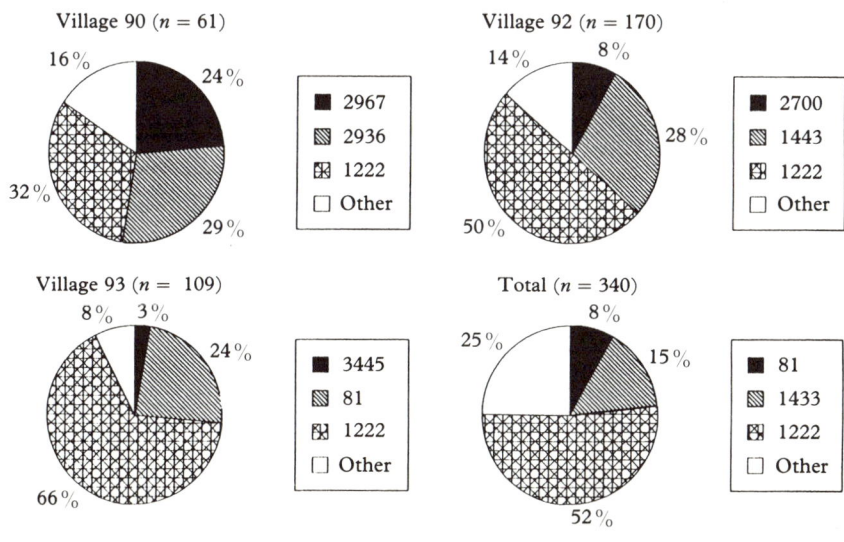

Village 90 (*n* = 61)

16% 24% 32% 29%

- ■ 2967
- ▨ 2936
- ▨ 1222
- ☐ Other

Village 92 (*n* = 170)

14% 8% 28% 50%

- ■ 2700
- ▨ 1443
- ▨ 1222
- ☐ Other

Village 93 (*n* = 109)

8% 3% 24% 66%

- ■ 3445
- ▨ 81
- ▨ 1222
- ☐ Other

Total (*n* = 340)

25% 8% 15% 52%

- ■ 81
- ▨ 1433
- ▨ 1222
- ☐ Other

31

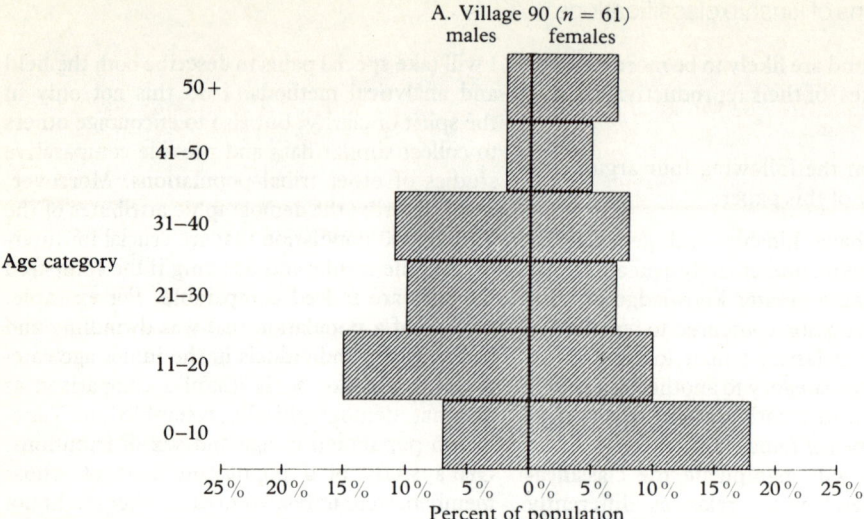

A. Village 90 (n = 61)

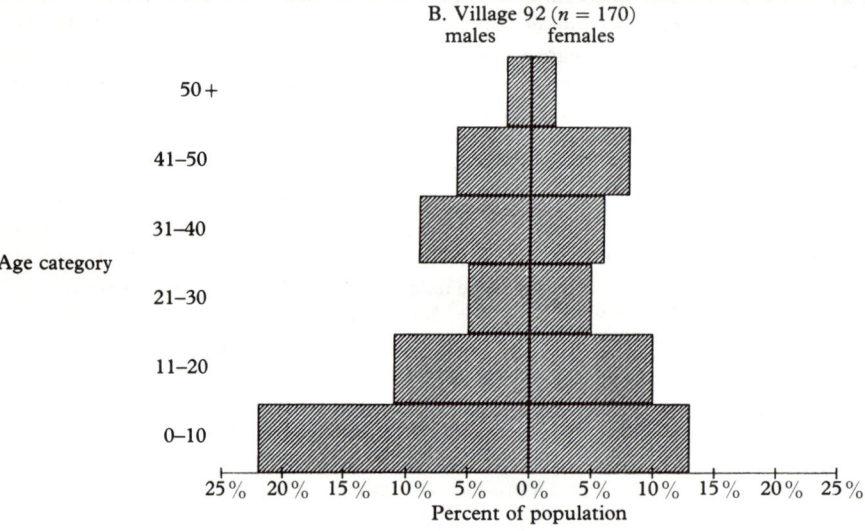

B. Village 92 (n = 170)

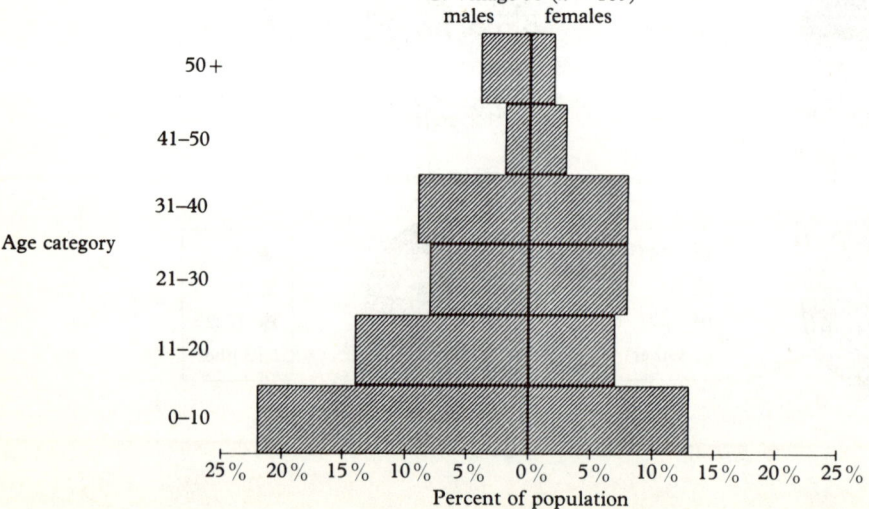

C. Village 93 (n = 109)

come from the same 'mother' population: their ancestors were all residents of the same village several generations back in time. Fissions divided them into their current villages (see Chagnon 1974, 1979). However, the members of Villages 90 and 92 were living together as recently as 1975, the approximate date of the fission that separated them. Members of Village 93 had split away much earlier, perhaps 40 or 50 years earlier. Second, the common history of the several villages is reflected in the fact that descent group '1222' dominates the composition of all three villages. This is the descent group of the Shamatari-Yąnomamö known as 'Shinbone' (viz. Chagnon 1974, 1979). Third, the degree to which a single descent group dominates, numerically, the composition of any particular village varies somewhat markedly. In particular, the composition of Village 93 is very heavily dominated by the lineal descendants of the founder of 1222: 66% of the residents belong to that one descent group. I have never come across a Yąnomamö village whose composition was so heavily dominated by representatives of a single descent group (cf. Chagnon 1979). The projected analyses will determine if this special composition has had any unusual effect on the nature of the kinship classification data from members of this village. It is possible that a few individuals, especially if they came from the same descent group and are full brothers, could bias the outcome of the kinship study: brothers tend to support each other in claims each makes about custom, rules, history of events, etc., and this carries over into the classification system as well (see Fredlund 1985, for an excellent analysis of the importance of close kinship in classifying marriages).

Age and sex distributions of the study populations

Figure 1.4 gives the age/sex distribution of the three villages in the current study. As is clear, the distribution is skewed in the smaller villages. Village 90, for example, had very few juvenile

Figure 1.4 Age and sex distributions of the three study villages by individual village. The general shapes of the distributions indicate that the population is still 'typical' for the primitive world.

males and Village 92 had relatively few individuals in the age category 21–30. This made it difficult to match ages of opposite-sex informants in Village 92, since there were many more boys between infancy and 10 years of age than there were girls.

The age/sex distribution in the three study villages in 1985 does not appear to differ markedly from what was found in earlier studies (cf. Chagnon 1974:158–9). The pooled age/sex distribution (not illustrated) shows a population 'pyramid' that is broad at the base and narrows rapidly. There are more males than females, especially in the junior age categories; this pattern reverses in the more senior age categories.

Age and sex distributions of the informants

Figure 1.5 gives the age and sex distributions of the 100 individuals whose classifications were solicited for co-villagers (pooled). As is clear, the majority of informants are above 11 years of age and there is a slight preponderance of male informants, reflecting the slightly higher proportion of males in the overall population. An attempt was made to get approximately equal numbers of male and female informants for all age categories, but this was not always possible for a number of reasons. Some villages had more individuals of one sex in certain age categories than others (see Figure 1.4). The exigencies of the field situation also complicated matters. For example, I was only able to spend approximately one week in Village 93 and had to work very rapidly: the residents had miscalculated the amount of food being produced by their new garden at that site and abruptly decided to move back to their previous village site where their gardens were more productive, thus terminating my investigation in that village. Nevertheless, the overall sex distribution of informants compares well with the population characteristics and the data are not unduly biased by sex. A more desirable sample for some purposes would have included proportionately more young informants in the youngest age category (0–10 years). The results reported here, however, focus primarily on classification of female kin by adult males or otherwise do not depend on a distribution of informants' ages and sexes that accurately reflects the population's age/sex characteristics.

Relatedness of co-villagers among each other

In general, the members of the three villages were highly related among themselves and the villages contained relatively few 'strangers'. One measure of within-village relatedness is the distribution by quartiles of every individual's co-resident kin (Chagnon 1982:295ff). Figure 1.6 provides the quartiles of relatedness for the members of the three villages. It is clear that most members of the three villages are related to more than three-quarters of all village residents. For example, more than 90% of the members of Village 92 are related to the members of that village in some genealogically-demonstrable way (shown in the 0.76–1.00 'quartile'). In this region of the Yąnomamö tribe, this is very characteristic as a pattern of relatedness in villages (Chagnon 1974, 1975, 1979).

While it was not possible to determine in the field how many relatives each informant had in the village, I did avoid using informants who were strangers or relative strangers in the village, such as recently abducted females or in-married young men from distant villages. Otherwise, informants were selected rather randomly, save for their ages and sexes.

The relatedness of informants to the co-villagers they were asked to classify, measured by the 'quartile' method, was similar to that

between co-villagers in general. Thus informants were a representative sample of the village.

Most of the informants are related to a very high fraction of the people they classified (see Table 1.2): if any genealogical connection could be demonstrated between the informant and the person classified, they were, by definition, 'related.' In some cases, the degree of relatedness was very high and complex (many close genealogical connections between them); in other cases, the relatedness was low. I will discuss this in more detail below.

Distribution of kin terms used by informants

The informants used a large number of different kinship terms to classify their relatives. Many of these were synonyms, such as the terms *shoriwä* and *heriya* used by males to classify their male cross-cousins and brothers-in-law, or the terms *suaböya*, *hesioböya*, and *sioböya* used by males to classify their female cross-cousins and wives. Over 40 distinct terms were used by all informants (cf. Chagnon 1974: Appendix C). These were combined in such a way to lump synonymous terms together: individual terms were given numbers, and those that were synonyms were lumped into a single letter designation. Therefore, the exact response of each informant for each co-villager still exists in the original data, as well as the 'lumping' convention used to reduce the large number of terms into the minimal discrete number of different terms. The analyses provided in this paper are based

Figure 1.5 Age and sex distribution of 100 informants (pooled) used to collect the 11 000 kinship responses from the members of the three study villages.

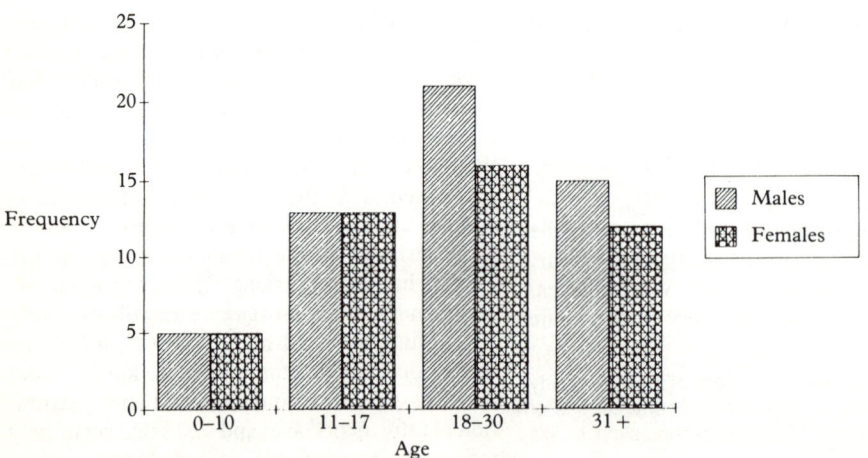

on the larger, more comprehensive categories; on the 'lumped' terms.

In addition to the kinship terms used by informants, I added categories for the following two kinds of cases. Informants were shown their own photographs and they generally responded by saying 'It is me!' (*kamiya*). I defined this as 'Ego' and represented it with the letter 'X' in the data set. In a few cases, particular co-villagers were not classified by some informants, usually because the tape cassette ran out and I did not allow sufficient overlap after putting a new tape in the recorder, or, I accidentally turned two pages at a time in the field book that contained the ID photographs, inadvertently skipping over the co-residents on one of the pages. These were coded as '?' or 'Not Asked' in the data set. Table 1.1 summarizes the kinship classifications and provides short glosses that define the Yąnomamö kinship term with regard to meanings they have in our own kinship terminology. In addition, Table 1.1 gives the frequencies of usage of the terms for both male and female informants.

Figure 1.7 breaks the distribution of kinship terms down by ages of informants: 'adults' are defined as individuals 18 years old or older, and 'sub-adults' as individuals 17 years old or younger. Approximately two-thirds of the kinship responses were by adults (see Table 1.1).

Figure 1.6 Quartiles of relatedness among co-villagers by village. In all three villages, most members of the village were related to 76% or more of their co-villagers (fourth quartile, right side of diagram), while less than 10% were related to 25% or fewer of their co-villagers (first quartile, left side of diagram). In general, an individual is related to most of the village residents and only a small minority of individuals have few or no kin.

There were 10 675 responses by the 100 informants. Table 1.2 gives the distribution of these terms by sex of informant and sex of person classified, and indicates the numbers of individuals to which the informants were genealogically related. Approximately 90% of all individuals classified were related in some genealogical way to the classifiers. Note that females tended to be related to classifiers slightly less frequently: this is due to the fact that all three villages contained a few abducted females (and their children).

Several features of the distribution are worth noting here. First, the most commonly used type of kinship term was 'sibling' (Type 'I'). Second, some terms are used only by males (e.g. the term for 'wife' [E]) and some terms are used only by females (e.g. the term for 'husband' [F]). Note also that there is a category, 'P', for which there are no instances. This was due to the adoption of the convention that the term *iba* would be treated as a separate entry, a term that simply means 'mine' or 'my.' I subsequently moved the relatively few cases in this category into other categories to which they legitimately belonged: e.g. 'my actual son,' 'my actual wife,' 'my actual daughter.' The term was invariably used for an immediate relative and there were very few instances of it to begin with. Differences in frequencies of kin term use given in Figure 1.7 correspond to differences in ages of informants. One would expect, for example, that older informants would have proportionally fewer 'grandmothers' than younger informants, or that younger informants would have fewer 'nieces' than older informants. In general, most of the

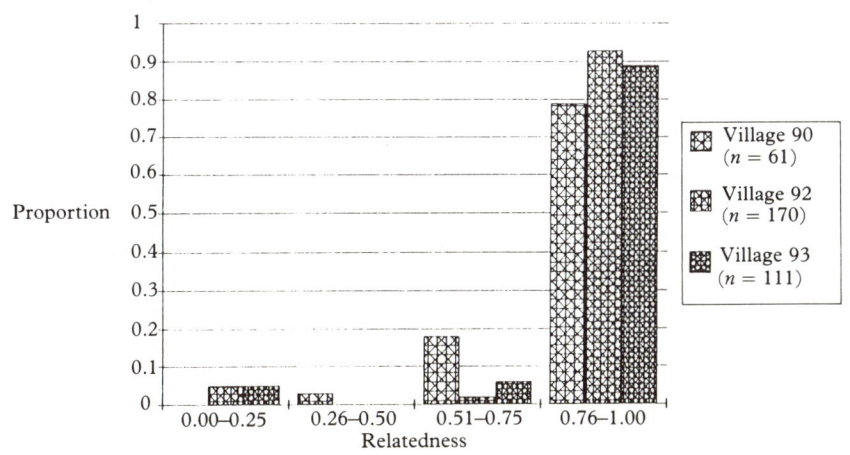

Proportion

Village 90 (n = 61)

Village 92 (n = 170)

Village 93 (n = 111)

Relatedness

Table 1.1 *Frequencies of male and female kin term usages and short English glosses for kinship terms*[a]

Kin term	Male usage		Female usage		
	Adults	All	Adults	All	
? Not asked	9	14	8	12	
A *Shoaya*	169	330	95	251	Father-in-law, grandfather
B *Yaya*	198	407	140	301	Mother-in-law, grandmother
C *Haya*	102	259	115	237	Father, father's brother
D *Naya*	153	316	127	275	Mother, mother's sister
E *Suaböya*	436	583	—	—	Wife, female cross-cousin
F *Hearoya*	—	—	351	599	Husband, male cross-cousin
G *Shoriwä*	388	613	—	—	Brother-in-law, male cross-cousin
H *Nadohiya*	—	—	301	468	Sister-in-law, female cross-cousin
I Sibling terms	676	939	450	712	[Many terms exist for siblings]
J *Ihiruya*	308	354	217	290	Son
K *Tääya*	246	282	183	220	Daughter
L *Yuhaya*	330	368	344	401	Niece
M *Hekamaya*	512	586	474	550	Nephew
N 'Vague' (females)	65	181	155	324	Vague terms for female kin
O 'Vague' (males)	60	122	195	331	Vague terms for male kin
P 'Mine'	1	1	0	0	'Mine'
Q *Kuwi*	12	183	14	66	'I don't know'
R *Shomi*	0	1	1	3	'Some non-relative'
X Ego ('Me')	35	52	27	45	Self
Totals	3700	5591	3197	5084	

All male/female informant totals	10 675
Adult male/female informant totals	6 897

[a] See Chagnon 1974, Appendix C, for more comprehensive discussion of Yąnomamö kinship classification and additional meanings of the above terms

Figure 1.7 Frequency distribution of 11 000 kinship terms used by 100 informants for co-villagers for informants 0–17 years old and informants 18 years old and older by sex of informant. (See Table 1.1 for English glosses of the terms.)

classified kin of all informants fall into 'own' or 'descending' generation, reflecting the relatively high mortality rates and the 'youngness' of the population: most living Yąnomamö are below

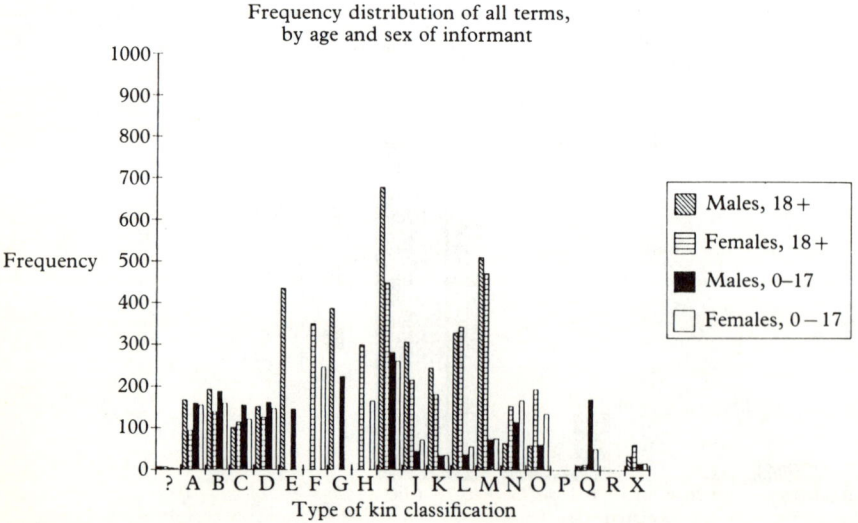

Frequency distribution of all terms, by age and sex of informant

Males, 18 +
Females, 18 +
Males, 0–17
Females, 0 – 17

Frequency

Type of kin classification

Table 1.2 *Percentage of co-villagers related to male and female classifiers by sex of classifiers and classified*

	Number (N) classified	Number (N) related	Percentage related
Males/males	3035	2782	91.7
Males/females	2619	2260	86.3
Females/females	2357	1955	82.9
Females/males	2729	2496	91.5
Totals	10740	9493	88.4

age 25, few people have many living, co-resident ascending generation kin.

'Vague' or 'endearing' kinship terms

I must mention one category of terms that are somewhat unique. I will hereafter call them 'vague' terms for sake of a better name. These are terms that simultaneously emphasize 'affect' while at the same time are inspecific regarding the genealogical connection between the classifier and classified. An example is in order. The term *nakami* can be translated as 'my darling [younger?] female relative,' or the term *mokawa* can be translated as 'my darling [younger?] male relative.' They often mean 'my daughter' or 'my son,' but they can also mean 'my little sister'

Figure 1.8 Proportion of 'vague' kin terms used by adult male and female informants by generation of kin classified with vague terms. Data from all villages are pooled. Females use vague terms more often than males, and most vague terms are for own-generation or descending generation relatives. Note that the range of vague terms is from two ascending to two descending generations.

or 'my little brother' – or 'my granddaughter' or 'my grandson.' During most of my early field research (1964–70) I thought that such terms were applied only to extremely young members of one's own generation or to kin of the first or second descending generations. The results of my 1985 field research show that the range of meaning is somewhat wider than this. I also thought that such terms (and there are a relatively large number of them) were used with approximately equal frequency by both males and females: that turns out not to be the case.

Figure 1.8 shows the distribution of 'vague' kin term use by sex of informant and generation of the classified relative with reference to the informant. Three features stand out. First, and most obvious, is the disproportionately high use of such terms by females. Second, the person classified might fall into any of five different generation levels with reference to the classifier, although most instances are for own generation ('0' in Figure 1.8) or the first descending ('−1' in Figure 1.8) generation. Third, but not readily

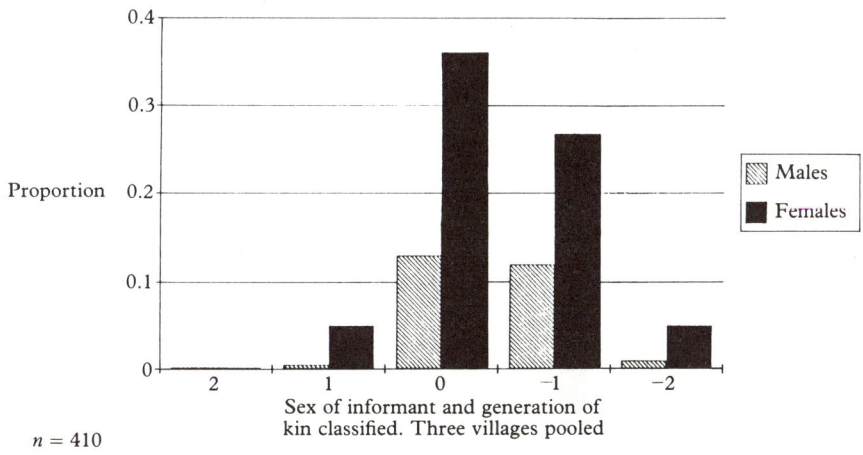

Proportion

Males
Females

Sex of informant and generation of kin classified. Three villages pooled

n = 410

37

apparent in Figure 1.8 (but will be in the sections below), is the fact that adults use such terms much less frequently than children.

My original interpretation was that these terms were primarily 'endearing' terms used by adults for very young relatives; the new data implies that the terms also function to conceal specificity, i.e. are perhaps deliberately 'vague' as well as being 'endearing.' They might serve, for example, to enable very young individuals to indicate that particular co-residents are 'close' (but yet unspecifiable) kin, or, might enable adults to conceal a specific genealogical connection when it is to their advantage to do so. An example of the latter function might be in reference to a consanguinal kin who should be called by a very specific term on the basis of genealogical relationship and the 'rules' of classification, but to do so would reveal an act of incest by some other very close relative, such as a brother. One can, by using a deliberately vague term, avoid drawing attention to such controversial issues.

One final feature of these terms is worth mentioning. Figure 1.9 gives the distribution of the use of 'vague' or 'endearing' terms by village and sex of informant. The somewhat startling feature of the distribution is that (adult) males in Village 93 *never once* used such terms for any relative, and that the females used them relati-

vely infrequently compared to females in the other two villages.

As mentioned above, the members of this village had miscalculated the productivity of their new garden and, during my stay in this village, people became increasingly hungry as each day passed. Since it is the men who 'own' the gardens and therefore decide who can legitimately ask for a 'share' of their cultivated staples, one could conclude that the men were, in effect, avoiding the use of 'endearing' terms to be better able to deny young supplicants a share of their temporarily scarce resources. The use of kinship classification in the village at this specific point in time might have been 'skewed' toward the 'formal' end with the deliberate intention of constraining whatever 'altruistic' implications might inhere in the use of endearing kinship terms. If this is true, and it can be verified by collecting the kinship classifications again under more economically salubrious conditions, then this is a rather surprising and unanticipated finding on how kinship classifications are utilized under varying conditions. One might characterize the situation as follows: hungry classifiers are less nepotistic than sated ones. It should be emphasized that the sample size, while being larger than what is commonly found in anthropological works on kinship classification, might be insufficiently large to arrive at this conclusion. I cannot think of a single 'traditional' kinship study that would predict that the overall 'profile' of the kin classification in a specific society (village, band) varied with the abundance or scarcity of

Figure 1.9 Proportion of all terms represented by vague terms, by sex of adult informant and village. Adult males in Village 93 did not use vague terms at all.

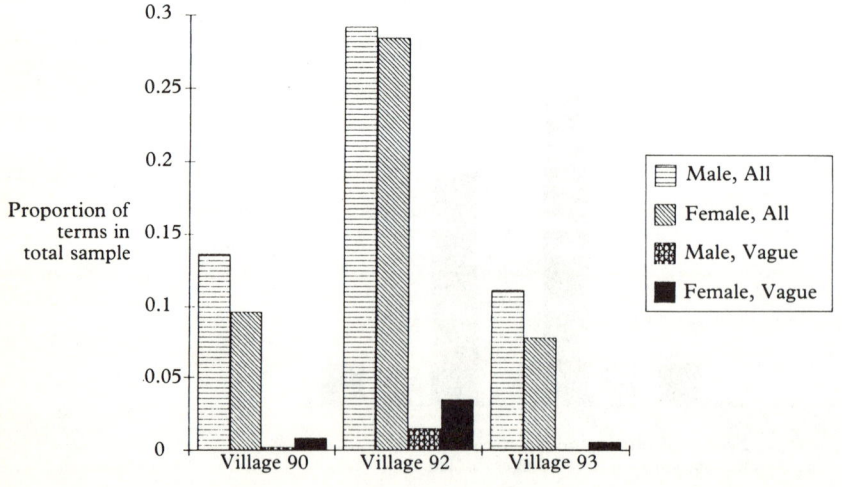

Table 1.3 *Y̨nomamö response rates in identifying kin by age and sex categories of informants*

Age	Male informants				Female informants				t	df
	N	Mean[a]	SD	SE	N	Mean[a]	SD	SE		
5–10	7	17.4	3.3	1.3	6	15.3	2.6	1.2	1.2	11
11–15	6	20.6	4.6	2.1	11	18.6	2.7	0.8	0.9	15
16–25	23	22.4	5.1	1.1	14	20.2	3.3	0.9	1.1	35
26+	16	21.6	3.1	0.8	14	19.1	2.9	0.8	2.3*	28
All	52	21.3	4.5	0.6	45	18.8	3.3	0.5	3.1†	95

* p. 025
† p. 005
[a] 'Mean' refers to numbers of kin classified per minute

resources over a short span of time – a month, season, year, or even the lifetime of the classifiers. We know from studies such as those conducted by Firth and Spillius (Firth 1959, Spillius 1957) on Tikopia, that natural disasters and ensuing food shortages dramatically affect the distributional/sharing aspects of a kinship-organized economy. That this sort of situation has an effect on *classification behavior* is, I believe, a new observation at the level of kinship taxonomy studies.

Results

Speed of response of informants by sex

The speed of response of all informants is given in Table 1.3. The responses of several of the informants were not timed; therefore, the total number of informants is less than 100. The age categories were chosen so as to focus on those categories where differences are likely to begin to emerge in the overall knowledge of individuals regarding classifications for their kin. For males, this would be approximately 15 years of age, that time in their youth when they are approaching marriageable age.

Males classified their relatives more quickly than did females. An examination of response time by each age category indicates that males are faster than females in all categories, but the differences in speed of response are not significant for the two youngest age categories. The 'fastest' rates for both males and females occurs in the age category 16–25 years.

While this is not a direct test of the hypothesis that males 'know more' about kinship and genealogy than females, speed of response could possibly indicate the amount or accuracy of knowledge. I would expect that having information 'at the tip of the tongue' reveals that the individual has an immediate command of the information and can reveal it quickly – does not have to search his mind for the answers. Many informants, particularly younger informants, in fact, pondered aloud the genealogical information that ultimately went into their responses. This took them additional time and lengthened their response times. While it was not apparent in the field that female informants did this more often or longer than male informants, the above data suggests that this is the case. But speed of response is different from accuracy of response and it is not yet clear that, although males are faster at classifying kin than females, males are more accurate than females in their kinship/ genealogical knowledge.

To test directly the hypothesis that males know more about kinship/genealogy or are more accurate in their knowledge will require comparing the individuals' kinship responses to the same individuals' genealogical connections to all classified kin, a time-consuming exercise that lies ahead. For the moment, I can only speculate that if speed of response correlates with knowledge, then it is possible that Y̨nomamö males 'know' more than females about kinship and genealogy.

There are a number of alternative explanations of the fact that males classify more relatives per unit of time than females. One of them is that my instructions were given more clearly to males than to females and that they understood the task more thoroughly. This was unlikely for several reasons. First, it became rapidly apparent to all residents what I was doing and how I wanted it done: it became the subject of village discussion and therefore widely known. Indeed, in not a few instances did residents shout, as a new informant took his/her seat. 'Do it fast – he likes it that way!'. Second, if there was any bias, it probably favored female informants: I probably explained more often and more repetitiously to females that I wanted it done fast and to let me know immediately if they did not know the answers. I also probably turned my tape recorder off more times to repeat my instructions to female informants who seemed to be responding more slowly than others (the 'off' time, of course, was not counted in the analyses).

A third possibility is that a male anthropologist will get a different degree of cooperation from male informants than he will from female informants. I cannot dismiss this on empirical grounds; the only certain answer would be for a female anthropologist to repeat this research. However, it is also likely that the sex of the anthropologist might lead to other biases and exaggerate the differences more: it is quite possible that male Yąnomamö informants would 'try harder' to please a female than a male anthropologist, whatever difference the sex of anthropologist might make on the speed of female informants' responses. The potential benefits for a male informant for so doing would be, in Yąnomamö terms, obviously higher – and probably consciously in mind. I rather suspect, however, that the opposite sex of anthropologist would not lead to conclusions opposite to what I report here.

A fourth possibility is that females, in general, are less cooperative informants or are more bashful as informants for all kinds of information and that their slower responses to kinship/genealogy questions do not necessarily reflect a difference in reproductive striving within which such knowledge is advantageous. This is a thorny question, since it deals with a host of other issues, including knowledge by sex for all things that males and females do, the division of labor and who should know what, and the ultimate function of knowledge in general for survival and reproduction. Obviously it would not be a useful test to compare what males and females know about the habits of game animals given that males do almost all of the hunting. Nor would it be especially revealing to compare the abilities of males and females in plaiting large baskets, since females do almost all of that kind

of work. It is not intuitively obvious, at least to me, that one sex should know more than the other in this society about kinship or genealogy. One might make the argument that males should know more about genealogy than females, since, in some fashion, this has something to do with political relationships between villages and men putatively 'control' politics. But can the same argument be posed about kinship classification? One could just as persuasively argue that since women have the babies, they ought to know more about both genealogy and kinship classification than males, and they should therefore reveal their knowledge in a manner quite the opposite of what they have done – unless their gender in this culture compels them to be less cooperative for reasons I do not know and therefore cannot describe. I suspect that if there would be any intuition among anthropologists regarding which sex knows more about kinship and genealogy, most of us would probably guess that women know more. It would be instructive to test this suggestion with a population of anthropologists who are unfamiliar with the arguments put forth in this paper.

At this juncture parsimony suggests that the interpretation put forth here is a reasonable one and accounts for the observed facts in an efficient manner. It was not intuitively obvious from the generally accepted view of kinship in anthropological theory that one sex should be faster at classifying kin than the other, nor was it obvious that this was even a relevant or useful question. However, male Yąnomamö do indeed classify their kin faster than female Yąnomamö, a finding that I predicted from hypotheses derived from the general theory of evolutionary biology. I think this finding is as useful and interesting to anthropology and kinship studies as it is to biology.

Manipulations of female classification by male informants

The Iroquois–Dravidian kinship classification system used by the Yąnomamö, along with their emphasis on patrilineal descent, was used to generate a set of expected usages. For extremely close kin, the Yąnomamö generally conform to the expected; they call their genetrix by the term for 'mother,' their genitor by the term for 'father.' As one progresses further out through genealogical links, the observed and expected begin to deviate. Precisely how much individual deviation exists will be the subject of other publications. Here it is sufficient to say that a set of expected kinship usages were generated from the kinship and descent rules and these, in turn, were compared to the actual genealogical connections that characterized each informant's relationship to the persons classified. The genealogical relationships (e.g. MFFSSD) are called 'Muddles' (cf. Schneider 1965). Some 250 such genealogical 'muddles' were defined for male relationships to female kin and all were given numerical codes.

Each informant's relationship to the individuals they classified was determined by computer analysis of the genealogies with the program KINDEMCOM (Chagnon and Bryant 1984). Thus, every informant was systematically compared to all members of the village and, if a demonstrable genealogical link was found for any 'ALTEREGO' in the computer search, that link was recorded. The link, of course, is a 'muddle.' Because of the systematic exchanges between members of different descent groups over many generations, most of the individual informants were related to their kin in multiple ways, and many different 'muddles' characterized the relationship between an informant and individual kin in most cases. Needless to say, this resulted in a large data set – scores of thousands of comparisons were made and an even larger number of 'muddles' resulted.

Genealogical complexity and reducing it

In general, the Yąnomamö pay most attention to the cloest genealogical connections and base their kinship classifications on these. For the moment, I am concerned with the broadest picture of classification as it relates to genealogy. To do so requires a methodological decision to reduce the enormous complexity to a manageable problem.

The multiple genealogical connections between related individuals have been reduced to a single closest genealogical connection. There were a large number of cases in which the first and second closest links were equally close; these invariably resulted from the fact that the dyads were, for example, full siblings, full first cousins, full second cousins, as distinct from half-

siblings, half first cousins, half second cousins.

Thus, analyses were made on a data file in which each informant was related to the individual he/she classified in one genealogical way – the closest genealogical connection between them. Individuals who were not related to their classifiers were excluded from analyses. Table 1.2 indicates that the informants were, in general, related to nearly 90% of the people they classified, so the number of cases excluded is relatively small.

The genealogical connection – the 'muddle' – was then used to establish the 'expected' kinship term usage. That is to say, the muddle was compared to the list of 'expected' usages that were made on the basis of the kinship and descent rules. In this fashion, the 'expected' usage of the informant for each kin was established. The expected usages were then compared to the actual kinship usages as recorded in the field interviews.

Male informants classify all their female relatives into seven distinct categories (see Table 1.1). For ease of description, I will hereafter adopt a single term that will stand as a shorthand reference for the taxon under question.

1. Daughters (*Täaya*).
2. Mothers-in-law (*Yesiya*).
3. Mothers (*Naya*).
4. Nieces (*Yuhaya*).
5. Sisters (numerous terms).
6. Wives (*Suaböya*).

And, as described above, there is a seventh category that cannot be analysed in the same fashion, since the genealogical specifications are too numerous to be predictable:

7. 'vague' – not predictable from genealogical connections.

It is possible to compare observed and expected for the first six of these categories, since the muddles are very specific about the predicted usage, while the observed usage is an actual datum collected in the field. Vague terms, however, had no predicted usage.

The hypothesis that males should be expected to classify more females as wives than is genealogically expected was then examined. Initially, I thought this could be adequately tested by examining only those muddles and kinship classifications that pertained to a male informant's 'wives' (all female cross-cousins). While males do classify more females as wives than was genealogically expected, it was not clear if they were treating 'wives' in a different fashion to the way they were treating all non-wife kin. In order to make certain that men were preferentially misclassifying female kin into wife categories I examined how male informants classified *all* female relatives.

Three classification 'cases' defined

Three distinct 'cases' were defined for each of the six types of female relatives all men have. The cases were defined as follows: Case 1: the 'expected' classification term, based on genealogical connection and the rules of classification, was identical to the actual kinship response given by the informant for that relative. For example, the genealogical connection between a male and a female was such that the man should have used a 'sister' term for the female and, in fact, actually did use a sister term – the 'expected' and 'actual' were identical. Case 2: the 'expected' and 'actual' terms differed for a particular taxon (e.g. 'sister') and the informant was characterized as moving a non-sister into the sister category when the sister category was the subject of analysis. Case 3: the 'expected' and 'actual' terms differed, as in Case 2, but the informant was characterized as having moved a genealogically expected sister into a non-sister taxon. Thus, for each of the six taxons that males put female relatives into, it was possible to determine how many female relatives were accurately classified (Case 1), how many were 'moved into' the taxon (Case 2) and how many were 'moved out' of the taxon (Case 3).

Table 1.4 summarizes the Cases for adult male informants (18 years or older) for all their female kin. Informants for all three villages are pooled. The column identified as 'W act.' gives the number of women from Case 3 that were misclassified into the wife category in all of the six genealogically specifiable kin taxons (except, of course, the 'wife' taxon). One of the possible kinship taxons is the 'vague' category, which cannot be 'predicted' by genealogical criteria. I have eliminated this category from statistical consideration. If misclassification of female kin were random, then the classifiers should misclassify any particular set of female relatives (mothers, nieces, sisters, etc.) in such a way that

Table 1.4 *Manipulations of classifications of female kin by adult males*

Relative	Case 1	Case 2	Case 3	W act.	1/5 exp.
Daughters	168	36	72	28	14
Mothers-in-law	115	43	26	6	5
Mothers	92	33	47	12	9
Nieces	189	57	108	42	22
Sisters	229	34	88	29	18
Totals	793	203	341	117	68[a]
Wives	236	121	39	—	—
'Vague'	—	48	—	—	—

Total number of classifications 1781
Percentage of classifications that are 'vague' 2.8%

[a] χ^2 likelihood ratio = 42.96, df = 5, $p < 0.001$; comparisons based on Case 3 totals for calculating expecteds

they would place approximately one-fifth of them into each of the remaining five categories. For example, for the 72 instances of genealogically predicted daughters who were classified as some other kind of (non-daughter) kin (Case 3) – 14.4 should have been moved into each of the remaining taxons. Thus, the column '1/5 exp.' of Table 1.4 is the number of misclassified female kin who would be expected to be put into the wife category if misclassifications were random.

The actual number of female kin reclassified as wives exceeds the expected in all taxons, and the overall pattern shows that adult males are far from random in reclassifying female relatives. This supports the hypothesis that adult males are moving female kin from categories of less reproductive utility (e.g. sisters) into the reproductively most useful category: wife. The results are statistically very significant.

An examination of the three cases for the term 'wife' in Table 1.4 indicates that adult males are moving proportionately more non-wife kin into the 'wife' category (Case 2 for wife) and moving proportionately fewer 'wives' into 'non-wife' taxons (Case 3 for wife). This pattern, compared to what they are doing with other taxons for female relatives, is summarized in Figure 1.10.

The 'Case 1' figures for each taxon in Figure 1.10 are defined as unity, and Cases 2 and 3 are plotted as proportions of Case 1 to make the taxons more readily comparable to each other. The higher the middle bar of the histograms, the more is the tendency for that taxon to 'create' relatives of that taxon; the lower the right-hand bar, the less the tendency to move relatives of that category into some other category. It is clear that the adult male informants are 'creating' more wives than other kinds of kin through their classificatory manipulations and are more reluctant to move 'wives' into other categories than they are for other kinds of female kin. A similar pattern obtains for the category 'mother-in-law.' It would appear that when a male Yąnomamö reclassifies a relative by the term for 'wife,' he has a tendency to reclassify her mother into the category 'mother-in-law.' This is an extremely sensitive 'taboo' relationship – mother-in-law – and it appears that the Yąnomamö 'extend' the manipulation for wives to the mothers of these wives. Whether they also do it in other manipulations (e.g. sisters, nieces, etc.) remains to be seen.

The data provided in Figure 1.10 can be shown also as a ratio of Observed/Expected. Table 1.5 gives the data in this form. The value of 1.00 can be interpreted in the following way. If the several different kin taxon O/E ratios are below the value 1.00, the male informants are 'getting rid of' relatives in that taxon. If the value is above 1.00, they are 'creating' more relatives of that type than is genealogically warranted.

The distribution of the O/E values indicates that Yąnomamö males are redefining many of their sisters, nieces and daughters as some other kind of female kin, while simultaneously putting many non-wife and non-mother-in-law kin into these two categories. As we shall presently see, the nieces, sisters and daughters are being redefined as wives.

Figure 1.10 Manipulation of female kin classification by adult male informants showing proportion of Case 1 represented by Cases 2 and 3. Case 1 (horizontal axis) is defined as unity and represents instances where the actual and expected kinship classification were the same. Case 2 represents instances where kinswomen should have been classified as some other type of relative. Case 3 represents instances where kinswomen were moved out of the category and defined as some other type of relative. Note in the sixth box adult males show a strong tendency to move non-wife kinswomen into the wife category; Case 2 for the wife taxon represents a large fraction of all wife classifications. These are women who were redefined as wife.

Classification by sub-adult males

The classificatory behavior of sub-adult male informants shows a very different pattern. Table 1.6 provides the statistical distribution of the same types of data that were shown for adult males in Figure 1.10. While it might be appropriate to consider the misclassifications of females by adult males as 'manipulations,' it is probably more reasonable to interpret misclassifications by sub-adult males as simply 'mistakes.'

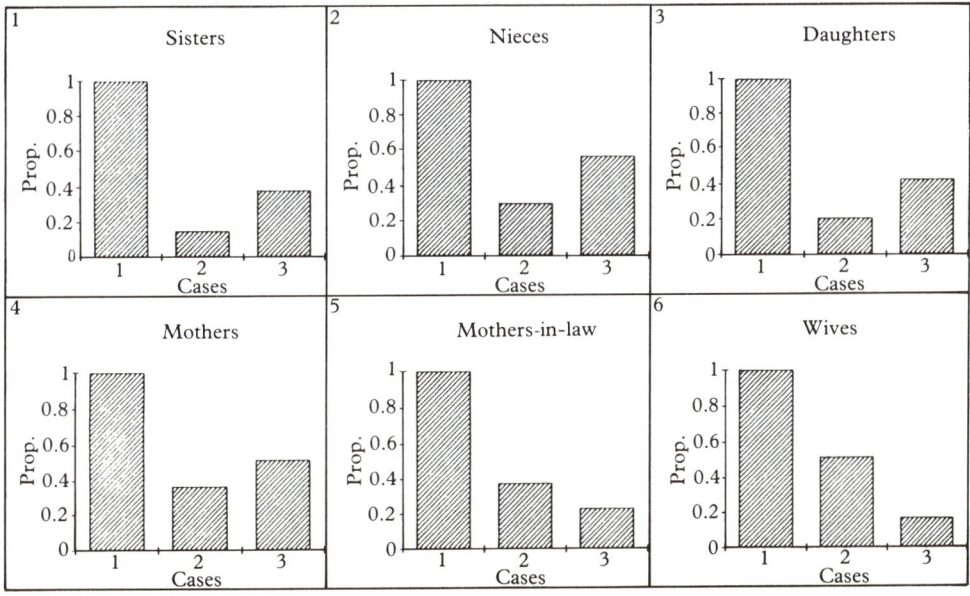

43

Table 1.5 *Ratio of Observed/Expected[a] for female classifications by adult male informants, 3 villages pooled*

Relative	Cases 1 + 3 (Expected)	Cases 1 + 2 (Observed)	Ratio O/E
Sisters	317	263	0.83
Nieces	297	246	0.83
Daughters	240	204	0.85
Mothers	139	125	0.90
Mothers-in-law	141	158	1.12
Wives	275	357	1.30
'Vague'	—	—	

[a] Observed is defined as all women correctly classified (Case 1) plus women misclassified as that type of relative (Case 2). Expected is defined as all women correctly classified (Case 1) plus women who should have been so classified, but were not (Case 3)

Table 1.6 *Misclassifications of female kin by sub-adult males*

Relative	Case 1	Case 2	Case 3	W act.	1/5 exp.
Daughters	25	9	36	6	7
Mothers-in-law	133	27	26	5	5
Mothers	107	42	27	3	5
Nieces	19	16	13	3	3
Sisters	62	30	101	6	20
Totals	346	124	203	23	40
Wives	109	24	42	—	—
'Vague'	—	104	—	—	—
Total number of classifications					952
Percentage of classifications that are 'vague'					11.0%

Many of these informants are children who may not yet know all the aspects of the kinship terminology and/or all the appropriate genealogical connections between them and their co-resident relatives.

Figure 1.11 shows the data for sub-adult male classifications that were shown in Figure 1.10 for adult males.

Note how different the patterns are for the taxons for 'mothers-in-law' and 'wives' compared to those characterizing adult male informants. The pattern among sub-adults that most resembles what adult males are doing with wives is the pattern describing mothers: sub-adults create relatively large numbers of mothers and seem reluctant to move genealogically definable mothers into other taxons. This is clear in Table 1.7, which provide the O/E ratios for all kin taxons. The mother taxon exceeds 1.00 by the widest margin, followed closely by nieces. Sub-adult males appear to make less of an effort to 'create' more wives.

Where the additional wives come from

Table 1.4 and Figure 1.10 above gave some indication of the provenience of the additional wives created by manipulation of kinship taxons by the adult males. Figure 1.12 summarizes this and provides a graphic comparison of categories from which the 'new' wives are drawn.

The most significant feature of the pattern is that additional wives are created by taking female kin out of 'younger' generational categories: nieces, sisters and daughters. Very few of the additional wives come from ascending generation categories – mothers and mothers-in-law. The average age of women who were moved from the niece, sister and daughter categories is 14.8 years whereas the average ages of the women from the mother and mother-in-law categories is 29.5 years. This supports the hypothesis that men are preferentially redefining as 'wife' those groups of females such as younger female kin who have the highest reproductive value and only rarely do they move generationally superior, older females (mothers, mothers-in-law) into the wife category.

Summary

The analysis of the approximately 11 000 kinship classifications made by the 100 Yąnomamö informants, along with the accompanying genealogical data that described how each informant was related to the individuals classified, shows the following patterns:

1. Male informants are 'faster' at classifying kin

than female informants are. Adult male informants manipulate their classifications for female kin in such a way as to 'create' more potential mates (cross-cousins) than is warranted by the genealogical relationships they have to the same women. They do this both by moving female kin from categories that are less useful reproductively into the single-most useful reproductive category and by 'creating' more mothers-in-law than is genealogically warranted.

2. While adult male informants show a pronounced tendency to move female kin from non-wife categories into wife categories, sub-adult males do not. Sub-adult males tend to reclassify females into the mother category. It is tempting to suggest that having more 'mothers' is better for the potential fitness of parentally dependent youngsters than having more 'wives.'

Figure 1.11 Misclassification of female kin classifications by sub-adult male informants showing the proportions of Case 1 that are represented by Cases 2 and 3. As in Figure 1.10, Case 1 (horizontal axis) is defined as unity and represents instances where the informant correctly classified the kinswomen. Case 2 represents instances where kinswomen were moved into the taxon. Case 3 represents instances where kinswomen were moved out of the category and defined as some other type of relative. Note that sub-adult males 'create' relatively few wives and seem less reluctant than adult males to move legitimate wives into other categories.

3. The females who are redefined by adult males as wives are drawn primarily from younger generation categories and are physiologically young and, therefore, probably have high reproductive value.

4. Males use 'vague/endearing' terms less often than females do, perhaps to conceal manipulations by close kin. Adult males use such terms less often than sub-adult males, the latter using them frequently possibly because they as yet do not know the more specific classifications for their kin. It is also possible that relative abundance or scarcity of cultivated food affects the usage of such terms, with men deliberately emphasizing formality in kinship classifications so as to be better able to deny requests for scarce food from other relatives.

5. While most contemporary theory in social and cultural anthropology acknowledges that there will always be a discrepancy between models based on the 'ideal' rules and what individuals or groups of individuals actually do, very little effort has been spent on documenting the magnitude of the discrepancy between ideal and actual, particularly with regard to kinship classification. Furthermore, such discrepancies have never previously been shown to be consistent with Darwinian predictions.

Whether these findings can be duplicated in

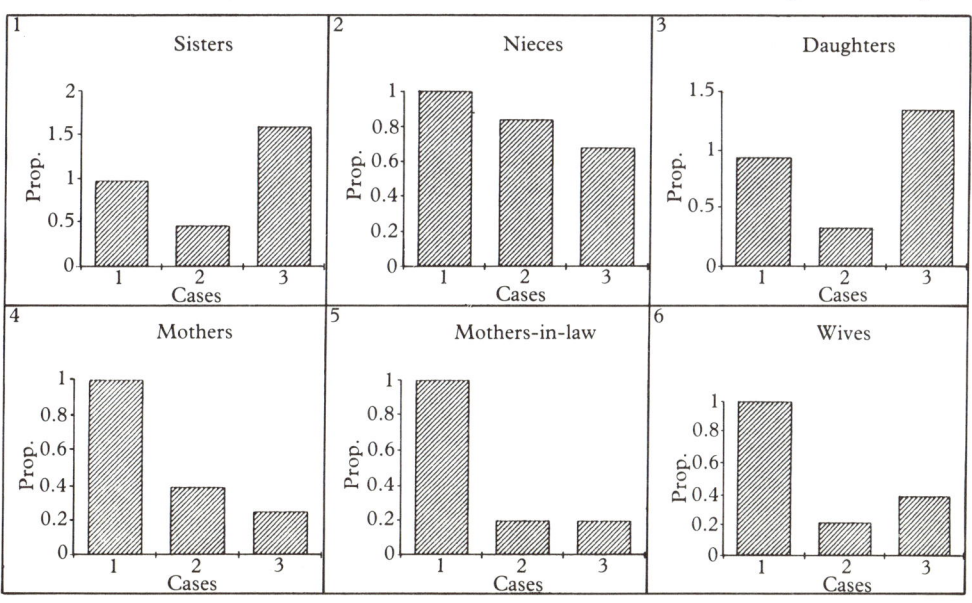

Table 1.7 *Ratio of Observed/Expected[a] for female classifications by sub-adult male informants, 3 villages pooled*

Relative	Cases 1 + 3 (Expected)	Cases 1 + 2 (Observed)	Ratio O/E
Sisters	163	92	0.56
Nieces	32	35	1.09
Daughters	61	34	0.56
Mothers	134	149	1.11
Mothers-in-law	159	160	1.00
Wives	151	133	0.88
'Vague'	—	—	—

[a] Observed and Expected as defined in Table 1.6

other societies remains to be seen. Comparative studies should, however, pay careful attention to the methods used here and should keep in mind the demographic features of the population as described in the text. It is possible that the only strictly comparable studies will have to be done on kinship/marriage systems that are 'prescriptive,' i.e. on societies whose marriage rules are bound up with kinship category specifications and where the prescribed marriage partner is some sort of consanguine. Otherwise, it would not be possible to predict the 'expected' classification on the basis of genealogies (viz. Needham 1963).

Figure 1.12 Where the additional wives come from. An analysis of the Case 2 instances for adult male classification of wives reveals the expected kinship categories of those women who were misclassified as wives. The frequencies of cases for these taxons is shown in this figure.

Acknowledgements

I would like to thank the editors of this volume – former students and, now, able and cherished colleagues – first, for their patience and, second, for the many helpful comments they provided on earlier drafts of this paper.

This paper is a continuation of many years of field research among the Yąnomamö Indians and the data analysis that follows the field trips. Several granting agencies and foundations supported my work at various stages and it is impossible to adequately express my gratitude to them and identify which made it possible for me to complete what aspect of my ongoing work. Most recently, the US National Science Foundation has supported my field trips and data analyses (1985 to the present, Grant Number BNS83-19644) and has supported my research several times in the past. This paper has been developed largely on data collected on my current NSF Research Grant. Many of the computer analyses and some of the field research and data analyses were made possible by the generous

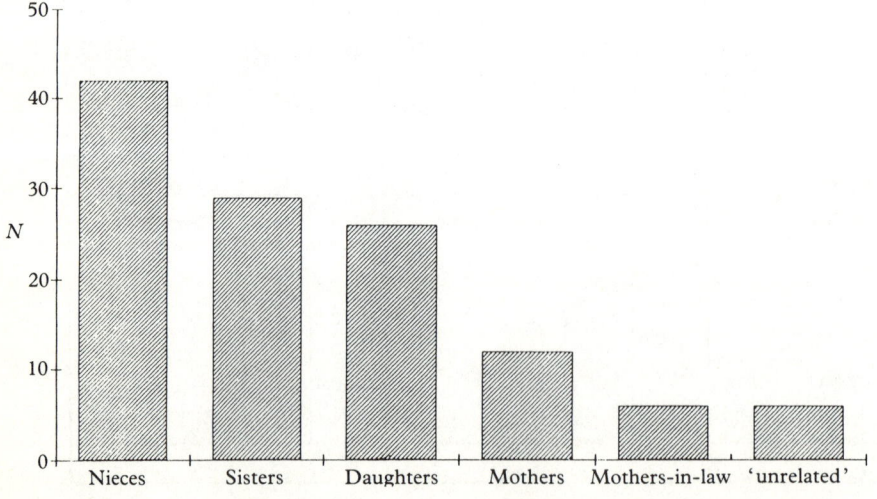

support of the Harry Frank Guggenheim Foundation for several of the past ten years; this support was crucial, since it came at a time when many funding agencies were reluctant to support the kind of research described here because it was then controversial. Some of my earlier work was funded by the National Institute of Mental Health and the Wenner-Gren Foundation for Anthropological Research.

I am grateful to many colleagues who spent considerable amounts of time reading earlier drafts of this paper and commenting on them. These include Donald Brown, Robin Fox, Harold Scheffler, Elman Service, Thomas Harding, Charles Erasmus, Elvin Hatch, Brian Fagan, Donald Symons, Keith Kintigh, Raymond Hames, Barry Hewlett, and Albert Spaulding – in addition to the editors of the volume. I am grateful to all of them and apologize if I have not modified the paper to meet all criticisms – most of them poignant and well-considered – they provided me. I would especially like to thank Albert Spaulding and Keith Kintigh for the useful advice and help they provided on statistical tests of some of the results.

I am grateful to my enthusiastic and diligent computer programmers, Dante DeLucia and Tony Rodoni, for producing from my files – often on very short notice – the data that went into the many tables and figures that are in this paper.

Finally, I am indebted to my many Yąnomamö informants and friends who patiently sat through the tedious sessions that led to the collection of the genealogical data and kinship classifications discussed here.

Endnote

In 1979 I designed a field research project for Giovanni Saffirio, a Catholic Priest who had spent many years among the Yąnomamö of the Catrimani River Basin in Brazil. He was then a Ph.D. candidate at the University of Pittsburgh. Saffirio conducted the field portion of the project as designed and provided me with the genealogical data, which I analysed for him in the same fashion as I did for the data in this paper. His subsequent Ph.D. thesis (1985) utilized somewhat different methods to those used in this paper. His data base is substantially smaller than the one one presented here, but his general conclusions, differences in analytical methods notwithstanding, are similar regarding male manipulations of female kinship classifications for reproductive advantage.

References

Chagnon, N. A. (1966) Yąnomamö warfare, social organization and marriage alliances. Ph.D. Thesis, University of Michigan.

Chagnon, N. A. (1968) Yąnomamö: The Fierce People. New York: Holt, Rinehart and Winston.

Chagnon, N. A. (1974) Studying the Yąnomamö. New York: Holt, Rinehart and Winston.

Chagnon, N. A. (1975) Genealogy, solidarity and relatedness: limits to local group size and patterns of fissioning in an expanding population. Yearbook of Physical Anthropology, 19, 95–110. Washington: American Association of Physical Anthropologists.

Chagnon, N. A. (1979) Mate competition, favoring close kin, and village fissioning among the Yąnomamö Indians. In Evolutionary Biology and Human Social Behavior: An Anthropological Perspective, ed. N. A. Chagnon and W. Irons, pp. 86–132. North Scituate, MA: Duxbury Press.

Chagnon, N. A. (1982) Sociodemographic attributes of nepotism in tribal populations: man the rule-breaker. In Current Problems in Sociobiology, ed. King's College Sociobiology Group, pp. 291–318. Cambridge: Cambridge University Press.

Chagnon, N. A. (1983) Yąnomamö: The Fierce People, 3rd edition. New York: Holt, Rinehart and Winston.

Chagnon, N. A. and Bryant, J. (1984) KINDEM-COM: The fourth style in the study of human kinship relationships. New York: Report to the Harry Frank Guggenheim Foundation (Mimeo).

Chagnon, N. A. and Hames, R. B. (1984) The social effects of mortality and divorce on the Yąnomamö nuclear family: kinship, fosterage, and marriage choice implications for tribal societies. Research Proposal funded by the National Science Foundation, Washington.

Eyde, D. and Postal, P. (1961) Avunculocality and incest: the development of unilateral cross-cousin marriage and Crow–Omaha kinship systems. American Anthropologist, 63, 747–71.

Faron, L. (1961) The Dakota–Omaha Continuum in Mapuche society. Journal of the Royal Anthropological Institute, 91, 11–22.

Firth, R. (1959) Social Change in Tikopia: Re-study of a Polynesian Community After a Generation. London: Allen and Unwin.

Fortes, M. (1969) Kinship and the Social Order: The Legacy of Lewis Henry Morgan. Chicago: Aldine.

Fox, R. (1967) Kinship and Marriage: An Anthropological Perspective. Baltimore: Penguin.

Fox, R. (1982) Principles and pragmatics on Tory Island. In Belonging: Identity and Social Organization in British Rural Cultures, ed. A. Cohen, pp. 50–71. Manchester University Press.

Fredlund, E. (1985) The use and abuse of kinship when classifying marriages: a Shitari Yąnomamö case study. Ethology and Sociobiology, 6, 17–25.

Gray, J. P. (ed.) (1984) A Guide to Primate Sociobiological Theory and Research. New Haven: HRAF Press.

Lane, R. and Lane, B. (1959) On the development of Dakota–Iroquois and Crow–Omaha kinship terminologies. *Southwestern Journal of Anthropology*, **15**, 254–65.

Leach, E. (1961 [1955]) The structural implications of matrilateral cross-cousin marriage. Reprinted in *Rethinking Anthropology*. London: Athlone Press.

Levi-Strauss, C. (1949 [1969]) *The Elementary Structures of Kinship*. Boston: Beacon Press.

Lizot, J. (1971) Remarques sur le vocabulaire de parenté Yąnomamö. *L'Homme*, **11**(2), 25–38.

Murdock, G. (1967) Ethnographic Atlas. *Ethnology*, **6**, 109–236.

Murdock, G. and White, D. (1969) Standard cross-cultural sample. *Ethnology*, **8**, 329–69.

Needham, R. (1962) *Structure and Sentiment*. Chicago: University of Chicago Press.

Needham, R. (1963) Some disputed points in the study of prescriptive alliance. *Southwestern Journal of Anthropology*, **19**, 186–207.

Saffirio, G. (1985) Ideal and actual kinship terminology among the Yąnomamö Indians of the Catrimani River Basin (Brazil). Ph.D. Thesis, University of Pittsburgh.

Schneider, D. (1965) Some muddles in the models: or, how the system really works. In *The Relevance of Models for Social Anthropology*, ed. M. Banton, pp. 25–85. London: ASA Monographs. Tavistock.

Service, E. (1971 [1962]) *Primitive Social Organization: An Evolutionary Perspective*, 2nd edition. New York: Random House.

Spillius, J. (1959) Natural disaster and population crisis in a Polynesian society: an exploration of operational research. *Human Relations*, **10**, 1–27.

Redistribution: equity or exploitation?

Introduction

'Everywhere in the world the indigenous category for exploitation is "reciprocity"' (Sahlins 1972:134). This may or may not always have been true everywhere in the world; it does seem, though, to have been true almost everywhere in anthropology. In any society, resources are at some point collectively procured and/or pooled, and then, either on the spot or at a later date, redistributed. And everywhere, at least on the surface of things, the redistributor seems inclined to skin the fat off the top.

On, for instance, the small Fijian island of Moala, Sahlins himself found that 'Chiefs and visitors of status are usually given items of some-what better quality and a slightly better than proportionate share' (Sahlins 1962:199). Also characteristically, 'If the amount given to a group of people is not enough to divide among them, senior houses take precedence and junior houses go without' (ibid.; pp. 346–7).

This pattern looks consistent on every continent. Typically, after everyone else had received their fair share, Nama Hottentot leaders in southern Africa took the best portions of meat at communal feasts (Schapera 1930:334); in informal divisions after a kill, Shavante headmen in Brazil 'acted for themselves and for their

[1] Museum of Zoology University of Michigan, Ann Arbor, MI 48109, USA

closest kin,' with the result that 'the chief's household thus invariably came off best' (Maybury-Lewis 1967:202, cf. p. 203); and important North American Huron chiefs, according to their Jesuit critics, took advantage of ritual redistributions of furs to appropriate the largest shares (Trigger 1969:86). And these are just the beginnings: in larger, more hierarchical groups men in authority liberally levied both tribute and labor on a regular basis from their subjects (see e.g. Betzig 1986). In, for instance, Inca Peru, 'The entire land belonged to the Sun [the king] and his descendants, whether they occupied public office or not; this permitted them to choose whatever they wanted, throughout the Empire, without it being possible to refuse them' (Garcilaso de la Vega 1961:25).

Three theories

In spite of all of which, to some, redistributors seem to have been lacking in economic self interest. Two philosophies stand squarely behind this position: 'substantivism' and Marxism. For Polanyi, who formally defined substantivism, 'The oustanding discovery of recent historical and anthropological research is that man's economy, as a rule, is submerged in his social relationships. He does not act so as to safeguard his individual interest in the possession of material goods; he acts so as to safeguard his ... social assets. He values material goods only in so far as they serve this end' (1944:46). To Polanyi the effect is that, in such societies, there is 'a continuous supply of want satisfying material means' (1957:248), that is, plenty of everything to go around. As a result, men and women are supposed to be without a motive to seek material gain.

After that fashion, Sahlins, too, has stressed the social function of redistribution. He has acknowledged that in the 'orginal affluent' societies resources are, again, always ample; accordingly, people with power in such groups are without a motive to exploit. To Sahlins, leadership always incorporates both rights and obligations; 'the dues and duties fall to both sides, both high and low have their claims' (1972:205). But, though in historic, including feudal, groups, *noblesse oblige* may hardly have cancelled out *droits du seigneur*, 'in primitive society social inequality is more the organization of economic equality[!] Often, in fact, high rank is only secured or sustained by overcrowding generosity: the material advantage is on the subordinate's side' (ibid.). To Sahlins, the 'primitive' chief is the the allegorical 'father' of his people, his relationships with them characterized by the generalized reciprocity usual among close kinsmen (cf. Alexander 1975, 1979), in which giving occurs without anticipation of any specified return.

This emphasis upon collective not individual benefit in pre-market/pre-state economies is of course anticipated by the Marxist tradition. As Morgan (1877) long ago maintained, primitive society was supposed to have been *gentile* society, based on the family, in which every resource necessary to sustain and perpetuate life, including members of the opposite sex, was held by communal right. In the 'consanguine' family, inferred from a form of classificatory kinship terminology, 'all my sisters are my wives, as well as the wives of my several brothers;' still earlier, promiscuity was further inferred to have been the general state of affairs. Once upon a time, then, the mode of *re*production was supposed to have been held in common; to a possibly great extent by implication, 'communism in living must, of necessity, have prevailed ..., because it was a requirement of their condition' (Morgan 1877 [1978]:410, 416; see, too, p. 418).

To Engels, to whom, as to Marx, Morgan stood as the final authority on prehistoric societies, *gentile* society was of course the original socialist society. In *The Origin of the Family, Private Property, and the State*, a presumed fall from grace was attributed, as it had been by Morgan, to an increase in accumulable, heritable, wealth (Engels 1884 [1964]; see especially pp. 144–53). For Marx and Engels, exploitation, that is, 'surplus–labour, labour beyond the time required for the labourer's own maintenance, and appropriation by others of the product of this surplus-labour' (from the *Anti-Dührung*, quoted in Terray 1975:94), was, again, supposed to have been absent before the emergence of the state.

This dichotomous view of pre-state versus state society has essentially withstood the onslaught of a century of evidence. There are, though, a few new voices of dissent. In an extensive discussion of Meillassoux's *Economic Anthropology of the Guro* (1964), Terray (1972) has been forced to defend an absence of class and exploitation in that society, following a contrary assertion by Dupré and Rey (in Terray 1972; see also Godelier 1978). For Dupré and Rey, 'Prestige-giving goods amount to a diversion of the produce by the elders, who make special use of it to reinforce the dependence of the direct producers'. That is, 'exploitation does, then, take place in traditional society' (Terray 1972 : 166–7).

An alternative to the substantivist and Marxist positions, on the contrary, *predicts* that, wherever present environments are enough like the environments we evolved in, people with power will try to exploit it to their productive and *re*productive advantage (Darwin 1859, 1871, and, e.g., Fisher 1958, Williams 1966, and Alexander and Borgia 1978). Individuals might maximize their genetic representation in future generations both by parenting children and by assisting other close genetic kin (Hamilton 1963, 1964). Where it is to the advantage of all concerned to equitably share the wealth, all are expected to do so (see e.g. Trivers 1971, Alexander 1979, Axelrod and Hamilton 1981). Where, however, subjects are sufficiently 'circumscribed' (see Carneiro 1970, Betzig 1982, 1986, Vehrencamp 1983) that their best option is to yield them, men and women in power might take whatever productive advantages they can get, and translate the 'fat' into reproduction.

Meillassoux himself has said, 'This discipline should cease to be a pretext for exotic fantasies' (1981 : x). To the end, at least, of discerning the relative empirical validity of the substantivist, Marxist, and Darwinian positions on exploitation, the following evidence of redistribution on a small Micronesian island is adduced.

The site

Ifaluk is a nearly circular atoll of two inhabited and two small uninhabited islets, totaling altogether just over half a square mile in land area, and supporting a full-time resident population in 1983 of just 446. It is located in the Western Carolines at 7° 15′ north latitude and 147° east longitude, 30 miles east of the nearest other inhabited island, about 350 miles east of the nearest 'high' island, Yap, and about 400 miles south of the nearest economic center, Guam (Figure 2.1). Its size and physical isolation have in many

ways allowed it to remain, over centuries of usually *laissiez-faire* Spanish, German, Japanese, and United Nations colonization, a political, social, and economic isolate as well.

To what extent could Ifaluk, at the time of the study, be considered a pre-market, pre-state society? The most important Western influences in evidence in 1983 were introduced at the end of the (Second World) War, with the institution, by the US-administered United Nations Trust Territory government, of formal education, and the proselytization, by Methodist and Catholic missionaries posted on other islands, of the Christian religion (see Lutz 1980). In 1983, all but 31 holdouts sat in an average thatch hut with a cross on it, or by an incomplete concrete edifice, every Sunday; and ten native men had been hired full-time to teach in Ifaluk's concrete and corrugated-iron elementary school. Three other native men were employed full or part-time as a health care worker, dental nurse, and builder of the small, new, concrete dispensary on the island. The only other source of cash income was from the sale of copra, at about one or two sacks per household with the arrival, roughly every six weeks, of the field trip ship from Yap. The coming of that ship is erratic, supplies it brings for sale, mainly luxuries like vodka and tobacco, and staples like sugar, flour, and rice, are extremely limited and unreliable; and storage/hoarding of them is virtually impossible. It may be important to note that, in 1983, the sale of an average amount of copra was the only source of cash available to any Ifaluk chief.

Figure 2.1 The western Pacific.

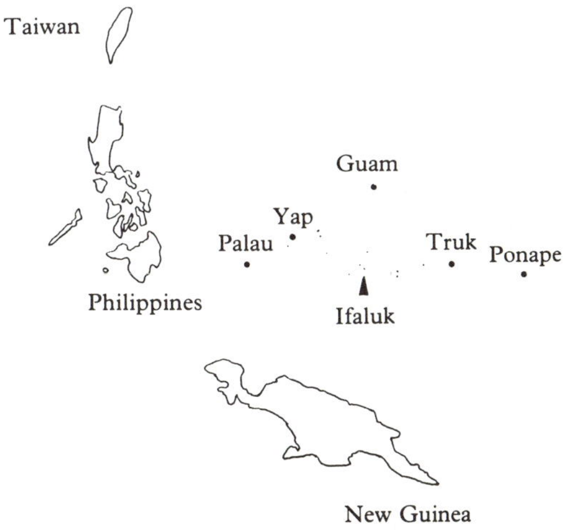

51

Early in the present century, Sarfert (in Damm 1908–1910) still found shell tools regularly in use on the island. At least that late, then, the Ifalukese might still have practiced a pristine 'shell age' economics. Since the first known European stop in 1797, Ifaluk was visited at long intervals by whalers and traders in the 19th century. Early in this century, it was visited by Germans, and later Japanese, who came briefly to stimulate the production of copra, and sometimes to conscript men's labor in phosphate mines on other islands, and by a Japanese agriculturalist, sent to establish a copra 'plantation' on Falalop island, but recalled with the end of the war (see Burrows and Spiro 1957, Lutz 1980). And in the last 40 years, Ifaluk has been intruded upon by a handful of American biologists and anthropologists (e.g. Tracey *et al.* 1956, Burrows and Spiro 1957, Bates and Abbott 1958, Lutz 1980, Turke 1985), none of whom have stayed more than a year.

At present, a subsistence economy still obtains: women cultivate taro, men fish and collect coconuts, and both women and men harvest breadfruit, bananas, and papayas, to support themselves. People still live in thatch houses they continually build and repair; women weave their own lava lavas on handmade looms with purchased thread or their own banana fiber; and men fish in outrigger canoes with nets and traps, all of their own construction. Politically, too, the people have largely retained their autonomy. Although Ifaluk has been since 1981 a part of the State of Yap of the Federated States of Micronesia, that authority is remote; most immediately, the people live under their traditional system of matrilineally inherited chiefly rank.

There are, and for at least half a century have been (Burrows and Spiro 1957), five major matriclans on Ifaluk. These are ordered according to rank. Each clan is generally headed by a man, who inherits his status from his mother's brother, or from an older brother. At the time of this study, the highest ranking clan, Hofalu, was headed by an elder woman, who had been allowed to succeed for a lack of suitable male heirs. A younger man from the Hofalu clan acted, however, as her executor. Also at the time of this study, the third ranking clan, Manauglifach, had no head at all, reportedly for a lack of suitable male or female heirs. Each of these chiefs is ranked according to the rank of his or her clan. They are, and traditionally have been, the most powerful people on Ifaluk atoll (cf. Burrows and Spiro 1957, Lutz 1980, Turke 1985). Historically, that power was so great that chiefs could take, or ask a sorcerer to take, a 'bad' subject's life (Wichimai, pers. comm.).

In 1983, three informants identified a total of eight people as clan chiefs' likely successors, seven of them men. In 1986, during a follow-up study, several informants came to a concensus as to which four men will most likely succeed as heads of their clans.

What follows assesses costs and benefits accorded the highest ranking men on Ifaluk. It looks at some of the rights and obligations of the three male clan chiefs, the male executor of the Hofalu clan, and their four probable successors compared to the 85 men over 15 who have never had a salaried job or traditional rank.

Results

Chiefly income

Traditionally, men of rank on Ifaluk enjoyed a control over resources characteristic of most ranked societies. The fishing area, both reef and lagoon, belonged collectively to clan chiefs; they also had the last word regarding use of the land (Burrows and Spiro 1957:188; cf. Alkire 1974). Clansmen of the highest ranking chief alone were given all prized sea turtles; and members of the second ranking clan had an exclusive right to all yellowfin tuna (Burrows and Spiro 1957:128). Even now, the chief of the second highest clan on Ifaluk gets ten baskets of breadfruit per household, one bottle of palm wine per man who cuts it, and fish from trolling expeditions, once yearly from Falachig village. Fines levied as punishment go directly to chiefs. And privileges in etiquette also persist. During our stay, whenever prepared food was collectively pooled among men, having been prepared by the apparently about evenly distributed hard labor of all the island women, chiefs were served first, big bowls of breadfruit and taro being brought to them by men deferentially bowed; and chiefs alone would be allowed, on such occasions, to drink wine.

In addition, chiefs were consistently allowed to skim the fat off the catch. Whenever fish were collectively caught, by all able-bodied men and boys either in a village or on one or the other inhabited island, they would be immediately redistributed by chief's advisors, under the attentive eyes of chiefs. Between August and November, 1983, five collective catches of schools of *pati*, a kind of mackerel, just off the shore of Falalop islet, and subsequent redistributions were witnessed. At least that many again, both of *pati* and of combinations of fish caught on the outer lagoon reef, were known to have occurred but were not or were incompletely observed. Chiefs and everyone else present generously allowed an intrusion with cameras, notebooks, and pens, with which proceedings were recorded in detail. Consistent with Sahlins' (1958) and others' (Burrows and Spiro 1957:116) assertions, fish *was* equitably distributed to every untitled household. In addition, also consistent with general impressions (ibid.), men of rank often got extra fish, and clan chiefs took the choicest and the largest amounts (Figure 2.2). In each case, we were able to weigh the share given the highest ranking chief on Falalop islet, the chief of the second highest clan. On these occasions, he generally came away with almost twice as much fish in pounds per person for his own household as was sent to other households on the island (Table 2.1). This is a significant difference (goodness of fit $\chi^2 = 35.75$, df $= 4$, $p < 0.001$).

It is interesting to add that, in conducting their most apparent administrative function, that is,

Table 2.1 *Perquisites allotted to the highest ranking male chief on Ifaluk in redistributions of collectively caught fish. Pati weigh eight to a pound; eight people, including children, lived in this chief's house*

Redistribution number	*Pati* per person	Chief's perks	Net of equity (%)
1	8	30 *pati*; 6 lb fish	222
2	10	83 *pati*; 2 lb fish	224
3	4	10 *pati*	131
4	8	30 *pati*	147
5	13	33 *pati*; 5 lb fish	170

$\bar{X} = 179\%$

addressing village- and island-wide meetings every few months, chiefs over and over again asked: that people keep the island clean; that women remain productive, and not steal from each other's taro patches; and (and this is the relevant point) that the men not fish individually, but wait for a chance to help bring in a communal catch (cf. Burrows and Spiro 1957). Such an admonishment, to the extent that cooperative fishing and redistribution are optimal for every islander, may be to the benefit of the group; to the extent that that cooperation is in fact *most* beneficial to chiefs, the admonishment may be self-interested as well.

Chiefly outflow

It is quite possible, though, that what productive edge Ifaluk chiefs gain in tribute and fish they eventually give up, or more than give up. Consistent with the general cross-cultural impression (Sahlins 1972), Burrows and Spiro suggested that on Ifaluk 'generous giving, to be sure, is chiefly behavior, part of a chief's expected role' (1957:173). Over the long run, does chiefly generosity effecively tip, as Sahlins (1972:205) suggests, the material balance in favor of subjects?

Over a period of four months in 1983, chiefs' households were never observed to contribute more than an equal share to resources pooled on any public occasion. But, the households of chiefs, as well as all households on the island, did take part in another kind of ongoing redistribution, in which subordinates could have netted

Figure 2.2 *Pati*-equivalents in pounds per person allotted to the highest ranking chief on Falalop islet (solid bars) vs. all other households (dotted bars), following five collective catches.

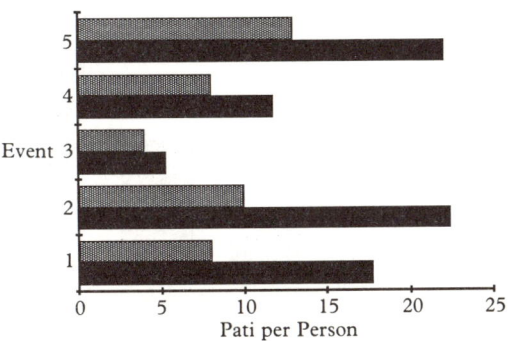

Pati per Person

a greater share. On average, households on Ifaluk take food to or receive food from other households every other day; chiefly households are no exception. Do chiefs use such occasions to reallocate whatever they gain in tribute and greater than equal shares of communal catches?

To study food sharing systematically, the heads of ten widely dispersed households on Ifaluk were asked to record food outflow to and intake from other households over the course of 12 consecutive days in October, 1983 (Betzig and Turke 1986a). In every case, the food shared was indigenous, usually breadfruit, taro, or fish, carried in a large coconut-frond basket or an iron pot. Altogether, a total of 84 food-sharing events involving 42 pairs of households were recorded.

In order to find out how closely households were related to those with which they shared food, these data were supplemented by genealogies. With the help in each case of one of three fluent English speaking Ifalukese, a census of each of the 56 households on Ifaluk was made. For every man, woman, and child, an exhaustive list of all lineal genetic ancestors remembered was recorded. Each item of genealogical data was checked by at least one independent source. These data were later fed into a computer program, generously provided by Napoleon Chagnon, designed to estimate the proportion of genes identical by descent shared by every pair of individuals on the island (details in Chagnon and Bryant 1984).

Altogether, over the course of our food sharing study, food flowed from unsalaried, untitled households to the households of the five highest ranking men on Ifaluk seven times, and from these chiefly to non-status households three times. These numbers are of course too small to be conclusive about the directionality of food sharing. The significant fact *is* that, while all food sharing households were more closely related to one another genealogically than were households on Ifaluk on average, households *giving* food to clan chiefs were more distantly related (Figure 2.3). In other words, unlike people without rank, Ifaluk chiefs appear on a continuous basis to be receiving food from everybody on the island, irrespective of their kinship distance from them.

On the other hand, chiefly houses do not appear to *give* food without respect to genealogical relationship. In fact, members of chiefly

households tend to be even more closely related, on average, to those to whom they give food than are food-sharing households on average (Figure 2.3). Chiefly households are much more closely related to households to which they give food than to those from which they receive food ($t = 3.92$, df = 8, $p = 0.0044$, two-tailed, for chiefly versus non-status households; $t = 3.37$, df = 10, $p = 0.0071$, two-tailed, for chiefly versus all other households; note that even on samples this small, the t-test is generally robust [Havlicek and Peterson 1974]). In other words, on a daily basis, *Ifaluk chiefs appear to get food from everybody and dole it out selectively to households closely related genealogically*. In this way, their actions look consistent with Hamilton's (1963, 1964) prediction: they offer material benefits to close kin.

The possibility exists that the food-sharing sample was in some important way biased. There is no evidence to suggest that it was. The ten households targeted for the food-sharing study were selected for the study on two major criteria, general location on the island, and the willingness and ability of at least one household member to communicate the relevant information. One result was probably a fair geographic representation: each of the four villages on Ifaluk is represented by at least two households, and altogether 32 of the 56 households were recorded as donors or recipients of food at least once. This precaution may have been irrelevant; no geographic differences in food-sharing patterns are apparent. Another result, a tradeoff for soliciting

Figure 2.3 Average relatedness ($\bar{r}$) among four samples of households. (1) All 56 Ifaluk households (1540 pairs); (2) chiefs' households to those giving them food; (3) all 42 pairs of food sharing households; (4) chiefs' households to those to which they gave food.

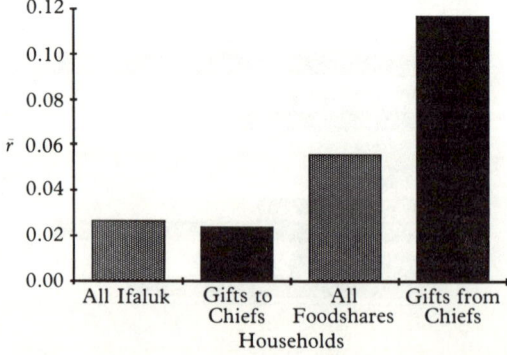

reliable information from those judged most likely to provide it, is that households with exceptionally good English speakers are probably overrepresented. There is no reason, though, why these men and women should have had an unusual propensity to give food to chiefs. On the contrary, the standard wisdom in anthropology seems to be that both kinship and traditional systems of status become less important to those exposed to Western influence (e.g. Sahlins 1972).

It is also possible that the sample was biased in time. Neither ethnographic accounts (e.g. Burrows and Spiro 1957, Bates and Abbott 1958, Lutz 1980) nor our own extensive interviews as to variability in the food-quest and food-sharing activity over the course of the year suggest any reason to suspect that the pattern recorded over this 12-day period was not the common one. But does the pattern vary between years? Ifaluk, like many other island societies, *is* occasionally devastated by severe natural disasters, especially typhoons (e.g. Lutz 1980). Do chiefs in such a situation effectively act to stave off starvation on the part of their subjects? No evidence exists for Ifaluk itself; but Sahlins' (1972: 127–30) own citing of the case of a Tikopian famine suggests a contrary conclusion. According to Firth (1959), a hurricane-precipitated famine on that island resulted in the 'atomization' of island economy into household economy. The pooling and sharing of resources stopped; and there was an estimated five-fold increase in theft. Overall, in Sahlins' words, 'The household proved a fortress of self-interest which in the crisis cut itself apart' (p. 129).

It is probably fair to conclude, then, that the material advantage in sharing food on Ifaluk is not on the subordinates' side (cf. Sahlins 1972: 205). Nor, in this respect, is access to these life-sustaining resources equal (cf. Engels 1884 [1964]). Rather, consistent with the Darwinian prediction, chiefs appear to gain productively by their positions. In collecting annual tribute, in skimming the fat off the catch, and in sharing food, Ifaluk chiefs appear to reap the fruits of the labors of everybody; they appear, then, to redistribute them selectively, in a manner consistent with their own reproductive interests.

Chiefly labor

The possibility remains that chiefs compensate, at least in part, for material benefits in redistribution by putting forth a greater than average effort to help procure them. Chiefly 'generosity' might take the form of extraordinary productivity. Sahlins, for example, suggests that this might be the case in some smaller societies, for example, among Melanesian big men, whom he credits with 'autoexploitation' (1972: 139).

To test for this possibility, quantitative data on activity budgets were gathered by an instantaneous scan (see methodological discussion in Betzig and Turke 1985). Behaviors were observed on a circuit of the larger of Ifaluk's two inhabited islands, Falalop, once every day over a period of 48 consecutive days from September to early November, 1983. On each circuit, time, ID number, and behavior of individuals seen were recorded on sight. Observations were made during daylight hours: scans were *begun* at randomly determined half-hour intervals from eight o'clock in the morning, late enough not to embarrass people unduly by catching them asleep or 'washing up' in the lagoon, to three thirty in the afternoon, in time to allow an up to two hour circuit to be done before dark. Exactly three circuits were made for every sampled time of day.

This circuit covered every area of major activity on the islet; it went through the taro swamp and coconut groves and beside every one of the household estates, or *bugot*, and canoe houses on Falalop (ibid). As it turns out, an atoll environment may be an ideal one in which to conduct an instantaneous scan. First and most importantly, the site of every kind of activity done on Ifaluk was within sight of this walk. An important result is that all data collected were actually based on observations; interview data about activities relatively inaccessible in other cultures, such as herding or hunting, were not merged with observational data. Second, virtually all activities conducted on Ifaluk during the day are open-air activities. Although sick or unusually tired individuals sometimes spend part of the day inside closed thatched huts, everyone else stays outdoors, either in the open air, or under open-sided huts along the shoreline, or open-sided huts on the *bugot*. Finally, because the population of Ifaluk is so small, all individuals seen on the circuit were very soon known by sight and by name.

As is evident in Figures 2.4 and 2.5, the two clan chiefs resident on Falalop islet spent much less time physically engaged in productive activities than did other men over 50 living on the same islet ($n = 12$). These two chiefs spent 72.73% and 67.86% of observed activity non-productively (i.e. physically resting, eating and drinking, bathing and grooming, or walking); other men over 50 on Falalop spent on average almost 60% of scanned activity *productively* (Table 2.2). This is a significant difference ($\chi^2 = 10.37$, df = 1, $p = 0.0013$). When these two chiefs are compared to the seven men in this cohort without any salary or title, the differences remain significant ($\chi^2 = 9.48$, df = 1, $p = 0.0021$).

Several alternatives to the interpretation that chiefs enjoy more leisure time than do other older men are conceivable; none of them are convincing. First, it might be argued that the study

is affected by seasonal bias: chiefs at different times of the year could compensate by working harder. This is unlikely, because the only important shift in activity on Ifaluk comes with the breadfruit season (see Burrows and Spiro 1957, Lutz 1980), roughly six months in duration, which was gradually coming to an end during the period scanned. Second, it could be supposed that chiefs work harder than other men over 50 off the scan circuit, or off scan hours. Because the scan covered the whole islet, though, the first possibility is unlikely; chiefs would literally have to have gone out of their way to hide their productive activity. Neither does it seem likely that chiefs waited to do their work after dark. Last, it could be argued that chiefs compensate for doing less manual work by more 'managerial' effort. This is possible, of course. The point still stands that Ifaluk chiefs do not contribute to the general material good by spending an exceptional amount of time at physical labor. Instead, an exemption from physical labor appears to be yet another perquisite of chiefly office.

Figure 2.4 Activities of two clan chiefs resident on Falalop islet.

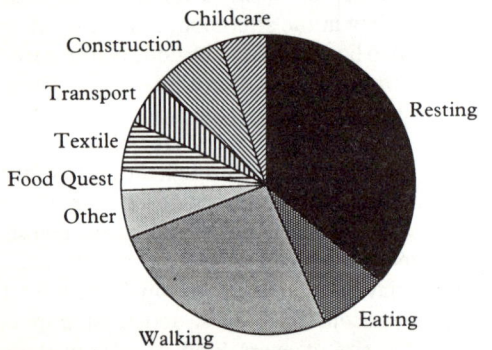

Figure 2.5 Activities of 12 other men aged over 50 resident on Falalop islet.

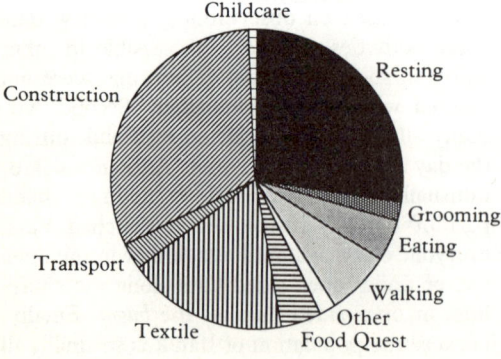

Chiefly reproductive success

Darwinian theory, as stated above, predicts that individuals may maximize their genetic representation in descendant generations both by assisting close collateral kin and by parenting children themselves. The evidence above suggests that chiefs convey at least some of their resources upon kin. The question remains: do Ifaluk chiefs, like men in almost every other preindustrial society (see Betzig 1986), translate their productive advantages into direct reproduction by having children?

It is likely that, more than anything else, direct reproduction among men has been facilitated by polygyny (e.g. Borgerhoff Mulder 1987). Like men in almost all the world's societies (e.g. Murdock 1967, Betzig 1986), those on Ifaluk formerly took more than one wife at a time whenever they were able. Although chiefs still recall those times with interest, harem polygyny has not been practiced in the Western Carolines since early in this century (Burrows and Spiro 1957:302).

In the absence of harem polygyny, do Ifaluk chiefs still father more children than men with

Table 2.2 *Observed labor and leisure activities of 2 clan chiefs vs. 12 other men over 50 resident on Falalop islet*

ID	Status[a]	Year of birth[b]	Labor activities	Leisure activities	% labor
1	C	1925	3	8	27.27
2	C	1933	9	19	32.14
3	v	1920	8	11	42.11
4	v	1920	18	13	58.06
5		1925	25	11	69.44
6	a	1927	14	12	53.85
7		1926	8	4	66.67
8		1925	16	9	64.00
9	e	1930	17	11	60.71
10		1925	15	9	62.50
11		1920	19	10	65.52
12	vs	1920	24	9	72.73
13		1920	9	15	37.50
14		1920	11	12	47.83

[a] Status symbols include: C (clan chief), v (village chief), a (advisor), vs (village chief's successor), e (formerly employed). Blank indicates never titled or paid
[b] Year of birth 1920 was the earliest recorded; it was used for men and women who were born 'before Japanese time,' that is, before the end of the First World War

less to give them? Taken alone, the three male clan chiefs on Ifaluk and the male executor for the chief of Hofalu clan have in fact fathered significantly more children than have the other men on the atoll over 15. However, older men must be expected to have fathered more children, and chiefs tend to be older men. There is also the possibility of a secular trend: members of the elder generation may, because of some contextual change, have produced more or fewer children on average compared to younger men. In Table 2.3, year of birth is used to control for both. In this way, the fertility to date of these five men of rank is determined to be slightly higher, but statistically indistinct, from that of other men over 15.

On the other hand, Table 2.3 also shows that chiefs' successors *have* had significantly higher fertility to date compared to unranked, unsalaried men over 15, even with year of birth controlled (cf. Turke and Betzig 1985). This is consistent with the Darwinian prediction. One possible reason why the prediction works for successors, that is, for chiefs of the next generation, but not for chiefs of this generation, may be involuntary infertility. Two of the four highest ranking men (incidentally, chiefs of the lowest ranking clans) are supposed to have fathered only one child each, both at early ages, although one of them was married twice. Hunt, Schneider, Kidder, and Stevens (1949)

have documented drastic depopulation on Yap over the past century, and attributed it, largely, to disease-induced sterility. If, as both theory and evidence (e.g. Kaplan and Hill 1985, Hill and Kaplan this volume (Chapters 17 and 18), Betzig, 1986) suggest, chiefs generally have enjoyed privileged sexual access historically, they might have been especially at risk of infertility.

In the absence of harem polygyny, several mechanisms might account for the greater fertility of chiefs and successors as a group. The most obvious might be serial polygyny. Compared to the 85 adult men without title or salary, the eight clan chiefs and succesors have had more, but not significantly more, previous spouses (4 for chiefs and successors vs. 13 for others, $\chi^2 = 1.249$, $p = 0.2638$ for presence or absence of previous spouses), and they have failed to produce significantly more children *by* previous spouses (2 for chiefs and successors vs. 10 for others; $\chi^2 = 1.092$, $p = 0.2960$ for presence or absence of children by previous spouses).

Other mechanisms appear to be more important. In an earlier study (Turke and Betzig 1985), a group of 18 high status men was found to have fathered children at somewhat, though not significantly, shorter birth intervals than men without status. They were also found to have failed altogether to reproduce significantly less often.

Table 2.3 *Number of children fathered to date regressed on status (measured dichotomously) and year of birth. Chiefs include the five men at the head of their clans*

Variable	Partial	Coefficient	Significance
I. Chiefs ($n = 4$) vs. non-status men ($n = 85$) ($R^2 = 0.2370$)			
Constant		6.5186	0.0005
Status	0.0046	0.0591	0.9659
Year of Birth	−0.4859	−0.0923	0.0000
II. Chiefs and successors ($n = 8$) vs. non-status men ($n = 85$) ($R^2 = 0.2771$)			
Constant		4.8956	0.0017
Status	0.1623	1.5757	0.1222
Year of Birth	−0.4710	−0.0899	0.0000
III. Successors ($n = 4$) vs. non-status men ($n = 85$) ($R^2 = 0.2975$)			
Constant		3.4310	0.0536
Status	0.2364	3.0594	0.0266
Year of Birth	−0.4868	−0.0904	0.0000

Chiefs and their successors appear to enjoy other reproductive advantages which might contribute to their fitness in later generations. Present *wives* of clan chiefs and successors have had slightly, though not significantly, fewer previous spouses than other men's wives (1 for chiefs' and successors' wives vs. 18 for others'; $\chi^2 = 0.001$, $p = 0.9890$ for presence or absence of previous spouses); neither have they produced significantly fewer children *by* previous spouses (3 for chiefs' and successors' wives vs. 13 for others'; $\chi^2 = 0.064$, $p = 0.7998$ for presence or absence of children by previous spouses). Women who have had previous spouses might contribute less to a man's reproductive potential than women who have not, whether or not they bore children by their former husbands. Those who have not borne children might be more likely to be infertile, while those who have borne children by other men might divert investment from present husbands to raise them.

Stronger than these demographic differences are differences in association patterns. The two pre-menopausal wives of a clan chief and successor resident on Falalop spent significantly more time together with their husbands than did the eight fertile wives of men without status. (Fertile wives of high status men were together with their husbands during 9 of 33 and 4 of 13 observations, respectively; fertile wives of non-status men were with their husbands during 7 of 82 observations as an aggregate; $\chi^2 = 4.94$, df $= 1$, $p = 0.0262$.) Presumably, wives who spend more time together with husbands may have less opportunity to produce children by other men (cf. Flinn 1987, this volume (Chapter 11)). A serious qualifier of such a conclusion, however, is that the scan data on which it is based were not collected at night.

Finally, evidence from yet another study (Betzig and Turke 1986b) suggests that men of high status might, tentatively, be spending time with their children in a way that may increase the number of their grandchildren. Consistent with Trivers and Willard's (1973) prediction, chiefs, advisors, and successors were found to spend about twice as much time with their sons as with their daughters, while fathers without salary or status were found to spend about twice as much time with their daughters as with their sons. This is again a significant difference.

Discussion

Ifaluk chiefs and their successors appear to enjoy a number of productive and reproductive advantages over men without status. Clan chiefs enjoy privileges in etiquette, tribute, and greater than equal shares of communally caught fish; they take in food on a daily basis from distantly related households, and redistribute it to closer kin; and they spend less time physically at work than other men of the same age. As an aggregate, clan chiefs and their successors enjoy a number of potentially reproductive advantages. But, looked at separately, chiefs in this generation are not outreproducing their subordinates, while successors are.

This raises two important questions. First, *why* are chiefs, who enjoy these productive advantages, not reproductively successful to the same extent? Again, the best guess seems to be that two of them have, since early in adulthood, been unable to father children. Evidence that chiefs tend to have had on average more wives, though not more children by them, is consistent with the idea that they tried unsuccessfully to find a fertile union.

Second, *how* do successors produce so many children? None of the productive advantages to chiefs in tribute, food sharing, and leisure appear to accrue now to their successors. Successors take equal shares of collectively caught fish; they give and receive food with roughly equal frequency to households related about equally (non-status households gave food to successors' households six times, $\bar{r} = 0.0559$, while successors gave food to non-status households eight times, $\bar{r} = 0.0512$; $t = -0.22$, df $= 13$, $p = 0.8315$); and they spend about as much time as non-status men of comparable age productively engaged. (The labor:leisure ratio for the single Falalop successor was 11:6.).

There are at least three other ways, though, in which successors might be outreproducing men without status. First, being members of chiefly lineages, they are likely to have privileged access to the fruits of atoll property. Though the size, quality, and tenure hierarchy associated with every patch of island has yet to be determined, it is likely that people of rank on Ifaluk, as elsewhere in the Pacific (see especially Alkire, 1974), enjoy productive advantages in these respects. Second, being heirs apparent, successors may have been able to attract wives with higher reproductive potential. Though, again, the data have yet to be analyzed on this point, successors' wives may have more material resources at their disposal in the form of property, more human resources at their disposal in the form of kin (Berté this volume (Chapter 4)), and more personal resources in the form of fat (Borgerhoff Mulder this volume (Chapter 3)). Third, and data are available on this question, successors with large families might be better able to get others to invest in their children through adoption. More than half

of all Ifalukese are adopted at birth (cf. Lutz 1980); though this arrangement can amount to very little (Carroll 1970, Brady 1976, Silk 1980), adopted children are sometimes taken in and raised for years by their adoptive parents. Compared to men without status, successors with large families were, at the time of our census, more likely to have children living with adoptive parents (Betzig 1988). Through adoption, then, they draw on larger pools of parental investment, and by that means are able to bring up more children.

In short, though the fit between rank, production, and reproduction is not always tight, Ifaluk chiefs and their successors do overall enjoy more productive and reproductive advantages than their subordinates.

Sanctions

None of this means that redistribution is not to some extent to the benefit of everybody in the group. This may be for the reason Polanyi suggested. 'The explanation, in terms of survival [read, reproduction?], is simple .... All social obligations are reciprocal, and their fulfillment serves also the individual's give-and-take interests best' (1944:46).

There is no argument that social conditions vary; some societies, especially smaller societies, may be characterized by sharing more than others. But in all societies, even one as small as that on Ifaluk, common interest seems to have been insufficient to eclipse conflicts of interest completely; accordingly, people in power exploit their positions to productive, and eventually reproductive, ends. The point made here is a point of emphasis: To the extent that they have no option but to yield to them, subjects will sacrifice the fruits of their labor to leaders.

Two things make this sort of exploitation an option (see Betzig 1986:101–2). First is an inability of the exploited to be extricated from their 'social obligations.' Ifaluk, as much as anywhere else on earth, is geographically circumscribed (Carneiro 1970). The nearest atoll is 30 miles west; the nearest 'high' island, Yap, is 350 miles west; and, traditionally, people on both were likely to have welcomed a visitor with hostility: Ifalukese were often at war with other archipelago atolls (e.g. Burrows and Spiro 1957), and were subservient to the tribute-extracting Yapese (e.g. Lessa 1950, Lingenfelter 1975). Even where islanders were friendly, the Pacific itself is a hostile environment (e.g. Gladwyn 1970). Even now, emigration is a difficult task (e.g. Levin 1976).

Second, an inability to live and reproduce as well without *benefits* afforded by leaders must be expected to raise tolerance levels. As much as redistribution itself, by ensuring an equitable share to the majority, ups the benefit to subjects of leadership, it may also lower the cost to leaders of exploiting it. Nor, of course, is redistribution the only advantage chiefs might offer their subjects. Chiefs might reciprocate in a number of ways for productive and reproductive benefits. The point is, they predictably extrapolate this form of payment. Consistent with the Darwinian prediction, men with power seek and find productive and reproductive rewards.

Substantivism, Marxism, and Darwinism

Contrary to Sahlins' (1972) suggestion, the balance in redistribution on Ifaluk appears not to be on the subordinates' side; contrary to the broader version of substantivism (e.g. Polanyi 1944, 1957), Ifaluk chiefs appear to seek, and to find, material gain. And, contrary to Marxist assertions that exploitation is absent in 'primitive' groups (e.g. Engels 1888 [1964], Terray 1972), the fruits of the extra efforts of men of low status appear to be successfully appropriated by chiefs. That is, the balance, as in more familiar societies, is on the side of people with power. And, productive perquisites of chiefly office appear to be, at least in part, successfully translated into reproduction.

Again, for Terray (1972), as earlier for Engels (in Terray 1975), exploitation exists, essentially, when some work harder than they have to in order to support themselves, and, presumably, their dependents, and the products of their labors are then appropriated by others. By this definition, contrary to their own arguments, exploitation *does* seem to exist in at least one pre-state society. This is consistent with the arguments of contrary Marxists, including Dupré and Rey. It is hardly contradictory to the more general Marxist conception that conflicts between classes with and without privileged access to the resources necessary to production and reproduction is an important determinant of political organization.

And again, for Polanyi (1944, 1957), as later for Sahlins (1972), material gain is not sought in pre-market societies, where there is supposed to be an absence of insufficiency of means. But in any society, if the goal of economic action is *re*production, as well as production, there must necessarily be such an insufficiency (Chagnon 1979). Even *if* no other resource were limiting, there would always be, for men, a shortage of women. Again, this does not call into question the broader substantivist contention that, in Polanyi's phrase, the economy is an 'instituted process,' best considered in the whole context of social relations. In fact, it argues that economies could hardly be understood otherwise, since social as well as material resources are essential to reproduction.

What then does Darwinism contribute? Darwinian theory predicts both that people in power will have a motive to exploit, and that resources thereby gained will be used as means to reproduction, both by helping close genealogical kin, and by parenting children. The extent of exploitation should coincide with realized reproduction. Such a prediction is less than intuitively obvious in a society such as ours. The evidence, however, suggests that it holds up strongly in preindustrial societies (Betzig 1986).

Napoleon Chagnon (1979) set the precedent for these conclusions when he asked, 'Is reproductive success equal in egalitarian societies?' The answer, of course, is that it is not. If a large family is considered to be an asset, then all men are not in fact equal in any society. As Chagnon points out, differential reproduction necessitates differences, if not in access to strategic resources, at least in consumption of them. 'Out of the reproductive inequalities also come economic inequalities' (p. 378). Clearly, a man with ten times as many children must have ten times the resources to feed them; and there are just two solutions to this problem. 'Either he alone works ten times as hard as his peers, or he controls the productive efforts of others around him who assist him' (ibid.). Pending empirical data distinguishing between these options, Chagnon's 'best guess' was that the latter was generally the case, and that helpers were most often close affines and kinsmen (cf. Berté this volume (Chapter 4)).

The results here suggest that at least somewhere in the world, in at least one traditional society, exploitation of the fruits of others' productive labor may be an important means to differential reproduction. And on Ifaluk, the direct beneficiaries, rather than the targets of that exploitation, are close genealogical kinsmen.

It may be important to conclude that the lack of a precedent of a lack of exploitation *in no way* precludes the possibility of its evolution. In fact, as conditions arise to promote common interest, equal access to both the modes of production and reproduction must be expected to go up (see Alexander 1979, 1987, Betzig 1986). Contrary to the very unfortunately widespread misconceptions of many (e.g., Lewontin, Rose and Kamin 1984), Darwin's theory no more precludes the evolution of an equitable society, including a socialist society, than does Marx's. And, being a *descriptive*, rather than a *prescriptive* theory (Symons 1979), it does not even preclude the desirability of that possibility.

Summary

On Ifaluk, an atoll in the Western Caroline Islands, chiefs and their likely successors reap productive and reproductive advantages over others. Clan chiefs:

1. Take home nearly twice as much in fish in pounds per person after communal catches;
2. Take in food on a regular basis from distantly related households, and redistribute it to closer kin; and
3. Spend just over half as much time physically at work as other men of the same age.
4. By a number of mechanisms, chiefs and their successors have fathered more children.

These results contradict both Sahlins' version of substantivism and Engels' and others' versions of Marxism. They are consistent with a Darwinian explanation.

Acknowledgements

My debt to Napoleon Chagnon for starting up this line of research is obvious. Thanks too to Richard Alexander, Monique Borgerhoff Mulder, Mildred Dickemann, and Paul Turke for comments, to Gene Mesher and Ron Schneider for computing help, to Malcom Dow for statistical advice, and to Paul Turke for helping collect the data. Support from the Wenner-Gren Foundation, The National Geographic Society, the University of Michigan Museum of Zoology, and an NIMH training grant from the University of Michigan Department of Psychology are all gratefully acknowledged, as are the warm assistance and forebearance of the people of Ifaluk, including its chiefs.

References

Alexander, R. D. (1975) The search for a general theory of behavior. *Behavior Science*, **20**, 77–100.

Alexander, R. D. (1979) *Darwinism and Human Affairs*. Seattle: University of Washington.

Alexander, R. D. (1987) *The Biology of Moral Systems*. Hawthorne, NY: Aldine.

Alexander, R. D. and Borgia, G. (1978) Group selection, altruism, and the levels of organization of life. *Annual Review of Ecology and Systematics*, **9**, 449–74.

Alkire, W. H. (1974) Land tenure in the Woleai. In *Land Tenure in Oceania*, ed. H. P. Lundsgaarde, ASAO Monograph No. 2. Honolulu: University of Hawaii Press.

Axelrod, R. and Hamilton, W. D. (1981) The evolution of cooperation. *Science*, **211**, 1390–6.

Bates, M. and Abbott, D. (1958) *Coral Island*. NY: Scribner's.

Betzig, L. L. (1982) Despotism and differential reproduction: a cross cultural correlation of conflict asymmetry, hierarchy, and degree of polygyny. *Ethology and Sociobiology*, **3**, 209–21.

Betzig, L. L. (1986) *Despotism and Differential Reproduction: A Darwinian View of History*. Hawthorne, NY: Aldine.

Betzig, L. L. (1988) Adoption by rank on Ifaluk, *American Anthropologist* (in press).

Betzig, L. L. and Turke, P. W. (1985) Measuring time allocation: observation and intention. *Current Anthropology*, **26**, 647–50.

Betzig, L. L. and Turke, P. W. (1986a) Food sharing on Ifaluk. *Current Anthropology*, **27**, 397–400.

Betzig, L. L. and Turke, P. W. (1986b) Parental investment by sex on Ifaluk. *Ethology and Sociobiology*, **7**, 29–37.

Borgerhoff Mulder, M. (1987) Reproductive success in three Kipsigis cohorts. In *Reproductive Success*, ed. T. H. Clutton-Brock. Chicago: University of Chicago Press.

Brady, I. (1976) *Transactions in Kinship*. Honolulu: University of Hawaii Press.

Burrows, E. G. and Spiro, M. E. (1957) *An Atoll Cul-

ture. Westport, CN: Greenwood Press. (Originally published in 1953 by HRAF Press.)

Carneiro, R. L. (1970) A theory of the origin of the state. *Science*, **169**, 733–8.

Carroll, V. (1970) *Adoption in Eastern Oceania*. Honolulu: University of Hawaii Press.

Chagnon, N. A. (1979) Is reproductive success equal in egalitarian societies? In *Evolutionary Biology and Human Social Behavior: An Anthropological Perspective*, ed. N. A. Chagnon and W. Irons. North Scituate, MA: Duxbury Press.

Chagnon, N. A. and Bryant, W. (1984) KINDEM-COM: A fourth style in the study of kinship. Report to the Harry Frank Guggenheim Foundation.

Damm, H. (1908–1910) Ergebnisse der Südsee-Expedition. In *Zentralkarolinen*, ed. G. Thilenius. New Haven: HRAF.

Darwin, C. (1859) *On the Origin of Species*. London: John Murray.

Darwin, C. (1871) *The Descent of Man and Selection in Relation to Sex*. London: John Murray.

Engels, F. (1884 [1964]) *On the Origin of the Family, Private Property, and the State*. New York: International Publishers.

Firth, R. (1959) *Social Change in Tikopia*. London: Allen and Unwin.

Fisher, R. A. (1958) *The Genetical Theory of Natural Selection*. New York: Dover.

Flinn, M. V. (1987) Mate guarding in Trinidad. *Ethology and Sociobiology*, **8** (in press).

Garcilaso de la Vega. (1961) *Royal Commentaries of the Yncas*. New York: Orians Press. (Original date 1609–1617.)

Gladwyn, T. (1970) *East is a Big Bird*. New York: Columbia University Press.

Godelier, M. (1978) The concept of the 'Asiatic mode of production' and Marxist models of social evolution. In *Relations of Production*, ed. D. Seddon, pp. 209–57.

Hamilton, W. D. (1963) The evolution of altruistic behavior. *American Naturalist*, **97**, 354–6.

Hamilton, W. D. (1964) The genetical evolution of social behavior. *Journal of Theoretical Biology*, **7**, 1–52.

Havlicek, L. L. and Peterson, N. L. (1974) Robustness of the *t* test: A guide for researchers on effects of violations of assumptions. *Psychological Reports*, **34**, 1095–1114.

Hunt, E. E., Schneider, D. M., Kidder, N. R. and Stevens, W. D. (1949) *The Micronesians of Yap and Their Depopulation*. Report of the Peabody Museum Expedition to Yap, 1948–1949. Washington, DC: Pacific Science Board, National Research Council.

Kaplan, H. and Hill, K. (1985) Hunting ability and reproductive success among male Ache foragers. *Current Anthropology*, **26**, 131–3.

Lessa, W. (1950) Ulithi and the outer native world. *American Anthropologist*, **52**, 27–52.

Levin, M. J. (1976) Population structure on Eauripik atoll. Ph.D. Dissertation, University of Michigan.

Lewontin, R., Rose, S., and Kamin, L. J. (1984) *Not in Our Genes*. New York: Pantheon.

Lingenfelter, S. G. (1975) *Yap: Political Leadership and Culture Change in an Island Society*. Honolulu: University of Hawaii Press.

Lutz, C. (1980) Emotion words and emotional development on Ifaluk atoll. Ph.D. Dissertation, Harvard University.

Maybury-Lewis, D. (1967) *Akwe-Shavante Society*. Oxford: Clarendon.

Meillassoux, C. (1964) *The Economic Anthropology of the Gura*. Paris.

Meillassoux, C. (1981) *Maidens, Meals, and Money*. Cambridge: Cambridge University Press.

Morgan, L. H. (1877 [1978]) *Ancient Society*. Palo Alto: New York Labor News.

Murdock, G. P. (1967) *Ethnographic Atlas*. New Haven: HRAF Press.

Polanyi, K. (1944) *The Great Transformation*. New York: Rhinehart.

Polanyi, K. (1957) The economy as instituted process. In *Trade and Market in the Early Empires*, ed. K Polanyi, C. Arensberg, and H. Pearson, pp. 243–70. Glencoe: Free Press.

Sahlins, M. D. (1958) *Social Stratification in Polynesia*. Seattle: University of Washington.

Sahlins, M. D. (1962) *Moala: Culture and Nature on a Fijian Island*. Ann Arbor: University of Michigan.

Sahlins, M. D. (1972) *Stone Age Economics*. Chicago: Aldine.

Schapera, I. (1930) *The Khoisan Peoples of South Africa: Bushmen and Hottentots*. London: Routledge and Sons.

Silk, J. B. (1980) Adoption in Oceania. *American Anthropologist*, **82**, 799–820.

Symons, D. (1979) *The Evolution of Human Sexuality*. NY: Oxford.

Terray, E. (1972) *Marxism and 'Primitive' Societies*. New York: Monthly Review.

Terray, E. (1975) Classes and class consciousness in the Abron Kingdom of Gyaman. In *Marxist Analyses and Social Anthropology*, ed. M. Bloch, pp. 85–135. New York: Wiley and Sons.

Tracey, J. Abbott, D., and Arnow, T. (1956) *Natural History of Ifaluk Atoll*. Bernice P. Bishop Museum Bulletin 222. Honolulu: University of Hawaii Press.

Trigger, B. G. (1969) *The Huron*. NY: Holt, Rinehart and Winston.

Trivers, R. L. (1971) The evolution of reciprocal altruism. *Quarterly Review of Biology*, **46**, 35–57.

Trivers, R. L. and Willard, D. E. (1973) Natural selection of parental ability to vary the sex ratio of offspring. *Science*, **179**, 90–2.

Turke, P. W. (1985) Fertility determinants on Ifaluk and Yap: tests of economic and Darwinian hypotheses. Ph.D. Dissertation, Northwestern University.

Turke, P. W. and Betzig, L. L. (1985) Those who

can do: wealth, status, and reproductive success on Ifaluk. *Ethology and Sociobiology*, **6**, 79–87.

Vehrencamp, S. L. (1983) A model for the evolution of despotic versus egalitarian societies. *Animal Behaviour*, **31**, 667–82.

Williams, G. C. (1966) *Adaptation and Natural Selection: A Critique of Some Current Evolutionary Thought*. Princeton: Princeton University Press.

Kipsigis bridewealth payments

Introduction

Bridewealth is a major contribution of parents to the mating effort of their sons. In this chapter I examine variations in bridewealth payments among the Kipsigis of Kenya in order to determine whether the amount of bridewealth parents give or demand at the marriages of their offspring is affected by reproductive considerations.

Rights to women and their progeny (Radcliffe-Brown 1950:53) are acquired through the payment of valuables, services or symbolic items (Fortes 1962:9), the quantity of which varies both between and within societies (Schneider 1964:42). Intense bargaining over bridewealth is reported in many societies (Goldschmidt 1974:325, 328) and this suggests that intracultural variability in bridewealth may result in part from each party seeking to maximize some value, be it material or social, often at the expense of the other party (Spiro 1975:98, Kressel 1977). Variability in bridewealth payments may therefore arise from the relative advantages or costs accrued by either party as a consequence of the marriage. Simply put, where the groom enters into a marriage that, for some material or social reason, is advantageous to him and his family a high bridewealth is paid, and where the bride

[1] Department of Zoology Large Animal Research Group, University of Cambridge, Cambridge, CB3 0DT, UK

enters a marriage that benefits herself or her family a low bridewealth is demanded. Conversely, marriages are characterized by low bridewealth where the groom's family suffers, and by high bridewealth where the bride's family suffers. On this premise, I propose that quantitative study of intracultural variability in bridewealth will reveal the critical qualities that parents seek in the spouses of their progeny.

In particular, I examine whether higher payments are made for brides who are likely to increase their husband's reproductive success, testing specific predictions from evolutionary theory. First, men are expected to pay inflated

bridewealth for women of high reproductive value, defined as those who will make an above-average contribution to the ancestry of future generations (Fisher 1930). Age at menarche, physique, health and evidence of fecundity are used as indicators of reproductive value. Other hypotheses are tested: first, men are predicted to pay highly for women who are nulliparous as opposed to those who have borne and are caring for other men's children, to avoid the costs of raising unrelated children. Second, men are likely to pay highly for women who will provide reliable economic contributions to the household. Third, the status or other characteristics of the prospective bride's kin group may influence a man's willingness to pay high bridewealth, if affinal alliances between kin groups affect his fitness.

Three general points should be noted. First, the predictions tested here are specific to the

Figure 3.1 Location of the study site in Rift Valley Province, Kenya. Kericho District is delineated, with its central town Kericho marked as a dot. A star marks the study site, lying on the border of Kericho and Narok Districts.

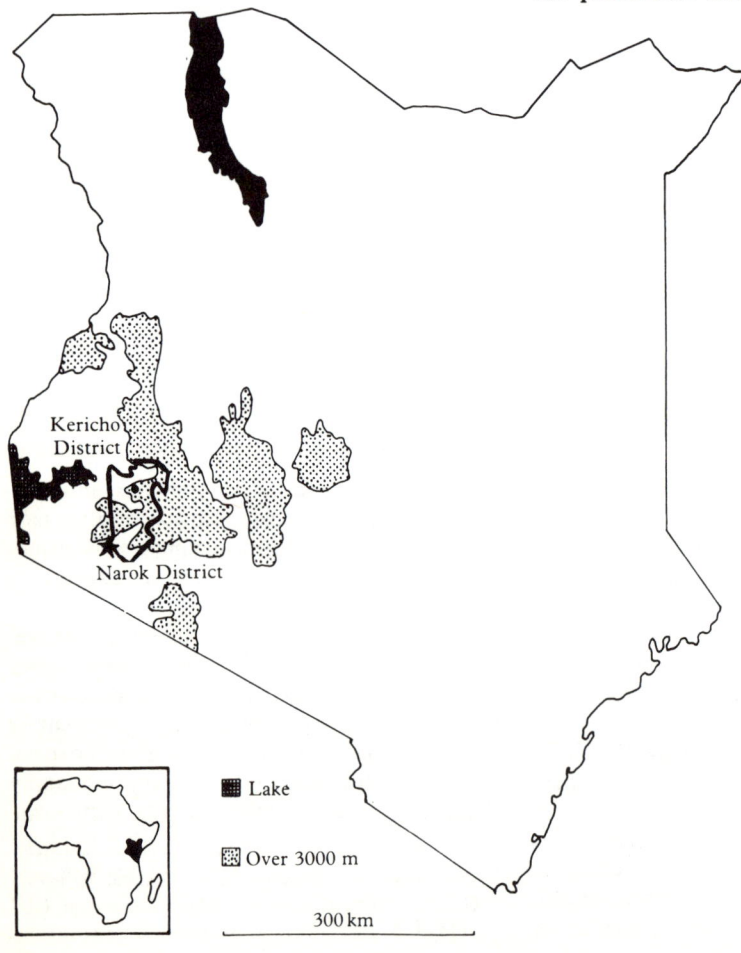

Kericho District

Narok District

▓ Lake

▒ Over 3000 m

300 km

Kipsigis marriage system, where divorce is prohibited and paternal investment high. Bridewealth payments may be affected by different factors in societies where the systems of marriage, production and alliance are differently organized, as discussed in the final section. Second, bridewealth can be studied both as parental and mating effort, because payments for first marriages are the responsibility of the groom's parents. This chapter focuses on bridewealth as mating effort, irrespective of whether the payment is made by the groom or his father. Third, the amount of bridewealth transferred is a consequence of protracted negotiations during which both parties retain the right to retract offers. For this reason, results are discussed from both the groom's and the bride's parents' points of view.

Ethnographic background

The Kipsigis are a Kalenjin-speaking, agro-pastoralist people living in Rift Valley Province, Kenya (Figure 3.1) They practise patrilineal inheritance and usually settle virilocally, not in villages but socially demarcated neighbourhoods known as *kokwotinwek* (singular *kokwet*, Peristiany 1939), approximately 2 kilometres ($1\frac{1}{4}$ miles) in diameter. Since the 1930s Kipsigis have increasingly adopted an agricultural way of life, selling maize for cash (Manners 1967). Women are responsible for agricultural and domestic work, while animal husbandry is shared by men, women and children (Borgerhoff Mulder 1985).

The prospective groom's father (subsequently referred to as GF) initiates marriage negotiations by making an offer of cows, goats or sheep, and (since 1960) cash to the father of the potential bride. Invariably, by all accounts, the bride's father (BF) counters by demanding a higher price than that offered by any of the suitors. After several months of deliberation and bargaining, BF decides, together with his wife and close kin, between the competing offers made for his daughter and the final bridewealth is negotiated with the father of the successful suitor. The preferences of the boy and girl concerned are relatively unimportant to the wishes of their parents, even nowadays. Only a few individuals are ineligible for reasons of age or relatedness (Peristiany 1939:107, Orchardson 1961:76).

While it is difficult to specify how many suitors a potential bride might attract, BF is generally in a position to choose among and reject prospective sons-in-law (Peristiany 1939:59, Orchardson 1961:69). Women are seen as being in short supply, partly because they marry at a modal age of 16 years whereas boys are first married at a modal age of 23 years and partly because of high levels of polygyny (Borgerhoff Mulder 1988a). As in traditional times girls are married within one or two years of the clitoridectomy 'circumcision' operation (Orchardson 1961:69) that all girls undergo on reaching menarche. A small proportion of the sample (4% of 612 women married after 1959) pursued secondary education after circumcision, thus delaying their marriages by several years.

The majority of marriages are negotiated before girls become pregnant (96% of 1226 married women in my sample). If a girl is pregnant, her father will try to force the man responsible into marriage. If this cannot be arranged, the father of the pregnant girl has two options. First, his daughter may remain at home and bear illegitimate children throughout her reproductive career. This option is not relished by a father unless he has no sons of his own. Second, his daughter can marry after she has given birth to one (or more) illegitimate offspring. She takes these illegitimate offspring to the house of the groom, who not only assumes total responsibility for the children he did not father but, in the case of boys, must provide inheritance and bridewealth. Such marriages are termed *kimut lakwet* ('accompanied' by children), and occurred in 2% of all marriages.

In this study the mean bridewealth payment for marriages occurring after 1959 was 6 cows, 6 goats and 800 Kenyan shillings, in total equivalent to £450 (sterling). For a man of average wealth this constitutes one-third of his herd of cows, half of his herd of goats and 2 months' salary (only 5% of adult men with offspring have any regular employment). Unlike some East African pastoralists, the groom's father is solely responsible for providing the bridewealth for his son's first marriage. Second and subsequent marriages are generally the responsibility of the groom himself. The sources of bridewealth are the natural increase of the family herd, the livestock received at the marriages of sisters and daughters, cash earnings and cattle raiding, which still occurs in remote areas (including the study area) despite its illegality. The livestock are subject to meticulous inspection (*suet ab tuga*) by the bride's kin and are handed over with the cash before, or immediately after, the major marriage ceremony (*katunisiet*). The speed with which Kipsigis make, and have always made payments (Peristiany 1939:59, 86), greatly facilitates the quantification of bridewealth, as debts do not persist over generations (cf. Kuper 1982:35).

Payment of bridewealth procures a man rights to all his wife's children, legitimate or not (Peristiany 1939:86), and to her labour services. Marriage is highly stable, and divorce almost unknown (Peristiany 1939:89, Orchardson 1961:79), with only one reported case in the sample. Maltreated wives may desert, generally on a temporary basis (5% of all 1226 women in my sample), but neither the bridewealth nor any portion thereof is ever returned to the groom. The reproductive opportunities of men who fail to marry are low because there are heavy sanctions against adultery. Moreover, unmarried circumcised girls are rarely encountered (due to the short interval between circumcision and marriage). Furthermore, any child born to an uncircumcised girl was traditionally strangled at birth. Unmarried men therefore have few reproductive chances, little secure economic support and tend to leave the community for cash employment elsewhere.

Relations between affines are characterized by equality, friendship and respect (Komma 1981:119). If living nearby, affines help each other with agricultural work and preparations for large ceremonies but this cooperation probably derives more from their common *kokwet* membership than affinity *per se* (Peristiany 1939). Thus affinity does not tightly prescribe a relationship but it can constitute the basis of a highly cooperative and supportive alliance between different families.

Methods

Information on the payments made at 267 marriages was collected between June 1982 and December 1983 through informal interviews with 150 families to whom I made regular visits as part of a behavioural study (Borgerhoff

Table 3.1 *Kipsigis bridewealth amounts 1934–1983[a]*

Years	Mean units	n	SD	Range
1934–1943	5.59	5	1.51	3.6– 8.2
1944–1953	6.92	16	2.14	3.4–12.5
1954–1963	8.42	66	1.78	5.6–12.0
1964–1973	8.30	68	2.05	1.0–12.5
1974–1983	8.55	112	1.96	3.5–12.5

[a] The differences between bridewealth payments in the first and second, and second and third periods were significant ($t_{5,16} = 2.10$, $p < 0.05$; $t_{16,66} = 4.11$, $p < 0.001$, respectively)

Mulder and Caro 1985) or in whose *kokwet* I was living. The behavioural sample was randomly selected and the *kokwet* did not differ in any obvious way from other *kokwotinwek*. Rapport with these families was particularly high, and this permitted detailed questioning about bridewealth payments and rigorous cross-checking between families.

For each marriage, a record was made of the number of cows, sheep or goats (interchangeable in value), and Kenyan shillings paid by GF to BF. Using the current value of a cow and sheep/goat *at the time of the marriage* a unitary scale was devised by means of which payments could be compared, standardized for their current commercial value (see Laughlin 1974:134 for a similar bridewealth index). Bridewealth values increased radically between 1930 and 1960, after which there was no significant change in the mean value by decade (Table 3.1). All analyses presented here are restricted to marriages occurring after 1959 to control for inflationary effects. They are also restricted to first and second marriages; whether a bride was the first or second wife of a man did not confound any of the results presented here.

'Recollected' payments are open to bias (Goody 1969:55). In this study, reliability tests ($n = 117$) between the reports of BF and GF showed a mean discrepancy of 0.49 units (0.26 of a standard deviation (SD)) and a range of discrepancies from 0 to 1.5 (0.80 of a SD). Where discrepancies occurred that could not be resolved through cross-checking with both parties present, the mean of the two reports was used.

Demographic interviews (see Borgerhoff Mulder 1987a) were used to determine a bride's age at circumcision, her reproductive status and

3. Kipsigis bridewealth payments

parity at marriage, her education and the location of her natal and marital households. Dates of birth, circumcision and marriage were established by referencing these events to male circumcision ceremonies and other datable past local incidences such as droughts. Detailed cross-checks were made between individuals.

The number of acres owned by the bride's and groom's respective fathers was determined from a household census (Borgerhoff Mulder 1987b), and subsequently checked with the local Land Office maps. In order to assess relative wealth, fathers of the bride and groom were subsequently categorized according to whether they fell into the lower (<15 acres), middle (<30 acres), or upper third of the distribution. This measure of relative wealth was only available for 85 marriages, in so far as the wealth of the bride's and groom's fathers was only recorded for 140 and 116 marriages, respectively.

Scan samples (Borgerhoff Mulder and Caro 1985) combined with weekly interviews were used to measure the incidence of wives deserting their husbands, wife-beating and ill-health in the

behavioural sub-sample. As regards desertion and wife-beating, if a woman was either observed or reported to be temporarily living in another household, the reasons for her leaving her marital home were identified; women speak with surprising openness about cases of marital discord. Concerning health, the incidence of illness for each member of the household was recorded during weekly interviews with the mother.

Finally, of marriages that occurred while I was in the community, brides were classified according to their physique, a subjective assessment made by three or more unrelated villagers as to whether the bride was '*manerat*' or '*sagitat*'. These terms denote plumpness and skinniness, combining notions of fat deposition and stature; they are frequently used by women as evaluative statements about a person's general physical condition and were consistent between reporters.

For all statistics two-tailed probabilities are quoted.

Results

Reproductive value

The payment of bridewealth generally establishes the transfer, sale or hire of reproductive services between families (Radcliffe-Brown

Figure 3.2 Bridewealth and age of circumcision. A significant regression can be fitted $r = -0.24$, $Y = 13.21 - 0.32(X)$, $f_{1,159} = 9.36$, $p < 0.01$, where $X =$ bride's age at circumcision and $Y =$ bridewealth units.

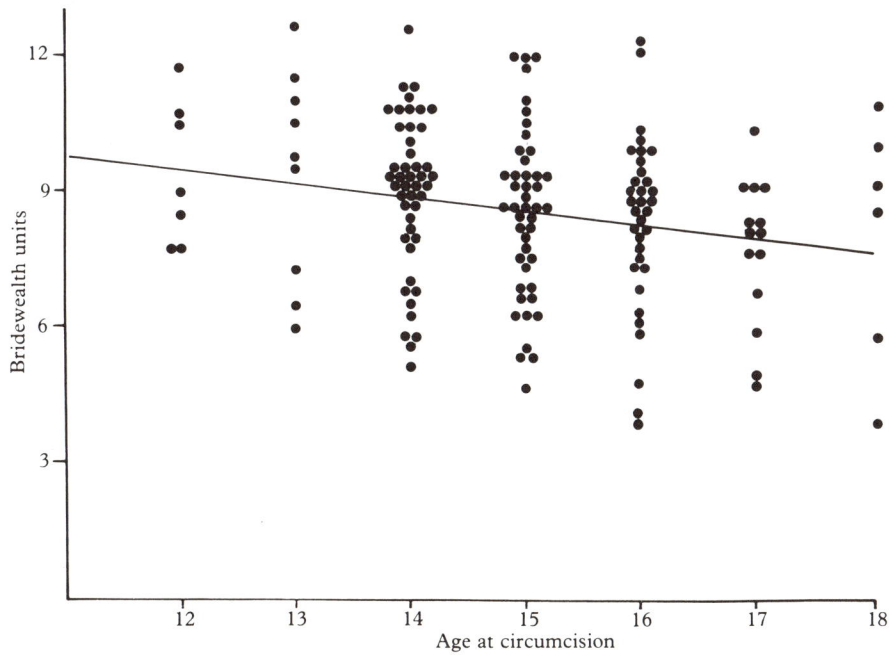

1950:50, Leach 1961:115, Lewis 1962:42, Goody 1973a:11, Schneider 1964:41) and yet the relationship between the reproductive value (probable future reproductive success, Fisher 1958) of the bride and the amount of bridewealth transferred has never been examined quantitatively. I first determine whether bridewealth varies as a function of the bride's reproductive value, using age at menarche, physical condition, health record and evidence of fecundity as indicators of reproductive value.

1. Age at menarche

For nulliparous, non-pregnant brides, bridewealth decreased with age at circumcision (Pearson $r = -0.24$, $n = 161$, $p < 0.01$, see Figure 3.2). This effect was independent of all other measured significant factors affecting bridewealth (see below).

Age at circumcision can be used as a measure of age at menarche because of the Kipsigis custom of sending girls for circumcision the December following first menses. Estimating menarcheal age in this way raises some problems. First, there are inevitably cases where the custom is not followed. Second, even when followed, the procedure results in separating women who may have been only a few weeks apart in age at first menses into different menarcheal age groups, and in lumping women who first menstruated almost 1 year apart into the same menarcheal age group. Because of this error on the X axis, a more rigorous statistical test entails dropping the median circumcision age category (15 years), and comparing women according to a dichotomous ranking of whether they were early maturers (circumcised between 12 and 14 years) or late (16–18 years) maturers. Such categories include only a few incorrectly ranked individuals for whom the usual clitoridectomy customs were not followed, constituting an unsystematic bias to both samples.

Testing the data in this way showed that the mean bridewealth paid for early maturers was significantly higher (9.00 units) than that paid for late maturers (8.1 units) ($t_{62,54} = 2.65$, $p < 0.01$).

2. Physical condition

Health and vigour are praised in Kipsigis women. For the 11 marriages that took place in the community while I was present, I classified the bride-to-be according to her health record over a 12-month period and her size (see Methods). Girls who had been ill ($n = 6$) on more than three occasions in the 12 months prior to their marriages were not significantly cheaper than brides with better health records (Fisher's Exact Probability, $n = 11$, NS). However, girls classified as 'plump' ($n = 4$) were more expensive than those classified as 'skinny' (Fisher's Exact Probability, $n = 11$, $p < 0.05$). These analyses were restricted to marriages of nulliparous, non-pregnant brides who were either 15 or 16 at circumcision, and were not therefore confounded by reproductive status or age at menarche.

Finally there were two physically handicapped brides, one hunchback and one with a clubfoot. No bridewealth figures were available, but I was told that they were 'almost free'.

3. Pregnancy

Brides who are already pregnant with the child of the prospective groom might be expected to be more expensive than those who are not, because they are clearly not barren. Such demonstration of fecundity is likely to be particularly valued in societies such as the Kipsigis, where bridewealth is never refundable, even in the case of childlessness. In contrast to the prediction, brides pregnant by their prospective husbands were significantly cheaper than those who were not pregnant at marriage ($t_{24,193} = -2.34$, $p < 0.02$).

Further analyses nevertheless suggested that the low bridewealth of pregnant brides was associated with the differential bargaining power of the two parties rather than the reduced intrinsic value of pregnant brides. Negotiations over marriages where the bride is known to be pregnant differ from those over other marriages in that the parties are not on an equal footing. BF has lost bargaining power and is seen as having been cheated. If he does not accept whatever the father of the man responsible offers, he has only the low bridewealth of an 'accompanied' marriage (see below) to look forward to, or no bridewealth at all (see Ethnographic Background). Where the bargaining power of BF is curtailed by his daughter's pregnancy, other inequalities between the two families may affect the outcome of negotiations. Specifically, the relative wealth of the two families may be a significant factor

3. Kipsigis bridewealth payments

in so far as large wealth differences are generally associated with considerable differences in influence and status (cf. Peristiany 1939:150, Borgerhoff Mulder 1987b). A man of lower social standing is usually unable to oppose the wishes of a more influential man, and this may account for the finding that pregnant brides were cheaper only where BF was poorer than or equal in wealth to GF ($t_{14,109} = -2.82$, using separate estimates of variance, $p < 0.01$, see Figure 3.3). Indeed where BF was richer than GF there was no significant difference between bridewealth paid for pregnant and non-pregnant brides ($t_{4,31} = 1.26$, NS, see Figure 3.3).

In sum, there is no evidence that demonstration of fecundity promotes high bridewealth payments. To the contrary, pregnant brides are relatively cheap, but this probably results from the poor bargaining power of their fathers.

Paternity certainty

Men should not be willing to pay high bridewealth for women who have already given birth

Figure 3.3 The effects of pregnancy on mean bridewealth according to the relative wealth of the bride's and groom's families. BF (bride's father); GF (groom's father); BF ⩽ GF (BF of lower or equal wealth category to GF); BF > GF (BF of higher wealth category than GF); 'poor', 'average' and 'rich' wealth categories defined earlier in text, see Methods.

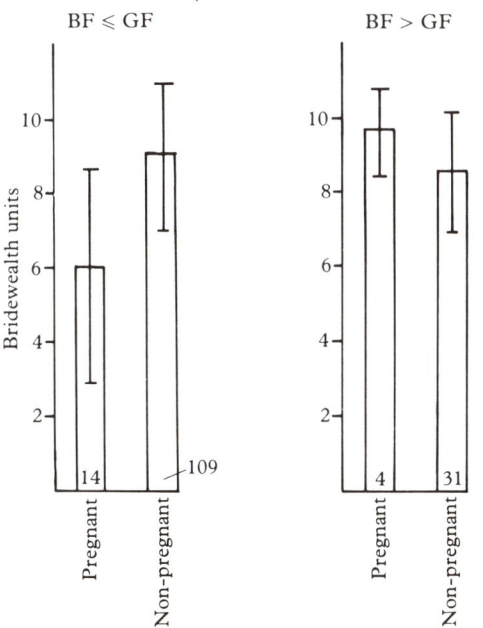

to the children of other men. Such illegitimate infants remain in the care of their mother and are 'adopted' by the husband at her marriage. Indeed, the mean bridewealth paid for brides who bring one or more infants ('accompanied' marriage) not fathered by the groom-to-be was significantly lower than that paid for brides of comparable age at circumcision (15 or over) in 'unaccompanied' marriages (($t_{19,99} = -2.81$, $p < 0.01$, Figure 3.4).

Given that an adopted son inherits land from his step-father it seems likely that brides accompanying infant sons would be less desirable, and thus cheaper, than those accompanying infant daughters. Infant's sex in fact had no effect on the bridewealth paid, although the sample was small, ($t_{5,8} = 1.12$, NS). Similarly there was no difference whether one or two infants were brought to the marriage ($t_{13,19} = 0.25$, NS). 'Accompanied' brides nevertheless ran away from their husbands more frequently than did 'unaccompanied' brides ($\chi^2 = 14.31$, df = 1, $n = 131$, $p < 0.001$), and they were more commonly beaten by their husbands ($\chi^2 = 3.88$, df = 1, $n = 131$, $p < 0.05$).

Marital distance

Bridewealth has been interpreted as a compensatory payment to the bride's kin for disruption of lineage solidarity (Radcliffe-Brown 1950:49) or for the loss of her labour (Goody 1973a:6, Divale and Harris 1976:523).

While a Kipsigis woman is almost completely incorporated into her husband's lineage, her natal family retains some rights over her labour (Orchardson 1961). A bride's mother expects and greatly values her daughter's assistance at harvest or at the birth of a new baby. In this study I used the distance between a bride's natal and marital homes (marital distance) as a measure of the extent to which her parents effectively lose rights to her labour, and predicted that a GF living far from BF will have to pay more for a bride.

The data support the hypothesis. There was a positive correlation between bridewealth and marital distance ($r = 0.20$, $n = 193$, $p = <0.01$), an association shown by regression analysis to be independent of both bride's age at menarche and the wealth of the fathers of the bride and groom (see below). The greatest difference between categories was found to lie between brides who come from within the *kokwet* (i.e. within 2 kilometres or 1¼ miles) and those who come from further away (3–128 kilometres (*c.* 2–80 miles) in this sample) ($t_{146,47} = -2.51$, $p < 0.05$, using separate estimates of variance, see Figure 3.5).

Data on labour cooperation in one *kokwet* showed that women were more likely to help their mothers if they were neighbours or if they lived in the same *kokwet* than if they belonged to different *kokwotinwek* ($\chi^2 = 10.45$, df = 1, $n = 32$, $p < 0.01$, see Figure 3.6). Grooms who marry within the *kokwet* are more likely to lose their bride's labour to their mothers-in-law.

An alternative explanation for the positive association between bridewealth and marital distance could be that a BF who gives his daughter to a family of the same *kokwet* can protect his daughter's interests by intervening in cases of marital discord and providing sanctuary for his daughter when she is in trouble. If this were so, incidences of wife-beating would be less likely to occur in marriages where the bride's

natal home lies within the *kokwet*. No association between the incidence of wife-beating and marital distance was found ($\chi^2 = 0.008$, df = 1, $n = 135$, NS), suggesting that a BF who lives near his daughter's marital home is no more able to protect his daughter's interests than one who lives far away. Furthermore, women whose natal homes were within the *kokwet* did not have a higher probability of deserting their husbands than those whose natal homes lay outside the *kokwet* ($\chi^2 = 0.47$, df = 1, $n = 135$, NS), indicating that BF is no more likely to provide sanctuary to his daughter if her marital home is nearby. Finally, no evidence was found that BF gains greater access to his son-in-law's labour by giving his daughter to a family in the *kokwet* rather than to a non-local family (Fisher's Exact Probability $n = 32$, NS), as suggested for the Gisu (La Fontaine 1962).

In summary, the data show that bridewealth increased with distance between the natal and marital households, and that brides from outside the *kokwet* less frequently help their mothers than do locally-married girls. There was no indication that non-local brides were more likely to be maltreated or to desert. Parents who give their daughters to a member of their *kokwet* benefit from continued access to their daughters' labour; parents who buy non-local brides for their

Figure 3.4 Mean bridewealth according to whether or not brides have given birth to illegitimate children. Data restricted to brides who were circumcised at 15 years or older.

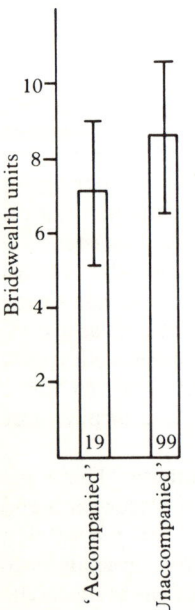

Figure 3.5 Effects of the marital distance on mean bridewealth.

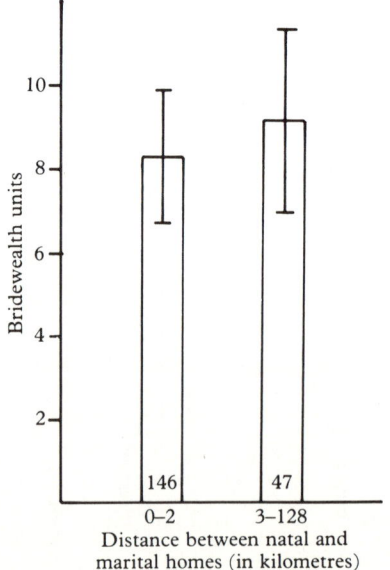

Distance between natal and marital homes (in kilometres)

sons can enjoy more constant labour services than can parents who buy local brides.

Affinal connections

Marriage is more than just a domestic issue (Radcliffe-Brown 1950:51, Fortes 1962:7, Irons 1981). Isolating marriage and its associated institutions (e.g. bridewealth) from the social and cultural context may restrict interpretation (Leach 1961:108, Needham 1971:6, Kuper 1982:164). Numerous studies have presented penetrating analyses of how marriages are arranged and negotiated so as to strengthen and expand a family's affinal connections within its own and other communities. The reasons for cultivating affinal alliances vary according to specific ethnographic circumstances: access to agricultural land and capital ventures for the Taita of Kenya (Harris 1962:79), succession to political office and entitlement to a wife's inheritance among the Tshidi of Southern Africa (Comaroff and Comaroff 1981:39), expansion of *moka* networks among the Melpa of New Guinea (Strathern 1980:52), securing future marriage partners for the Yąnomamö of Venezuela (Chagnon 1979a:106) and attainment of prestige among the Bedouin of Cyrenaica (Peters 1980:154) and the Ugandan Karimojong (Dyson-Hudson 1966:84). So does negotiated bridewealth among Kipsigis reflect potential social and economic benefits accrued from establishing affinal links with families of different status?

Because vicarious benefits (cf. Goody 1969:59) such as loans, assistance, access to a small field or a milking cow, can be acquired though ties of affinity among the Kipsigis, the poorer partner to a marriage may be expected to suffer materially from the negotiated bridewealth in expectation of future benefits. Thus a wealthy BF should charge high bridewealth, so as to discourage an affinal relationship that has few anticipated payoffs. Furthermore, a wealthy GF could probably acquire a bride for his son with only a modest offer, promising aid and cooperation in the future. If Kipsigis were making such calculations, bridewealth would be expected to vary negatively with GF's wealth and positively with BF's wealth.

The data do not support this prediction. First, there was no correlation between the number of acres owned by BF or by GF and the amount of bridewealth transferred ($r = -0.00$, $n = 140$, NS, $r = -0.08$, $n = 116$, NS, respectively). Furthermore, the relative differences in wealth between negotiating parties did not significantly affect bridewealth values ($f_{4,80} = 0.19$, NS, see Figure 3.7). These results were restricted to the marriages of nulliparous, non-pregnant brides, and were not affected by controlling for bride's age at menarche nor for marital distance. Finally, there was no evidence that bridewealth

Figure 3.7 Effects of relative wealth on mean bridewealth. = (both partners of same wealth category); »08 (first partner rich, second partner poor); > (first partner rich, second partner average; or first partner average, second partner poor).

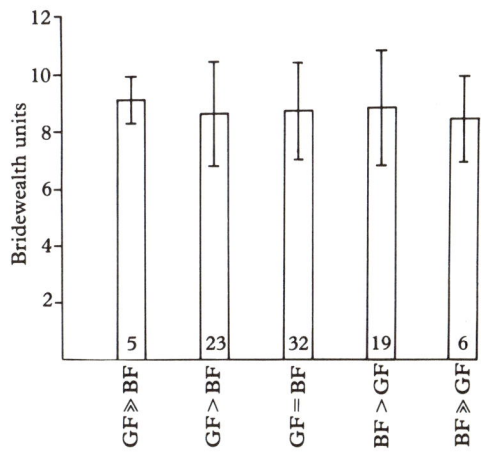

Figure 3.6 Effects of marital distance on the incidence of daughters helping their mothers. Shaded bars represent women who helped their mothers; unshaded bars represent women who did not help their mothers.

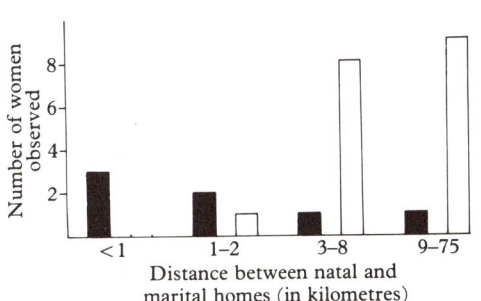

paid between families already related through marriage differed from that between non-relatives ($t_{48,71} = 0.01$, NS).

These results indicate that BF does not accept low bridewealth from a potentially powerful affine who is much richer than himself, nor does he demand high bridewealth from a very much poorer man who might become an economic liability. Similarly GF does not agree to pay a high bridewealth for an affine who is much richer than himself, nor does he offer low bridewealth to a much poorer affine. Finally, establishment of new affinal alliances is associated neither with particularly high nor low payments.

Summary of the results

Analysis of variance was conducted to establish the amount of variance in Kipsigis bridewealth payments that has been explained, and to determine the *independent* contributions of each variable. Brides who were either pregnant at marriage, or who had already given birth to another man's child(ren), were categorized together, because marriage negotiations in such cases were constrained by considerations of paternity and influence; in this way, zero cells were avoided. Bridewealth was associated negatively with bride's age at circumcision ($f_{1,198} = 18.43$, $p < 0.001$) and positively with marital distance ($f_{1,198} = 10.79$, $p < 0.01$); pregnant and non-nulliparous brides were cheap ($f_{1,198} = 4.31$, $p < 0.05$). These three variables explained 21% of the total variance.

Discussion

It is perhaps not surprising that only 21% of variance in bridewealth payments could be explained, given the complexity of social factors that determine both marriage choice and marital payments (e.g. Leach 1961). Recognition of this has led many anthropologists to eschew quantitative analyses of bridewealth (and other social phenomena). Nevertheless, in this study a number of factors are found to be significant determinants of bridewealth payments, demonstrating the value of a quantitative approach (cf. Borgerhoff Mulder and Caro 1985).

In this discussion I first review the major parental considerations associated with variability in bridewealth among the Kipsigis, and then examine whether parents pay highest bridewealth for brides who are likely to enhance the reproductive success of their offspring, particularly their sons. I conclude by suggesting some hypotheses that test the interpretation of the Kipsigis findings in other cultural contexts.

The husband's reproductive benefits

The high bridewealth that fathers pay for young wives for their sons has direct consequences on their sons' reproductive success, because women who reach menarche early have, on average, three more surviving offspring than women who reach menarche later. This is due to longer reproductive lifespans, higher fertility-per-year and enhanced offspring survivorship (Borgerhoff Mulder 1987c), reflecting similar findings of negative associations between age at first birth (or menarche) and subsequent female fertility in a number of societies (Bumpass *et al.* 1978, Aghajanian 1981, Udry and Cliquet 1982).

A possible explanation for the reproductive advantage of early maturing women is that they differ in important physiological respects from late maturing women. Menarcheal age is determined, in part, by weight (Frisch and McArthur 1974), although the particular physiological triggers are not yet clearly understood (Scott and Johnston 1985). The kinds of environmental conditions that favour fast growth and adequate fat deposition in adolescent girls (Garn and Bailey 1978, Tanner 1981) appear to be responsible for subsequent differences in fertility and offspring survival (cf. Udry and Cliquet 1982, Borgerhoff Mulder 1987c)

Kipsigis men do not usually know the exact age of potential brides (and hence their age at menarche), and yet bridewealth reflects such age differentials. This raises interesting questions about the cues used in assessing age and negotiating bridewealth. How do they know whether or not a girl is an early maturer with high reproductive value? Plumpness is associated with high bridewealth among the Kipsigis. It is possible that men use plumpness as an indicator of reproductive value, in that increased fat deposition in adolescence is associated with early menarche (Frisch 1972, Frisch and McArthur 1974). By choosing recently-circumcised girls who are fat, men are more likely to select early-maturers, even if they are unaware of the exact age of the girl at menarche.

Men may value plump women for reproductive reasons other than as a signal of early menarche. First, there is growing evidence that nutritional status is associated with reproductive performance (e.g. Frisch 1975:344, Carael 1981:281, Lunn et al. 1984, Hill and Kaplan this volume (Chapters 17 and 18), reviewed in Borgerhoff Mulder (1987a), although some argue only severe nutritional stress inhibits fertility (e.g. Bongaarts 1980). Maternal nutritional status may contribute to the commonly found association between wealth and female reproductive success (e.g. Bean and Wood 1974, Chagnon 1979b, Irons 1979, Turke and Betzig 1985, Borgerhoff Mulder 1987a). Second, the Kipsigis state that plump women stay healthier during the long dry season before the harvest, and are able to undertake heavier work with less strain. Unfortunately, the terms *manerat* and *sagitat*, used in this study, confound fat with stature; Kipsigis may choose women on physical frame rather than fat deposits because of the difficulties small women face in childbirth. Prior to the introduction of Western medicine, death during childbirth is likely to have constituted a strong selective pressure, with males favouring large-statured women. Data on the association between anthropometric differences among women and subsequent reproductive performance are required before the reasons why men pay more for *manerat* brides can be determined. Finally, the token bridewealth paid for evidently physically handicapped women may also reflect considerations of reproductive value in that no severely handicapped woman in the study (all aged over 35) had more than three children.

Concerning the reproductive status of the bride, it seems contrary to a man's reproductive interests not to pay a high bridewealth for brides who are of proven fecundity. The explanation is perhaps that the groom cannot be very sure of his paternity of a child conceived prior to marriage. He is therefore not prepared to pay a high bridewealth, despite the evidence of fecundity of his bride, because of the risk to his fitness in raising and, in the case of sons, providing inheritance for another man's child.

Preference for investing paternal resources in genetic as opposed to adopted offspring may also account for the low bridewealth paid for women who bring children of other men to the groom's household. Kipsigis are well aware of the economic stress entailed in such 'accompanied' marriages, mentioning, in particular, the strain on family resources in bringing up additional children and the jealousies that arise between real and adopted sons over inheritance.

It is, however, surprising that neither the sex nor the number of adopted children affect the bridewealth payment in 'accompanied' marriages. In so far as sons inherit land, cows and bridewealth from their fathers whereas daughters ultimately fetch a bridewealth at marriage, the costs of rearing sons to reproductive independence are probably higher than those of rearing daughters. These results suggest that other factors may be important in lowering bridewealth for 'accompanied' brides. Traditionally, giving birth prior to circumcision was the most heinous of crimes (Peristiany 1939:58) and even nowadays a girl who conceives before her father finds her a husband is viewed as somewhat unruly, although not shameful. A man married to such a girl may be less certain of his paternity than if he were married to a bride who had been more discreet in her pre-marital affairs. Such a proposition is difficult to test, but is suggested by the finding that brides married in 'accompanied' marriages run away from their husbands more frequently than do brides in 'unaccompanied' marriages; accusations of infidelity are often involved. While running away cannot be taken as a direct measure of marital infidelity it does indicate low levels of marital trust and harmony. In short, it is difficult to separate the interdependencies between unruly behaviour, runaway wives and the bringing of an illegitimate child to the marriage, but the latter may serve to identify a certain kind of less desirable girl.

In many societies the youth, attractiveness, beauty, fidelity, health, plumpness, strength and reproductive potential of the bride are cited as influencing how much the bride's father is likely to demand for his daughter, and how much the groom expects to pay (La Fontaine 1962:99, Lewis 1962:13, Schneider 1970:118; Laughlin 1974:132, Strathern 1980:58; but see Goody 1969:58). Sebei, of eastern Uganda, pay significantly lower prices for old widows, stating explicitly that this is because they have few fecund years left (Goldschmidt 1974:320). Among the Turu of Tanzania, when bridewealth is refunded for a divorced woman, deductions are made for the physical 'depreciation of the wife's body' (Schneider 1964:53). Such anecdotal references suggest that paying highly for qualities that are possibly associated with reproductive potential is not unique to the Kipsigis. Further, they indicate that negotiating parties are conscious of the importance of reproductive potential in determining a bride's price.

The argument that men maximize progeny through the payment of bridewealth was first made by Goldschmidt (1969, see also Laughlin 1974:138) but no substantive data were presented to support the hypothesis. The data presented here suggest that an underlying consideration influencing how much a Kipsigis man is prepared to pay for a bride for his son is the number of children she will bear. These data support the prediction that men should be more attracted to women of high reproductive value than to women of high current reproductive capacity (Williams 1975), given the evidence for adolescent sub-fecundity in this population (Borgerhoff Mulder 1988a). They also show that variations in human behaviour may, in part, reflect strategies that increase the number of offspring and grandoffspring an individual leaves (cf. Alexander 1979).

The labour contributions of women

The positive correlation between bridewealth and distance between the bride's natal and marital homes may be associated with the finding that women who settle further from their natal homes are less likely to help their mothers, since women travel little. An alternative explanation is that the high payment compensates the bride for the poor treatment she is likely to receive from her husband when her father is too far away to protect her interests (Cunningham 1966:17). This explanation was rejected because incidences of wife-beating and running away were no more common in distant than local marriages.

The high bridewealth demanded of a distant husband, who is likely to receive his wife's undivided labour, is probably related to the major economic role of Kipsigis women (Borgerhoff Mulder and Caro 1985). In addition to domestic

housework and secondary processing of food products, they weed and harvest maize and millet, assist with ploughing, milk the cows and share responsibilities for herding, while men undertake many fewer daily tasks. A husband whose wife is frequently at her own mother's house is likely to experience domestic and economic problems, thus justifying the lower bridewealth offered for a wife from within the *kokwet*. Furthermore, a woman constantly at the call of both her marital and natal home may experience more stress, although it is difficult to know to what extent this is offset by any possible advantage of having her mother nearby. While it is not known whether labour stress inhibits a woman's reproductive performance, there is some evidence that it may be associated with a decline in the quality of infant care (Kumar 1978, but see Borgerhoff Mulder and Milton 1985). Directly questioned on these matters, Kipsigis men express little preference over the distance of their spouses', or offsprings' spouses' natal homes, but in daily life they exhibit annoyance with wives who are constantly visiting their mothers, proclaiming that such a wife is 'useless'.

The present study therefore shows that within a society in which females play a critical role in production, labour alienation may account for some of the intracultural variability in bridewealth. Whether the constant availability of a wife's labour increases a man's reproductive success cannot be conclusively determined in this study. Nevertheless, in a labour-intensive mode of production, a hard-working wife will contribute to the wealth of the family and independent evidence shows that the wealth available to a woman is positively associated with the survivorship of her offspring (Borgerhoff Mulder 1987a). There are some grounds therefore for arguing that in paying highly for wives who will provide reliable labour service in the marital home Kipsigis men are behaving in a way that is likely to increase their reproductive success, particularly the survivorship of their offspring.

The bride's and bridegroom's families

There is no evidence that bridewealth is positively associated with the wealth of BF or negatively associated with the wealth of GF. More importantly, even the relative wealth differences between families do not affect payments. The hypothesis that variations in bridewealth are, in part, reflections of parental strategies to acquire affines who are more powerful and wealthy than themselves is not confirmed among the Kipsigis. Indeed, the way the Kipsigis view marriage negotiations suggests that such a hypothesis is inappropriate. Kipsigis claim that it would be unwise for a rich BF to demand high bridewealth from a poor suitor; such greed merely impoverishes the son-in-law's home (Orchardson 1961:70) and increases the chances that the bride will suffer in her new home and consequently run away. Furthermore they argue that a rich GF should not force the payment of a low bridewealth, in effect stealing a bride from a poor family, because this will earn him a reputation of meanness which might hinder the marriage prospects of his other sons. Similar cases of the apparent generosity of wealthy parents are reported for a number of East African pastoralists (e.g. Gulliver 1955:236), the Taita of Kenya (Harris 1962:71) and some Bedouin groups (Kressel 1977:444).

These results are nevertheless directly at odds with evidence from some other societies where the party that gains through vicarious affinal connections is generally reported to suffer materially from the bridewealth transaction *per se*. Among the Swazi of Southern Africa, for example, rich men at the top of the social hierarchy pay little or nothing for their wives but charge extortionate amounts for their daughters, for whom lesser men are willing to pay so as to obtain a prestigious link with a wealthy family (Kuper 1978:568, 576). A similar pattern is reported for the Hageners of New Guinea (Strathern 1980:58) and LoWiili of Ghana (Goody 1969:59).

So why are powerful affines sought through the manipulation of bridewealth in some societies, but not among the Kipsigis? This may be due to the nature of stratification. Among Kipsigis, wealth differentials are relatively unstable compared to some other societies: cattle are subject to raids and disease, and land until recently was not owned by statutory title. It may therefore be unwise for Kipsigis to assume that currently wealthy affines will necessarily be able to provide economic assistance in the future. This interpretation can be tested cross-culturally. Alliances with particular families will be

highly valued where families are stably differentiated in their access to critical resources, wealth or power, but will be less important where socioeconomic differences between families are not marked. This does not suggest that in egalitarian societies ties of affinity are unimportant – indeed affines may be of critical importance in settling disputes as among the Nuer (Evans-Pritchard 1940) – but simply that the relative status of affines may be of less importance in determining negotiated bridewealth outcomes in egalitarian societies. Thus affinal considerations should influence the outcome of bridewealth negotiations in societies characterized by rigid stratification, not in more egalitarian societies. There is some supportive evidence for this hypothesis. Among the hierarchical Swazi, men will pay high bridewealth for an aristocrat's daughter, thus enlisting a guarantee of protection in the future (Kuper 1978). In more egalitarian societies of East Africa, such as Turkana (Gulliver 1955:236), Nuer (Evans-Pritchard 1951:84), Samburu (Turton 1980:87) and Dassanetech (Almogor 1978:194), negotiations are based on what the bride's father thinks the groom's father can afford, as with the Kipsigis. Further evidence comes from reports on bridewealth variation within societies: among the Gisu of Kenya and the Kachin of Burma, the socially differentiated upper strata emphasize the reputation and status of the proposed affinal contact and pay high bridewealth, whereas the less socially demarcated lower strata are more concerned with the sexual and domestic services of women (Leach 1961:118, La Fontaine 1962:116).

Another reason why the Kipsigis do not buy powerful affinal connections may be because affinity is not the sole institutional basis for establishing a network of people to whom a man can turn in time of trouble. The lineage, the solidarity of the *kokwet*, the age set system, *kimananga* (cattle loaning) and, in the past, the regimental organization for warfare each provide critical support networks that are more binding than those of affinity. Families were, until recently, highly mobile, and affines were too dispersed to act as effective allies. A further hypothesis is therefore suggested: if marriage is the critical institutional means of establishing potentially supportive links in the community, then characteristics of the new affines (e.g. their wealth) will strongly affect the bridewealth settlement. Some evidence for this comes from New Guinea. Among the Melpa, for whom marriage is the major way of extending *moka* partnerships, bridewealth offers function as critical signals of willingness to reciprocate generously in the future (Strathern 1980:58). Alternatively, among the Wiru, neighbours of the Hageners among whom *moka* is less developed and marriage has less political significance, bridewealth is viewed more as a payment for the 'skin' or 'body' of the bride (essentially a child payment, Strathern 1980:60). These observations suggest that bridewealth payments are influenced by political considerations only where relations of affinity are of major social and economic importance. Where alternative institutions exist, as among the Kipsigis and to a lesser extent the Wiru, bridewealth payments are more strongly influenced by reproductive and labour considerations than by political factors.

Reproductive, labour and affinal value: some further predictions

The reasons given for why Kipsigis fail to consider affinal value in their marriage negotiations derive from a simple principle: if affinal ties procure access to scarce resources which are likely to confer reproductive advantage on the family in present or future generations (cf. Hartung 1985), affinal value will influence the outcome of bridewealth negotiations. Contexts in which affinal value may be important were proposed. Among the Kipsigis, affinal ties are unlikely to confer reproductive advantage because of the relative instability of wealth differentials, the lack of binding obligations between affines and the availability of other support systems. Indeed affinal value does not appear to be an important parental consideration in determining bridewealth settlements among relatively egalitarian pastoralists or agro-pastoralists.

This same principle can be extended to the discussion of the reproductive value and labour services of brides. The effort males exert in procuring brides of high reproductive value will vary both between societies and over time, and will depend, in part, on the extent to which the quality of the bride contributes to male reproductive success (Borgerhoff Mulder 1988a). Thus in the Kipsigis case, where wealthy men anticipate no particular problem in bringing up large numbers of children (80 in one case), high bridewealth payments are made for brides of high reproductive value. However, the costs and benefits of producing very large families will vary between societies. Goody (1971, 1973b) has discussed the socioeconomic and ecological factors that influence strategies of reproduction and inheritance (see also Boserup 1970). These include the mode of production (whether production is labour or capital intensive), the extent of off-spring mortality, the costs of raising children and the availability of women. This suggests that in societies where it is important to produce a large number of children, for example where off-spring mortality is high, or where children are not excessively costly to raise, for example in labour-intensive systems of production, female reproductive potential will be highly valued (see Figure 3.8A, line X). Alternatively, where production of a large family is not feasible, either because children constitute a net cost or because production is limited by capital rather than labour assets, women of high reproductive value may not be more expensive than those of lower reproductive value (see Figure 3.8A, line Y). In short, if a man can support, at most, four children, he does not benefit from paying more for a wife who is likely to produce eight rather than four children.

There is some evidence for this: for example, Laughlin suggests that the recent deflation of

Figure 3.8 Differential effects of (A) reproductive value and (B) alienation of female labour on bridewealth. (A) Using age of bride at menarche as a measure of reproductive value, lines X and Y describe how the differential evaluation of reproductive value in different cultures might affect negotiated bridewealth. (B) Using distance between natal and marital homes as a measure of alienation of female labour services, lines X and Y describe how the differential evaluation of female labour in different cultures might affect negotiated bridewealth.

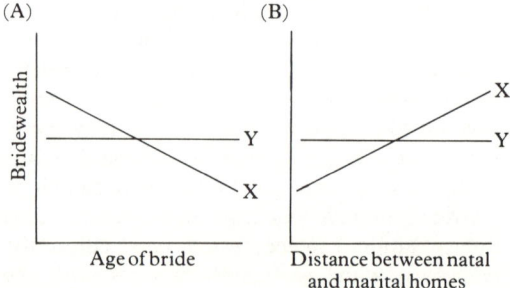

bridewealth payments among the So of Uganda are related to a decline in the productive role of children (Laughlin 1974:138). More generally, the variability with which reproductive and domestic rights in women are distinguished among different East African coastal peoples appear to reflect the relative scarcity of women and the different ways of acquiring rights to children (Parkin 1980:210).

In sum, while evolutionary biological theory suggests that men should exert considerable mating effort to procure mates of high reproductive value, the magnitude of this effort would be expected to vary cross-culturally (Borgerhoff Mulder 1983) and would depend, in part, on the extent to which quality of mate contributes to variance in male reproductive success.

Similarly, the importance of women's economic roles differs between societies and may be associated with bridewealth variability (see Figure 3.8B). Where women play a critical role in a labour-intensive mode of production, men will pay highly for total control over their wives' labour (line X). Alternatively, where women's labour inputs are less important, differential access to a wife's labour services may not be associated with any variability in bridewealth (line Y). The evidence for this in cases other than the Kipsigis is ambivalent: in some present-day Middle East towns bridewealth is increasing while the economic contributions of women are declining (Kressel 1977:442). Moreover, bridewealth is stable in some parts of southern Africa despite radical shifts in the division of labour (J. Comaroff, pers. comm.). The initiation of bridewealth payments among northwest coastal American Indians may, however, be related to a recent increase in the economic role of women (Kressel 1977:443); and a similar explanation has been given for the recent inflation of bridewealth in Kenya (Kitching 1980). To date, both cross-cultural and intracultural studies of bridewealth variability have been insufficiently controlled for secular factors affecting the availability and fluidity of bridewealth valuables, and this issue cannot yet be resolved.

Summary

This chapter focuses on the importance of four factors, (1) the reproductive value of the bride, (2) the paternity of her children, (3) her labour services and (4) her family connections, in determining variation in negotiated bridewealth payments among the Kipsigis of Kenya.

1. High bridewealth is paid for early-maturing brides and for plump brides. Kipsigis demographic data demonstrate that early-maturing women have higher lifetime reproductive success than late-maturing women. It is proposed that plumpness is also likely to be associated with high reproductive success among Kipsigis women.

2. Lower bridewealth is paid for brides who have previously given birth to the child(ren) of another man than for similarly-aged nulliparous women. It is argued that Kipsigis men are unwilling to adopt unrelated children, given high paternal investment in a patrilineal society.

3. Bridewealth payments are positively associated with the distance between the natal and marital homes of the bride. It is argued that brides whose natal homes lie outside the local community are more available for domestic and agricultural duties in their husbands' households than are those whose natal homes lie in the community, because the latter frequently help their mothers.

4. Wealth differences between intermarrying familes have no effect on negotiated bridewealth settlements. Comparison with other ethnographic examples suggests that in labour-intensive egalitarian societies the reproductive and labour services of women are more highly valued than are their family connections.

Acknowledgements

My thanks to the Office of the President, Nairobi, for permission to conduct research in Kenya. Sostin arap Mibei, Paulo arap Kurui and David arap Koskei assisted me greatly in the collection and verification of the data on marriage payments. Tim Caro offered constant advice on problems arising throughout the analysis and writing of this study. Steve Albon, John Hartung and Martin Major gave invaluable help with the statistical analysis. Richard Alexander, Laura Betzig, Tim Clutton-Brock, John Comaroff, Martin Daly, Mildred Dickemann, Malcolm Dow, Paul Turke and Margo Wilson commented on an earlier manuscript. To all these people I am very thankful, and most of all to the people of Abosi, Kamerumeru and Tabarit for their warm and friendly welcome.

References

Aghajanian, A. (1981) Age at first birth and completed family size in western Malaysia. *Journal of Biosocial Sciences*, **13**, 197–201.

Alexander, R. D. (1979) *Darwinism and Human Affairs*. Seattle: University of Washington Press.

Almogor, U. (1978) *Pastoral Partners*. Manchester: University of Manchester Press.

Bean, E. D. and Wood, C. G. H. (1974) Ethnic variations in the relationship between income and fertility. *Demography*, **11**, 629–40.

Bongaarts, J. (1980) Does malnutrition affect fecundity? A summary of the evidence. *Science*, **208**, 565–9.

Borgerhoff Mulder, M. (1983) Social organisation and biology. *Man*, **18**, 786–7.

Borgerhoff Mulder, M. (1985) Polygyny threshold: a Kipsigis case study. *National Geographic Research Reports*, **21**, 33–9.

Borgerhoff Mulder, M. (1987a) Resources and reproduction in women with an example from the Kipsigis. *Journal of Zoology* (in press).

Borgerhoff Mulder, M. (1987b) On cultural and reproductive success: Kipsigis evidence. *American Anthropologist* (in press).

Borgerhoff Mulder, M. (1987c) Low reproductive performance and women's age at the onset of reproduction. In *Anthropologiai Kozlemenyek*, ed. O. G. Eiben. Budapest: Hungarian Academy of Sciences (in press).

Borgerhoff Mulder, M. (1988a) Reproductive success in three Kipsigis cohorts. In *Reproductive Success: Studies of Individual Variation*, ed. T. H. Clutton-Brock. Chicago: University of Chicago Press (in press).

Borgerhoff Mulder, M. (1988b) Reproductive consequences of sex-biased inheritance. In *Comparative Socioecology of Mammals and Man*, ed. R. Foley and V. Standen. London: Blackwells (in press).

Borgerhoff Mulder, M. and Caro, T. M. (1985) The use of quantitative observational techniques in anthropology. *Current Anthropology*, **26**, 323–35.

Borgerhoff Mulder, M. and Milton, M. (1985) Factors affecting infant care among the Kipsigis. *Journal of Anthropological Research*, **41**, 231–262.

Boserup, E. (1970) *Women's Role in Economic Development*. London: Allen and Unwin.

Bumpass, L., Rindfuss, R. and Janosik, R. (1978) Age and marital status at first birth and the pace of subsequent fertility. *Demography*, **15**, 75–86.

Carael, M. (1981) Child-spacing, ecology and nutrition in the Kivy province of Zaire. In *Child Spacing in Tropical Africa*, ed. H. J. Page and R.

Lesthaeghe, pp. 275–86. London: Academic Press.

Central Bureau of Statistics (1980) Kenya Fertility Survey 1977–78. Nairobi: Central Bureau of Statistics, Ministry of Economic Planning and Development.

Chagnon, N. A. (1979a) Mate competition, favoring close kin and village fissioning among the Yạnomamö Indians. In *Evolutionary Biology and Human Social Behavior: An Anthropological Perspective*, ed. N. A. Chagnon and W. G. Irons, pp. 86–132. North Scituate, MA: Duxbury Press.

Chagnon, N. A. (1979b) Is reproductive success equal in egalitarian societies? In *Evolutionary Biology and Human Social Behavior: An Anthropological Perspective*, ed. N. A. Chagnon and W. G. Irons, pp. 86–132. North Scituate, MA: Duxbury Press.

Comaroff, J. L. and Comaroff, J. (1981) The management of marriage in a Tswana chiefdom. In *Essays on African Marriage in Southern Africa*, ed. E. J. Krige and J. L. Comaroff, pp. 24–49. Capetown: Juta and Co Ltd.

Cunningham, C. E. (1966) Categories of descent in a Timor village. *Oceania*, **37**, 13–21.

Divale, W. T. and Harris, M. (1976) Population, warfare, and the male supremacist complex. *American Anthropologist*, **78**, 521–38.

Dyson-Hudson, N. (1966) *Karamojong Politics*. London: Oxford University Press.

Evans-Pritchard, E. E. (1940) *The Nuer*. London: Oxford University Press.

Evans-Pritchard, E. E. (1951) *Kinship and Marriage among the Nuer*. Oxford: Clarendon Press.

Fisher, R. A. (1958) *The Genetical Theory of Natural Selection*. Oxford: Clarendon Press.

Fortes, M. (1962) Introduction in *Marriage in Tribal Societies*, ed. M. Fortes, pp. 1–13. Cambridge: Cambridge University Press.

Frisch, R. E. (1972) Weight at menarche: similarity for well-nourished and undernourished girls at different ages, and evidence for historical constancy. *Pediatrics*, **50**, 1445–50.

Frisch, R. E. (1975) Critical weights, a critical body composition, menarche and the maintenance of menstrual cycles. In *Biosocial Interelations in Population Adaptation*, ed. E. S. Watts, F. E. Johnson and G. W. Lasker, pp. 319–51. The Hague: Mouton.

Frisch, R. E. and McArthur, J. W. (1974) Menstrual cycles: fatness as a determinant of minimum weight necessary for their maintenance and onset. *Science*, **185**, 949–51.

Garn, S. M. and Bailey, S. M. (1978) Genetics of maturational processes. In *Human Growth*, vol. I, ed. F. Falkner and J. M. Tanner, pp. 307–30. London: Plenum Press.

Goldschmidt, W. (1969) Game theory, cultural values and the bride price in Africa. In *Game Theory in the Behavioral Sciences*, ed. I. R. Buchler and H. G. Nutini, pp. 61–74. Pittsburg: University of Pennsylvania Press.

Goldschmidt, W. (1974) The economics of bridewealth among the Sebei in East Africa. *Ethnology*, **13**, 311–33.

Goody, J. (1969) 'Normative', 'recollected' and 'actual' marriage payments among the LoWiili of northern Ghana, 1951–1966. *Africa*, **39**, 54–61.

Goody, J. (1971) Class and marriage in Africa and Eurasia. *American Journal of Sociology*, **76**, 585–603.

Goody, J. (1973a) Bridewealth and dowry in Africa and Eurasia. In *Bridewealth and Dowry*, ed. J. Goody and S. J. Tambiah, pp. 1–58. Cambridge: Cambridge University Press.

Goody, J. (1973b) Strategies of heirship. *Comparative Studies in Society and History*, **15**, 3–20.

Gulliver, P. and Gulliver, P. H. (1953) *The Central Nilo-Hamitics* London: International African Institute.

Gulliver, P. H. (1955) *The Family Herds: a Study of Two Pastoral Tribes in East Africa; the Jie and the Turkana*. London: Routledge and Kegan Paul.

Harris, G. (1962) Taita bridewealth and affinal relations. In *Marriage in Tribal Societies*, ed. M. Fortes, pp. 55–87. Cambridge: Cambridge University Press.

Hartung, J. (1985) Matrilineal inheritance: New theory and analysis. *Brain and Behavioral Sciences*, **8**, 661–88.

Irons, W. G. (1979) Cultural and biological success. In *Evolutionary Biology and Human Social Behavior: An Anthropological Perspective*, ed. N. A. Chagnon and W. G. Irons, pp. 257–72. North Scituate, MA: Duxbury Press.

Irons, W. G. (1981) Why lineage exogamy? In *Natural Selection and Social Behavior*, ed. R. D. Alexander and D. W. Tinkle, pp. 476–89. New York: Chiron Press.

Kitching, G. (1980) *Class and Economic Change in Kenya*. London: Yale University Press.

Komma, T. (1981) The dwelling and its symbolism among the Kipsigi. In *Themes in Socio-cultural Ideas and Behaviour among the Six Ethnic Groups of Kenya*, ed. N. Nagashima. Tokyo: Hitotsubashi University.

Kressel, G. M. (1977) Bride-price reconsidered. *Current Anthropology*, **18**, 441–58.

Krige, E. J. and Comaroff, J. L. (1981) *Essays on African Marriage in Southern Africa*. Capetown: Juta and Co Ltd.

Kumar, S. K. (1978) *Role of the Household Economy in Child Nutrition at Low Incomes: A Case Study in Kerala*. Occasional Paper No. 95. Ithaca, New York: Department of Agricultural Economics, Cornell University.

Kuper, A. (1978) Rank and preferential marriage in Southern Africa: the Swazi. *Man*, **13**, 567–79.

Kuper, A. (1982) *Wives for Cattle: Bridewealth and Marriage in Southern Africa*. London: Routledge and Kegan Paul.

La Fontaine, J. (1962) Gisu marriage and affinal relations. In *Marriage in Tribal Societies*, ed. M. Fortes, pp. 88–120. Cambridge: Cambridge University Press.

Laughlin, C. D. (1974) Maximization, marriage and residence among the So. *American Ethnologist*, **1**, 129–42.

Leach, E. R. (1961) *Rethinking Anthropology*. New York: Athlone Press.

Lewis, I. M. (1962) *Marriage and the Family in Northern Somaliland*. Kampala: East African Institute for Social Research.

Lunn, P. G., Austin, S. Prentice, A. M. and Whitehead, R. G. (1984) The effect of improved nutrition on plasma prolactin concentrations and postpartum infertility in lactating Gambian women. *American Journal of Clinical Nutrition*, **39**, 227–35.

Manners, R. A. (1967) The Kipsigis of Kenya: Culture change in a 'model' East African tribe. In *Contemporary Change in Traditional Societies* vol. 1, ed. J. Steward, pp. 207–359. Urbana: University of Illinois Press.

Needham, R. (1971) Remarks on the analysis of kinship and marriage. In *Rethinking Kinship and Marriage*, ed. R. Needham, pp. 1–34. Tavistock, London: ASA Monograph No. 11.

Orchardson, I. Q. (1961) *The Kipsigis*. Nairobi: Kenya Literature Bureau.

Parkin, D. (1980) Kind bridewealth and hard cash: Eventing a structure. In *The Meaning of Marriage Payments*, ed. J. L. Comaroff, pp. 197–220. New York: Academic Press.

Peristiany, J. G. (1939) *The Social Institutions of the Kipsigis*. London: Routledge and Kegan Paul.

Peters, E. L. (1980) Aspects of Bedouin bridewealth among camel herders in Cyrenaica. In *The Meaning of Marriage Payments*, ed. J. L. Comaroff, pp. 125–59. New York: Academic Press.

Radcliffe-Brown, A. R. (1950) Introduction in *African Systems of Kinship and Marriage* eds. A. R. Radcliffe-Brown and D. Forde, pp. 1–85. London, Oxford University Press.

Schneider, H. K. (1964) A model of African indigenous economy and society. *Comparative Studies in Society and History*, **7**, 37–55.

Schneider, H. K. (1970) *The Wahi-Wanyaturu: Economics in an African Society*. New York: Viking Publications Fund, No. 48, Wenner-Gren Foundation.

Scott, E. C. and Johnston, F. E. (1985) Science, nutrition, fat, and policy: Tests of the critical-fat hypothesis. *Current Anthropology*, **26**, 463–73.

Singer, A. (1973) Marriage payments and the exchange of people. *Man*, **81**, 80–92.

Spiro, M. E. (1975) Marriage payments: a paradigm from the Burmese perspective. *Journal of Anthropological Research*, **31**, 89–115.

Strathern, A. J. (1980) The central and the contingent: bridewealth among the Melpa and Wiru. In *The Meaning of Marriage Payments*, ed. J. L. Comaroff, pp. 49–66. New York: Academic Press.

Tanner, J. M. (1981) *A History of the Study of Human Growth*. Cambridge: Cambridge University Press.

Turke, P. W. and Betzig, L. L. (1985) Those who can do: wealth, status and reproductive success on Ifaluk. *Ethology and Sociobiology*, **6**, 79–86.

Turton, D. (1980) The economics of Mursi bridewealth: a comparative perspective. In *The Meaning of Marriage Payments*, ed. J. L. Comaroff, pp. 67–92. New York: Academic Press.

Udry, J. R. and Cliquet, R. L. (1982) A cross-cultural examination of relationships between ages at menarche, marriage and first birth. *Demography*, **19**, 53–63.

Williams, G. C. (1975) *Sex and Evolution*. Princeton: Princeton University Press.

K'ekchi' horticultural labor exchange: productive and reproductive implications

Introduction

Developments in evolutionary biological theory as it applies to social behavior have led to a reassessment of productive practices, or strategies of resource acquisition, in light of their reproductive implications (Chagnon 1979, Hames 1979, Irons 1979, Berté 1983, Flinn 1983, Turke and Betzig 1985). The simple reason behind this marriage of productive and reproductive concerns derives from the expectation that individuals will expend both somatic and reproductive effort towards the broader goal of maximizing inclusive fitness (Hamilton 1963, 1964, Alexander and Borgia 1979).

In this chapter, predictions are made concerning the productive and reproductive consequences of horticultural labor, a key factor in the swidden productive system of a community of K'ekchi' Mayans. In swidden horticultural systems like that of the K'ekchi' of San Miguel village in Belize (see Figure 4.1) which require periodic intensive labor investment in crop cultivation, labor exchange becomes an important pivot for social interaction because it affects both resource acquisition and mating, and, therefore, reproduction. The predictions made here suggest that labor exchange is (1) part of a

[1] Department of Anthropology, Northwestern University, Evanston, IL 60201, USA

strategy for acquiring subsistence resources, and (2) a factor in determining (a) the acquisition of mates, and (b) the type of post-marital residence, which in turn affects the availability of kin, that is, potential nepotists, within the local population. Finally, (3) the consequences that access to the labor potential of others has on the fertility of individual farmers is assessed.

These predictions are:

1. The intensity of domestic production of the staple crop, maize, is determined by (a) domestic need (number of consumers in the household) and by (b) the number of adult male workers that a household head can enlist from other households to work his fields.
2. Parents and marriageable offspring will expend effort to find mates within the village in order to maintain productive relationships with local kin.
3. Fertility of male household heads (plot 'owners') is positively affected by the presence of related males who are productive workers in the village.

Figure 4.1 Map of Belize (Central America)

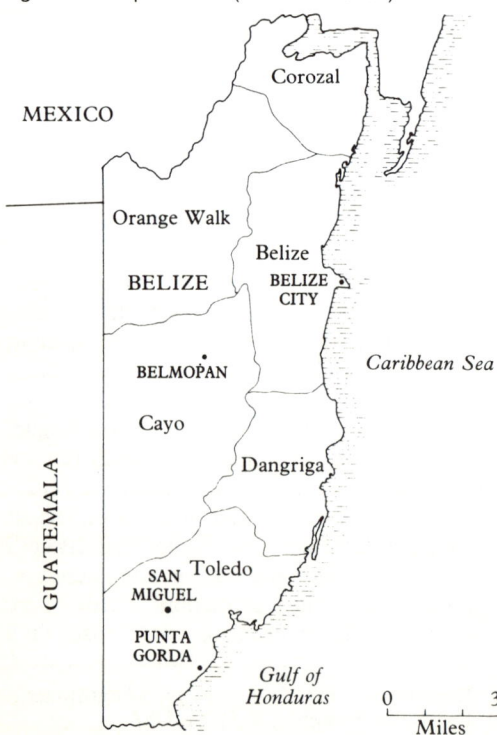

Subsistence agriculture

The organization of domestic productive activities in non-industrial communities has received much attention in recent years (Kerblay 1971, Sahlins 1971, 1972, Cancian 1972, Ortiz 1973, Minge-Kalman 1977, Durrenberger 1979, Smith 1979, Tannenbaum 1984 and papers in Barlett 1980a and Durrenberger 1984). Such studies are to varying degrees concerned with the efficacy of Chayanov's (1966) theory of peasant production. Chayanov proposed that productive behavior in non-industrial societies cannot be understood using formal economic theory since (1) such theory bases its predictions on economic factors such as capital, wages, interest, and rent, which are rarely all present in traditional productive systems, and (2) translating the costs and benefits of peasant productive activities, in particular, human energetic investments in farming (labor), into monetary ones distorts the decision-making process within the farm family. These two arguments are echoed by a generation of substantive anthropologists, most notable among them, Sahlins (1972). Chayanov predicted instead that among peasant farm families, household production levels are determined by a balance between (a) the subjective drudgery of agricultural labor, which increases exponentially as a farmer's work load increases, and (b) the marginal utility of production output, which decreases as output increases. The marginal utility of production output is largely determined by the amount necessary to support consumers in a household as deemed suitable by a particular society, and the consumer/worker ratio within that household. Sahlins (1972:87) simplified this prediction as 'the greater the relative working capacity of the household, the less its members work,' or 'Chayanov's Rule.'

Barlett (1980b) criticized Chayanov's second assertion that imputing monetary costs and benefits to agricultural decisions in peasant farm families is inappropriate. She suggested instead that the best approach might be to combine formal economic methods of quantitatively assessing the costs and benefits of peasant production practices with some evaluation of the subjective value of labor effort proposed by Chayanov. But the issue of whether to use 'Chayanov's Rule' in conjunction with, or in place of, formal economic methods is not the only one. The empirical question remains as to whether Chayanov's Rule can be generalized to all peasant farm systems, in particular, to those systems in which domestic productive groups do not function independently from one another. In addition, analyses of productive decisions based solely on economic rationality as prescribed by Western economists may ignore issues beyond whether, for example, labor should be measured using objective criteria (monetary cost-benefit) and/or subjective criteria (returns on individual labor weighted by assessments of labor 'drudgery'). Either or both may be too simplistic to account for the complex and multi-faceted interrelations which commonly bind together members of traditional productive systems. It is suggested here that it may be more appropriate, and enable us to better understand economic behavior in traditional societies, if we view such behavior as part of a general evolutionary strategy involving the acquisition, control, distribution, and consumption of resources, including *both* productive and reproductive resources.

Methods

Data concerning productive and reproductive activities were gathered over an 11-month period in 1980 on a population of 235 K'ekchi' Mayan Indians inhabiting the foothill region of southern Belize's Mayan Mountain chain in Central America. Since the K'ekchi' and Mopan Mayans first began migrating into this area from Guatemala as early as the late 19th century, the region has provided a suitable environment for the cultivation of maize, the staple dietary crop, using swidden horticultural techniques. Although the residents of the village of San Miguel, the study population, have more recently added dry rice cash cropping to their horticultural activities, their reliance on maize farming for subsistence remains intact.

Although most of the acreage on 'milpas' is used for maize, milpas also support a host of subsidiary crops including, but not limited to, beans, cassava, and yams. Such intercropping common to swidden gardening may improve the nutrient condition of the soil, while providing a varied diet. Maize accounts for the major part of the dietary regime of the San Miguel K'ekchi', as shown in Table 4.1. While it was impractical to collect accurate estimates of the volume of

Table 4.1 *Frequency of occurrence of food types in 831 meals*

Food	% occurrence
1. Locally procured	
A. Grains	
(1) Maize	94.9
(2) Rice	6.4
B. Legumes	4.7
C. Animal sources	
(1) Chicken	13.7
(2) Other	<0.1–7.7[a]
D. Vegetable	1.6–7.8[a]
E. Fruit	5.5–7.3[a]
2. Non-locally procured	
A. Wheat flour	7.3
B. Fish	0.2
C. Processed imported foods	0.8–2.0[a]

Summarized from Tables XII and XIII, Berté 1983:169–70.
[a] Ranges reflect condensed categories. For example, in the category of 'other' animal sources, a species of antelope occurred in the diet less than 1% of the time, whereas eggs were consumed 7.7% of the time

each food consumed, since food was often eaten from a common pot or dish, data on the incidence of a food consumed at each meal show that *in almost 95% of all meals in the sample, maize was consumed.* Sharing meals daily with the K'ekchi' made it clear to me that the majority of kilocalories consumed during each meal derived from some type of food processed from maize, most commonly, tortillas. Data on food consumption were collected from the 40 households in the village by observing each household for a randomly selected week during a three-month period which covered both pre-harvest and harvest conditions. I attended the main evening meal each day a household fell into the observation sample during which time the contents of that meal were recorded, and all household members were questioned about what foods they consumed throughout the day. Table 4.1 reflects information from a total of 831 recorded meals, as well as foods consumed outside of the household while visiting other households, and wild foods collected 'on the road,' such as that consumed by men while walking to the fields, or by children while playing in the forest surrounding the village.

Land available for milpas is determined by governmentally instituted reservations which run adjacent to each of the Mayan villages in the Toledo District of southern Belize. Plot 'ownership' is established through usage rights rather than private property and inheritance rules. A farmer marks a boundary around an intended plot site and clears it of small trees and brush, thereby asserting his right to use that tract of land for as many consecutive years as he chooses. He relinquishes that right only when he allows the milpa to lie fallow, although occasionally a farmer may be forcibly denied access to local reservation land by his fellow villagers. One young farmer, for example, having angered several unrelated household heads in the village, was physically and hostiley prevented from clearing an intended plot sight in 1980. As a consequence, he planted only 0.2 acres of maize (the smallest plot size in the village that year) directly adjacent to his house on the outskirts of the village. The average milpa size in 1980 was 3.72 acres (range, 0.2–8.0), and the estimated average distance traveled between the village and a milpa was 3.8 miles (range, 0.3–9.0).

At the time of the study land was owned by the government and could not be inherited as private or corporately owned family property (although subsequent to 1980 the Belizean government began to sell reservation lands to private buyers). Because villagers had no absolute control over land and its disposition, even though *land* was and still is essential for subsistence production and therefore survival, it did not strongly direct or influence relations within the productive community at the time of the study. Investment of *capital* in securing a subsistence livelihood was also not a major factor influencing social relations within San Miguel, despite the fact that an incipient cash economy derived largely from the cultivation and sale of rice was on the rise at the time of the study. Although a number of men did purchase seed from the government agricultural station, most relied very little if at all on monetary investments for a successful milpa harvest.

Although San Miguel farmers in 1980 could not directly control land with private ownership and/or inheritance rights, they could exercise indirect control through another factor of production – *labor*. Controlling labor was the primary key to controlling land since a farmer could at least temporarily control as much land through usage rights as he could work.

Milpa cultivation, like swidden gardening in general in tropical habitats, requires intensive labor inputs periodically throughout the year. Cooperative labor teams are necessary to relieve the burden of labor-intensive tasks such as clearing a milpa site, and time-limited tasks such as planting and harvesting. Maize must be planted just when the first rains of the season are anticipated. If fields are planted too early or late they can succumb either to rapid weed regrowth or to flooding of immature seedlings. Similarly, crops must be harvested just as they mature, otherwise pests, predators, or rotting may spoil them. The use of cooperative labor for clearing an intended milpa site, however, does not arise so much out of time constraints, as it does with planting and harvesting. It is more related to the laborious nature of the task. Most farmers used some help from men outside the domestic group, while others preferred to rely solely on the energies of grown sons within the household. Farmers have a far greater time latitude in preparing a field. Field sites can be cleared for many weeks at the latter part of the dry season which lasts roughly from January to the end of March or beginning of April. In summary, *periodic cooperation in agricultural tasks is important for the successful production of maize*. Not surprisingly, then, exchanges of agricultural labor are important in molding village social organization in San Miguel during each cultivation season, and from year to year. During the dry season, or the first few months of the year, plot 'owners' negotiate labor alliances with other villagers. Agricultural work among the San Miguel K'ekchi' is almost exclusively the province of men. Data collected on labor exchange were gathered by questioning plot 'owners', members of their assisting crews of workers, and wives of plot 'owners' about who assisted a plot 'owner' with agricultural work in his field that season. This interview information was corroborated (1) by observing groups of men heading to and returning from the fields in groups, as is customary, and (2) by personally visiting a sample of fields during working hours and observing the men cooperatively working.

A summary of the labor exchanges for the agricultural tasks of clearing a milpa site and planting the maize shows that 69.3% of all labor exchanges took place between related individuals (57.3% cognates, 12.1% affines) and

30.7% between unrelated co-villagers. The pool of potential laborers was defined as all adult men and older boys who participated in these labor exchanges during the 1980 season, which comprised all physically able male workers who permanently resided within the village at that time.

Having many relatives in the local pool of potential laborers should be advantageous to a subsistence farmer on grounds consistent with kin selection theory (Hamilton 1963, 1964). That is, rather than having to negotiate exchanges of labor with unrelated men, he should be able to utilize the labor energies of more men by virtue of genealogical relatedness shared directly between them, and by virtue of the mutual reproductive interests (i.e. the survival of related dependent offspring to reproductive maturity) shared with both cognatic and affinal kinsmen belonging to the labor pool. A lack of genealogical relatedness and mutual reproductive interests could possibly inflate the energetic costs of labor exchange in the long run, because labor alliances between unrelated men should be more exacting and concerned about reciprocity in kind only. *The sum of a plot 'owner's' relationship coefficients* (as measured by Chagnon's (1975) F_g statistic) *to all potential laborers in the local population*, measuring how related a farmer is to those who could potentially help him, was found to correlate significantly with *the number of laborers who actually assisted a plot 'owner' plant his milpa*, a productive task critically demanding labor cooperation between members of different households within the village (Pearson $r = 0.3712$, $n = 40$, $p = 0.009$). Reciprocal exchanges of labor for either clearing the bush or planting the milpa were found to be twice as frequent as one-way flows of labor (Berté 1983:234).

For the purposes of this study, *acres of maize planted* was used as a measure of agricultural intensity. Acres planted was measured primarily by interviewing both household heads and several assisting laborers on separate occasions concerning the size of a milpa. These estimates were consistent from individual to individual, and proved reliable when cross-checked against measurements from a sample of fields. Acres planted reflects a compromise between a domestic group's targeted or desired productivity level given its subsistence needs, and the production level a male household head (plot 'owner') was

actually able to attempt given his control over available labor within the local village. Acres planted was deemed a preferable measure to, for example, volume of maize harvested, since the latter can be biased by unpredictable or uncontrollable factors in the natural environment. Insect devastation, patchy local rainfall patterns, and incursions by predators such as birds, rodents, and jaguars can all reduce the effective milpa size by the end of the crop cycle independent of labor considerations. Minge-Kalman (1977:273–4) criticized Sahlins' (1972) and Evans' (1974) use of indirect measures of labor intensity, such as surface area under cultivation or kilograms harvested, since, he suggested, these measures could not account for differences in labor inputs needed for different crops. Acres planted was nevertheless deemed a suitable albeit indirect measure of labor intensity in this study since all San Miguel farmers cultivated the same staple crop – maize.

The household, or domestic group, is defined as the unit of production and consumption in this study. The household comprises a residential group most commonly consisting of a nuclear family and sometimes one or both elderly dependent parents or recently married offspring who have not yet established their own household. Although Wilk (1984:217–44) has described several types of residental units as 'household clusters' in three other Mayan villages in southern Belize, the single dwelling household is a suitable analytic unit for the purposes of this analysis. Households in San Miguel, as in the other three villages studied by Wilk, are indeed spatially arranged into various types of groupings based on relationships between male and female household heads (i.e. the parents of the core nuclear family within the co-resident domestic group). For example, patrilocal clusters might comprise a nuclear family domicile with neighboring domiciles belonging to several married sons. Such clusters do generally reflect intense interaction in social and economic matters. Nevertheless, the establishment of a physically separate domicile is contingent upon the new male household head having established his own network of labor allies, and thereby, his own milpa. The household is therefore a production unit not in the sense that its members singularly perform all the requisite productive activities involved in swidden horticulture, since in fact they depend largely on help from outside of the domestic group. Rather, it is a production unit in the limited sense that a household head is responsible for soliciting and organizing the assistance of non-domestic workers within the village for the success of his family's milpa.

Although maize is sometimes loaned, bartered or sold between households, especially as the next harvest approaches and food supplies from the previous season dwindle too early for some, food consumed by members of a household is largely derived from the food grown on its own milpa. The household is therefore an appropriate unit of consumption.

Results

The first prediction mentioned at the beginning of this chapter concerns the influence of agrarian labor exchange on the acquisition of subsistence resources and, therefore, on survivorship:

> The intensity of domestic production of the staple crop, maize, is determined by (a) domestic need (number of consumers in the household) and by (b) the number of adult male workers that a household head can enlist from other households to work his fields.

Intensity of production, as mentioned above, was measured as acres of maize planted, *domestic need* as the number of consumers in a household, or the full-time residents of a domestic group (excluding temporary visiting kinsmen from other villages, as occurred in only two cases), and *assisting male workers* as the number of laborers enlisted by a household head to plant his milpa *excluding* members of his own household (e.g. himself and co-resident older sons). A stepwise regression procedure was used in predicting acres of maize planted for the 40 household heads in the village in 1980, with domestic need and assisting laborers as the independent variables in the equation:

$$A = 0.14831 + 0.14434 N_a + 0.36994 C$$
$$(0.0021) \quad (0.0001)$$

$$R^2 = 0.493$$

where A = acres of maize planted, N_a = number of assisting planters outside of the domestic group, and C = number of consumers in the household.

Both variables N_a and C were found to be significant predictors of productive intensity as measured by acres of maize planted. Interestingly, when a third independent variable was included in the equation, that is, *the number of laborers within the household* (N_d), this variable was removed from the equation because its significance level was too low. In other words, the production of a subsistence crop in this population of horticulturalists is dependent upon assistance from outside of the group of domestic producers.

This prediction was then compared with an alternative based on Sahlins' (1972) interpretation of Chayanov's theory of peasant production, which, in its simplest form, suggests that intensity of production is determined primarily by the domestic ratio of consumers to producers. The larger the value of the ratio, that is, the more consumers there are per worker in a household, the more work per capita the workers will have to do, or the greater will be the intensity of their energies invested in agricultural production. While this may work well in situations where the domestic group is an autonomous labor unit, as may be the case for the Russian peasants studies by Chayanov, it falls short when considering populations in which inter-domestic cooperation in farming is an important component of productive strategies, at least in this case. To illustrate this, using the same stepwise regression procedure as above, acres of maize planted was predicted by the ratio of domestic consumers to domestic producers with the following results:

$$A = 2.96552 + 0.18272 C/N_d \quad R^2 = 0.046$$
$$(0.1860)$$

where A = acres of maize planted, C = number of consumers in the domestic group, and N_d = number of workers assisting within the domestic group.

Clearly, the first regression equation using domestic consumers and assisting planters from outside of the domestic group as independent variables is the better predictor of productive intensity. Had Chayanov incorporated into his theory situations in which inter-domestic labor alliances are an integral component of the productive system, he might have simply summed N_a and N_d in the denominator of the ratio. But the number of workers within the domes tic group (N_d) was not found to be a significant predictor in this case-study. Furthermore, N_a is not a relatively fixed variable as is N_d since the number of assisting laborers from outside the domestic group can vary depending upon the success of a farmer's solicitations, whereas domestic labor is relatively consistent over a long period of time. By the time younger sons enter the work-force, older sons have often married and moved into their own households, thus keeping a constant supply of domestic workers between the time that an eldest son is old enough to work and a youngest son sets up his own household.

Mate acquisition and reproductive success

Picking up Hamilton's (1964) gauntlet on kin selection Alexander (1979:46) stated that 'in sexually reproducing organisms, reproductive effort (calories expended and risks taken in the effort to reproduce) is evolved to be expended entirely as nepotism, including (1) parenthood, (2) assistance to relatives other than offspring, and (3) mating effort or the effort involved in placing one's gametes in the best possible environment... Sexually reproducing organisms literally evolve to be... altruists of a very special sort whose altruism, whatever form it takes, is ultimately channeled to genetic relatives.' Consistent with the first two of these expectations I have argued that (1) expending male energy and time toward staple crop production is important for insuring survivorship of offspring, a major component of parenting for males, and have shown that, (2) cooperation in subsistence horticultural work among males from different households is important in meeting domestic productivity needs, and that related individuals are twice as likely to assist one another in this pursuit than are unrelated individuals. In this section, the relationship of nepotistic effort expended in subsistence horticulture to mate acquisition and direct reproduction will be addressed.

Chagnon (1979) clearly established the important link that exists between economic and reproductive realities while dispelling the notion that social relations and social status are inherently egalitarian in primitive society. Contrary to the materialist assumption that equal access to local resources in primitive society results in egalitarianism (Fried 1967, Harris 1975), Chagnon points out the asymmetry in the utilization of strategic material resources which results from differential reproductive success. 'Out of the reproductive inequalities also come economic inequalities' (Chagnon 1979:378). Among the Yąnomamö, variability in reproductive success among males, which is largely due to differential success in polygyny, means that some males can amass the political support of relatively large numbers of patrilineally related kinsmen. Such kinsmen are important in a politically competitive social environment as that described for the Yąnomamö. Kin-based political power can be used to gain preferential access to mates for a man and his offspring, and to 'obligate younger male kin to contribute labor and the fruits of that labor to the consumption requirements of the polygynous household' (Chagnon 1979: 400). In short, reproductive inequalities beget economic inequalities, and perpetuate reproductive variance in heretofore assumed egalitarian societies (Chagnon 1979:378, see also Betzig this volume (Chapter 2)).

Given the absence of polygyny among the K'ekchi', reproductive variance among K'ekchi' males is low compared to that among Yąnomamö males. Nevertheless, an analogous relationship between reproductive and productive realities exists for the K'ekchi'. High paternal investment, particularly in terms of the labor effort required to obtain subsistence resources, may indeed account for monogamy among the K'ekchi', as Chagnon (1979:400) suggests, since men are limited reproductively by how many offspring they can support to reproductive age (cf. Hewlett this volume (Chapter 16)). Nevertheless, a man's ability to support offspring is directly affected by his ability to solicit help from within his village for productive tasks. It is expected, therefore, that related adult males will choose to live near each other in order to gain access to each other's productive energies. Married sons, for example, should attempt to live close to productively active kinsmen such as fathers, brothers, and other collateral male relatives within their own and parental generations. Similarly, parents should attempt to maintain married daughter's access to the potential nepotistic effort of local kinsmen. The best way to do this is to marry village endogamously. Labor is almost never exchanged with farmers, relatives or otherwise, from other nearby villages, probably because of the added costs of traveling the additional distance to the milpas of relatives in other villages.

Having many children who remain in the village after marriage breeds productive security for children and grandchildren. Individuals with large families (daughters are also important to the successful rearing of large families since they provide important help in the laborious work of food preparation and child-care), should have greater reproductive success within the limits set by low male reproductive variance, since large families breed expanding nepotistic networks, including networks of labor exchange. Offspring can tap into or 'inherit' upon reproductive maturity those labor ties established by their father, and add to these their own networks of related laborers among peers of their own age. Securing mates for offspring within this milieu of potential nepotists, therefore, is expected to be the goal of both parents and marriageable offspring. With this in mind, let me present data concerning the interrelationship between K'ekchi' mating and productive effort, and finally, the consequence on the reproductive success of farmers.

Methods

Agrarian labor is not invested solely towards productive ends. Marriageable young men, and sometimes their fathers, make presents of their labor to farmers with marriageable daughters. This informally exchanged but customarily anticipated brideservice is an important overture in attempting to attract and obtain a bride. Should a marriage be contracted, labor relations often continue between the newly established affines.

K'ekchi' marriage is uniformly monogamous. Apparently high paternity certainly is supported by strong social sanctions against sexual permissiveness, particularly for women, and a strong religiously sanctioned adherence to monogamous unions. Further, the intense paternal investment in offspring evident especially in terms of subsistence production as described above might not be expected if paternity were uncertain. Serial monogamy does occur but usually only between widowed women beyond their reproductive years and older widowed men, and therefore accounts for little of the reproductive variance among males. Marriage dissolution is uncommon. Only two cases of divorce occurred in the reproductive histories of adults in the 1980 San Miguel population. Both marriages ended after just one year of cohabitation, and neither with any resulting children. Although it cannot be verified, infertility was a plausible cause of these divorces since, with one exception, all other couples in the population conceived within the first year of marriage, and since interviews with divorced individuals were suggestive of such a cause. A strong preference for patrilocal post-marital residence was established through interviews, and was in fact the most frequently practiced form of post-marital residence.

A man's ability to perform agricultural labor is considered a highly desirable quality in a potential son-in-law/husband, just as a woman's ability to process and prepare food, keep house, and bear and raise children are highly regarded and the source of much comment. The cost of marriage is incurred by the groom's family in the form of a feast given for the entire village. The food consumed at the feast, a gift of clothes and traditional K'ekchi' jewelry to the bride, and the farming labor donated by a potential son-in-law and other adult male kin in his family add up to a considerable cost to the groom's family.

As mentioned above, village endogamy is advantageous for the groom, as well as his family, because it allows him to continue working relations in the fields with his primary source of labor, that is, kinsmen, particularly agnatic ones. A young married couple commonly remains in the household of the groom's father (patrilocal marriage) until sometime after the birth of their first child. Later they build a separate nuclear family hut often next to or nearby that of the groom's parents, and continue to assist each other in agricultural work. Both the bride's and groom's families profit from endogamous marriage by having created new labor allies in addition to securing spouses for their children.

Results

The second prediction mentioned at the beginning of this paper specified that:

Table 4.2 *Average cost of wedding feast by residential type of marriage*

Type[a]	n	%	Livestock	Cash[b]
1	27	61	2.5	386
2	11	25	2.6	491
3	3	7	0.5	83
4	3	7	0.9	121

Based on data from 44 first marriages for males in San Miguel; marriage costs for five older men could not be determined
[a] Type:
1. Endogamous, patrilocal – bride is from same village as groom; post-marital residence is in groom's natal household
2. Exogamous, patrilocal – bride is from a different village than the groom; post-marital residence is in groom's natal household
3. Exogamous, matrilocal – groom is from a different village than the bridge; post-marital residence is in bride's natal household
4. Neolocal – bride and groom are either from the same or different villages and reside in new and separate household immediately after marriage. *Note:* Most neolocal unions occurred between elder generation couples back when they first migrated to Belize from Guatemala
[b] In Belizean dollars. $1.00 BZ = 0.50 US

Parents and marriageable offspring will expend effort to find mates within the village in order to maintain productive relationships with local kin.

Table 4.2 shows the average cost of a wedding for the 44 marriages active in 1980 according to the residential type of the marriage. Livestock represents the number of pigs slaughtered for the meal, and cash includes money spent on the purchase of the bridal trousseau, and on other non-local consumer items incorporated into feasts in recent years (e.g. Coca Cola, wheat flour for breads, and sweets), and purchased from the coastal Garifuna (Black Carib) community some 30 miles away.

Clearly, village endogamy, which is always patrilocal in this population, is the most common marital choice (61% of the marriages), and parents are willing to pay in cash and livestock for local wives for their sons. The apparently slightly higher costs of bringing a bride from another village, the second most frequent marriage pattern (25% of the marriages), if significant at all, may be attributed to the fact that these wedding feasts must provide not only for the entire local village of the groom, as is the custom, but also for many of the bride's kinsmen from outside the village.

San Miguel, then, poses a contrary situation to that which Boserup (1970) expects: where women do little agricultural work, dowries are the custom rather than brideprice (cf. Borgerhoff Mulder, this volume (Chapter 3)). It appears, rather, that K'ekchi' parents, in securing a son's reproductive future, are willing to indulge in costly wedding feasts in order to maintain a lien on his labor and keep him with his kinsmen, perhaps the most reliable labor sources in the village.

In only three cases did a groom move to his bride's village. In one case, the man, who remarried exogamously and matrilocally after the death of his first wife, claimed to have few relations in his former village. Another case represents the first marriage of a young man from Santa Teresa, the smaller, related parent village of San Miguel, who had difficulty finding a mate of the appropriate age and relatedness status in his natal village.

The average age of marriage is approximately 18 for males and 14 for females. Cousin marriage was not found in this population, a pattern which is supported by prohibitions against cousin marriage imposed by the various Christian religions they now practice. (It is possible that further genealogical information in ascending generations, which is difficult to collect on immigrant populations such as this one, might show that some of the unions in San Miguel are actually between remotely distant cousins.)

Although migrations of entire families between K'ekchi' villages in the Toledo District do take place, San Miguel has remained fairly stable in composition since it separated from its parent village, Santa Teresa, further south early in 1952. A fairly stable population plus the large number of village endogamous marriages means that fewer potential mates are available to those males and females entering the mate pool who have extensive genealogical ties within the village. In short, there are many first-cousin relations within the village, and, therefore, not an abundance of potential mates for those individuals with many local relatives. Those with few local kinsmen, on the other hand, such as the few recent immigrants in the village, have comparatively many legitimate potential mates in the local population.

Table 4.3 *Relatedness to the San Miguel population of exogamously versus endogamously married men*

A. All men in the population:
 $t = 2.10$, df $= 44$, $p = 0.041$
(using two-tailed t-test comparing endogamous and exogamous unions)
Mean relatedness within San Miguel population (i.e. the average of the relatednesses between all possible pairs 0.033)
Relatedness to the Miguel population of exogamously married men Mean $= 0.022$ SD $= 0.018$
 Range: 0.000–0.056
Relatedness to the San Miguel population of endogamously married men Mean $= 0.037$ SD $= 0.021$
 Range: 0.11–0.075
B. Men under age 35 in the population:
 $t = 2.12$, df $= 26$, $p = 0.044$
(using two-tailed t-test comparing endogamous and exogamous unions)
Relatedness to the San Miguel population of exogamously married men Mean $= 0.022$ SD $= 0.016$
Relatedness to the San Miguel population of endogamously married men Mean $= 0.037$ SD $= 0.019$

Table 4.3 shows the relatedness to the local population of those men who married exogamously (types 2 and 3 in Table 4.2 – exogamous patrilocal and exogamous matrilocal, respectively). These data reflect the residential form that characterized all currently active or most recent unions (two men were widowed) when the unions first began for men who lived in San Miguel in 1980. Average relatedness uses Chagnon's (1975) version of Wright's (1922) inbreeding coefficient in measuring the sum of an individual's total relatedness to each other individual in the village divided by the population size less self ($n - 1$).

The mean relatedness among all villagers (or the average of all average relatednesses of all villagers) was 0.033 in the population in 1980. Only two men who brought women from other villages to marry (11.2% of these unions) were found to have an average relatedness above the population mean. All other exogamously married men fell at or below the population mean. The average relatedness to the local population for this group was 0.022, whereas it was 0.037 for endogamously married men. Eleven endogamously married men (37.9% of these unions) fell well above the population mean (between 0.054 and 0.075 average relatedness).

The potential mate pool for individuals near or just entering marriageable age by the end of 1980 was quite variable. In addition to being related by less than first cousins, potential mates were defined as falling within a certain age range, reflecting the age differences found between mates in the marital histories in the village geneaology. Potential male mates, for example, were defined as being no more than four years senior to, and never younger than potential female mates. Among the thirteen females aged 11 through 15, for example, potential mates for the 1980 male population (i.e. unwed males between the ages of 15 and 19) were as few as one and as many as ten. Among the ten unmarried males aged 15 to 19, potential mates varied between four and eleven.

Men with few kinsmen in their natal village tend to find more marriageable females in the local population than do men of comparable age who have many local kinsmen, and therefore, many female first-cousins in the same generation. Nevertheless, there is a positive association between degree of local relatedness and local endogamy. A two-tailed t-test comparing observed differences in degree of relatedness to the local population in 1980 between endogamously and exoga mously married men is significant (see Table 4.3). This significant difference pertains even when calculated only on men under 35, or those who do not have married sons and grandchildren to inflate their relatedness figure (see Table 4.3). Unfortunately, it was impossible to fully re-create the precise composition of the village at the time each man was married, and, therefore, potential mates could only be inferred from degree of relatedness to the local population.

Having many genealogical relatives within the local population means, of course, having many potential laborers who are kinsmen, as demonstrated in a Pearson correlation coefficient calculates between (1) *the total genealogical relatedness of plot 'owners' to all other persons in the population* and (2) *the total genealogical relatedness of plot 'owners' to all local potential laborers in the population:*

$$r = 0.8704, n = 40, p = 0.000$$

A regression analysis of the relationship between (a) *the marital status of a plot 'owner's'* current union and (b) *his total relatedness to all local potential laborers* illustrates that having many kinsmen in the local pool of potential laborers significantly increases the probability of maintaining contact with them after marriage:

$$M = 1.790 - 0.223\,L \qquad R^2 = 0.172$$
$$(0.0087)$$

where M is residential form of marriage (1 = endogamous, 2 = exogamous patrilocal, and 3 = exogamous matrilocal – five neolocal cases were excluded from this test since they were marriages contracted during migration into Belize, and L reflects the total genealogical relatedness of a plot 'owner' to all potential laborers in the local population. A significant ($p = 0.0087$) negative *beta* coefficient (-0.223) for L suggests that when relatedness to local laborers is large, marriage type is coded low, the lowest coded marital type being the most preferred type: endogamous patrilocal.

Earlier I discussed the use of agrarian labor exchange as an important aspect of male parenting and a principal example of general nepotism within the village. But the contention of this chapter is that labor exchange is also a part of mating effort, or, as Alexander (1979:46) put it, the effort involved in placing one's gametes in the best possible environment. Above I have discussed the benefit that endogamous marriage confers on a man in maintaining access to potential nepotists, particularly in terms of agrarian labor, and speculated as to possible advantages some men might have in gaining local mates despite disadvantages derived from demographic conditions.

But an assessment of the efficacy of the Darwinian theory underlying this discussion of labor exchange, nepotism, and mating must ultimately address the effect that these behaviors have on individual reproductive success. The third prediction made at the start of this paper specified that:

> Fertility of male household heads (plot 'owners') is positively affected by the presence of related males who are productive workers in the village.

In other words, does having access to local labor translate into biological fitness? The following regression equation predicts a measure of the (F) *reproductive success of K'ekchi' plot 'owner'* by their (L) *relatedness to the local pool of potential laborers*, as defined earlier, and weighted by the (A) *current age of plot 'owner'*:

$$F = -6.506 + 0.310\,A + 1.097\,L$$
$$(0.0007) \quad (0.0000)$$
$$R^2 = 0.781$$

where F was measured as the number of offspring who survived the first half-year of life (after which the probability of surviving to adulthood increases greatly) ever sired by a plot 'owner', A was measured as the current age of a plot 'owner' (except that if he had completed his reproductive history his age was calculated as 50, that is, the latest age of any man in the population when his last child was born), and L was measured as the summed coefficients of genealogical relatedness pertaining between a plot 'owner' and the local pool of potential laborers, as described above.

This equation combines a variable which is synchronic, that is, relatedness to potential laborers in the 1980 population, and a diachronic or cumulative variable, fertility up until 1980. Nevertheless, since the population remained fairly stable in composition over this time, it is not unreasonable to assume that the relationship between the two variables can be generalized beyond the 1980 situation in San Miguel.

For men with grown sons who belong to the local pool of potential laborers, however, fertility and relatedness to the local pool of laborers are not independent. The following equation recalculates the regression of the previous equation predicting male fertility only for those men with no offspring in the pool of potential laborers:

$$F = -5.217 + 0.285\,A + 0.668\,L$$
$$(0.0005) \quad (0.0694)$$
$$R^2 = 0.477$$

It appears, then, that living in a village with potential nepotists, particularly those who can provide assistance in the production of a stable crop, may offer reproductive advantages to men.

Conclusions

The findings presented here support the predictions made at the beginning of this chapter based on Darwinian models of sociality. Chayanovian theory, a prominant traditional anthropological approach to explaining productive activities and decision-making in farming societies, specifies the material and energetic costs and benefits of labor invested in farming, but does not account for the effect that sources of nepotism (of labor) outside of the domestic group can have on domestic production. Explaining patterns of agrarian labor exchange as a component of a broader Darwinian model, as I have attempted to do here, may permit an understanding of practices related to subsistence production beyond that which purely economic models can provide. A Darwinian model also permits an examination of the possible consequences that productive decisions (the donation of labor in this case) can have on reproductive success.

According to our present understanding of Darwinian theory, individuals should strive to invest and obtain those material and energetic resources which prove important to survival and mating in particular social, technological and ecological environments such that they maximize their inclusive fitness. The data presented here suggest that the way in which agrarian labor is exchanged has much to do with productive success (amount of maize planted per capita by a household), mate choice (preference for keeping men together after marriage), and reproductive success (fertility of farmers). Where cooperation among men in subsistence production is important for the success of farming, men attempt to maintain proximity with their kinsmen, and to favor assisting kinsmen in horticultural activities. Remaining in one's natal village is the best way to stay around kinsmen, or potential nepotists.

While the findings are preliminary and but suggestive at this point, it may be that local kinsmen assist each other in marrying endogamously. This would not only keep related men around to help one another in farming, a mutual benefit to both the marrying man and his kinsmen, but would also keep his future children near those potential nepotists among their maternal relatives. It may also be that parents find it attractive to marry daughters into local families which have many kinsmen among the pool of potential laborers. This would also improve the probability that men with many local kinsmen and thus few local potential mates marry endogamously. A detailed behavioral study beyond the scope of this paper would clarify such strategies.

The utility of Darwinian theory in uncovering strategies for achieving productive and reproductive success, and the relationship between these strategies, is just beginning to be realized by social scientists. In particular, it may be useful, if not essential, for economic studies in anthropology to take into consideration the reproductive as well as productive consequences of individual social behavior in order to achieve a truly holistic understanding of rational economic man.

Summary

To summarize the findings in this paper concerning somatic effort expended by K'ekchi' farmers, or the effort to insure survivorship of offspring, and other genealogical relatives, we have seen that:

1. The success of maize cultivation, which is critical to insuring a subsistence food base to members of a household, and therefore critical to the survivorship of dependent offspring, is largely dependent upon the ability of a household head to gain access to the labor energies of productively active men within the village but outside of his household.

2. The number of assistants a plot 'owner' can enlist to help plant his milpa is positively affected by the number of genealogical relatives he has in the local pool of potential laborers; approximately two-thirds of all labor exchanges occur between individuals who are related either genealogically or affinally.

Summarizing the findings concerning mating effort and reproductive success of K'ekchi' farmers we see that:

3. Parents of marriageable sons expend resources in the form of livestock and money in an effort to find them mates within the village, or at least to insure that sons remain in the village after marriage.

4. Men who are highly related to the local population may have fewer potential mates, as defined by relative age and

94

genealogical relatedness, but nevertheless marry local women more often.

15. Married men who are highly related to the local pool of potential laborers have higher reproductive success as measured by age-weighted fertility.

Acknowledgements

I wish to thank the National Science Foundation and the Hill Fund for Anthropological Research for their financial support, and my friends and colleagues, Laura Betzig, Paul Turke, and Monique Borgerhoff Mulder for their helpful comments on earlier drafts of this paper.

References

Alexander, R. D. (1979) *Darwinism and Human Affairs*. Seattle: University of Washington.

Alexander, R. D. and Borgia, G. (1979) On the origin and basis of the male–female phenomenon. In *Sexual Selection and Reproductive Competition in Insects*, ed. M. F. Blum and N. Blum, pp. 417–40. New York: Academic Press.

Barlett, P. F. (1980a) *Agricultural Decision Making*. New York: Academic Press.

Barlett, P. F. (1980b) Cost–benefit analysis: a test of alternative methodologies. In *Agricultural Decision Making*, ed. P. F. Barlett, pp. 137–60. New York: Academic Press.

Berté, N. A. (1983) Agricultural production and labor investment strategies in a K'ekchi' village, Southern Belize. Ph.D. Dissertation, Northwestern University, Evanston, IL.

Boserup, E. (1970) *Women's Role in Economic Development*. London.

Cancian, F. (1972) *Change and Uncertainty in a Peasant Economy: The Mayan Corn Farmers of Zinacantan*. Stanford: Stanford University Press.

Chagnon, N. A. (1975) Genealogy, solidarity and relatedness: limits to local group size and patterns of fissioning in an expanding population. *Yearbook of Physical Anthropology*, **19**, 95–110. Washington, DC: American Anthropoligical Association.

Chagnon, N. A. (1979) Is reproductive success equal in egalitarian societies? In *Evolutionary Biology and Human Social Behavior: An Anthropological Perspective*, ed. N. A. Chagnon and W. Irons, pp. 374–401. North Scituate, MA: Duxbury Press.

Chayanov, A. V. (1925 [1966]) *The Theory of Peasant Economy*, ed. D. Thorner, R. E. F. Smith and B. Kerblay. Homewood, IL: Richard D. Irwin. American Economic Association.

Durrenberger, E. P. (1979) An analysis of Shan household production decisions. *Journal of Anthropological Research*, **35**, 447–58.

Durrenberger, E. P. (ed.) (1984) *Chayanov, Peasant, and Economic Anthropology*. New York: Academic Press.

Evans, M. (1974) A note on the measurement of Sahlins' social profile of domestic production. *American Ethnologist*, **1**, 269–79.

Flinn, M. V. (1983) Resources, mating, and kinship: the behavioral ecology of a trinidadian village. Ph.D. Dissertation, Northwestern University, Evanston, IL.

Fried, M. H. (1967) *The Evolution of Political Society*. New York: Random House.

Hames, R. (1979) Relatedness and interaction among the Ye'kwana: a preliminary analysis. In *Evolutionary Biology and Human Social Behavior: An Anthropological Perspective*, ed. N. A. Chagnon and W. Irons, pp. 238–49. North Scituate, MA: Duxbury Press.

Hamilton, W. D. (1963) The evolution of altruistic behavior. *American Naturalist*, **97**, 354–6.

Hamilton, W. D. (1964) The genetical evolution of social behavior, I, II. *Journal of Theoretical Biology*, **7**, 1–52.

Harris, M. (1975) *Culture, People and Nature: An Introduction to General Anthropology*, 2nd edition. New York: Crowell.

Irons, W. (1979) Natural selection, adaptation, and human social behavior. In *Evolutionary Biology and Human Social Behavior: An Anthropological Perspective*, ed. N. A. Chagnon and W. Irons, pp. 4–38. North Scituate, MA: Duxbury Press.

Kerblay, B. (1971) Chayanov and the theory of peasantry as a specific type of economy. In *Peasants and Peasant Societies*, ed. T. Shanin, pp. 150–60. New York: Penguin.

Minge-Kalman, W. (1977) On the theory and measurement of domestic labor intensity. *American Ethnologist*, **4**, 273–84.

Ortiz, S. (1973) *Uncertainties in Peasant Farming*. London: Athlone Press.

Sahlins, M. (1971) The intensity of domestic production in primitive societies: social inflections of the Chayanov slope. In *Studies in Economic Anthropology*, ed. G. Dalton, pp. 30–51. Anthropological Studies No. 7, Washington, DC: American Anthropological Association.

Sahlins, M. (1972) *Stone Age Economics*. Chicago, IL: Aldine–Atherton.

Smith, A. E. (1979) Chayanov, Sahlins, and the labour–consumer balance. *Journal of Anthropological Research*, **35**, (4), 477–80.

Turke, P. and Betzig, L. L. (1985) Those who can do: wealth, status, and reproductive success on Ifaluk. *Ethology and Sociobiology*, **6**, 79–87.

Tannenbaum, N. (1984) The misuse of Chayanov: 'Chayanov's Rule' and empiricist bias in anthropology.

Wilk, R. R. (1984) Households in process: agricultural change and domestic transformation among the Kekchi Maya of Belize. In *Households: Comparative and Historical Studies of the Domestic Group*, ed. R. McC. Netting, R. R. Wilk and E. J. Arnold. University of California Press.

Wright, S. (1922) Coefficients of inbreeding and relationship. *American Naturalist*, 56, 330–8.

John H. Crook[1]
Stamati J. Crook[2]

Tibetan polyandry: problems of adaptation and fitness

Introduction: basic premises

The attempt to relate the biology of human species to its cultural expression by self-aware individuals has moved from a strongly reductionist beginning (Wilson 1975) to a greater awareness of the complexity of the relationship between the human organism and its cultural environment. Irons (1979), following the pioneering lead of Haldane (1956), remarked that the most reasonable hypothesis is that the behavioural differences shown by contrasting human groups 'are environmentally induced variations in the expression of basically similar genotypes' and that the ability to vary behaviour in response to environmental differences is itself the prime

human adaptation to a social world. Evidence that the social expressions of human phenotypes are often strategic in the sense that they maintain the inclusive fitness of individuals in ways formally comparable to those of animals without culture has been interpreted in several ways (Berghe and Barash 1977, Alexander 1979, Durham 1979, Irons 1979, Crook 1980, Lopreato 1984). We therefore wish to begin by stating the basic premises with which we approach these issues in human sociobiology.

The basic social unit of almost all human

[1] Department of Psychology, University of Bristol, Bristol, BS8 1HH, UK
[2] St Catherine's College, Oxford University, Oxford, UK. Present address c/o John H. Crook

populations is the family; a small group of people integrated around the marital alliance of one or more men with one or more women and their children and which may extend to a greater size by a continuing association with more distant relatives – uncles, nephews. The marital family functions in two modes facing inwards upon the reproduction of children, the cultivation or acquisition of resources for family maintenance and child rearing, and the inheritance of possessions, skills or rights, where such exist, from one generation to another; and outwards upon its relations as a unit with other families, some of which will be kin groups and some of no known kinship affiliation, within a wider network of the population and its structural organization. In this outward-facing regard competition between families as units may have important outcomes with respect to their economic and reproductive prosperity and that of the individuals comprising them (Figure 5.1).

Human societies show a range of marital types from monogamous through polygynous or polyandrous to complex forms of polygynandry. These types are often specific to particular socioeconomic conditions. The adaptive relationships between marital systems and their environments arise, we argue, because the behaviour of the individuals comprising them is flexible with respect to the types of sexual union and labour imposed by contrasting systems.

The central prediction made in a Darwinian perspective is that humans are endeavouring consciously or unconsciously to optimize their reproductive success. It is then a matter of research to discover whether individuals marrying in contrasting ways in different contexts are in fact showing behaviour that does promote their genetic fitness. Where strategic behaviour maintaining fitness is demonstrable it may be argued that humans, like for example gelada baboons (see Kummer 1975, Crook 1980:236, Dunbar 1985), have dispositions to interact in ways that create social organizations in which they reproduce successfully. We know that humans live in tightly controlled, culturally constrained, value systems that determine such things as marital choice often very precisely (but see Chagnon this volume (Chapter 1)). These systems may ensure the fitness of parents as much as that of the marrying couple and express long-term historically successful adaptations of communities to circumstances. The culturally dictated rules for behaviour often seem to maintain or enhance personal fitness in each generation just as the dispositions to behave of lower organisms without culture may do.

Any demonstration of a strategic property in individual human behaviour does not lead immediately to the naive conclusion that a genetic involvement in determining the behaviour has been demonstrated. What may have been demonstrated is that the value systems of the individuals concerned have been shaped by adaptive learning to match the socioeconomic context in ways that are functionally effective with regard to reproduction. It follows that over generations a selective process operating at

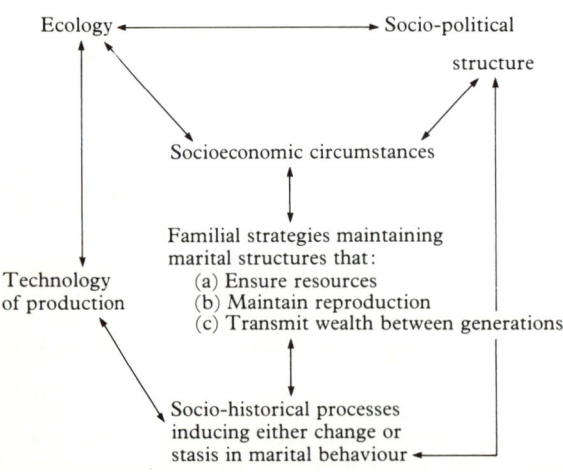

Figure 5.1 The context of human marital systems.

several levels (Plotkin and Odling-Smee 1981) is likely to have been at work both in the historical elimination of family lineages that fail to maintain themselves and in the differential elimination of poorly functioning individual phenotypes. While the genetic basis for a disposition to learn adaptively can certainly undergo selection in this way, we do not opt for any argument supposing that marital strategies are as such genetically inherited. In our own study we know that children of one marital type can opt for another under changed circumstances. The genetic adaptation consists in the provision of a flexibility that allows reproductively optimizing behaviour to vary with context. What remains remarkable and open to research is the context-related precision with which behaviours in marital relations are reproductively successful. It is this strategic precision that calls forth comparisons with the behavioural adaptations of non-cultural animals and the suggestion that common ground rules, albeit manifested through very different mechanisms, are often at work.

Polyandry is a rare phenomenon occurring infrequently in birds (Jenni 1974) and in no mammal other than man. Several authors have attempted explanations of human polyandry. Suggestions range from an imagined shortage of women due to infanticide, latent homosexuality, to a supposed imposition of monastic dominance (reviewed in Crook and Crook 1988). The closest theoretical proposal to the viewpoint advocated here is owing to Alexander (1974: 372) who saw it as functional in situations of low agricultural productivity with a need for a high labour input. Since 1971 the major contributions of Goldstein (1971a, 1971b, 1973, 1976) based on his extensive fieldwork, have transformed the picture by taking a broad perspective interpreting fraternal polyandry as an aspect of major sociocultural adaptations to precise economic and ecological circumstances. On a basis of these studies and in the light of Dickemann's analysis of hypergynous stratified societies (1979a, 1979b), Crook (1980: 216) proposed that Tibetan polyandry as witnessed by him in Ladakh could be explained in the following way. In brief, a set of brothers marries the same spouse and the children in common are raised as a single family under the same roof. The co-husbands collaborate on their agricultural estate both in crop raising and animal husbandry. The estate is handed down by a rule

of primogeniture to the eldest son but when he marries some of his younger brothers may also marry the same wife, along with him. The estate thus passes from generation to generation from sets of paternal co-husbands to their sons. In the classical situation this is the only marriage in the family in each generation – a rule named by Goldstein as the 'monomarital principle'. Daughters either marry out – or in many cases remain unmarried as additional labourers on the estate. In a family without sons the estate passes to the eldest daughter who marries a *mag.pa* husband. The estate remains in the stem family and passes to her children. Sometimes two such sisters marry the same incoming male. Families are often large, posing problems for younger brothers; while some marry out as *mag.pas* others become monks affiliated with the local monastery which is therefore very much part of the local community. In Zangskar, Ladakh, we found in 1980 that some 30% of brothers were monks – clearly a very important demographic fact (Crook and Shakya 1988b).

Goldstein's demographic work at Limi in Nepal (1976) had shown that because of polyandry 31% of potentially reproductive women there do not bear children in wedlock. A total of 38% of marriages were polyandrous with married and non-married women bearing 3.3 and 0.7 children on average, respectively. Goldstein argued that were the population to become wholly monogamous there would be a 16% increase in numbers.

Crook (1980) supported the view that for these high-altitude farmers working in harsh conditions there is always both a risk of labour shortage and a risk of over-population in remote areas without transportation for food, and a requirement to store supplies for long winters. There is thus a tension between the need for labour to maximize production and tendency to leave the land. The polyandrous domus with the monomarital principle is interpreted as a response to an ecology where the carrying capacity of the land is not only restricted but subject to severe seasonal constraints. 'K selection' for a mode of subsistence increasing collaboration so that at least a maximum possible number of young can be raised seems to be operating at this cultural level in similar ways to its effect in non-cultural animals (MacArthur and Wilson 1967, Pianka 1974).

The monomarital principle ensures that estates are not divided in each generation. Were this to happen, there can be no doubt that without some system of redistribution estates would rapidly become agricultural inviable. A family with a daughter is likely to seek to place her in a polyandrous household where the collaborating husbands can ensure sufficient welfare for her to rear a family. Furthermore, under many social situations that obtained in traditional Tibet, the farm-owning families had numerous duties with respect to their overlords. To meet these demands a collaborating team of labouring men and women was essential if the estate was to remain in the family lineage.

This paper discusses the limited factual material available to support this model. Much of the data has been derived from studies based on the verbal reports of Tibetan refugees no longer living on their traditional estates (e.g. Goldstein 1971a, 1971b, Aziz 1978, Dhargyay 1982). Goldstein's further work (1976) was, however, collected from fully functioning villages in Nepal and our own data from Ladakh is likewise first-hand. Limitations in this material are its relatively small scope, its lack of historical depth and its collection in a period of rapid socioeconomic change. It is nonetheless questionable whether much more data of equal accuracy could be collected; some remote areas may still provide information of value. We believe that, given these limitations, the material we have assembled (for further details see Crook and Crook, 1988) does allow us to explain fraternal polyandry in a comprehensive and highly plausible manner even where proof of some of our contentions, in the sense of sufficient statistical analyses, cannot be secured. Our evidence allows us to discuss:

1. The precise socio-ecological circumstances to which fraternal polyandry of the Tibetan type is an adaptation.
2. A model of the demographic consequences of polyandry and its theoretical history in a particular Ladakhi ecology.
3. The effects of change in socioeconomic circumstances on household structure and marital organization over 40 years.
4. Quantitative assessments of the reproductive success of women and men marrying either polyandrously or monogamously.

5. A discussion of the question as to what extent polyandrous marriage maintains the reproductive fitness of individuals as compared with alternative marital situations on agricultural land.

The socioeconomic context of Tibetan polyandry

Crook and Crook (1988) provide a comprehensive survey of the contexts in which Tibetan polyandry has been reported. Drawing on the work of Prince Peter of Greece (1963), Fürer-Haimendorf (1964), Goldstein (1971a, 1971b, 1976, 1979), Aziz (1978), Dhargyay (1982), and Grist (1980), we have examined studies in Nepal, on refugees from southern Tibet and Kham and research in the Indus valley of Ladakh (Figures 2 and 3). These reports are taken in conjunction with our own field results from Zangskar (Crook and Osmaston 1988).

The monomarital principal of co-fraternal polyandry operates on agricultural estates which are either owned by the farming family or held on long inalienable tenancies. These estates are passed from generation to generation through a primogeniture in which other siblings are associated in marriage. Typically the parental family leaves the main house of the estate (*khang.chen*) as soon as the son(s) marries and occupies a lesser building on the estate known as the *khang.chung*. There may be additional *khang.chung* which are

Figure 5.2 Location of the study area.

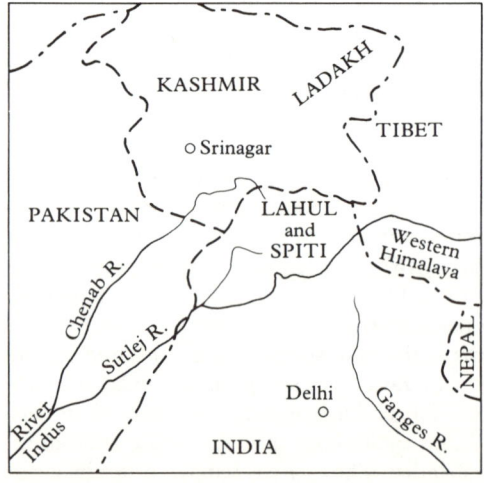

residences for other relatives, uncles, grandparents, normally of the generation preceding the current reproductive one. These *khang.chung* are dependent upon the estate as a whole and may have certain rights within it – but the overall direction of the estate is under the control of the eldest brother of the *khang.chen*. Traditionally the only marriage on the estate is that of the *khang.chen* together with those of the parental and grandparental *khang.chung*. Marriages by brothers, uncles, etc. within the estate are not possible within the ideal system. However, they do sometimes occur when negotiations for the formation of a new estate with separate lands and a new branch patrilineage can begin. This will be commonly resisted by the existing estates of a community unless new land can be broken and the water supply is sufficient to allow an extension of the agricultural area.

At our research village, sTongde in Zangskar,

in 1980 the situation was of an almost classical simplicity; virtually the whole population of the valley consisted of estate owning farmers (Crook 1988a). This is however a secondary effect of the invasions of the last century, particularly the Dogra invasion, which effectively removed the influence of old aristocratic families. The same is largely true of the Indus valley further north in Ladakh. The prime difference between the farming estates we studied in Zangskar and the estates tenanted to aristocratic religious or governmental institutions in pre-1959 Tibet is the absence of taxation and other duties which bore so heavily on the old farming communities of Tibet.

The reconstructions of life in southern Tibetan villages reveal a complex structure. Land was owned by large government estates, aristocrats or religious houses to whom the farmers were tenanted under strict obligation

Figure 5.3 Sketch map of Ladakh.

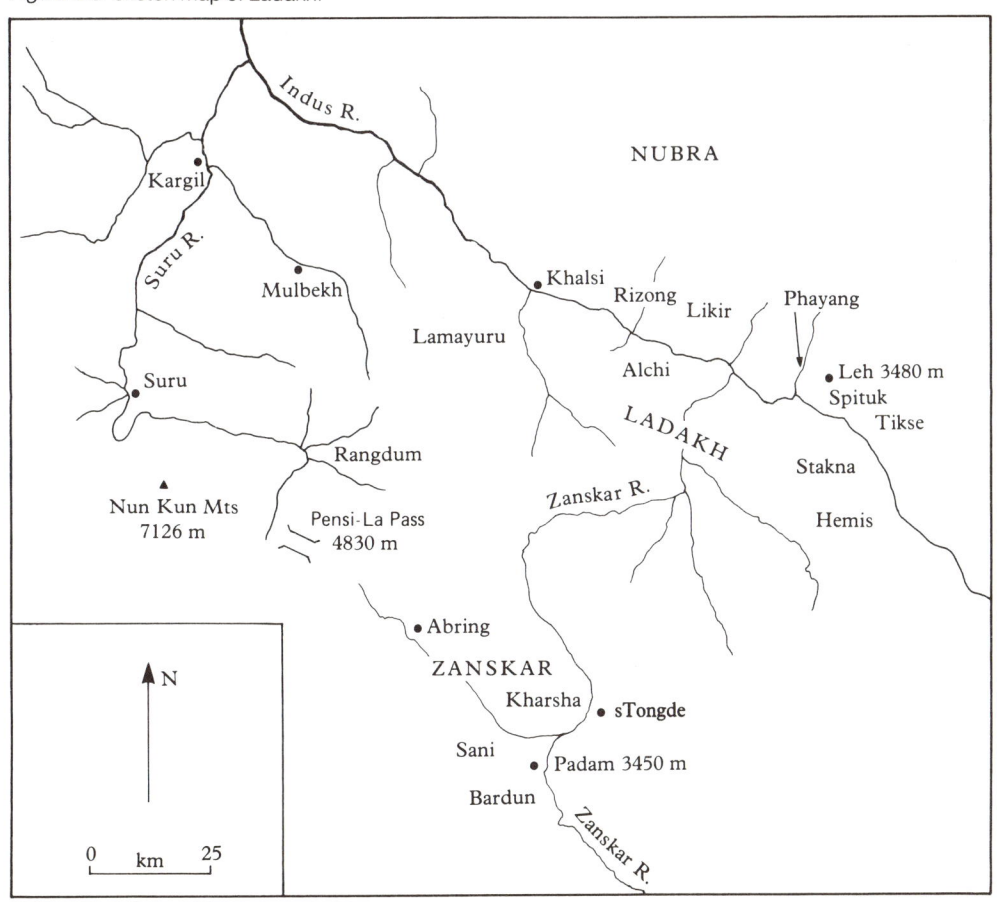

although with inalienable right to pass their tenancy on to their children. In these developed communities there was also a sizeable population of non-land holding peasants who derived income from working the land of others or as artisans. Aziz (1978) also reported on the social structure of the small town of Ding.ri. The results of these studies show that apart from the owned or tenanted estates almost all ways of life adopt monogamy with division of inherited property on the death of parents. The monomarital system with non-division of the estate is thus highly correlated with the ownership or tenancy of a productive farming estate.

Modelling the socio-ecological system of polyandry in Zangskar

The simplicity of the communal structure in Zangskar allows a particularly direct relationship between ecology and farming to exist there. The demographic relationship between polyandry and resources in Zangskar can be modelled without much difficulty.

In Zangskar, villages are established on alluvial fans where springs or meltwater from glaciers emerge from the sides of the mountain range. Agricultural productivity is determined by a relationship between:

(a) The area of cultivatable land on the alluvium.
(b) The flow of water to the cultivatable area.
(c) The seasonablity of the water flow.
(d) The slope of the alluvium and the soil quality.

Only a limited number of farming families can be established on an alluvium and between the alluvia are wide stretches of montane desert. In modelling these relationships we argue that population pressure will tend to drive farm size down to that area upon which a family can effectively maintain itself and rear children. The farm work is heavy, although less so in the snowbound winter when little work other than feeding and watering livestock is possible. Farm work divides into animal husbandry and cereal production. The subsistence economy utilizes only a primitive although effective technology which is labour intensive. The number of workers on an estate bears directly upon its pro-

ductivity and upon the extent to which it can husband reserves. A family with many growing children could easily strain its resources.

In our simulation, only a handful of families are able to settle initially on an alluvium as arable land is limited until irrigation works are built so that the water may be exploited to the full. The village then expands allowing more estates and households to be established. This period is labour intensive and eventually the population and the number of households are strictly limited by the small amount of irrigable land available. At some stage the full potential of the water resource is realized and the area of alluvium utilized ceases to grow. A restriction on the number of estates is soon established as inter-generational divisions of farming units cause them to reach the minimum size for economic viability. To prevent an increase in the number of households there can now be only one marriage per estate per generation. The numbers of families must be limited and, since irrigation works have been completed, non-agricultural labour is no longer at a premium. Some growth may occur as agricultural techniques become more labour intensive, but again a plateau is reached limiting further increases in numbers. Given these constraints, individual reproductive interests are best served when the one marriage-per-generation rule is enforced on the estate and population controlled, or exported. The functional role of polyandry as a means of limiting family reproduction can be envisaged in the context of this village evolution. We see several stages in progression:

1. The initial settlement with a very small amount of land has a strict limit on population but a demand for labour (surplus to agricultural requirements) for building irrigation channels. Taking a population of *100 males and 100 females* as a basis for computer modelling (Table 5.1), we can see how an increased level of polyandry limits population while increasing the labour force per household, thus solving the labour versus population problem. Each farming unit, or household, is able to spare some of its members from agricultural duties to build irrigation works.

2. As irrigation channels are dug and more arable land becomes available new households may be established and the limit on population

5. Tibetan polyandry

Table 5.1 *Effect of increasing polyandry in a population of 100 men and 100 women. Reproduction rates per generation given as 3.0 and 0.5 for married and unmarried women, respectively. As polyandry increases labour per household grows concomitantly with a decrease in the number of households, a lower population and an increase in children per household*

Polyandry level	Monog. men	Poly. men	Monog. women	Poly. women	Single women	Legitim. children	Illegitim. children	Marriages (household)	Children per household	Total population	Total persons household
Monog.	100	0	100	0	0	300	0	100	3.0	500	5.0
Diandry	80	20	80	10	10	270	5	90	3.1	475	5.3
	60	40	60	20	20	240	10	80	3.1	450	5.6
	40	60	40	30	30	210	15	70	3.2	425	6.1
Triandry	70	30	70	10	20	240	10	80	3.1	450	5.6
	40	60	40	20	40	180	20	60	3.3	400	6.7
	10	90	10	30	60	120	30	40	3.7	350	8.8

Table 5.2 *Effect of increasing polyandry with constant number of marriages (100). The increasing population is absorbed into a social structure without increasing the number of households. Labour availability is high*

Polyandry level	Monog. men	Poly. men	Monog. women	Poly. women	Single women	Legitim. children	Illegitim. children	Children per household	Total population	Total persons household
Monog.	100	0	100	0	0	300	0	3.0	500	5.0
Diandry	90	20	90	10	10	300	5	3.0	525	5.3
	80	40	80	20	20	300	10	3.1	550	5.5
	70	60	70	30	30	300	15	3.2	575	5.8
Triandry	90	30	90	10	20	300	10	3.1	550	5.5
	80	60	80	20	40	300	20	3.2	600	6.0
	70	90	70	30	60	300	30	3.3	650	6.4

is raised in relation to the amount of new land under cultivation. Available labour per household remains relatively high and one should expect a lower level of polyandry as the settlement expands. We can see from Table 5.1 that a gradual reduction in the level of polyandry would allow for a slow increase in the number of households without a drastic increase in population.

3. Eventually the full potential of the spring will be realized and, barring any improvements in the level of technology available, the village will cease to grow. Soon, farm units will have reached minimum size to support a family and as no further cultivatable land is available a strict limit must be placed upon the number of households. In Table 5.2 we see how the increasing polyandry allows population increases to be absorbed into the prevailing marital structure while the *number of marriages* (i.e. households) *remains constant.* Labour per household increases and agricultural techniques may be intensified, crafts produced, trade indulged in, or some other activity introduced to exploit the excess labour. Without polyandry families in such a community would have to export population, or large numbers of men and women would have to remain unmarried, in order to ensure a constant number of households.

4. As population continues to increase due to inadequate contraception and illegitimacy, the limit on household numbers can only be maintained by increasing levels of polyandry. We assume, for the purposes of the model, that the village is isolated and that excess population, as seems to be generally true in Ladakh, does not migrate to other areas. Eventually, population will have increased to such an extent that a further increase in polyandry will be unable to cope with population control. Population cannot be exported and there can be no increase in households, as the land available will not support new estates. Family size on estates can now only be controlled by limiting the number of married, and therefore more fertile, women. Up to this point polyandrous marriage has absorbed surplus men while the corresponding single women remain in their natal households. At this stage, however, polyandry is unable to soak up the surplus men and a minority of single men arises. With both single men and single women in the population, couple formation would be hard to prevent and one would expect a situation where there were more marriages than there were farming estates.

5. Two possible consequences could follow. First, the landless couples might marry monogamously and, as elsewhere in Tibet, form a class of landless labourers (*mi.bo*) who would be available for employment on the estates (see Aziz 1978, for example). This development would require local resources being available for non-agricultural work and an agricultural production somewhat in excess of estate requirements. Alternatively, where men were recruited and exported as soldiers under a national system, as used to be the case in ancient Tibet, a simple control of household numbers would arise. Alternatively, single men and women could be segregated, as in recent Tibet, through the establishment of monastic institutions to which younger persons would be sent. In a poorly endowed locality the reproductive exclusion of a minority of socially isolated males would allow the number of local marriages to be kept constant and the population levels to stabilize at a low level. Without some such social device the population would inevitably continue to increase unless effective methods of control could be found through contraception, through abstinence, infanticide, emigration, war, etc. In Zangskar we do in fact find 30% of brothers are monks and there is a large number of unmarried women with some religious status.

Our model depicts the functional significance of polyandry in relation to an ecology of limited carrying capacity. This is however a simplified picture because throughout Tibetan history most agricultural households have been subjected to intense pressure from landlords, the government and religious houses to produce sufficient resources to:

(a) Meet taxation in agricultural kind.
(b) Meet labour taxes in the form of providing through-transportation for government in a district.
(c) Contract labour to landlord in addition to that on own farm.
(d) Meet other forms of labour taxation, military service, obligatory services to monasteries etc.

This means that the actual carrying capacity of each estate must have been substantially larger than that attributable to eco-demographic relations alone. There would have been pressure to maintain an optimally large area under agricultural production, a large enough herd of animals and enough labour not only to work the farm but to meet the demands of obligatory work for landlord, government, etc. These pressures would have had the effect of intensifying the need for a balance between labour availability and the number of mouths to be fed on an estate. They also therefore increased those factors that promoted the maintenance of a monomarital principle.

There is in fact evidence from both Tibetan and Ladakhi history that rulers sought to regulate the size of estates through distributing it in equable proportions (see Crook and Crook 1988). While such moves were undoubtedly in part an effort by a ruler to contain the power of aristocratic houses a deeper implication is that such redistribution could produce estate sizes closer to the optimum size for agricultural production. Estate size could be regulated to fit the average family size under the monomarital principle so that the carrying capacity was fully taken up. Regulation could also ensure a system of taxation and service through stabilizing the socio-demographic relation with the ecological base. Finally, such regulation would attend to the welfare of the farming people so that their work was effective and not unduly disturbed by emigration, estate desertion, dissension or breakdowns in the rule of law.

The above considerations imply that it is probably not a sufficient explanation to relate the functions of polyandry solely to the features of a limiting ecology. While polyandry could well have originated in such an adaptation and while this relationship is currently visible in contemporary Zangskar lacking a political superstructure, the interference of the state and the landlord has been massive throughout much of Tibetan history. The long duration and fixity of the monomarital principle is undoubtedly in large measure a response to these socioeconomic pressures.

Socioeconomic change and alterations in household structure

The hypotheses of the last section can be tested through close examination of those 'natural experiments' that arise when external factors stimulate change in the socioeconomic conditions that maintain the monomarital system.

Crook and Shakya (1983) have analysed changes in family structure on six agricultural estates near Leh, Ladakh. In 1938 Prince Peter of Greece described the known genealogies of these families. These were brought up to date in 1981 and will be published shortly (Crook and Shakya 1988a). While genealogical reports are not as reliable as actual demographic censuses, it is possible to see in them the way in which family organization has changed over 40 years.

The Crook/Shakya analysis showed that household size has markedly increased since 1938 and that this increase has been accommodated by an increase in the percentage of family members occupying the *khang.chung*. The frequency of polyandrous marriages has dropped dramatically since 1938.

In terms of structure, the families by 1980 had largely ceased to follow the old monomarital principle and an increase in the occurrence of monogamous marriages additional to the marriage in the *khang.chen* can be seen in the *khang. chung*. This increase can be related to improved job opportunities outside agriculture, freeing brothers and uncles of estate owners to make their own economically independent marital liaisons while still living upon and doubtless contributing to the estate. In addition the old father often remains in the *khang.chen* so that the passing of the estate to the eldest son is now more delayed than previously and a waning authority of the older generation replaces the clear-cut shift in estate direction of the earlier times. An estate is becoming a loose conglomeration of potentially independent, mostly monogamous, nuclear family units, still however based upon the functioning agricultural unit and living in the set of buildings basic to it. The economic release from the traditional constraints on agricultural family life clearly renders polyandry obsolete near Leh where monetization and urban development have driven the increase in new job opportunities. A similar story may account for the changes in marital practices and system of inheritance among Sherpas which correlate with modifications to their mode of livelihood in recent years (Fürer-Haimendorf 1964, Ortner 1978, Crook 1988b).

Assessing the reproductive success of polyandrous marriage

This section addresses two major questions concerning the fitness of individuals marrying in contrasted ways in Ladakh. First, are polyandrous marriages as reproductively successful as monogamous ones? Second, are differential effects of marriage type also apparent in the second generation as reflected in a comparison of grandparental fitnesses?

The most direct way of assessing fitness when field data are available is the comparison of reproductive success between categories. The genealogies of Prince Peter updated in 1981, provide us with unique evidence on completed family sizes in Ladakh over a period of some 40 years with the majority of family completions prior to the most recent economic changes in the Indus valley. Families in these genealogies were assessed as to their completeness by determining the age of the mother and the age of her last recorded child. Table 5.3 compares completed family sizes on six estates according to their residence in the *khang.chen* or in a *khang. chung* and according to marital type. All *khang. chung* families were monogamous; all polyandrous families were in *khang.chen*. In accordance with a faulty application of the monomarital principle a minority of non-stem family marriages (30%) occurred in *khang.chung*. Only families growing up on the actual six estates sampled are assessed; the families of out-marrying women and *mag.pa* husbands are not included since our concern here is the comparison of residence and marital type within estates. Since positive and negative influences between marriages on the same estate have not been quantified no attempt at measuring inclusive fitness is made here although this would become significant if more extensive modelling were to be attempted (Grafen 1982).

A one way ANOVA on data in Table 5.3 showed that significant contrasts between categories existed ($F_{2,26} = 4.28$, $p < 0.05$). Post-hoc comparisons between means using the Sheffe procedure gave the following results:

(a) A comparison of means for completed monogamous and polyandrous families showed a significant difference ($p < 0.05$).

(b) A comparison of means from *khang.chung* with *khang.chen* showed a significant

Table 5.3 *Completed family sizes (number of children) on six estates near Leh. Data collated from genealogies established by Prince Peter of Greece (1963) in 1938 and updated by Crook and Shakya (1988a). Family sizes are listed according to marital type and residence*

Khang.chung families			*Khang.chen* families		
Monogamous	Monogamous	Diandrous	Triandrous		Tetrandrous
4	8	7	6		9
4	6	7	5		
3	6	6	3		
1	6	4			
1	5	3			
1	5	2			
0	3				
	2				
	2				
	1				
	1				
	0				
$\bar{x} = 2.0$	$\bar{x} = 3.75$	$\bar{x} = 4.8$	$\bar{x} = 4.7$		
$s^2 = 1.43$	$s^2 = 2.25$				
$n = 7.0$	$n = 12.0$	$n = 6.0$	$n = 3.0$		$n = 1$
Monogamy $\bar{x} = 3.10$			$\bar{x}$ Polyandry $= 5.2$		
$s^2 = 2.02$			$s^2 \quad = 1.8$		
$n = 19$			$n \quad = 10$		

difference ($p = 0.05$, two tailed).

(c) Comparison of means between monogamous families in *khang.chung* and *khang.chen* was not significant.

(d) Comparison of means between monogamous *khang.chen* families and polyandrous *khang. chen* families was not significant.

In spite of a considerable difference in mean family sizes it is not possible to conclude from these small samples that polyandry is more successful than monogamy *within khang.chens*. The overall argument that *khang.chen* life and economics support a more reproductively successful polyandrous marriage for a woman than a choice to marry monogamously in a *khang.chung* is, however, well supported. The result implies that a parent with a marriageable daughter interested in her reproductive success should seek to place her in a *khang.chen* wherein a polyandrous association with brothers would be quite acceptable.

How in fact are marital arrangements made? Traditional polyandrous marriages are arranged through consultations between the young people concerned and the family *pha.spun*. In Zangskar, although no longer in the Indus valley of Ladakh, the *pha.spun* is an association of patrili-

neally related families the heads of which get together to manage affairs of marriage and funeral rites for each participating household. Representatives of the patriline as a whole are thus traditionally involved in the choice of marriage partner for their kin and in the maintenance of the estate from one generation to another. Individual choices by men and women are thus restricted by considerations arising from consultations within the patriline as a whole. Individual monogamous liaisons breaking the monomarital principle are not likely to have been monitored or approved in this way. In the Indus valley where socioeconomic change has been greatest the *pha.spun* itself it no longer a specifically patrilineal association but more a mutual help association between families whose affairs may be economically diverse (Braun 1980, Crook 1988a).

Due to the monomarital principle there are relatively few opportunities for women to marry. In fact only a few women selected by male kin in a *pha.spun* patriline will end up as wives in *khang.chen*. Reproductive variance among women in this society, unlike that in hypergynous dowry societies (Dickemann, 1979), will be high and, due to polyandry, marrying

Table 5.4 *Grandmothers and grandchildren in the genealogies of six families of Leh, Ladakh (Crook and Shakya 1988a)*

Name of family	Name of grandmother	No. of grand-mother's husbands	No. of grand-mother's own children	No. of type of marriages by grandmother's children[a]	No. of grand-children (g)	Grandmaternal fitness (0.25g)
Tok.Tok	C. Dol.ma	2	7	1 P, 1 sororal Pg	10	2.5
	T. Panzom	2	2	3 M	14	3.5
	T. Yangzom	1 ⎫ same		1 P	7	1.75
	Lhadzom	1 ⎭ husband	8 1 monk	4 M, 1 P	21	5.25
Mahe	Putit	3	5	1 M, 2 P	12	3.0
Tsang.bi	YangsKid	1	1	1 M	6	1.5
	T. Rolma	1	6	2 M, 1 P	10	2.5
Goba.	T. Dzompa	2	7	5 M, 1 P	24	6
	Putit	2	6	3 M, 1 Pg	15	3.75
Od.Idan	Puntzog	1 (*mag.pa*)	6	3 M, 2 P	27	6.75
	T. Putit	2	6	6 M	22	5.5
Gad.pa.pa	T. Paldzan	1	6	1 P	9	2.25
	T. Chodan	4	9	8 M	24	6.0
Σ		13	22	71	36 M, 10 P, 2 other	201	$\bar{x} = 3.9$

[a] M = monogamy, P = polyandry, Pg = polygyny

brothers may have a rather low inclusive fitness (see below). Indirect intra-sexual competition is thus characteristic of this traditional system with large reproductive variance in each gender. The considerably higher reproductive success of the marrying woman and the importance of the senior husband's ability, with or without co-husbands, to support her may underlie, not necessarily explicitly, the choices made by *pha.spun*.

A further perspective on the success of marital strategies can be obtained by considering the reproductive fitness of grandmothers arising as a result of their children's marriages. Data were compiled on grandmothers from the genealogies of Prince Peter updated to 1981. These genealogies cannot be considered precise demographic records and such accounts constructed from group memory must inevitably be treated with caution. There is some evidence from the sex ratios in these genealogies as compared with our village demographic surveys (see Crook and Osmaston 1988) that some out marrying women have been forgotten but there is no evidence that this occurs with any particular bias within a family tree. There are, however, no other data available with which to approach this question and an analysis seems worth the attempt.

Table 5.4 provides the basic data from the updated genealogies. There are 13 grandmothers who at one time or another have had between them 22 husbands and 71 children. The children

Table 5.5 *Grandmother's children's marriages in relation to her family size and grandmaternal fitness*

Grandmaternal fitness	No. of grandmother's own children	% children's marriages (M–P)
6	9	100 (8–)
5.25	8	80 (4–1)
2.5	7	83 (5–1)
4.2 ($\bar{x}$ of 5 cases)	6	74 (14–5)
3	5	66 (2–1)
1.6 ($\bar{x}$ of 2 cases)	2	66 (2–1)
1.5	1	100 (1–)

married monogamously in 36 cases, in polyandry 10 times and two cases of two sisters marrying an incoming *mag.pa* husband are shown in the data. These marriages produced 201 children. This data set comprises not only the family sizes of marrying groups on the six estates but also the families of daughters and *mag.pa* who married out. The grandmaternal fitness calculated as one quarter the number of grandchildren (0.25g) ranges from 6.75 to 1.5 and averages 3.9.

Table 5.5 shows that the larger her own family the greater is grandmaternal fitness. It also shows that there is a higher proportion of monogamous marriages in the larger families.

Table 5.6 shows that grandmothers who themselves marry polyandrously have a (Mann-Whitney *U*-test not-significant) slightly higher

Table 5.6 *Grandmother's fitness in relation to her own marriage type*

Monogamy 1.5, 1.75, 2.25, 2.5, 5.25, 6.75	$\bar{x} = 3.33, s^2 = 1.76$
Diandry 2.5, 3.5, 3.75, 5.5, 6	$\bar{x} = 4.25, s^2 = 0.95$
Triandry 3	
Tetrandry 6	
All cases polyandry $\bar{x} = 4.32, s^2 = 1.37$	

average grandmaternal fitness than those marrying monogamously.

Table 5.7 shows the actual number of grandchildren born to completed families of three types resulting from the marriages of grandmothers' own children. The results indicate that the family sizes of the marital types and therefore the grandmaternal fitness derived from them does differ. Polyandrous family sizes, and hence the mean fitness contribution from such marriages, are greater than the family sizes and contributions of monogamous families. Ranking the fitness contributions in a Mann-Whitney U-test produces a significant result and a t-test for unrelated samples gives $t_{16} = 3.190$, $p < 0.01$. Although no statistical conclusions can be drawn it will also be noted that the two cases of sororal polygyny contributed well to grandmothers' fitness but not as well as the mean of the large number of polyandrous marriages studied. These findings are summarized in Table 5.8.

We may now attempt some account of grandpaternal fitness in the same data (Table 5.9). Since we can determine neither the proportion of their children sired by a named grandfather and his brothers in co-husbandry nor the proportion of children sired by 'full' sons and daughters and 'half' sons and daughters in their children's marriages the index of grandpaternal fitness used here is simply one quarter the number of grandchildren (g) divided by the number (f) of co-husbanding fraternal grandfathers ($0.25g/f$). Table 5.9 thus shows only a theoretical relationship between grandpaternal fitness and their own marriage type. On the above assumptions the mean fitness of grandfathers marrying monogamously is close to that for monogamous grandmothers. The theoretical mean fitness of individual polyandrous grandfathers is however much lower than that of their wife in common while a grandfather showing polygyny scores a very high fitness value. On reproductive grounds one would expect males to seek *mag.pa* or mono-

gamous marriages wherever these were socioeconomically possible and to accept polyandry only when their life circumstances constrained them to do so.

To what extent however do marrying males actually lose out reproductively by polyandrous marriage? The larger numbers of offspring born to polyandrous families suggests that to some degree the improved reproductive success of this liaison makes up for the theoretical deficit in fitness contingent upon the polyandrous choice. It is possible to calculate the extent to which a polyandrous stem marriage must be larger than a monogamous stem marriage assuming that under the monomarital principle brothers other than co-husbands do not marry on a traditional estate.

If the mean monogamous family size is x, individual fitness of a monogamous husband is $0.5x$ because he is related to each of his children by a half. A polyandrous husband sharing his wife as one of h *full* brothers will, assuming equal shares in paternity for all his brothers, have p/h children and $p(h-1)/h$ nephews and nieces (to whom he is related by 0.25) in a family of p children. This will give him a personal fitness of $0.5ph^{-1} + 0.25p(h-1)h^{-1} = p(h+1)(4h)^{-1}$. For the polyandrous husband to have fitness at least equal to that of his monogamous counterpart $p(h+1)(4h)^{-1}$ must be equal to or greater than $0.5x$. Rearranging this algebraically we have:

$$p(h+1)(4h)^{-1} > 0.5x$$
$$\Rightarrow p > 2hx(h+1)^{-1} \text{ where } p = \text{mean}$$

polyandrous family size with h co-husbands (*full* brothers) and $x = $ mean monogamous family size. In other words the family size under polyandry needs to increase at less than double the size of the monogamous equivalent if males are to do as well genetically. Consider a case in which an elder brother is likely to be the father of two children if he had his wife to himself but in which his younger brother would have none. If they both married the woman and had an equal opportunity of fathering children they would have to produce 2.66 children jointly for it to be genetically worth the elder brother's while to share his wife. By a similar argument, to benefit from joining a polyandrous marriage an otherwise unmarrying brother would need a family size of greater than $hx(h+1)^{-1}$ – hence in diandry 66% of x, in triandry 75% of x.

Table 5.7 *Grandmaternal fitness attributable to marital types of her children*

Grandmaternal fitness (0.25g)	No. of grandchildren	No. of grandchildren from each marital type and (in brackets) mean fitness of grandmother attributable to marriages of each type					
		Monogamy (n = 36)		Polyandry (n = 10)		Sororal polygyny (n = 2)	
6.75	27	9,6,0	(1.25)	6,6	(1.5)		
6	24	6,4,4,3,3,2,1,1	(0.75)				
6	24	6,4,3,3,2	(0.9)	6	(1.5)		
5.5	22	8,5,4,3,3,0	(0.92)				
5.25	21	8,4,3,1	(1.0)	5	(1.5)		
3.75	15	4,4,1	(0.75)			6	(1.5)
3.5	14	8,4,2	(1.17)				
3	12	1	(0.25)	7,4	(1.38)		
2.5	10	4,3	(0.88)	3	(0.75)		
2.5	10			7	(1.75)	3	(0.75)
2.25	9			9	(2.25)		
1.75	7			7	(1.75)		
1.5	6	6	(1.5)				
Σ	201	132		60		9	
s²	6.3	1.7		1.2			
x̄ 3.87	15.5	3.66	(0.94)	6	(1.52)	4.5	(1.13)

Table 5.8 *Summary of grandmaternal fitness in relation to the marital types of her children*

Numbers of grandmothers	13
Number of grandchildren	201
Mean number of grandchildren (range)	15.5 (6–27)
Variance (s²) in grandchildren	6.3
Mean family size of children	4.3
Number of monogamous families	36
Mean size monogamous families	3.66
Variance (s²) monogamous families	1.7
Number of polyandrous families	10
Mean size polyandrous families	6
Variance (s²) polyandrous families	1.2
Number of cases sororal polygyny	2
Mean sororal polygynous family size	4.5
% grandchildren in sample from monogamy	66%
% grandchildren in sample from polyandry	30%
% grandchildren in sample from sororal polygyny	4%
Mean fitness derived by grandmothers (n = 9) from each of their children's monogamous marriages	0.94
Mean fitness derived by grandmothers (n = 8) from each of their children's polyandrous marriages	1.51
Mean fitness derived by 2 grandmothers from each of their daughters polygynous marriages	1.13
Mean fitness differential between monogamous and polyandrous marriages	0.57

Table 5.9 *Estimated grandpaternal fitness in relation to their own marital type assuming equal access to wife in polyandry*

No. of fraternal grandfathers (f)	No. of grand-children (g)	Fitness (0.25g/f)
1 (with 2 wives)	28	7
1	27	6.75
1	10	2.5
1	9	2.25
1	6	1.5
2	24	3
2	22	2.75
2	16	2
2	14	1.75
2	10	1.25
3	12	1
4	24	1.5
x̄ monogamous grandfathers' fitness		3.25
x̄ polyandrous grandfathers' fitness		1.89
one case successive monogamy		7

The data from the six estates near Leh show that for 13 completed monogamous *khang.chen* families the mean number of children was 3.7 while the average size of six diandrous, three triandrous and one tetrandrous families was 5.2. Applying our formula the polyandrous family sizes would have to be greater than 4.8, 5.4 and 5.8 for diandrous, triandrous and tetrandrous families respectively in order to prevent a loss of fitness by co-husbands. Furthermore from our data we see that the average family size under polyandry must be greater than $(6 \times 4.8 + 3 \times 5.4 + 1 \times 5.8)/10 = 5.1$. Since the actual mean value obtained was 5.2, co-husbands marrying polyandrously do not therefore on this use of evidence show a loss in fitness compared with a man marrying monogamously under the monomarital principle (one stem family marriage only, full brothers do not marry except within the stem family).

Unfortunately this inference, based upon a comparison of means, cannot be adequately supported since the analysis of variance on our small samples did not demonstrate that the populations from which these means derive are statistically different. If however we allow for the fact that the monomarital principle is often only faultily applied and that some marriages in *khang. chung* do occur, then, on this less stringent basis, we can calculate that from the mean of all monogamous marriages (3.1) polyandrous marriages would have to yield 4.4 children for co-husbands to achieve a comparable fitness. While this estimate ignores any possible inclusive fitness resulting from interactions between *khang.chen* and *khang.chung*, it is based on comparing means from significantly different samples. The actual figure (5.2) does greatly exceed the required one and our data does therefore support our general proposition.

The result of this analysis suggests that any loss of fitness for individual males under polyandry compared with monomarital monogamy could be much less than might be supposed. The actual value of a marital choice for an individual male is however constrained by many factors – his birth order position, his age, the size of the family of older relatives, the size of the land holding and its productivity. The prime concern of the *pha.spun* is to ensure a marriage to the elder son on an estate so that the estate lineage and farm occupancy may be continued. The number of brothers co-marrying under the traditional system may have been contingent upon *pha.spun* decisions relating potential resources on an estate to the labour needed to exploit them. Our results do suggest that for younger sons co-marrying with an elder brother the fitness that may result could, given equal access to the wife, be as good as that of a single son marrying monogamously. Of course if brothers are in some form of competition for

access to the wife their fitness differential might then be greatly increased. Furthermore, were all the brothers to marry monogamously their inclusive fitness under unconstrained circumstances could well exceed that in polyandry.

Data in Aziz' study (1978) show that age differences between co-husbands can often be large (see Crook and Crook 1988). If the older brother marries early in his reproductive years he is likely to be at least initially more mature socially and sexually than his brothers, especially the more junior ones. Furthermore, the wife is in some cases considerably older than her younger husbands. Since reproduction starts on marriage the advantages of age may imply that most of the early children in the marriage are sired by the eldest father rather than his teenage brothers. The tradition of ascribing equal paternity is probably a fiction to improve the family atmosphere. A wife probably has a good idea as to who the father of a child is but does not discuss this in public and certainly not with these investigators.

The reproductive advantage of the elder brother can also be increased by the elimination from co-husbandry of the brother nearest to him in age. We know that the most frequent birth order position for a monk in two Zangskari monasteries is the second place (Crook and Shakya 1988b). The reproductive dominance of elder brothers thus seems highly plausible and a tendency for his collaborators to opt for a second marriage later in life is not surprising. There are a number of records in our data both from Leh and from sTongde showing that younger brothers tend to separate from the polyandrous group later in life and may take wives of their own.

It seems likely, then, that the fitness of brothers in polyandry is not equal because the assumption of equal access to the wife may often be invalid. The social emphasis on primogeniture and the dominance of an elder brother may therefore correlate with his higher fitness as well as his greater responsibility in the running of the estate.

Concluding discussion: the comparative study of marital systems in stratified societies

Polyandry in Tibet probably arose in the context of the monomarital principle regulated, as at present in our research area of Zangskar, through the deliberations of elder kin in a patrilineal group of families. The provision of a single marriage in each generation ensures the continuity of an agricultural estate with sufficient labour in a community with a birth rate lowered by polyandry and monasticism. This adaptation to particular socioeconomic conditions of montane desert agriculture with a low carrying capacity and needs for over-wintering storage, breaks down with the provision of alternative additional sources of income to the estate which thus allows the emergence of separate monogamous households still held together in estate collaboration. Since polyandrous families tend to be larger than monogamous ones our analysis suggests that men who marry polyandrously may not necessarily lower their individual fitness greatly. Nonetheless between brothers fitness is likely to be biased in favour of elder brothers.

This examination of polyandrous marriage in Tibetan society complements Mildred Dickemann's study (1979a, 1979b) of polygyny in hypergynous stratified societies. Both in Tibet and in the traditional Indian and Chinese systems discussed by Dickemann complex late medieval systems of peasant agriculture supported a political superstructure of considerable complexity, yet the marital systems within these societies developed in very different ways.

Mildred Dickemann put forward a model of the socio-demographic process responsible for polygyny, social stratification and infanticide in medieval Indian, Chinese and European class ranked societies and based her arguments on socio-ecological considerations in ethological literature (Verner and Wilson 1966, Orians 1969, Trivers and Willard 1973). Under ecologically and sociologically insecure conditions powerful houses offered a buffer against bad fortune under poor conditions, and great wealth under good ones. The acquisition of positions of power enabled a man to offer conditions under which women could rear children safely and which would also maximize his own reproductive success through increasing the number of his wives. The wealth differential was associated with hypergyny (women marrying up society) and the payment of dowry enabling them to do so. The upward accumulation of women at the 'top' of the society led to the establishment in extreme cases of vast harems and the elimination of unwanted girls through infanticide. Hypergyny also produced a shortage of women in the lower regions of society where brideprice often had to be paid to obtain a wife. Many men never did so – producing a large population of low class unmarried males augmented by a fallout of unmarried men from the upper ranks. Dickemann pointed out that the underlying ground rules for the movement of women lay in the custom of controlling fertilizations by choosing for marriage males of households in which female reproductive success and that of their offspring could be at a predictable optimum. Male power to maximize their fertilization rate thus links with female choice of powerful males who provide reproductive security. In spite of the inevitable coercion and restriction on female behaviour and the massive amount of infanticide involved in such a system, it became the socially accepted norm of entire societies expressing the effect of wealth differential on intra-sexual competition in both genders.

The widespread occurrence of this medieval pattern of social stratification, hypergyny and male primogeniture in inheritance may also reflect the rather obvious fact that the inheritance of wealth, particularly of sources of production, is likely to enhance security for reproduction over several generations. In terms of Hamilton's (1964) inclusive fitness theory an individual can 'maximise the fitness enhancing potential of his wealth if he [sic] transfers it to descendants who have inherited the highest concentration of his genes' (Hartung 1976, 1982). Similarly among descendants of equal relationship to the ancestor the fitness enhancement provided by inherited wealth will maximize when transferred to descendants whose reproductive success is most dependent upon wealth. Hartung also suggests that, since males have potentially higher reproductive variance than females, inheritance will benefit the donor most if transferred to males – and gives reasons for supposing that a male's fitness may be most enhanced if inheritable wealth is passed down patrilineally.

We suggest that polygynous and polyandrous marital arrangements in stratified agricultural societies characterize two broadly different socioeconomic situations which are also in part contingent upon basic ecological contrasts. The polygynous system described by Dickemann is adapted to a hierarchically organized society in climates in which eco-climatic conditions produce periods of plenty with the recurrence of disasters (floods, famines, etc.) – a situation in which the possibility of rapid reproduction and expansion is produced by recurrent falls in population well below the carrying capacity of the environment in its friendlier phases. The polygynous family is part of a social system shaped by r selection – as evolutionary ecologists would express it. By contrast, the monomarital system with polyandry is adapted to a situation of low carrying capacity and, when compared to the polygynous one, can be said to be K selected. As with other K selected systems there is an emphasis on collaboration and altruism.

Jack Goody's work on medieval European society (1983) points to the effect of advanced agricultural techniques in a temperate Europe of socially stratified nation states, where rich agricultural resources surplus to subsistance requirements became available for marketing and storage within a commodity exchange economy. Here the emphasis focuses on monogamy and the splitting of inheritance between offspring of both genders on the death of the parents – a result also promoted by ecclesiastical policies aimed at draining wealth away from extended patrilineal families attempting the intergenerational maintenance of wealth.

We therefore now have comparative accounts of three types of marital organization in stratified societies suggesting a complex adaptive radiation of social form under economic and social constraints specific to particular ecological conditions. Further work may lead to a general theory of human marital systems in preindustrial societies.

Summary

1. Fraternal polyandry is a rare form of human marriage. In the Tibetan culture zone it is found only in populations of land-owning or tenanting farmers engaged in both crop agriculture and animal husbandry.

2. The system of farm inheritance follows a monomarital principle whereby one marriage is contracted per generation on the agricultural estate. In the traditional society such marriages are often polyandrous. On the marriage of the eldest son (with or without co-husbands) the parents move to a smaller house on the estate.

3. A model of the socio-ecology of estate families living under the monomarital principle with polyandry in Zangskar shows how this practice, together with monasticism, may function to control birth rate. The practice is interpreted as analogous to K adaptations in other animals in relation to an environment of low carrying capacity.

4. Circumstances that generate an economic release for a farming population lead to changes in marital and inheritance systems towards monogamy and estate division on the death of parents. A field-study from Ladakh is summarized.

5. Quantitative assessments based on recently updated genealogies from six estates originally surveyed by Prince Peter of Greece in 1938 show that completed polyandrous family sizes are larger than monogamous ones and that marriages in the main estate house produce more children than marriages elsewhere. It follows that a parental or patrilineal strategy marrying daughters into the main estate domus with polyandry is effective in maintaining reproductive fitness. We demonstrate that the effect continues into the grandparental generation.

6. Our assessments suggest that, due to the large size of polyandrous families, co-husbanding brothers with (theoretical) equal access to their wife in common may not show a loss in fitness when compared to a single brother marrying monogamously. However, the high probability of a differential access to the wife, contingent upon the greater age and maturity of the eldest brother early in the marriage, means that a substantial reproductive variance between marrying brothers is likely. A junior brother's strategy should thus be to prefer monogamous marriage wherever this is economically possible – and upon economic release this tends to be the case.

7. This system of polyandrous marriage is compared with polygynous and monogamous marital systems described for other stratified preindustrial societies. We now have a sound basis for further studies on the adaptive radiation of these culture-controlled systems in relation to economic and ecological conditions.

Acknowledgements

Without the heartfelt participation of our Ladakhi friends this analysis would not have been possible. To them we are greatly indebted. We also thank all members of the Bristol University expeditions to Ladakh in 1977, 1980 and 1981 for their ideas and company. Moonis Raza and Harjit Singh of the Centre for the Study of Regional Development at the Shri Jawaharlal Nehru University, New Delhi, aided us greatly with collaboration, advice and information without which our project could not have been successful. Clive Frankish helped us with the statistical analyses and Monique Borgerhoff Mulder drew our attention to the importance of grandmothers. We owe the inspiration for this paper to Peter, Prince of Greece and Denmark and Melvyn C. Goldstein whose valuable studies on Tibetan society are the basis for our work and to Mildred Dickemann's provocative analysis of Asian marital systems. The field research discussed here was generously supported by the Harry Frank Guggenheim Foundation, the Nuffield Foundation, Maison des Sciences de l'Homme, and Bristol University.

References

Alexander, R. D. (1974) The evolution of social behaviour. *Annual Review of Ecology and Systematics*, 5, 323–83.

Alexander, R. D. (1979) Evolution and culture. In Chagnon, N. and Irons, W. (ed.).

Aziz, B. N. (1978) *Tibetan Frontier Families*. New Delhi: Vikas.

Berghe, P. van den and Barash, D. P. (1977) Inclusive fitness and human family structure. *American Anthropologist*, 79, 809–23.

Braun, M. (1980) *Feste in Ladakh*. Gratz.

Chagnon, N. and Irons, W. (eds.) (1979) *Evolutionary Biology and Human Social Behavior: An Anthropological Perspective*. North Scituate, MA: Duxbury Press.

Crook, J. H. (1980) *The Evolution of Human Consciousness*. Oxford: Oxford University Press.

Crook, J. H. (1988a) Social organisation and personal identity in sTongde. In Crook, J. H. and Osmaston, H. (eds.).

Crook, J. H. (1988b) Zangskari attitudes. In Crook, J. H. and Osmaston, H. O. (eds.).

Crook, J. H. and Crook, S. J. (1988) Explaining Tibetan polyandry: socio-cultural, demographic and biological perspectives. In Crook, J. H. and Osmaston, H. O. (eds.).

Crook, J. H. and Osmaston, H. (eds.) (1988) *Himalayan Buddhist Villages*. Warminster: Aris and Phillips.

Crook, J. H. and Shakya, T. (1983) Six families of Leh. In *Recent Research on Ladakh*, eds. Kan-

towsky, D. and Sanders, R. Munchen: Schriftenreihe Internationales Asienforum. 1.

Crook, J. H. and Shakya, T. (1988a) Six families of Leh (with genealogico). In Crook, J. H. and Osmaston, H. D. (eds.).

Crook, J. H. and Shakya, T. (1988b) Monastic communities in Zangskar: location, function and organisation. In Crook, J. H. and Osmaston, H. (eds.)

Dhargyay, E. K. (1982) *Tibetan Village Communities: Structure and Change*. Warminster: Aris and Phillips.

Dickemann, M. (1979a) Female infanticide, reproductive strategies and social stratification. In Chagnon, N. and Irons, W. (eds.).

Dickemann, M. (1979b) The ecology of mating systems in hypergynous dowry societies. *Social Science Information*, 18(2), 163–95.

Dunbar, R. (1985) *Reproductive Decisions: An Economic Analysis of Gelada Baboon Social Strategies*. Princeton: Princeton University Press.

Durham, W. H. (1979) Towards a co-evolutionary theory of human biology and culture. In Chagnon, N. and Irons, W. (eds.)

Fürer-Haimendorf, C. von (1964) *The Sherpas of Nepal*. London: John Murray.

Goldstein, M. (1971a) Taxation and the structure of a Tibetan village. *Central Asiatic Journal*, 15, 1–27.

Goldstein, M. (1971b) The balance between centralisation and decentralisation in the traditional Tibetan political system. *Central Asiatic Journal*, 170.

Goldstein, M. (1976) Fraternal polyandry and fertility in a high Himalayan in N.W. Nepal. *Human Ecology*, 4(3), 223–33.

Goldstein, M. (1979) The circulation of estates in Tibet. Reincarnation, land and politics. *Journal of Asian Studies*, 32(3), 445–55.

Goody, J. (1983) *The Development of the Family and Marriage in Europe*. Cambridge: Cambridge University Press.

Grafen, A. (1982) How not to measure inclusive fitness. *Nature*, 298, 425–6.

Grist, N. (1980) Polyandry, marriage and land tenure. *Cambridge University Expedition Reports on Ladakh*, 1977–1979, pp. 230–44.

Haldane, J. B. S. (1956) The argument from animals to man: an examination of its validity for anthropology. *Journal of the Royal Anthropological Institute*, 86, 1–14.

Hamilton, W. D. (1964) The genetical evolution of social behaviour. Parts 1 and 2. *Journal of Theoretical Biology*, 7, 1–52.

Hartung, J. (1976) On natural selection and the inheritance of wealth. *Current Anthropology*, 17(4), 607–22.

Hartung, J. (1982) Polygyny and inheritance of wealth. *Current Anthropology*, 23(1), 1–12.

Irons, W. (1979) Natural selection, adaptation and human social behaviour. In Chagnon, N. and Irons, W. (eds.).

Jenni, D. A. (1974) Evolution of polyandry in birds. *American Zoology*, 14, 129–44.

Kummer, H. (1977) Rules of dyad and group formation among Gelada baboons (*Therapithecas gelada*). *Symposium 5th Congress International Primatogical Society*, 1975, pp. 129–60. Tokyo: Japan Science Press.

Lopreato, J. (1984) *Human Nature and Biocultural Evolution*. Boston: Allen and Unwin.

MacArthur, R. H. and Wilson, E. O. (1967) *The Theory of Island Biogeography*. Princeton: Princeton University Press.

Orians, G. H. (1969) On the evolution of mating systems in birds and mammals. *American Naturalist*, **103**, 589–603.

Ortner, S. (1978) *Sherpas Through Their Rituals*. New York: Cambridge University Press.

Peter, Prince of Greece and Denmark (1963) *A Study of Polyandry*. The Hague: Mouton.

Pianka, E. R. (1974) *Evolutionary Ecology*. New York: Harper and Row.

Plotkin, H. C. and Odling-Smee, F. J. (1981) A multiple level model of evolution and its implications for sociobiology. *Behavioural and Brain Sciences*, **4**(2), 225–68.

Surkhang, W. (1966) Tax measurement and Lag'don tax. *Bulletin of Tibetology*, **31**, 15–28. Gangtok.

Trivers, R. and Willard, D. (1973) Natural selection of parental ability to vary the sex-ratio of offspring. *Science*, **179**, 90–2.

Verner, J. and Wilson, M. F. (1966) The influence of habitats on mating systems of North American passerine birds. *Ecology*, **47**, 143–7.

Wilson, E. O. (1975) *Sociobiology: The New Synthesis*. Harvard: Belknafe Press.

Pathogen stress and polygyny in humans

Introduction

Environmental extremeness and unpredictability of various sorts have been argued to be important selective pressures on a variety of life history and behavioral traits (e.g. Levins 1968). The impacts of environmental extremeness (the ecological correlate of risk, as it increases the probability of failure) and unpredictability on reproductive variance are not yet well understood, perhaps because they have rarely been treated in a sufficiently well-defined or restricted way that allows hypotheses to be tested. In this paper, I test hypotheses about the effects of one set of biologically-imposed risks and uncertainties, risks imposed by particular types of serious pathogens, on the degree of polygyny in human societies.

Pathogens and the evolution of sexuality

Unpredictably changing environments seem likely to favor the production of variable offspring. Williams (1975) argued that when the environmental conditions to be faced by offspring cannot be predicted by parents (e.g. when offspring disperse to new habitats), the pressures favoring maximum genetic representation in each offspring – leading to the evolution of sexuality.

[1] Evolution and Human Behavior Program and School of Natural Resources, University of Michigan, Ann Arbor, MI 48109, USA

Bell (1982), in part based on Maynard Smith (1971), argued that the conditions producing the appropriate type of unpredictability were stringent: the only suitably unpredictable environments are those in which the fitness of parent and offspring genotypes are always correlated, but negatively (also see Jaenike 1978). Bell termed such environments *capricious*, and argued that they were rare.

Hamilton (1980) and Hamilton *et al.* (1981) proposed that these criteria were met by a particular source of unpredictability: that of serious parasites or pathogens with very short generation times. Such pathogens would produce rapid changes in the direction of selection favoring offspring genotypes different from parental genotypes in succeeding generations (cf. van Valen 1973). Bell (1982:143–57) constructed a similar argument for predators and prey.

Pathogens and sexual selection

Hamilton and Zuk (1982) advanced another possible role for certain kinds of pathogens in sexual selection. Mate choice, and thus signalling of fitness, acquire great importance in the presence of certain kinds of serious pathogens – those with: 1. a longer cycling time than those required for the evolution of sex (e.g. long enough to produce a positive parent–offspring fitness correlation but short enough to maintain genetic variance in fitness); and 2. an acute phase coupled with persistence in chronic form, either as an infection actually latent, or as prolonged debilitating after-effects. Death of potential mates obviates choice; complete recovery after the acute phase leaves no criteria on which to determine resistance. As Hamilton and Zuk noted, the available evidence suggests that pathogen resistance may be permanently heritable, and static equilibria due to fitness overdominance are unlikely. If this is true, variance in fitness as a mate should not diminish over time.

Their argument leads to two predictions:

1. The more prevalent and severe are serious pathogens, the more heritable variability should exist in potential mates. The importance of mate choice should lead in such cases to increased polygyny.
2. Signalling of fitness should be more strongly favored the more serious the pathogen stress.

Hamilton and Zuk tested the second hypothesis, using data for five genera of protozoan and one nematode blood parasites, in North American passerines. Considering both monogamous and polygynous species, they found a series of weak, but highly significant, associations, supporting the second hypothesis. Most of the passerines are monogamous, and this tends to restrict the variance on which natural selection can act. Because the effects of signalling and variations in health are greater for males in polygynous species than in monogamous ones (e.g. Wade and Arnold 1980), one expects a stronger pattern in polygynous species (hypothesis No. 1); however, this is not necessarily so. Polygyny opens the way for the full force of 'runaway' sexual selection, and this proceeds independent of utilitarian objectives (e.g. Wade and Arnold 1980). Thus the overall picture may be confounded. However, females are expected to convert monogamy to polygyny precisely when there are special advantages to mating with 'best' males, as will be the case, according to Hamilton and Zuk, when pathogen stress is severe.

Human ornamentation is more than simple augmentation of signals of health and sexual fitness. Many signals appear to be complex and send a variety of messages, including wealth and social status; few or none can be shown to relate directly and exclusively to physical condition and/or heritable pathogen resistance. Because humans do use ornaments to accentuate sexually attractive features, I include it in the analysis, but expectations of its correlation with pathogen stress for humans are, in fact, unclear.

In this paper I test the possibility that the predicted trends are detectable in patterns of human marriage system, mate choice and ornamentation, using data on polygyny, information in ornaments, and seven pathogens from 93 human societies.

Methods

The sample comprised the 93 odd-numbered societies of the standard cross-cultural sample (Murdock and White 1969; Figures 6.1 and 6.2; Appendix A). This sample is stratified for geographic distribution and language group, and represents a sample for which available ethnographies are by qualified ethnographers resident with the society for a substantial period of time.

6. Pathogen stress and polygyny

Initial choice of pathogens was determined by surveying the literature on serious pathogens for which good worldwide distribution maps were available, so that accurate codes could be derived for presence and severity of exposure for the societies in the sample. Pathogens were then examined for the following characteristics: acute, possibly fatal initial stage of infection; and long-term chronic effects, either in debilitation or in likelihood of repeated acute episodes. Only pathogens meeting both criteria were retained for analysis.

Pathogens chosen were: leishmanias (*Leishmania tropica, L. braziliensis, L. donovani*); trypanosomes (*Trypanosoma gambiense, T. rhodesiense*); malaria (*Plasmodium vivax, P. ovale, P. malariae, P. falciparum*); schistosomes (*Schistosoma japonicum, S. mansoni, S. haematobium*); the filariae, a group of blood- and tissue-dwelling nematodes (*Wucheria bancrofti, Brugia malayi*); spirochetes (*Borrelia duttoni, B. recurrentis, Treponema*); and leprosy.

For each pathogen, a three-level code was constructed: 1 = absent or not recorded; 2 = present, no indication of severity; and 3 = present and serious, widespread or endemic. Codes for each pathogen were constructed from data in Beaver *et al.* (1984), Markell and Voge (1981), Faust and Russell (1964), and maps of the American Geographical Society of New York (1950, 1955), constructed from WHO data. When data existed from more than one time period, data from the earlier period, closer to the time of the ethnographer records, were given preference. For all ethnographies since 1800, tests were run to see if there was any relationship among date of ethnography (i.e., time between ethnographic data and pathogen data), pathogen load, and degree of polygyny. Because there is no reason to predict a relationship with any particular pathogen

Figure 6.1 Marriage system (Low, unpublished) of the 93 odd-numbered societies of the standard cross-cultural sample. triangle = polygandry, diamond = monogamy, plus sign = <20% polygyny, open circle = 21–40% polygyny, filled circle = >40% polygyny.

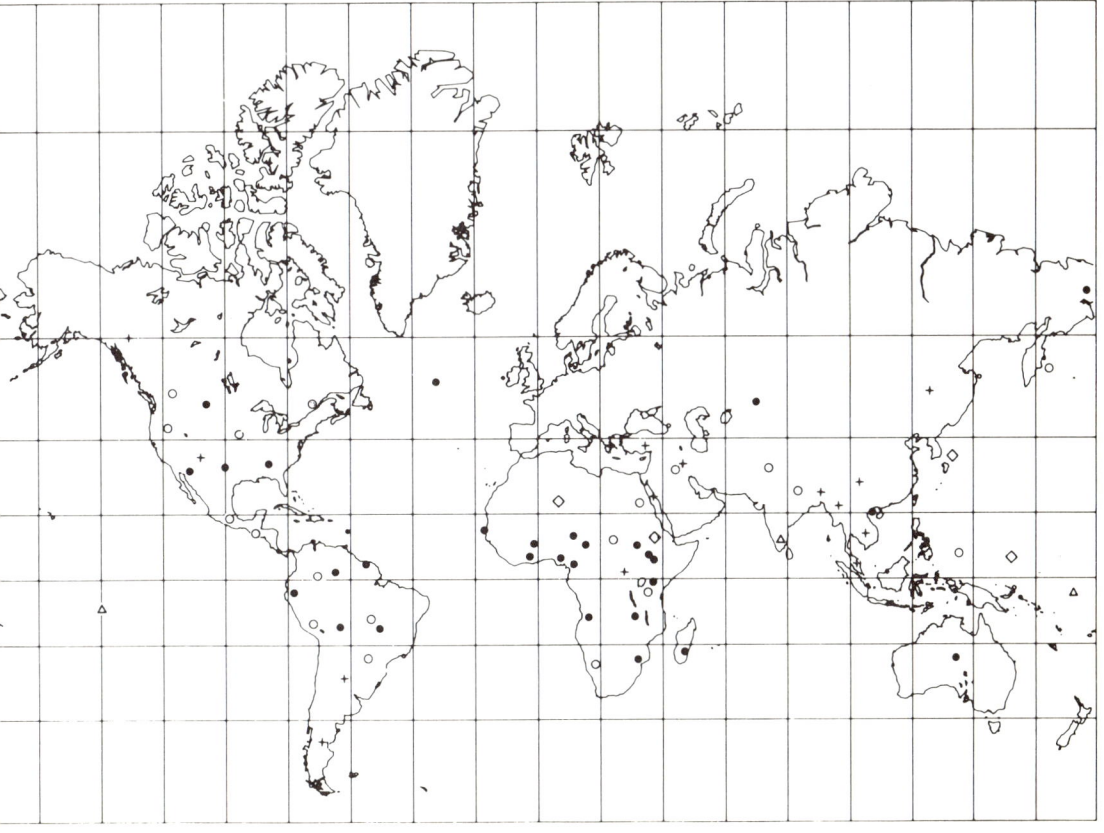

and signalling or polygyny, a combined measure of seriousness of total pathogen exposure was constructed; this measure was the sum of the codes for risk of each pathogen (Appendix B).

Several measures of polygyny exist for humans, nd although they correlate strongly with each other (Low 1987), their relationships to ecological variables are unknown. I therefore tested all available measures: whether multiple spouses occur, independent of the stated societal preference (Whyte 1978:V31); percentage of men polygynously married (Murdock and Wilson 1972, Whyte 1978:V32); percentage of women polygynously married (Hartung 1982); percentage of men and women polygynously married (Low 1987); and maximum harem size (Betzig 1986).

The amount of information in sexual signals was taken from Low (1979) or coded using the same rules by naive coders. These included information signalled about: male pubertal

Figure 6.2 Level of pathogen stress in the 93 odd-numbered societies of the standard cross-cultural sample. Triangle = low, diamond = moderate, plus sign = high.

status, female marital and pubertal status, and female ornaments reflecting the husband's status. Information given by male signals of own status were not used in analysis, because no societies were found in which men did not signal their power, wealth, or status in the group. A score summing all information given by signals was constructed to reflect the amount of information given by sexual signals in each society. Measures of women's ability to control resources or hold political office were taken from Whyte (1978).

Non-parametric statistical tests were used, as no assumption could be made about the distribution of the data. Spearman's ρ (Conover 1980) was calculated for each pathogen and the combined pathogen risk versus measures of polygyny and signalling. To test whether the seriousness of pathogen risk differed among societies with different marriage systems (polyandry, monogamy, polygyny) the Kruskal–Wallis test statistic was calculated (Conover 1980). To examine patterns of association, the Goodman–Kruskal

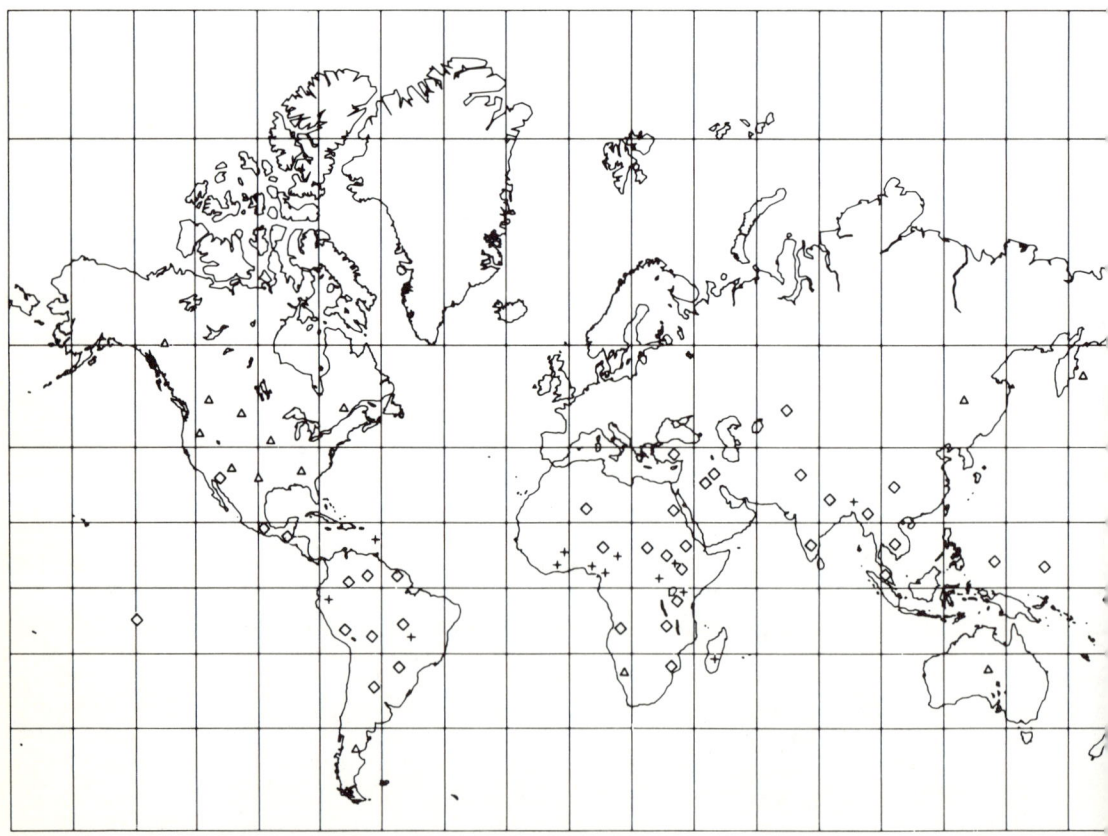

Table 6.1 *Relationship between pathogen stress and measures of polygyny. Whyte V31 and Murdock and Wilson are measures of preferred marriage form, reflecting percent of men married polygynously; Hartung measured percent of women polygynously married; Low is a combined measure of percent of men and percent of women polygynously married; Whyte V32 reflects whether multiple spouses are known regardless of marriage form preference; and Betzig measured maximum harem size. Differences in the sign of ρ simply reflect that some codes gave high values to polygyny and low values to polyandry, while others did the converse*

Variable	n	G–K γ	τ–β	SE	Signif.	ρ
Whyte V31	93	−0.2140	−0.1676	0.0837	0.0455	−0.2072
Murdock and Wilson	93	0.3157	0.2363	0.0853	0.0055	0.2934
Hartung	37	0.3186	0.2767	0.1285	0.0317	0.3536
Low	93	−0.1975	0.1614	0.0820	0.0492	0.2104
Whyte V32	92	−0.4644	−0.2703	0.0874	0.0019	−0.3279
Betzig	50	0.1440	0.1130	0.1161	0.3366	0.1553

Table 6.2 *Relationships between group size and polygyny, and group size and pathogen risk*

Variable	G–K γ	τ–β	SE	Signif.	ρ
Whyte V31	0.0803	0.0619	0.1099	0.5798	0.0692
Murdock and Wilson	−0.1093	−0.0790	0.1117	0.4854	−0.0964
Hartung	0.0463	0.0375	0.1606	0.8353	0.0423
Low	−0.0797	−0.0634	0.1072	0.5610	−0.0879
Whyte V32	−0.1025	−0.0595	0.1145	0.6110	−0.0679
Betzig	0.4426	0.3407	0.1405	0.0152	0.3831
Pathogen stress (analytic)	0.1119	0.0977	0.1026	0.3465	0.1299
Pathogen stress (3-level code)	0.1518	0.1081	0.1144	0.3504	0.1328

γ was divided by the standard error for each relationship, and the distribution of the measure was examined. On a null hypothesis of no association, a standard normal distribution with a mean of zero is expected (Goodman and Kruskal 1963).

Results and discussion

Pathogens and polygyny

There is a significant positive relationship between the total seriousness of pathogen exposure and the degree of polygyny, no matter how it is measured (Table 6.1). The ρ values range from 0.35 (percent of women polygynously married; Hartung 1982) to 0.207 (percent of marriages polygynous; Whyte 1978). The sign of the ρ value is irrelevant; it merely reflects the fact that some authors (Whyte V31, V32) assigned low values to polygyny and high values to polyandry, while others did the reverse.

There is no relationship between the total seriousness of pathogen risk and the intensity of polygyny (maximum harem size) (Table 6.1).

In non-stratified non-human polygynous species, this result would be surprising. In humans, however, large maximum harem size is associated with stratification, perquisites, and societal constraints resulting in a small proportion of men monopolizing the reproduction of the majority of women (Betzig 1986). It would indeed be unexpected for pathogen stress to create a situation in which all but a small proportion of men were rendered unsuitable as mates.

The modes of transmission of these pathogens suggest a possible alternative hypothesis: that the parasites may be correlated with large group size, or high population density. If polygyny also correlates with large group size, the reported correlations, even if reasonable, may not reflect any causal relationship. However, pathogen stress shows no significant correlation with group size (Table 6.2). Further, no measure of degree of polygyny increases with group size (Table 6.2); maximum harem size, which shows a relationship with group size, shows no pattern with pathogen stress.

Another possibility is a historical one. Perhaps the patterns of contact between Europeans and

Table 6.3 *Patterns of polygyny and pathogen stress. Both show important geographic patterns, but they do not co-vary*

	Polygyny ranks	n	Pathogen ranks
Africa	5	20	5
Mediterranean	1	6	2
Insular Pacific	2	33	3
North America	3	18	1
South America	4	16	4
	K–W = 26.5 93		K–W = 44.8
	p = 0.0000		p = 0.0000

1 = lowest
5 = highest

non-technological societies result in a meaningless correlation: Europeans discouraged polygyny in all societies with which they established contact, and they tended both to establish contact in less parasitized areas of the world earlier than in more heavily parasitized areas, and to introduce medical countermeasures. Although this hypothesis is more difficult to test, an examination of the dates of earliest available ethnographies does not suggest any pattern. There is no correlation between the date of the ethnography and the marriage system reported, even when only ethnographies since 1800 are considered ($n = 83$, $\rho = -0.0614$, $p = 0.61$).

Finally, pathogen stress and polygyny might simply co-vary geographically. Both show important geographic patterns, but do not co-vary (Table 6.3).

Parasites and advertisement

Hamilton and Zuk (1982) argued that in the presence of unpredictability arising from serious diseases or parasites, individuals are favored who advertise their fitness as mates. In the bird species they tested, as well as in many vertebrates, sexual signals are likely to be morphological (e.g. color) or behavioral (e.g. song) and conspicuous in either case – implying both energy cost and risk. Human cultural augmentation is considerably more complex, and may be very subtle (e.g. Low 1979).

When the amount of information given by human sexual signals was tested against the degree of pathogen risk, the results were only marginally significant ($n = 53$, $\rho = 0.255$, $\pi = 0.07$). These results may reflect the fact that,

in complex human societies, there are a variety of reasons why an individual may be more or less suitable as a mate, in addition to simple health and vigor. Inspection of the codes suggests that this may be true: a large part of the reason there is little trend in signalling is that men in almost all societies signal wealth or power status, whether or not pathogen risk is high (Low 1979). Thus, while pathogens may be a selective force favoring advertisement, they are clearly only one of several forces. Advertisement signalling worth as a mate (wealth, status) directly, independent of any heritable resistance to pathogens, appears to have been strongly favored.

When the measures were distributed in the same way as Hamilton and Zuk's data (Goodman–Kruskal gamma divided by standard error, and grouped), male marital pubertal status and female reflection of male wealth/power are not distributed with a mean of zero – suggesting that a positive relationship may exist. These data should be interpreted cautiously, however, as the measure was designed for large samples (Goodman and Kruskal 1963), and data were only coded for seven pathogens.

Mate choice: for what?

The results suggest non-random patterns of mate choice. Mate choice exists in both resource-based and non-resource-based animal mating systems (reviewed by Trivers 1985). In resource-based non-human systems, the choice appears to depend largely on the quality of the resource; a female seal, for example, chooses an area of beach on which to give birth and, willy-nilly, is mated by the male controlling that area (Le Bouef 1974). In some resource-based polygynous systems, the resource (e.g. territory) provides benefits for offspring as well as functioning to attract mates, and thus represents parental as well as mating effort. Female choice in such systems is even more stringently tied to the quality of the resource: it is not uncommon for some males, holding rich resources, to be polygynous, while other territorial males can attract no females, or only one. This 'polygyny threshold' (Verner and Willson 1966, Orians 1969) is set by territory quality. Maximum harem size is limited by the costs of resource defense.

6. Pathogen stress and polygyny

Association between polygyny and pathogen stress leaves unresolved the questions of whether choice is made on the basis of (1) heritable true fitness in pathogen resistance alone, (2) resource control ability as a result of such fitness, or (3) resource control as a favored trait in its own right for reasons independent of heritability of pathogen resistance (i.e. because offspring can be better endowed). In the first case, we expect a pattern with polygyny and pathogen stress, but not resource control; in the second, we expect pathogen stress, polygyny, and unequal resource control to co-vary; in the third case, we expect a pattern between resource control and polygyny, but not pathogen stress. It is difficult to test directly for these relationships, but some inferences are possible.

If the variance in men's number of wives arises from choice based on resource control, then use of resources in reproductive effort should increase with the degree of polygyny. The use of some form of payment by men (bride price or bride service), as opposed to the exchange of goods or women, or the use of dowry, is associated with the occurrence of polygyny ($n = 77$, K–W $= 7.94$, $p = 0.019$). Within polygynous societies, bride price is used more than predicted in highly polygynous societies, and less than expected in low and moderately polygynous societies ($n = 71$, df $= 4$, $\chi^2 = 9.46$, $p = 0.05$, $\varphi = 0.258$). These results are consistent with Hartung's (1982) findings that inheritance is male-biased in polygynous societies, and suggest that when men can accumulate resources, they use those resources for mating effort (cf. Dickemann 1982, Hartung 1983, Flinn and Low 1986).

If resource control simply reflects the variation in men's health (i.e. healthy men can garner more resources) then the use of some form of marriage payment (demonstration of resource control as mating effort) should be positively associated with disease and/or pathogen stress; if resource control is, in and of itself an advantage, no such association is predicted. There appears to be no association ($n = 70$, $\chi^2 = 8.42$, $p = 0.39$, $\varphi = 0.24$).

In some non-human animals, quite specific preferences by females for males of particular genotypes have been demonstrated (Partridge 1980, Lenington 1983); females act as if choosing males with 'good genes.' It is also generally assumed that in non-paternal species, male control of resources reflects a successful genotype and good current health of males, though few or no appropriate tests have actually been done, and heritability of ability to control resources, predicted by the theory, is not clear (cf. Taylor and Williams 1982).

In humans, preference for particular males resulting in polygyny is associated both with existence of serious pathogens and with the use of resources. As just noted, resource use does not appear to be directly associated with pathogen risk. Selection of mates with considerable resources seems likely to be favored not simply because resource control can only be accomplished by a male with 'good genes' but for other reasons – the most obvious being increased investment in offspring. In fact, the complexities of human societies (reciprocity, friendship, coalitions, etc.) make it unlikely that resource control ever functions, as it may in non-human lekking systems (in which only symbolic resources are controlled), simply as a reflection of heritable resistance to pathogens.

Mate choice: who chooses?

The specificity of mate choice is extreme in humans (e.g. Alexander 1979, Flinn and Low 1986). In a majority of societies for which data exist, a man's 'preferred' mate is specified as one of several types of cross-cousin or a specific parallel-cousin. Further, while females in other species appear simply to choose mates, in humans it is seldom clear that a woman independently chooses a man she prefers among competing males; in many societies, a woman's parents or a coalition of her male relatives are involved in the alliance negotiations (Whyte 1978, Flinn and Low 1986). In fact, in many societies, men control the reproductive destinies of not only their mates (as in many polygynous species), but their daughters, sisters, and nieces (Flinn and Low 1986); in such societies, while mate choice exists, *female* choice may be virtually absent, or strongly compromised.

To some degree, a woman's reproductive interests and those of her male kin overlap, but they are unlikely to converge completely. In societies in which there are few resources, the convergence of interests should be more complete. In societies in which men control considerable resources, a woman's best interests are served when her mate's resources are concentrated on her and her own children; a conflict exists if he chooses to expend resources on other wives and their children or if her male relatives can, in the marriage arrangements, divert some of those resources to their own ends (Flinn and Low 1986).

If polygyny results from the simple exertion of mate choice by women, one predicts it to be associated with evidence of women's ability to be independent. The degree of polygyny is not associated with women's ability to hold political office ($n = 74$, $\chi^2 = 7.5$, $p = 0.47$, $\varphi = 0.23$), to be active in community affairs ($n = 62$, $\chi^2 = 4.18$, $p = 0.38$, $\varphi = 0.26$), or to control the use of dwellings ($n = 72$, $\chi^2 = 13.99$, $p = 0.30$, $\varphi = 0.25$). Further, it is not associated with women's authority in domestic matters ($n = 89$, $\chi^2 = 6.86$, $p = 0.87$, $\varphi = 0.16$) or women's ability to hold leadership positions in the kin group ($n = 53$, $\chi^2 = 2.01$, $p = 0.73$, $\varphi = 0.19$). The degree of polygyny is negatively associated with women's ability to inherit property ($n = 63$, $\chi^2 = 20.89$, $p = 0.002$; $\varphi = 0.33$; $\rho = -0.255$, $p = 0.03$). On the other hand, as noted above, payment of some kind by the prospective bridegroom to the bride's family shows a positive relationship with the degree of polygyny, suggesting that no general pattern of simple choice by females exists (cf. Hartung 1982, Flinn and Low 1986).

Conclusions

These results suggest that the greater the risk of exposure to serious pathogens (a major biological uncertainty), the greater the degree of polygyny, measured as percent of men, women, or both sexes polygynously married. In humans, with complex societal patterns and custom amounting to cultural inheritance, it is difficult to interpret this simply as the result of choice for heritable pathogen resistance. The extraordinary degree of resource control exerted by humans complicates matters.

The results of this paper suggest, consistent with several previous analyses, that when resources are available they are used by men in the context of sexual selection. Hartung (1982)

found that inheritance tends to be male-biased in polygynous societies. Flinn and Low (1986) found that the exchange of women, or only a token exchange of goods, is significantly more likely in societies without rules of inheritance, and without stratification of wealth or hereditary class. Borgerhoff Mulder (this volume, Chapter 3) found that Kipsigis men paid higher bride prices for women of higher reproductive value, and thus likely to produce more children, although reciprocal relationships and societal complications could modify the price. Betzig's review (this volume, Introduction) makes it clear that in the majority of societies for which data exist, resources contribute to reproductive success.

The correlation between use of resources as mating effort by men (e.g. bride price) and the degree of polygyny is also consistent with the restriction of monogamous societies to two conditions: poor resources bases and large nation-states in which laws restrict the number of current spouses to one. It appears that when resources and custom permit, men tend toward polygyny, and when any factor (e.g. health, resources) makes some men much better mates than others, women too, can profit reproductively from polygyny (cf. Verner and Willson 1966, Orians 1969). Even in 'monogamous' societies, monogamy is far from absolute, and male reproductive success appears to be related to status or resource control. In Kalahari Bushmen, living in a resource-limited and harsh environment, 5% of the men (the best hunters) still manage to have two wives (Lee 1979). Similarly, good Ache hunters appear to have more wives and extramarital affairs than other men (Hill and Kaplan, this volume, Chapters 17 and 18). In a socially imposed monogamous situation like most modern technological societies, if the rate of remarriage and second families is higher for men than for women, the society is rendered effectively polygynous.

The use and control of resources by men in the context of mating effort do not appear to be simply analogous to the use of resources in the same context by males of other species. In non-humans, female choice seems to be common, and appears to be relatively straightforward. If women in human societies made the same sort of choices, one would expect to find polygyny, as a result of open female choice, associated with reflections of female independence, both socially and with regard to resources. The results of this paper suggest no such associations. In fact, in some societies it is not clear that the bride has much choice: male relatives negotiate alliances, using both women and resources to bargain (e.g. Flinn and Low 1986). No societies in this sample are reported as giving a greater role to older female relatives in arranging marriages, and only in three societies is the bride reported to have more say than the groom in initiating or refusing a match. Thus we have the curious result that women's contribution to the subsistence base is associated with increased polygyny, and with some enhancement of women's ability to control certain resources (cf. Whyte 1978, 1979, Low, unpublished) – but women appear to use those resources almost exclusively parentally, to feed their children, rather than to gain independence in mating choices. This, too, argues that women enhance their reproductive success not by choosing for pathogen resistance but by directing resources to their offspring; it is entirely consistent if women or their relatives choose mates using resources as a guide.

In sum, while there are similarities in the general ecology of human and non-human polygyny, there are important differences. Unpredictability arising from the risk of serious parasites is positively associated with polygyny and, to some extent, with sexual selection characteristics, as it is with sexual advertisement in birds (Hamilton and Zuk 1982). The major differences appear to be in the matter of who chooses mates. In many human societies, women apparently have little formal voice in the choice of mates; coalitions of their male relatives frequently determine this choice. Resource acquisition and control are important in mate choice.

Summary

1. This paper test hypotheses about relationships between the occurrence of seven serious human pathogens with both acute and chronic effects (cf. Hamilton and Zuk 1982), and the degree of polygyny, sexual advertisement, and patterns of mate choice.
2. The sample comprised the 93 odd-numbered societies of the standard cross-cultural sample, stratified for geographic location and language group, and for which ethnographies are by qualified ethnographers resident within the society for a considerable period of time.
3. The greater the risk of exposure to serious pathogens, the greater the degree of polygyny ($p < 0.05$), no matter how degree of polygyny is measured. No relationship is apparent between the intensity of polygyny and pathogen stress.
4. A marginally significant correlation exists between the risk of exposure to serious pathogens and the amount of information in sexual signals ($p = 0.07$).
5. The causal relationships giving rise to these patterns are not simple, as they appear to be in many other species, in which males may advertise heritable pathogen resistance and females choose healthy males (who, if the distribution of resources permits, may control resources). In humans, non-random mate choice resulting in polygyny is associated with male control of resources independent of pathogen risk, and in many societies, female choice appears to be non-existent or seriously compromised.

Acknowledgements

Many people were helpful in the development of the ideas in this paper. The idea that degree or intensity of polygyny in humans might correlate with severity of parasites was originally suggested by William D. Hamilton at the 1981 meeting of the Conference for the Study of Evolution and Human Behavior at The University of Michigan. Later, he was most helpful in discussing the selective impact of pathogens, and choice of appropriate pathogens. Kathryn Noonan helped develop the combined polygyny measure. Dick Alexander, Laura Betzig, Mildred Dickemann, Steve Frank, and members of the Study of Evolution and Human Behavior Program at The University of Michigan provided helpful criticism and comments.

Appendix A. Cross-cultural sample: odd-numbered societies

The number of the culture is used as it appears in the Murdock and White sample. The specific group and time to which the information refers and the names of the authors of the main sources used are included. In most cases these also correspond to those indicated by Murdock and White, and may include additional authorities drawn from the Ethnographic Atlas published periodically in the journal *Ethnology*. Full bibliographical citations of all the sources used can be obtained from the author upon request.

1. Nama Hottentot: The Geillkhauan tribe reconstructed from 1860.
   A. W. Hoernle, L. Schultze, I. Shapera
3. Thonga: The Ronga subtribe around Lourenco Marques in 1895.
   H. A. Junod
5. Mbundu: The Bailundo subtribe in 1890.
   W. Hambly, G. M. Childs
7. Bemba of Zambia in 1897.
   A. I. Richards
9. Hadza in 1930.
   D. F. Bleek, J. Woodburn
11. Kikuyu of Metume or Fort Mall district in 1920.
    J. Kenyatta, L. S. B. Leakey
13. Mbuti: The Epulu net-hunters of the Ituri forest in 1950.
    C. M. Turnbull
15. Banen: The Ndiki subtribe in 1935.
    I. Dugast
17. Ibo of the Isu-Ama division in 1935.
    T. Northcote, M. Green, V. Uchendu
19. Ashanti of Kumasi state in 1895.
    R. S. Rattray, M. Fortes
21. Wolof of Upper and Lower Salum in Gambia in 1950.
    D. W. Ames, D. P. Gamble
23. Tallensi in 1934.
    M. Fortes
25. Wodaabe Fulani of Niger in 1951.
    M. Dupire, D. J. Stenning
27. Massa of Cameroon in 1910.
    I. de Garine, G. von Hagen
29. Fur around Jebel Marra in 1880.
    A. C. Beaton, R. W. Felkin
31. Shilluk in 1910.
    D. Westermann, E. E. Evans-Pritchard
33. Kaffa in 1905.
    M. Gruhl, G. W. B. Huntingford
35. Konso in the vicinity of Busc in 1935.
    C. R. Hallpike, R. Kluckhohn
37. Amhara of the Gondar district in 1953.
    S. D. Messing, H. Lhote, J. Nicolaisen

39. Kenuzi Nubians in 1900.
    R. Herzog
41. Tuareg of Abaggar in 1900.
43. Egyptians of the town and environs of Silwa in 1950.
    H. Ammar
45. Babylonians of the city and environs of Babylon in 1750 BC.
    H. Suggs, G. Contenau
47. Turks of the Anatolian plateau in 1950.
    M. Makal, P. Stirling, J. E. Pierce
49. Romans of the city and environs of Rome in AD 110.
    J. Carcopino, L. Friedlander, M. Pellison
51. Irish of Kinvarra parish in 1955.
    R. Cresswell, C. Arensberg
53. Yurak Samoyed in 1894.
    K. Donner, A. Engelhardt
55. Abkhaz in 1880.
    M. Dzhanashvili, L. J. Luzbetak, Ya. S. Smirnova
57. Kurds in and near the town of Rowanduz in 1951.
    E. Leach, W. Masters
59. West Punjabi of the village of Mohla in 1950.
    M. Darling, Z. Eglar
61. Toda of the Nilgiri hills in 1900.
    M. B. Emeneau, W. H. R. Rivers
63. Uttar Pradesh in and near Senapur village in 1945.
    B. S. Cohn, M. Opler, R. Singh
65. Kazak of the Great Horde in 1885.
    N. I. Grodekov, A. E. Hudson
67. Lolo of Taliang Shan mountains in 1910.
    H. M. D'Ollone, Y. Y. Lin, C. L. Tseng
69. Garo of Rengsanggri and neighboring villages in 1955.
    R. Burling, C. Nakane
71. Burmese of Nondwin village in 1960.
    M. Nash, J. G. Scott
73. North Vietnamese of the Red River Delta in 1930.
    P. Gourou
75. Khmer Cambodians circa 1860.
    E. Aymonier, J. Delbert, G. Poree, E. Maspero
77. Semang of the Jahi subtribe in 1925.
    I. Ivans, P. Schebesta
79. Andamanese of the Aka Bea tribe in 1860.
    E. H. Man, A. R. Radcliffe-Brown
81. Tanala of the Menabe subtribe in 1925.
    R. Linton
83. Javanese in the vicinity of Pare in 1955.
    H. Geertz, A. Dewey, R. R. Jay
85. Iban of the Uli Ai group in 1950.
    J. D. Freeman

87. Toradja of the Bar'e subgroup in 1910.
    N. Adriani, A. C. Kruijt
89. Alores of Atimelang in 1938.
    C. DuBois
91. Aranda of Alice Springs in 1896.
    T. G. H. Strehlow, B. Spencer, F. J. Gillin
93. Kimam of the village of Bamol in 1960.
    L. M. Serpenti
95. Kwoma of the Hongwam subtribe in 1937.
    J. W. M. Whiting
97. New Irelanders of Lesu village in 1930.
    H. Powdermaker
99. Siuai of the northeastern group in 1939.
    D. L. Oliver
101. Pentecost Islanders of Bunlap village in 1953.
    R. B. Lane, B. S. Lane
103. Ajie of Neje chiefdom in 1845.
    J. Guiart, M. Leenhardt
105. Marquesana circa 1860.
    E. S. C. Handy, R. Linton, R. C. Suggs
107. Gilbertese of Makin Island in 1890.
    B. Lambert
109. Trukese of Romonum Island in 1947.
    W. H. Goodenough, F. Lebar, T. Gladwin, S. Sarason
111. Paulauans of Koror Island in 1873.
    H. G. Barnett, A. Kramer
113. Atayal in 1930.
    Y. Okada, Y. F. Rueh, C. L. Chen
115. Manchu of the Aigun district in 1915.
    S. M. Shirokogoroff
117. Japanese of southern Okayama prefecture in 1950.
    R. Beardsley, G. DeVos
119. Gilyak in 1880.
    L. Shternberg
121. Chukchee of the Reindeer group in 1900.
    W. Bogoras
123. Aleut of the Unalaska branch in 1778.
    G. Sarytschew, I. Veniaminov
125. Montagnais of the Lake St John and Mistassini Bands in 1910.
    F. Speck, J. E. Lips, J. A. Burgess
127. Salteaux of the Berens River, Little Grand Rapids, and Pekangekum Bands in 1930.
    A. I. Hallowell, A. Skinner
129. Kaska of the Upper Liard River in 1900.
    J. J. Honigmann
131. Haida of the village of Masset in 1875.
    J. R. Swanton, G. P. Murdock
133. Twana in 1860.
    M. Eells, W. W. Elmendorf
135. Eastern Pomo of Clear Lake in 1850.
    S. A. Barrett, E. W. Gifford, E. M. Loeb
137. Wadadika Paiute of Harney Valley in 1870.
    F. A. Riddell, B. B. Whiting

139. Kutenai of the Lower or Eastern branch in 1890.
    A. F. Chamberlain, H. H. Turney-High
141. Hidatsa of Hidatsa village in 1836.
    A. W. Bowers, W. Matthews
143. Omaha in 1860.
    J. W. Dorsey, A. Fletcher, F. LaFlesche
145. Creek of the Upper Creek division in 1800.
    J. R. Swanton
147. Comanche in 1970.
    E. A. Hoebel
149. Zuni in 1880.
    F. H. Cushing, M. C. Stevenson
151. Papago of the Archie division in 1910.
    R. Underhill
153. Aztec of the city and environs of Tenochtitlan in 1520.
    F. B. de Sahagun, J. Soustelle, G. C. Vaillant
155. Quiche of the town of Chichicastenango in 1930.
    R. Bunzel, L. S. Schultze-Jena
157. Bribri tribe of Talamanca in 1917.
    A. Skinner, D. Stone
159. Goajiro in 1947.
    G. Bolinder, V. G. de Pineda
161. Callinago of Dominica in 1650.
    R. Breton, D. Taylor
163. Yanomamö of the Shamatri tribe in 1965.
    N. A. Chagnon
165. Saramacca of the upper Suriname River in 1928.
    A. M. Coster, M. C. Khan, M. J. Herskovitz, F. S. Herskovitz
167. Cubeo of the Caduiaria River in 1939.
    I. Goldman
169. Jivaro in 1920.
    R. Karsten, M. W. Stirling
171. Inca in the vicinity of Cuzco in 1530.
    P. de C. de Leon, B. Cobo, R. Rowe
173. Siriono near the Rio Blanco in 1942.
    A. Holmberg
175. Trumai in 1938.
    R. Murphy, B. Quain
177. Tupinamba in the vicinity of Rio de Janiero in 1550.
    A. Thevet, A. Metraux
179. Shavante in the vicinity of São Domingo in 1958.
    D. Maybury-Lewis
181. Cayua of southern Mato Grosso in 1890.
    J. B. Watson, V. D. Watson
183. Abipon in 1750.
    M. Dobrizhoffer
185. Tehuelche in 1870.
    G. C. Musters

Appendix B. Codes and coding rules

V1–V6: Type and intensity of pathogen risk.
V1 (*Leishmania*), V2 (*Trypanosoma*), V3 (malaria), V4 (*Schistosoma*), V5 (filaria), V6 (spirochetes), V7 (leprosy):

1 = no record of occurrence
2 = occasional records, or present with no indication of severity
3 = serious or endemic levels of occurrence

V8 (Pathogen stress) = sum of V1 through V7

V9 (reduced pathogen stress):
1 = V8 = 0 to 9
2 = V8 = 10 to 16
3 = V8 = 17 through 21

		1	2	3	4	5	6	7	8	9
ID	Name	*Leish*	*Tryp*	Malar	Schist	Filar	Spiroch	Lepros	Apropar	Path
1	Nama	1	1	1	1	1	1	2	8	1
3	Thonga	1	1	3	2	1	1	2	11	2
5	Mbundu	1	2	3	1	3	2	2	15	2
7	Bemba	1	3	3	3	3	1	1	15	2
9	Hadza	1	1	3	3	3	3	2	16	2
11	Kikuyu	1	3	3	3	3	3	3	19	3
13	Mbuti	1	1	3	3	3	3	3	17	3
15	Banen	3	2	3	3	3	3	3	20	3
17	Ibo	3	1	3	3	3	3	3	19	3
19	Ashanti	3	1	3	3	3	2	3	18	3
21	Wolof	3	1	3	3	3	3	3	19	3
23	Tallensi	3	3	3	3	3	3	3	21	3
25	Fulani	1	1	3	3	3	3	1	15	2
27	Massa	3	3	3	3	3	3	3	21	3
29	Fur	1	1	1	2	3	3	2	13	2
31	Shilluk	3	1	3	3	3	1	2	16	2
33	Kaffa	3	1	3	3	3	3	3	19	3
35	Konso	1	1	3	2	3	1	1	12	2
37	Amhara	1	1	3	1	3	3	3	15	2
39	Nubian	3	1	3	1	3	3	1	15	2
41	Tuareg	1	2	1	3	3	3	3	16	2
43	Egypt.	1	1	2	3	3	3	3	16	2
45	Babylon.	1	1	2	3	1	3	2	13	2
47	Turks	1	1	3	1	1	3	2	12	2
49	Romans	3	1	1	1	1	3	1	11	2
51	Irish	1	1	1	1	1	3	1	9	1
53	Yurak	1	1	1	1	1	1	1	7	1
55	Abkhaz	1	1	3	1	1	3	1	11	2
57	Kurd	3	1	3	1	1	3	2	14	2
59	Punjabi	3	1	3	1	1	2	2	13	2
61	Toda	1	1	3	1	3	3	3	15	2
63	Uttar Prad.	3	1	3	1	1	3	3	15	2
65	Kazak	3	1	1	1	1	1	3	11	2
67	Lolo	1	1	3	1	1	3	2	12	2
69	Garo	3	1	3	1	3	3	3	17	3
71	Burmese	2	1	3	1	3	3	3	16	2
73	N. Viet.	1	1	3	1	3	3	2	14	2
75	Khmer	1	1	3	1	3	3	2	14	2
77	Semang	1	1	3	1	3	3	2	14	2
79	Andaman.	1	1	3	1	3	3	1	13	2
81	Tanala	1	1	3	3	3	3	3	17	3
83	Java.	1	1	3	1	3	3	2	14	2
85	Iban	1	1	3	1	1	1	1	9	1
87	Toradja	1	1	3	3	3	3	2	16	2
89	Alorese	1	1	3	1	3	3	3	15	2
91	Aranda	1	1	1	1	1	3	1	9	1
93	Kimam	1	1	3	1	3	1	1	11	2
95	Kwoma	1	1	3	1	3	1	1	11	2
97	Lesu	1	1	3	1	3	2	3	14	2
99	Siuai	1	1	3	1	3	3	3	15	2
101	Pentecost	1	1	3	1	3	3	3	15	2
103	Ajie	1	1	2	1	3	3	3	14	2
105	Marquesan	1	1	2	1	3	1	2	11	2
107	Gilbertese	1	1	3	1	3	1	2	12	2
109	Trukese	1	1	3	1	3	3	2	14	2
111	Palauan	1	1	3	1	3	1	2	12	2
113	Atayal	1	1	3	1	3	3	2	14	2
115	Manchu	1	1	1	1	1	1	2	8	1
117	Japanese	1	1	3	3	3	3	2	16	2
119	Gilyak	1	1	1	1	1	1	2	8	1
121	Chukchee	1	1	1	1	1	1	2	8	1
123	Aleut	1	1	1	1	1	1	1	7	1
125	Montagnai	1	1	1	1	1	1	1	7	1
127	Salteaux	1	1	1	1	1	1	1	7	1
129	Kaska	1	1	1	1	1	1	1	7	1
131	Haida	1	1	1	1	1	1	1	7	1
133	Twana	1	1	1	1	1	1	1	7	1
135	Pomo	1	1	1	1	1	1	1	7	1
137	Paiute	1	1	1	1	1	1	1	7	1
139	Kutenai	1	1	1	1	1	1	1	7	1
141	Hidatsa	1	1	1	1	1	1	1	7	1
143	Omaha	1	1	1	1	1	1	1	7	1
145	Creek	1	1	1	1	1	3	1	9	1
147	Comanche	1	1	1	1	1	1	1	7	1
149	Zuni	1	1	1	1	1	1	1	7	1
151	Papago	1	2	3	1	1	1	2	11	2
153	Aztec	3	1	3	1	1	1	2	12	2
155	Quiche	3	3	3	1	1	2	2	15	2
157	Bribri	3	3	3	1	1	3	2	16	2
159	Goajiro	3	3	3	1	3	1	2	16	2
161	Callinago	2	1	3	3	3	3	2	17	3
163	Yąnomamö	3	1	3	1	3	1	1	13	2
165	Saramacca	2	1	3	3	3	1	1	14	2
167	Cubeo	3	1	3	1	1	1	1	11	2
169	Jivaro	3	3	3	3	1	3	2	18	3
171	Inca	3	1	3	1	1	1	2	12	2
173	Siriono	3	3	3	1	1	3	2	16	2
175	Trumai	3	3	3	2	1	1	1	14	2
177	Tupinamba	3	3	3	3	3	1	2	18	3
179	Shavante	3	3	3	2	3	3	3	20	3
181	Cayua	3	1	3	1	1	1	2	12	2
183	Abipon	1	3	3	1	1	1	2	12	2
185	Tehuelche	1	1	1	1	1	1	1	7	1

126

References

Alexander, R. D. (1979) *Darwinism and Human Affairs*. Seattle: University of Washington Press.

American Geographical Society of New York. (1950–1955) *Atlas of Distribution of Diseases*. New York: American Geographical Society.

Beaver, P. C., Jung, R. C. and Cupp, E. W. (1984) *Clinical Parasitology*, 9th edition. Philadelphia: Lea and Febiger.

Bell, G. (1982) *The Masterpiece of Nature: The Evolution and Genetics of Sexuality*. Berkeley: University of California Press.

Betzig, L. B. (1986) *Depotism and Differential Reproduction: A Darwinian View of History*. Hawthorne, NY: Aldine Press.

Conover, W. J. (1980) *Practical Nonparametric Statistics*, 2nd edition. New York: Wiley.

Dickemann, M. (1982) Comment on Hartung's 'Polygyny and the inheritance of wealth.' *Current Anthropology*, 23 (1), 8–9.

Faust, E. C. and Russell, P. F. (1964) *Clinical Parasitology*. 7th edition. Philadelphia: Lea and Febiger.

Flinn, M. V. and Low, B. S. (1986) Resource distribution, social competition, and mating patterns in human societies. In *Ecological Aspects of Human Social Systems*, ed. D. Rubenstein and R. Wrangham. Princeton: Princeton University Press.

Goodman, L. A. and Kruskal, W. H. (1963) Measures of association for cross classifications III: Approximate sampling theory. *Journal American Statistical Association*, 53, 310–64.

Hamilton, W. D. (1980) Sex versus non-sex versus parasite. *Oikos*, 35, 282–90.

Hamilton, W. D. and Zuk, M. (1982) *Heritable true fitness and bright birds: a role for parasites Science*, 218, 384–7.

Hamilton, W. D., Henderson, P. A., and Moran, N. (1981) Fluctuation of environment and coevolved antagonist polymorphism as factors in the maintenance of sex. In *Nature Selection and Social Behavior: Recent Research and Theory*, ed. R. D. Alexander and D. W. Tinkle. New York: Chiron Press.

Hartung, J. (1982) Polygyny and inheritance of wealth. *Current Anthropology*, 23 (1), 1–12.

Hartung, J. (1983) In defense of Murdock: A reply to Dickemann. *Current Anthropology*, 24 (1), 125–6.

Jaenike, J. (1978) Ecological genetics in *Drosophila athabasca* – its effect on local abundance. *American Naturalist*, 112 (984), 287–99.

Le Bouef, B. J. (1974) Male–male competition and reproductive success in elephant seals. *American Zoologist*, 14, 163–76.

Lee, R. B. (1979) *The !kung San: Men, Women and Work a Foraging Society*. Cambridge: Cambridge University Press.

Lenington, F. (1983) Social preferences for partners carrying 'good genes' in wild house mice. *Animal Behavior*, 31, 325–33.

Levins, R. (1968) *Evolution in Changing Environments: Some Theoretical Explorations*. Princeton: Princeton University Press.

Low, B. S. (1979) Sexual selection and human ornamentation. In *Evolutionary Biology and Human Social Behavior*, ed. N. A. Chagnon and W. Irons. Boston: Duxbury Press.

Low, B. S. (1987) On measuring polygyny in humans. *Current Anthropology* (in press).

Markell, E. K. and Voge, M. (1981) *Medical Parasitology*, 5th edition. Philadelphia: Saunders.

Maynard Smith, J. (1971) What use is sex? *Journal Theoretical Biology*, 30, 319–35.

Murdock, G. P. and White, D. R. (1969) Standard cross-cultural sample. *Ethnology*, 8, 329–69.

Murdock, G. P. and Wilson, S. (1972) Settlement patterns and community organization: Cross-cultural codes 3. *Ethnology*, 11, 254–95.

Orians, G. H. (1969) On the evolution of mating systems in birds and mammals. *American Naturalist*, 103, 589–603.

Partridge, I. (1980) Mate choice increases a component of offspring fitness in fruit flies. *Nature*, 283, 290–1.

Taylor, P. D. and Williams, G. C. (1982) The lek paradox is not resolved. *Theoretical Population Biology*, 22, 392–409.

Trivers, R. L. (1985) *Social Evolution*. Menlo Park, CA: Benjamin Cummings.

van Valen, L. (1973) A new evolutionary law. *Evolutionary Theory*, 1, 1–30.

Verner, J. and Willson, M. F. (1966) The influence of habits on mating systems of North American passerine birds. *Ecology*, 47, 143–7.

Wade, M. J. and Arnold, S. J. (1980) The intensity of sexual selection in relation to male sexual behavior, female choice, and sperm precedence. *Animal Behavior*, 28, 446–61.

Whyte, M. K. (1978) Cross-cultural codes dealing with the relative status of women. *Ethnology*, 17, 211–37.

Whyte, M. K. (1979) *The Status of Women in Pre-Industrial Society*. Princeton: Princeton University Press.

Williams, G. C. (1975) *Sex and Evolution*. Princeton: Princeton University Press.

Steven J. C. Gaulin[1]
Harol A. Hoffman[2]

Evolution and development of sex differences in spatial ability

'Is it not reasonable to anticipate that our understanding of the human mind would be aided greatly by knowing the purpose for which it was designed?'

(G. C. Williams 1966)

Introduction

The theory of sexual selection is an efficient model for analyzing and explaining sex differences, because it provides an evolutionary mechanism for the origin and maintenance of such differences. In its present form (e.g. Trivers 1972), it argues that adaptive differences between the sexes arise when males and females allocate their reproductive effort differently. The assumptions are few and simple. The total amount of reproductive effort that an individual can expend is finite, and reproductive effort expended in one way, for example nurturing zygotes, is not available to be expended in some other way, for example seeking additional matings. Furthermore, the specializations (anatomical, physiological, behavioral, etc.) that render one pattern of reproductive effort expenditure more efficient may render alternative allocation patterns less efficient. Thus, where the sexes differ in their optimal patterns of reproductive effort allocation, the evolutionary result often is disruptive selection for the traits most relevant to their divergent reproductive tactics.

The mediation of such sex differences is unlikely to be directly genetic. In obligately sexual species, males receive half their genes from a

[1] Department of Anthropology, University of Pittsburgh, Pittsburgh, PA 15260, USA
[2] Department of Anthropology, University of North Carolina, Greensboro, NC 27401, USA

female (their mother), and females receive half their genes from a male. Thus, over evolutionary time, the average autosomal (non-sex chromosome) gene spends half its time in male bodies and half its time in female bodies. Thus genes that made positive contributions to the formation of, say, female phenotypes but compromised the reproductive prospects of male phenotypes would be disfavored. The most likely outcome is that genes (and thus traits) will spread if and only if they respond facultatively to the sex and experience of the body in which they find themselves, producing one set of (advantageous) phenotypic effects in female bodies and a different set in male bodies. Because of this facultative mediation of sex differences, a complete analysis of any sexually dimorphic trait required a statement about both its evolutionary and more proximate developmental causes.

Evidence for sex differences in spatial ability

L. J. Harris (1978) introduced an exhaustive review of the spatial ability literature with the following summary:

> The spatial sense has been of particular interest to differential psychologists because the most persistent of individual differences on multifactor tests of psychological functioning is a sex difference in spatial ability. Males have decidedly better spatial skill than females. Indeed, on a number of tests, only 20% to 25% of females exceed the average performance of males (Harris 1978: 405).

Before the evidence for these assertions can be considered in detail we need to specify what we mean by 'spatial ability'. The present consensus is that spatial ability is not a unitary trait but rather a collection of competencies, subsumed under a single heading because of their common reference to the visuo-spatial domain. Thus, tests of spatial ability are diverse, requiring the subject to duplicate a pattern with colored blocks, to imagine the folding of a pattern or the rotation of an object, to recognize specified shapes when these are embedded in a more complex design, to read a map, or to solve a maze problem (e.g. Guilford and Lacey 1947; Witkin

1950; Gross 1959; Money *et al.* 1965; Porteus 1965). Factor-analytic techniques have been used to explore the relationships among the various tests said to measure spatial ability, and, typically, two factors emerge (French 1951; Michael *et al.* 1957). Spatial orientation measures the ability to judge the spatial position and relationship of stimuli relative to the observer (i.e. the subject), while spatial visualization measures the ability to manipulate stimuli mentally without distorting the spatial configuration of the stimulus elements. A few authors (e.g. Linn and Pulos 1983) have suggested a third factor. Regardless of how these abilities are partitioned, however, males consistently outperform females on all factors. Harris (1978), McGee (1979, 1982), Wittig and Petersen (1979), Burstein *et al.* (1980), and Rosenthal and Rubin (1982) all provide recent, critical literature reviews that substantiate the reliability and generality of this finding.

Although the reality of these sex differences is fairly well established, the timing of their emergence is not. Maccoby and Jacklin (1974) asserted that reliable sex differences do not emerge until adolescence. However, Oetzel (1966) reviewed 19 studies of sex differences in spatial ability in children and found that only five studies showed no significant sex differences. Of the remaining 14, all showed better performance by boys. It seems clear that the magnitude of the sex difference increases during adolescence (e.g. Witkin *et al.* 1967, Petersen 1976). Harris (1978) reviewed the developmental patterns test by test. For example, in the embedded figures test the subject looks at and is asked to remember a simple geometric shape. Then the subject attempts to find an example of the target shape in a more compex geometric pattern. Nine studies of 5- to 10-year-olds are cited, seven of which show no sex difference and two, a male superiority. But four studies of 12- to 18-year-olds, and eight studies of adults all yielded better performance by males (Harris 1978). Witkin *et al.* (1967) used embedded figures to study spatial ability longitudinally in two groups: 8 to 13 years old, and 10 to 24 years old. These authors report superior performance by males at all ages.

A variety of visual-maze tests have been devised which require the subject to move a pencil or other marker through a set of barriers to an objective. Porteus (1965) reviewed sex differences in performance in such studies. In 105 separate comparisons among groups of males and females (total sample size: 5282 males; 5086 females), aged 5 to adulthood, 99 studies yielded superior male performance and five superior female performance. However, McGinnis (1929) and Mattson (1933) found no sex differences in maze performance among 3- to 5-year-olds, and 5- and 6-year-olds, respectively.

Mental rotation tasks are typically the most difficult of spatial tasks, and yield the most dramatic sex differences. Such tasks typically depict a two- or three-dimensional object (e.g. a block construction), and require the subject to imagine what the stimulus would look like from some other perspective. Sex differences are noted from about 11 years of age (Vandenberg et al. 1968, Hartlage 1970), and by adulthood the effect size is huge. For example, Book (1932) found that in a large sample of college-age subjects, only 23.9% of the women exceeded the male mean. Wilson and Vandenberg (1978) examined cognitive abilities of parents ($n = 2961$) and offspring ($n = 2096$) among Japanese Americans and European Americans in Hawaii. They found maximal sex differences on a mental rotations task. Among the offspring group (14 to 20 years old) average male and female scores were 24.3 and 15.1, respectively; among the parent group (mostly 35 to 60 years old) male and female means were 16.6 and 6.4, respectively.

What little controversy there is in this literature can be traced to two sources. First, since spatial ability is loosely defined, and because it is said to be measured by such a wide array of tests, the comparability of studies using different measures is reduced. This can cause disputes over the particular age at which sex differences in spatial ability first emerge; they are detectable at different ages with different tests. Second, it does seem clear that sex differences in spatial ability increase at least through the pubertal years. This fact means that studies of older children will more likely yield statistically significant results than will studies of younger children, thus creating precisely the pattern of results one finds in the literature.

Remarkably, sex differences in spatial ability seem not to be restricted to *Homo sapiens*. Of course most of the tests used to evaluate spatial ability in humans are inappropriate for use with non-human subjects, but mazes have been used to investigate spatial learning in both groups. It has been known and reliably verified for over 70 years that, in both wild and laboratory rats, males perform significantly better than do females on maze-learning tasks (Hubbert 1915, Sadownikova-Koltzova 1926, McNemar and Stone 1932, Barrett and Ray 1970, Dawson 1972, Dawson et al. 1973, 1975, Stewart et al. 1975, Joseph et al. 1978). An efficient theory of sex differences in spatial ability would explain both the human and non-human data.

The evolution of spatial ability

To analyze spatial ability as an evolved trait, we need to postulate its adaptive function. This is risky, since an erroneously chosen function will produce an irrelevant and probably misleading analysis. The particular trait under consideration – the ability to collect, process, store and access spatial data – seems less problematic in this respect than many other sorts of traits. If we ask the adaptive function of a coloration pattern, for example, many possible answers present themselves. It might provide camouflage in certain environments. It might be attractive to potential mates. It might provide advantages in heat absorption or dissipation. It might not be an adaptation at all, but rather, an incidental side-effect of selection for some other trait, perhaps a particular metabolic pathway. However, if we look at a complicated and integrated system we are more likely to be able to deduce its function simply from its structure and organization (Williams 1966). Thus it would probably not be controversial to suggest that the olfactory system evolved to monitor the abundance of various volatile compounds. It simply does not do anything else, and such integrated complexity is unlikely to be an incidental by-product. In the same sense, spatial ability is intimately linked to the maintenance of a clear image of the spatial organization of the environment and a sense of one's own position in that environment.

Numerous authors have suggested that particular sorts of situations demand, and therefore select for, high spatial ability. Most involve resource acquisition and are assumed to have influenced males more than females as a consequence of sexual division of labor. For example,

Dawson (1969, cited in Dawson 1972) has emphasized the need to locate and relocate the family group 'in relation to food, water and the territorial restrictions imposed both by natural hazards and by enemies and predators.' Berry (1966) suggested that these spatial problems are more severe in 'undifferentiated', i.e. relatively featureless, environments, and Washburn and Lancaster (1968) have emphasized that human ranges are often very large, further compounding the difficulties. In addition, Vandenberg (1975) noted the spatial demands associated with making and using tools and constructing shelters. The striking thing about these ideas is that, while they emphasize that selective pressures fostering spatial ability could be strong in humans, and suggest that such selection might be stronger in human males than females, they provide no clear explanation of the evolutionary mechanisms responsible for maintaining any sexual division of labor. Such division of labor may itself be the consequence of sexual selection, males may hunt in order to harvest certain scarce or valuable nutrients that are attractive to females. Thus all these arguments beg the fundamental question of what evolutionary pressures might underlie sex differences in spatial ability.

If we return to the basic hypothesis that spatial ability evolved in response to the need for accurate internal representations of the spatial environment and of one's position in that environment, that is, in response to navigational demands, why might selection have produced sex differences in spatial skills? The simplest hypothesis is that the navigational demands on males exceed those on females. Such a hypothesis might seem unlikely; home range sizes should be adjusted to supply all the resources necessary for survival and reproduction. Within any given species, would this adjustment not tend to produce the same range size in both sexes, simply as a consequence of the strong ecological similarity between males and females? The answer seems to depend on the reproductive tactics of each sex. In species where females invest heavily in each offspring, a mother's reproductive success is highly dependent on her efficient use of ecological resources, because ultimately her investment must be harvested before it can be converted to offspring. If males make considerably smaller investments in offspring, and larger investments in mate acquisition, a father's reproductive success may depend on a rather different set of resources. In such cases, the distribution of potential mates may be as important as the distribution of the ecological precursors of investment (e.g. food), since both food and females ultimately limit male reproductive success (Wrangham 1980, Gaulin and Sailer 1985). In those species where both sexes invest heavily in the offspring, male and female reproductive success would tend to be limited by more similar resources, and disruptive selection for range size would be minimal.

Another possibility discussed by the editors in the Introduction and by Kurland and Gaulin (1984) is that males are competing with each other for resources that can be expended either nuturing offspring or courting additional mates. This situation would also produce an asymmetry in the reproductive tactics of the two sexes, since females lack such flexibility in the allocation of their effort.

The ethological literature supports this analysis. In most mammal species, males have larger home ranges or territories than do females, but monogamous species represent a systematic exception to this rule, with the members of a mated pair having similarly-sized, overlapping ranges throughout the year (Blair 1951, Brown 1966, Trivers 1972, Chivers 1974, Kleiman 1977, Gaulin and FitzGerald 1986). The strongest evidence that the 'surplus' ranging behavior of males in non-monogamous species should be regarded as a reproductive tactic comes from species with discrete breeding seasons. In such cases, male ranges shrink, virtually obliterating the sex difference outside the breeding season (Ferner 1974, Stamps 1977, Farentinos 1979, Webster and Brooks 1981). This change in ranging patterns presumably is a consequence of a shift in the limiting resource for males. During the breeding season, male reproductive success is limited by the availability of fertilizable females; once females stop ovulating, the limiting resource becomes the materials necessary for survival to the next breeding season. This association between mating system and the relative range sizes of males and females is not without exception. For example, in some effectively polygynous lek-breeding species, males are strongly territorial and persistently localized but females forage widely. Moreover, among highly migratory species the breeding ranges of both males and females are minute compared to the size of their annual range. This annual range, which is often very similar for the two sexes, is probably more important in selecting for navigation skills, and its effects could overshadow any consequences arising out of sex differences in breeding range. Nevertheless, these exceptions do not invalidate the model developed here, but merely define its sphere of relevance and suggest criteria for the choice of species used to evaluate it.

This analysis of selection for spatial ability can be summarized in terms of the general model of sexual selection. Where males commit a large proportion of their reproductive effort to the quest for mates, and the resources to court and support them, selection will often favor increased mobility (Trivers 1972:165), and as a facilitating and supporting cognitive base, increased ability to process spatial data. Conversely, where males invest heavily in particular offspring, committing little more reproductive effort to mate-seeking than do females, disruptive selection for sexually dimorphic range size and spatial ability is strongly reduced. Gaulin and FitzGerald (1986) have offered field and laboratory data in support of this model. Two species of microtine rodents were compared in their natural habitats. *Microtus pennsylvanicus* is ordinarily polygynous, and adult males exhibit little if any paternal care (Madison 1980), whereas *Microtus pinetorum* is monogamous with significant paternal care (Boyette 1966, FitzGerald and Madison 1983). Radiotelemetry revealed that, in the polygynous species, males range considerably more widely than do females. In contrast, identical methods yielded no sex differences in ranging pattern in the monogamous species. Laboratory tests of spatial ability produced the same pattern of results. In the polygynous species, males performed much better than did females on the maze-learning task. This is not surprising since it is the rule in both wild and laboratory rats, which are polygynous or have a polygynous ancestory. However, the monogamous species showed no sex differences in maze performance. These results are consistent with the idea that spatial ability is evolutionarily linked to ranging patterns and only differs between the sexes of a single species when their ranges differ (Gaulin and FitzGerald 1986).

The application of this model to the human case requires an assessment of human mating systems. A variety of kinds of evidence suggest that *Homo sapiens* has a mildly polygynous evolutionary heritage. For example, 708 of the 849 societies catalogued by Murdock (1967) practice polygyny. Secondly, humans exhibit an array of unambiguous sex differences that are characteristic of polygynous mammals, but absent in fully monogamous ones. Thus, relative to females, human males are larger (Harrison *et al.* 1977, Alexander *et al.* 1979, Gaulin and Boster 1985), are more active in courtship (Daly and Wilson 1983), have higher mortality rates (Shapiro *et al.* Kitagawa and Hauser 1973), and exhibit delayed onset of sexual maturity (Tanner 1962). This is not to say that human males contribute no paternal investment, but simply that, relative to females, their expenditures of reproductive effort are skewed away from nurturance of offspring and toward mate seeking. If the inference of polygyny is correct for *Homo sapiens* then the present hypothesis suggests a functional perspective on sex differences in spatial ability. The differences in the reproductive effort allocation patterns of males and females will put a selective premium on nurturant traits in females and a premium on traits that lead to the acquisition of additional mates in males. Superior male spatial skill should be viewed as one evolved tactic in the male's somewhat polygynous mate-seeking strategy. The developmental evidence suggesting that sex differences in spatial ability are maximal just after the attainment of sexual maturity is consistent with the interpretation that spatial ability is a reproductive tactic of differential value to males and females.

The proximate biology of spatial ability

Brain lateralization

The human brain comprises two hemispheres, connected at the cortical level by the corpus callosum. There are several kinds of evidence that, normally, the left hemisphere is somewhat more specialized for language functions whereas the right hemisphere plays a greater role in visuospatial processing. Such specialization, never complete, is called lateralization. The earliest evidence for lateralization comes from clinical studies, which have shown that specific linguistic functions such as speech production, comprehension and timing, and name-finding are localized in particular parts of the left hemisphere. (Weisenberg and McBride 1935, Penfield and Roberts 1959, Hecaen and Albert 1978). Clinical studies also provide evidence that visuo-spatial functions, such as puzzle assembly, physical or mental manipulation of geometric patterns, pattern completion, and the integration of form and space relationships, are more often disrupted by lesions in the right hemisphere (Weisenberg and McBride 1935, Benton *et al.* 1975, Inglis and Lawson 1981).

A second general category of evidence on the lateralization of cognitive processes derives from a relatively small set of subjects whose corpora callosa were wholly or partially severed (commisurotomy) as a treatment for severe epilepsy (Gazzaniga 1970). If a commisurotomy patient is asked to fixate on a point, and a stimulus is flashed briefly (tachistoscopically) to either the patient's right or left visual field, that stimulus only reaches the contralateral hemisphere. Such tachistoscopic presentation can thus be used to investigate the cognitive abilities of right and left hemispheres separately. The results of this 'split-brain' research have confirmed clinical findings. Sperry (1968) found that when pictures were tachistoscopically presented to the right visual field, patients could verbally report what was seen, presumably because the stimulus reached the linguistically competent left hemisphere. Stimuli presented to the left visual field (right hemisphere) produced verbal reports that nothing had been seen, although when asked to choose a similar object from a collection of objects out of view, the left hand, controlled by the right hemisphere, was highly competent. In other words, while both hemispheres knew what they had seen, only the left hemisphere could access the language functions necessary to produce a verbal report.

These data, together with those from auditory studies, suggest the expected left hemisphere bias for linguistic tasks (Milner *et al.* 1968, Springer and Gazzaniga 1975). A right hemisphere effect on spatial tasks is also apparent. For example, when patients were asked to match two- and three-dimensional shapes on the basis of their shared geometric features, the right hemisphere performed much better than did the left (Franco and Sperry 1977). Nebes (1972) presented exploded line drawings of geometric shapes as stimuli, and then asked patients to choose from an array of geometric solids out of sight, the one which had been depicted. Patients performed well with their left hands, but at the chance level (as if they were guessing) with their right. In summary, the split-brain literature corroborates the clinical literature and confirms the superior linguistic competence of the left hemisphere and the superior spatial competence of the right hemisphere (see Gazzaniga and LeDoux 1978 and Springer and Deutsch 1981 for good reviews). The final sort of evidence on hemispheric lateralization comes from studies of normal individuals. Bryden (1982) provides a comprehensive review of this literature. For reasons that are not yet fully understood, the hemisphere that first receives a stimulus has an advantage over the other hemisphere in processing that information, even in normal individuals. Thus the intact brain exhibits more weakly the same asymmetries seen in the commisurotomized brain. In language processing therefore, one would expect to find a right-visual-field (left-hemisphere) advantage. Tachistoscopic studies have overwhelmingly confirmed this expectation. Subjects are more accurate at reporting words in the right visual field (McKeever 1971, Kershner and Jeng 1972, McKeever and Gill 1972, Mackavey *et al.* 1975, Hines 1976).

Research on normal subjects indicates similar lateralization effects. For spatial tasks there is fairly good evidence of a left-visual-field (right-hemisphere) superiority (e.g. Witelson 1976). Kimura (1969) projected a single dot tachistoscopically and asked her subjects to indicate the position of that dot on a response card that depicted a matrix of possible dot locations. This task yielded a right-hemisphere advantage, and the effect has been replicated (Levy and Reid 1978). Subjects are also better at reproducing patterns of dots projected to the left visual field (McKeever and Huling (1970)). Young and Bion (1979) replicated Kimura's (1966) element enumeration study in grade-school children and similarly found a left-visual-field advantage.

Dichotic listening experiments were first devised to measure linguistic lateralization by Kimura (1961a, 1961b). Using subjects whose language lateralization was known, she used dichotic listening experiments to measure a right or left ear advantage for recognition of speech sounds. Consistent contralateral ear advantages were found: normal subjects with left hemisphere linguistic function showed a right-ear advantage whereas those subjects whose language functions were lateralized in their right hemisphere exhibited a left-ear advantage. This result has been replicated many times under a variety of conditions (Curry and Rutherford 1967, Satz *et al.* 1967, Studdert-Kennedy and Shankweiler 1970, Geffen and Caudrey 1981). Bryden (1982) in his thorough summary of this literature concludes 'there is little doubt that this right-ear effect is related to cerebral speech lateralization'.

In general, the results from clinical studies of brain lesion victims and from experiments with both split-brain patients and normal subjects all point in the same direction – left hemisphere dominance for linguistic functions and right hemisphere dominance on spatial tasks. The reverse is seldom reported. The absence of significant differences in some studies may be due in part to the fact that the differences are not always large, but probably more importantly to the fact that the sexes seem to differ in cerebral organization, with females tending to be less lateralized than males.

Sex differences in lateralization

A comprehensive literature survey by Inglis and Lawson (1981) on the effects of unilateral brain damage illustrates the sex difference in laterality, as well as the problems of investigating laterality in a population that is really two populations, males and females. They examined the extent to which verbal IQ and 'performance' IQ (the latter comprises mostly spatial measures) were affected by unilateral brain damage. They found a strong interaction between side of damage and type of deficit. Compared to intact subjects, those with left hemisphere damage showed reduced verbal scores while those with right hemisphere damage exhibited depressed performance scores; but this pattern was only apparent in studies where male subjects predominated. Looking across studies there was a clear reduction in the side-by-subtest interaction as the number of female subjects increased. This result is all the more telling because none of the studies

reviewed by Inglis and Lawson (1981) was designed to investigate sex differences.

In general, many of the same kinds of evidence that have been used to show overall patterns of cerebral specialization have also been used to show that these patterns differ to some extent in males and females. Clinical data on the effects of brain damage by sex have only recently been available. This is in part due to the fact that, for reasons that may ultimately spring from sexual selection, males are more likely to suffer brain trauma than are females. For example, most of the large-sample studies involve war veterans. Lansdell (1961) was the first to look for sex differences in the effects of head trauma. Much previous work, such as that summarized above, had led him to expect that left hemisphere damage would lead to impaired linguistic functioning and that right hemisphere damage would produce deficits in spatial ability. He found these effects only among his male subjects, and was led to speculate that the hemispheres of the female brain are typically less specialized, with verbal and spatial functions being more equally shared than they are in the male brain. Other studies have subsequently replicated these results with a variety of verbal and spatial measures (McGlone and Kertesz 1973, McGlone 1978, Hecaen *et al.* 1981); McGlone (1978), for example, noted that left-hemisphere damage is three times more likely to produce aphasia (loss of language production) in men than it is in women. Hecaen *et al.* (1981) note that *right*-hemisphere damage produced aphasia in only 3% of their male subjects but 13% of their female subjects, suggesting less left dominance for language functions in women. Right-hemisphere damage was, however, twice as likely to produce spatial disorders in males (53% of males as opposed to 27% of females; Hecaen *et al.* 1981).

Split-brain patients have not contributed to the literature on sex differences in laterality, apparently because of their very small numbers, but studies of normal individuals are increasingly common. Right-ear advantages are typical in dichotic listening tests using verbal material, and there is a trend for this right-ear advantage to be larger in males (McGlone and Davidson 1973, Lake and Bryden 1976). A number of studies involving tachistoscopic presentation of language material have shown significantly stronger right-visual-field effects in men than in women, again suggesting more dominant left-hemispheric language functions in males (Hannay and Malone 1976, Bradshaw et al. 1977, Bradshaw and Gates 1978, Kail and Siegel 1978). Tachistoscopic presentation of spatial material also frequently yields sex effects. The typical pattern is that men are more accurate when the stimulus is presented to the left visual field (right hemisphere), whereas women show no left–right bias, or a slight right-visual-field advantage (Kimura 1969, McGlone and Davidson 1973, Davidoff 1977). Among 5- to 12-year-olds, boys showed a stronger left-visual-field advantage than girls on a dot-enumeration task (Young and Bion 1979).

There is also anatomical evidence for sex differences in cerebral asymmetry. The left temporal planum, associated with one of the primary linguistic areas, is larger than the right, and this left–right difference is greater in males than in females (Wada et al. 1975). The corpus callosum comprises fibers that link the two hemispheres. The posterior part of the corpus callosum, the splenium, carries fibers linking visual areas of the cortex, and is larger in females (de Lacoste-Utamsing and Holloway 1982). The massa intermedia is another midline brain structure. In non-human primates it connects the left and right halves of the thalamus, but it is curiously absent in roughly one-third of all men and one-quarter of all women. Lansdell and Davie (1972) showed that the presence of a massa intermedia depressed spatial test scores among males but had no effect on females' performance on these same tests.

Although not all studies that have looked for sex differences in lateralization have found them, one feature of the literature is clear: almost no studies report greater lateralization for females. If the results reported above were cases of Type I error (accepting the observed differences as real when they are merely chance aberrations in the data), then we would expect to see an equal number of studies reporting greater lateralization in females (Springer and Deutsch 1981). Thus, it seems likely that the coherent pattern of results discussed above does reflect an actual sex difference, and that some studies may fail to uncover such differences because both their samples and the effects they attempt to estimate are small (Bryden 1982).

Levy (1969) attempted to build a model that explains the relationship between patterns of hemispheric dominance and patterns of cognitive abilities. Her working hypothesis was that the type of neural organization that best serves spatial processing differs from the optimal neural organization for verbal processing. Thus, the confinement of these two processing modes to the two separate hemispheres allows the patterns of neural connections to specialize, and therefore optimize, for the particular cognitive functions they serve. It follows from this that, when particular cognitive functions (partially) invade the opposite hemisphere, they compromise the efficacy of the processing mode normally served by the invaded hemisphere. Such a model has no problem explaining the sex difference in spatial ability, since females are known to be less lateralized for verbal tasks, and would therefore be expected to show the effects of neural 'competition' in the normally spatial right hemisphere. But this begs the issue since the model was developed, in part, to explain this sex difference. Levy (1969) has, however, carried out an independent test of her model. Independent of sex, left-handers are also known to be less lateralized for language functions (Subirana 1958, Bryden 1965). Thus, on average, they should also show a depression of spatial ability. In a comparison of right- and left-handers, Levy (1969) found no difference in verbal IQ, but a highly significant depression of performance IQ in the latter group, and this pattern has been verified in other studies (e.g. Miller 1971, Nebes 1971, McGlone and Davidson 1973).

Other indirect evidence for Levy's competition model comes from studies of head-injury patients and individuals with chromosomal aberrations. As noted above, left-hemisphere damage typically produces a verbal deficit. However, if such trauma is ontogenetically early it also produces non-verbal impairment, presumably because verbal processing is competing for neuronal space in the intact right hemisphere (Lansdell 1969). Moreover, women with Turner's syndrome, a chromosomal anomaly, are even less lateralized than normal females, and have very low spatial ability (Gordon and Galatzer 1980). However, some problems remain for Levy's competition model. If specialization of cognitive functions in separate hemispheres yields superior performance on spatial tasks, why does it not do likewise for verbal tasks; since males are more lateralized for both, they should, according to this hypothesis, outperform females on both sorts of tasks. It may be possible, with a more detailed neurological analysis of these two sorts of processing, to explain this apparent contradiction.

Hormonal effects on spatial ability

The apparent sex differences in cerebral organization discussed above must have a developmental basis. That is, some mechanisms within the developing soma must cue the body as to its sex, and thereby shift ontogenetic programs toward more masculine or more feminine outcomes. An early proposal was that the sex chromosomes themselves carry a major gene for superior spatial ability. Specifically, the gene was hypothesized to reside on the X-chromosome and to be recessive (Bock and Kolakowski 1973). Since males have only a single X-chromosome and females have two, the gene would be more likely to be expressed in males. This hypothesis has been rejected (principally because Turner's syndrome females have a 45,XO genotype and lack a second X-chromosome as do males, but have very low spatial ability) in favor of the view that the sex chromosomes affect cognitive differentiation in the same way that they shape many other facets of development, indirectly, through the influence of the sex hormones. This view is rendered plausible by the fact that the mammalian brain has receptors that are specifically responsive to gonadal hormones (MacLusky and Naftolin 1981).

Typically, the mammalian fetus has the potential to develop either a male or female phenotype. If a Y-chromosome is present, the fetal gonads develop into testes which in turn secrete large amounts of androgens. These androgens alter the subsequent course of development, yielding a male phenotype. In the absence of a Y-chromosome, the fetal gonads become ovaries, which secrete only small quantities of androgens. Without the testicular androgens, development follows a female path. A subsequent dose of either male or female sex hormones finishes at puberty the differentiation process begun *in utero*. It now appears that, together, the fetal dosage of androgens and the type and dosage of sex hormones at puberty shape not only anatomical sex differences, but cognitive ones as well. Such a possibility was initially suggested by the observation that sex differences in spatial ability become much more pronounced at adolescence and then decrease in middle age, thus paralleling the pubertal peak and subsequent decline in sex hormones (Petersen 1976, Harris 1978). But more direct sorts of evidence are available. Genetic or environmental accidents can produce various sorts of hormonal disorders, and the affected individuals often show atypical patterns of cognitive abilities. A comparison of these aberrant patterns with those of normal individuals can suggest the cognitive effects of the altered hormone. The earliest such evidence is from males with the protein-deficiency disease, kwashiorkor (Dawson 1967). This disease, through its effects on liver function, can perturb hormone balance such that affected males have abnormally high estrogen levels, leading, for example, to gynaecomastia. Dawson (1967) found that such kwashiorkor-feminized males had lower spatial ability than did normal controls. More extreme forms of feminization are known. Androgen insensitivity is a disorder not of hormonal metabolism, but of the target tissues. In these instances, males with a 46,XY genotype have normal levels of circulating androgens but defective receptor cells. As a result, they exhibit none of the normal signs of fetal or pubertal androgenization and are thus phenotypic females. Such individuals exhibit feminine cognitive profiles, with verbal IQs higher than performance IQs (Masica *et al.* 1969, Perlman 1973), but since they appear and act like normal females in virtually every respect it is likely that socialization into a female gender role has also shaped their development (Masica *et al.* 1971).

More decisive evidence comes from males with idiopathic hypogonadotropic hypogonadism. These individuals also have a 46,XY genotype but experience more or less normal fetal masculinization. They are raised as boys and their defect only manifests itself later, when the absence of a gonadotropin releaser prevents normal puberty. While affected individuals have normal verbal abilities, their spatial abilities are depressed (Bobrow *et al.* 1971, Buchsbaum and Henkin 1980, Hier and Crowley 1982). Hier and Crowley's (1982) study is especially informative because of its within-group comparisons. First, some of their subjects acquired hypogonadotropic hypogonadism only after they had already undergone a normal puberty. These individuals did not differ from controls on tests of spatial ability. Second, among those subjects with idiopathic hypogonadotropic hypogonadism, spatial ability was positively correlated with testicular volume, while verbal ability was not. These findings suggest that the masculinizing dose of pubertal androgens significantly elevates spatial ability, and that effects are dose dependent, since more extreme testicular hypotropy produces more extreme spatial deficits.

Klinefelter's syndrome occurs in males with a 47,XXY genotype, and though it retards sexual development and sometimes involves some degree of somatic feminization, affected individuals usually undergo a masculinizing puberty. Studies of spatial ability in this group have produced conflicting results; Ratcliffe *et al.* (1982) found that the performance IQ of 16- to 18-year-old boys ($n = 12$) with Klinefelter's syndrome was not significantly different from that of matched controls, but Nyborg and Nielsen (1981) found that, on 4 out of 5 tests of spatial ability, Klinefelter's men ($n = 20$) performed significantly worse than normal males, but no worse than normal females. This inconsistency in results is to be expected if the slight feminizing effect of Klinefelter's syndrome produces a slight reduction in spatial ability. Some studies would thus yield statistically significant results and some would not.

Turner's syndrome in women with 45,XO genotypes (or mosaic genotypes involving the absence of a second X-chromosome in some somatic cells) results in complete gonadal disgenesis. Thus these women lack even the low levels of androgens produced by the ovaries, and have a spatial ability below that of normal females, even though their verbal ability may be above average (Money 1963, Alexander *et al.* 1964, Garron 1977, Buchsbaum and Henkin 1980, Gordon and Galatzer 1980). Rovet and Netley (1982) found this same pattern, with Turner's syndrome patients performing as well as controls on verbal tasks but significantly worse on a spatial task. Moreover, these authors examined the performance of their subjects in a very detailed way, considering how both accuracy and response time changes with increasing difficulty of the spatial problem. Their conclusion was that

Turner's females differ from normal females in exactly the same way normal females differ from normal males. This finding is particularly important in the light of Gordon and Galatzer's (1980) conclusion that Turner's women are even less lateralized than normal females.

Congenital adrenal hyperplasia (CAH) is an endocrine disorder caused by a recessive autosomal gene. In affected individuals, the adrenal cortex secretes abnormally low levels of cortisol, thus elevating the rate of ACTH synthesis, and thereby increasing the level of androgen production. Girls with this syndrome are thus fetally androgenized and typically are born with some signs of masculinization such as clitoral hypertropy. These girls are usually surgically corrected shortly after birth, placed on regular cortisol-replacement therapy, and raised as normal females. At puberty they become reproductively capable women. Some early studies of affected females have produced conflicting results. Baker and Ehrhardt (1974) found that CAH girls engaged in more masculine sorts of play activity and were more often coded as 'tomboys,' but they did not differ from normal girls in either verbal or performance IQ. Conversely, Perlman (1973) found that CAH girls had high 'non-verbal' evaluative ability. Unfortunately, these studies involved a preponderence of preadolescent girls. Since the events of puberty are known to be important in establishing sex differences in spatial ability, these studies must be treated with circumspection. Resnick *et al.* 1986 have studied both childhood activities and cognitive abilities in a sample of adolescent and postadolescent women with CAH, and in a control group of their unaffected siblings and cousins. They found that females who had experienced such fetal androgenization had significantly higher spatial ability than did controls. Moreover, females with this endocrine disorder were somewhat more likely to have engaged in activities requiring spatial manipulation, but within-individual correlations between spatial activity and spatial ability were negligible and not significant. The authors thus conclude that 'differential hormone exposure influences both activity and cognitive variables, [but] its effects across the two domains appear to be unrelated' (Resnick *et al.* 1986).

In summary, much independent evidence suggests that male hormones, both *in utero* and at puberty, elevate spatial ability. There are also indications that female hormones may depress spatial ability. Diabetic women have low endogenous estrogen and progesterone levels, and thus are sometimes prescribed exogenous hormone treatment during pregnancy. Their male offspring, exposed to these exogenous female hormones *in utero*, exhibit a variety of feminine characteristics, including spatial ability below the male norm (Yalom *et al.* 1973). There may also be shorter-term effects of hormones on cognitive performance. Komnenich *et al.* (1978) found that women performed worst on a test of spatial ability during the ovulatory phase of their menstrual cycles, i.e. when their estradiol levels were maximal, and others have found a similar pattern (Wickham 1958, Klaiber *et al.* 1974, Dor-Shav 1976).

While our main focus is on *Homo sapiens*, experimental studies with laboratory animals are informative since they permit the manipulation of hormones while controlling for other factors. Sexual differentiation in laboratory rats is organized much as it is in humans, except that the critical stage of gonad differentiation and concommitant masculinization or feminization by gonadal hormones occurs neo-natally rather than *in utero*. Thus, perinatal gonadectomy eliminates the organizing effects of the gonadal hormones. Such manipulations may or may not be accompanied by replacement with the opposite-sex hormone. Alternatively, development can be allowed to proceed normally with hormone manipulations occuring only at puberty or in adulthood. In these subjects, spatial ability is measured by maze-learning performance. The general findings are clear. Normal males typically perform significantly better on maze tasks, but androgenization significantly improves female performance, and administration of female hormone depresses male performance. In both cases, the effects are strongest for the earliest hormone manipulations, with neo-natal manipulations typically producing a pattern of performance indistinguishable from that of opposite-sexed normals (Dawson 1972, Dawson *et al.* 1973, 1975, Stewart 1975, Joseph *et al.* 1978).

From the evidence summarized so far it might simply appear that spatial ability develops in proportion to the quantity of circulating androgens. This is a reasonable conclusion if one takes normal males as a baseline and compares them with progressively less androgenized individuals. Thus, males with Klinefelter's syndrome (who are slightly less androgenized than normal males) and CAH females (who are more androgenized than normal females) have spatial ability between that of typical males and females. Highly deandrogenized males with idiopathic hypogonadotropic hypogonadism have spatial ability which is lower than that of Klinefleter's males, and perhaps equivalent to that of typical females. Turner's syndrome females are even less androgenized and have lower spatial ability than normal females. All of this would lead to the expectation that highly androgenized males would have very high spatial ability. They do not. In fact, among normal males, there seems to be an inverse relationship between androgens and spatial ability. Thus, overall, there appears to be a curvilinear relationship between androgen production and performance on spatial tasks. Increasing androgens seem to elevate spatial ability through the normal female range and into the lower fringes of the male range (e.g. Klinefelter's), but then reverse in their effect, such that progressive increases in androgen levels depress spatial ability.

The first suggestion of this curvilinear relationship comes from the work of Petersen (1976). Petersen did not measure hormone production directly, but inferred its influence from measures of the secondary sexual characters. She examined males and females in three age groups (13, 16, and 18 years old) and found that the most masculine girls and the most feminine boys had the highest spatial ability. Berenbaum and Resnick (1982) attempted a replication of this work, and, although their results showed the same trend found by Petersen (1976), this trend did not reach statistical significance. More recently, Shute *et al.* (1983) were able to show the hypothesized curvilinear relationship between androgen levels and spatial abilities across the two sexes by measuring androgen production directly, rather than inferentially.

In an elegant series of experiments, Waber (1976, 1977a, 1977b) attempted to link hormone influences on spatial ability with lateralization. She did not measure hormone production directly but, like Petersen (1976) and Berenbaum and Resnick (1982), used ratings based on development of secondary sexual characters.

However, rather than ranking subjects on a masculine–feminine dimension, she grouped them by whether their sexual maturation was precocious or late. Waber found that, in a sample of 10- to 16-year-olds, maturation rate had a stronger effect on spatial ability than did sex. Within each sex, late maturers had higher spatial ability and were more lateralized than early maturers. According to Waber (1977b), her results support the curvilinear relationship between androgens and spatial ability found by Petersen (1976) and Shute *et al.* (1983) since, among males, early maturers are more masculinized, while among females, early maturers are more feminized. Thus she concludes that variation in hormonal state, through its effects on development, can account for individual differences in both hemispheric lateralization and spatial ability. The evidence for very low spatial ability and highly unlateralized cognitive organization in Turner's syndrome women (Gordon and Galatzer 1980) also suggests a causal pathway from sex hormones, through lateralization of function, to spatial ability.

Experiential influences on spatial ability

Regardless of the influence of endogenous factors, such as hormones, it is quite possible that spatial ability is fostered by certain kinds of experiences. Several studies have attempted to isolate the particular sorts of experiences that might foster the development of high spatial ability. Among the major themes of this research are the effects of specific training programs, and the effects of generalized experience with the environment.

Effect of training

Goldstein and Chance (1965) and Kato (1965) were the first to show that specific kinds of training could elevate spatial ability. This led Sherman (1967) to argue that sex-related differences in spatial ability might result from differential practice with spatial problems during childhood, as a consequence of cultural sex-typing. As a result, studies on the effects of training have focused on male *versus* female activity preferences, unfortunately, without attempting to identify the precise aspects of masculine activities that might enhance spatial skill. Thus, no

a priori model exists to suggest which experiential variables are critical to spatial learning, nor whether similar experiences produce differential learning depending on the sex of the subject.

A second problem that has hampered this research program is the possibility that 'a critical learning period' exists. Early childhood experiences, for example, may be more critical to spatial learning than later experiences despite the fact that sex-related differences in spatial ability tend to make their appearance in early adolescence (Vandenburg and Kuse 1979:68, 84). For example, Vandenberg (1975) found model building to significantly increase the spatial scores of sixth-grade girls but not of their male counterparts. Connor *et al.* (1977, 1978) obtained similar results among first-graders, using complex visual figures rather than models. As Goldstein and Chance (1965) also found, practice increased spatial scores for both sexes and, more importantly, eliminated the pre-test sex difference. This suggests that females gained proportionately more from the training experience (Saegert and Hart 1978:169). Both results indicate the importance of early learning experiences in the development of spatial ability. Further support for the importance of early learning experiences is found in the work of Coates *et al.* (1975), who found a positive relationship between block play and field-independence in pre-school girls.

Some studies have shown a relationship between particular sorts of coursework and performance on spatial tests. Blade and Watson (1955) demonstrated that coursework in engineering was related to increased spatial ability for college men. They also found differences in levels of mechanical and technical school experience between the males who scored lowest and highest in their spatial relations test. Likewise, an 11-month engineering program significantly increased spatial performance scores of females (Wittig *et al.* 1984). Unfortunately, neither study controlled for the possibility that, regardless of sex, students select courses on the basis of their prior ability to grasp spatial material.

Studies of the relationship between leisure activities and spatial ability have produced similar results. Tobin-Richards (1980) found no relationship between spatial ability and masculine or feminine activity preferences among high-school seniors. But, in a similar study by Newcombe *et al.* (1983) in which masculine and feminine activities were classified on the basis of their spatial content, significant correlations were obtained between spatial ability and participation in 'spatial' activities for males but not for females. Here again it may be that spatial aptitudes predispose individuals to particular activities.

In sum, the results of training studies are equivocal. There has been no attempt to measure whether the apparent training effects are transient and, more importantly, most studies lack control groups that would allow valid comparisons of changes in spatial ability over training *versus* non-training conditions, i.e. do all college women respond to spatial training in the same way as those who enrol in engineering programs. Furthermore, the precise 'spatial-ness' of many activities has remained nebulous and undefined, and we are left to question which common denominator other than sex-typing, underlies so-called 'spatial' activities. That such a common denominator may be environmental interaction in the form of ranging experiences, is suggested by the cross-cultural literature.

Developmental effects of ranging on spatial ability
Our hypothesis that sex differences in spatial ability are an evolutionary consequence of sex differences in ranging assumes that the adaptive function of spatial ability is navigational. Evidence for this assumption comes from cross-cultural studies in which spatial ability was found to vary with both subsistence type and the availability of environmental cues. Witkin *et al.* (1962), Berry (1966, 1971, 1973, 1976) and Berry and Annis (1974) for example, found both sex differences and cultural differences, as well as variation in sex differences across cultures on embedded-figures-test and rod-and-frame-test performance. In a comparison of Baffin Island Eskimo hunters and West African Temne agriculturalists, Berry (1966) found the usual sex difference in the latter society, but no statistically significant sex differences among the Eskimo. He attributed his findings to the different life styles of the two groups. Among the Eskimo, whose hunting economy and dispersed settlement pattern require much travel, the ability to make subtle visual discriminations in a relatively featureless (undifferentiated) environment was thought to be critical to survival for both men and women. For the Temne, whose environment

is much more visually differentiated, and whose agricultural subsistence pattern requires much less travel – especially for the relatively sedentary females – high spatial ability was not necessary. Unfortunately, no quantitative data on the actual ranging patterns of men and women are presented for either society. However, it is clear that two 'ecological' or environmental variables influencing spatial ability distinguish the two groups. The first, extensive travel, pertains to the amount of movement through an environment; the second concerns the nature of environmental perceptual cues which influence the ease or difficulty of such travel.

In further cross-cultural work, Berry (1971: 133) expanded on his initial ecological model, arguing that among traditional hunter–gatherer peoples, the possession of good visual discrimination and spatial skills is a necessity, and thus is fostered by the cultural system. This is accomplished, according to Berry, 'through the presence of a high number of 'geometrical spatial' concepts, a highly developed and generally shared arts and crafts production, and socialization practices whose content emphasizes independence and self-reliance and whose techniques are supportive and encouraging of separate development.'

Berry's idea that socialization practices influence cognitive abilities underlies many of the socio-cultural studies. Unfortunately, the logical structure of the socialization arguments has not always been consistent (e.g. Barry *et al.* 1959, Burton and Whiting 1961, D'Andrade 1966, Whiting 1968, Chodorow 1971, Dawson 1972, Witkin and Berry 1975). Two lines of argument are common. A particular environmental variable may create a demand for high spatial ability which is met by adjustment in the socialization process. Alternatively, socialization practices may be shaped by some extrinsic force, which incidentally affects cognitive organization. In spite of these inconsistencies, the available socialization data is valuable to our line of inquiry because it is useful to know which aspects of socialization affect spatial ability.

Van Leeuwen (1978) has thoroughly reviewed the cross-cultural literature dealing with the effects of socialization on psychological differentiation, and she suggests that observed sex differences are a function of socialization experiences. In the work she summarizes, Witkin, Berry and others used such tests as the rod-and-frame and the embedded figures to assess what they called cognitive styles or psychological differentiation (Witkin *et al.* 1962; Witkin and Berry 1975). It now seems clear from correlational studies that these early researchers were essentially measuring spatial ability (Sherman 1967, Harris 1978, McGee 1979).

The common variable found by Van Leeuwen to correlate with sex differences in cognitive style across cultures is the degree to which societies encourage conformity. Her hypothesis is that the socialization practices of restrictive societies encourage conformity and dependence more in females than in males. This limits the environmental experience of girls, and thus inhibits their development of field-independence, thereby producing strong sex differences in cognitive style. Van Leeuwen describes 16 studies of sex differences in performance on spatial tasks in societies rated for social conformity (Van Leeuwen 1978 : 104–5). Of these 16, only four showed no interaction effects; the remaining 12 lend support to Van Leeuwen's thesis. The strongest support comes from a 10-year, longitudinal study that measured embedded-figures-test performance of Mexican and Texan adolescents. The results revealed a significant sex-by-culture interaction. Among Mexican students, males scored significantly higher, while no significant sex differences were found in the US sample. Van Leeuwen notes that Mexican girls are typically house-bound; they are assigned the largest number of household tasks and report the fewest outside interests of the four sex-by-culture groups. Mitchelmore (1975), comparing Jamaicans and US whites, Chandra (1974, cited in Van Leeuwen 1978), studying Fijiians and Indians in Fiji, and Meizlik (1973) focusing on orthodox and less traditional Jewish students in New York, all have produced similar results. In each of the studies, females in the more restrictive group exhibited the lowest spatial ability.

Further evidence for an interaction among sex, restrictiveness and spatial ability comes from the work of Mebane and Johnson (1970). These authors found that psychological differentiation (i.e. spatial ability) was positively correlated with a variety of child-rearing practices for males, but that, for females, only the amount of independence experience positively correlated with performance on spatial ability tests. This suggests that independence experience may be a more important source of variability in female spatial ability than it is for males. Such an effect would also tend to produce maximal sex differences in spatial ability in the most restrictive societies.

Two novel studies (Munroe and Munroe 1971, Nerlove *et al.* 1971) conducted among children of the Logoli of Western Kenya and the Gusii of southwestern Kenya, assess the relationship between spatial ability and ranging experience directly. In both studies, sex differences were found in ranging as measured by 'children's distance from home,' with boys ranging farther. Secondly, when subjects were divided into age-matched pairs, consisting of one boy and one girl, performance on spatial tasks was higher for the pair member who had ranged farther from home, even where that pair member was female, with only one exception.

> Both Logoli females who were found to be more distant from home were more proficient on spatial ability tasks. In the Gusii sample as well, the two girls who were found to be more distant from home were more proficient on spatial tasks . . . Similarly, in the cross-cultural pairs, two of the three girls who were found to be farther from home than were male counterparts also performed better on all spatial tasks; one girl performed less well than did her less distant male partner. The authors conclude that environmental exploration may be one of 'several unintended learning experiences which contribute to the differential development of spatial abilities in males and females' (Nerlove *et al.* 1971: 9).

No studies have been conducted in Western settings which demonstrate a relationship between the specific environmental experience of ranging and the development of spatial ability, in the manner of the Munroe and Nerlove studies.

Further data possibly suggesting a relationship between ranging and spatial ability come from studies of cognitive mapping abilities. Sherman *et al.* (1979) investigated the effect of a person's pattern of travel within an environment on his/her cognitive representation of distances between locations. Opaque and transparent barriers were erected to separate some environmental locations but not others. Subjects learned about the environment by visual surveillance, but were allowed to walk only along certain prescribed routes. Subsequently, they were asked to recall the distances between certain pairs of locations. Subjects' recollection of distances was found to be significantly affected both by their movement patterns as well as by the type of barrier and actual separation between locations. Although this study did not consider spatial ability *per se*, its significance lies in the startling evidence it provides for the effects of travel on perceptual processes. The authors considered the travel effect remarkable 'given the relatively small distances involved and the immediacy of perceptual information available to a person while moving through the environment. In larger environments, where longer travel time and more circuitous routes might place greater memory demands on the person, the factors found to be operative here might have even greater impact' (Sherman *et al.* 1979:38–9).

A recent study by Matthews (1984) on the cognitive mapping abilities of young boys and girls, found that boys 'consistently revealed wider environmental knowledge.' Within each age group studied (ages 6–11), boys were aware of places farther from home than girls. After assessing students' awareness of place, Matthews asked the children to draw maps of their home areas. He found that boys demonstrated a much greater awareness of the spatial organization of their environments, and suggested that this is due to the freedom of movement that boys enjoy from an early age.

Sex differences in ranging

We began this paper by proposing an evolutionary model to explain sex differences in spatial ability. In that model, sex differences in range size is the key independent variable. The data on how both sex and mating system shape ranging patterns in non-human mammals have been reviewed above. Unfortunately, very few anthropologists have taken the animal behaviorists' approach and measured such basic biological parameters as home range. Nevertheless, many anecdotal accounts and some quantitative data exist. Typical of the anecdotal reports is Smole's (1976:82) for the Yanoama of Venezuela. He notes that 'On the whole, females stay close to home except for normal group travels. Men and older boys travel extensively ...' Many eth-

nographers give similar summaries, but few offer any sort of evidence to support their assertion, probably because humans are so mobile, and therefore hard to track, and perhaps because ethnographers regard this sex difference as so self-evident.

Much of the quantitative evidence that is available measures range only discontinuously. For example, Draper (1974) noted that among both bush-living and settled !Kung, girls spent a higher proportion of their time in camp than did boys. Working among another San group, the G//ana, Cashdan (1984) found that, when visiting away from home, women were more likely to visit within the central reserve where they lived and men were more likely to visit outside the reserve; this was true for all three of her sample periods.

Among the child-socialization studies, few have attended to the spatial ranges of either sex. Saegert and Hart (1978:159) recognized this limitation, and have called into question Maccoby and Jacklin's (1974) conclusion that the bulk of evidence indicates little or no differences in the socialization of boys and girls in Western societies for independence. Saegert and Hart point out that few of the socialization studies on parental restrictiveness available to Maccoby and Jacklin (Sears *et al.* 1957, Hatfield *et al.* 1967, Baumrind 1971, Radin [cited in Saegert and Hart 1978]), bothered to investigate parental restrictions and punishments regarding spatial range.

A study by Tindal (1971) of home ranges of black elementary school children reported boys' ranges to be significantly larger than girls' and the difference increased with age between second-graders (8 years old) and fourth-graders (10 years old). Similar findings were obtained by Landy (1965:136) in a study of child-socialization in rural Puerto Rico. On a scale measuring restrictiveness of physical mobility, where 4.0 represented 'extreme restriction,' Landy obtained a median score for boys of 2.5 and for girls, of 3.0. Data collected in New England by Hart in 1972 (cited in Saegert and Hart 1978), on ranging behavior of children aged 4 to 12, revealed significant sex differences. Hart (1979), in a study of children's use, knowledge and experience of the landscape, found clear sex differences in the parentally defined spatial range restriction of children over 6 years of age. Studies conducted in a Calgary suburb by Coates and Bussard (1974) and Payne and Jones (1977) found the ranges of girls to be more strictly controlled than boys, 'with their [i.e. girls'] range boundaries, such as roads, fences and streams, clearly defined. The environmental fear of many parents was seen to give rise to considerable sex differentiation towards children, with more protective attitudes evident towards girls.' (Matthews, 1984: 328).

Recent socialization research has suggested that boys and girls differ in environmental experience from the first year of life onward. Lewis (1972), for example, found that boys at 2 years of age were more willing to venture farther away from their mothers than girls. Draper (1974: 271) cites a study by Goldberg and Lewis (1969) in which males of one year were found to be more investigative of their environment than females. She concludes that the finding of superior environmental exploration for males, 'is apparently a forerunner of superior male performance on tests of spatial ability.'

Hewlett (this volume, Chapter 16) assessed the ranging behavior of men and women among the Aka pygmies of the Central African Republic. He found that men traveled significantly farther, and explicitly invoked a sexual-selection explanation for the observed difference. Betzig and Turke (e.g. this volume, Chapters 2 and 10) used a scan sampling technique (Altmann 1974) to record behavior, including location, on Ifaluk atoll. Although this material is not yet published they have generously allowed us to present it here. Ifaluk consists of four islands, only two of which are inhabited. These two, Falachig and Falalop, are separated by a channel which varies in width with the tide, but can always be waded. All observations were carried out on Falalop and thus the test consists of a comparison of the sex ratio of Falalop residents observed in the scans compared with the sex ratio of Falachig residents, who must have crossed the channel to appear in the scans. Among Falalop residents the observed ratio was 1320 males: 1236 females, i.e. only a slight sex bias. However, among Falachig residents the sex ratio was 47 males: 13 females, i.e. males were more than 3.5 times more likely to be observed. The χ^2 statistic shows this distribution to be significant at $p < 0.001$.

Flinn (e.g. this volume, Chapter 11) has used similar scan sampling techniques in Trinidad. He used four distance-from-household categories to code each individual's location. Flinn (unpublished) has broken down these data by sex and 10-year age classes. In seven of the eight age classes males were observed farther from home, on average, than were females. These differences are statistically significant ($p < 0.05$) in the two most reproductively critical age classes, 10–20, and 20–30 years. Borgerhoff Mulder also has generously made unpublished data available. She asked Kipsigis men ($n = 47$) and women ($n = 67$) what was the farthest distance they had ever traveled from home during their married life. The mean for males was 89.7 km, for females, 21.7 km. This difference is statistically significant with $p < 0.0001$. While it would be desirable to have quantitative data for more societies, with a variety of subsistence, sociopolitical and mating systems, the fact that none of the available evidence contradicts the hypothesized sex difference in range size, is strongly supportive of the proposed model linking spatial ability to ranging behavior.

Discussion

Our initial proposal was that we might profitably consider spatial ability as an evolved adaptation, and ask why it has been more strongly selected in males. The working hypothesis is that spatial ability is favored in direct proportion to the navigational demands placed on the organism by its ecology (that is, in proportion to its range size). We have suggested that in *Homo sapiens*, both sexes are subject to relatively high navigational demands. However, sex differences in spatial ability only make adaptive sense if the navigational demands also differ by sex. We argue that these differential pressures spring ultimately from the sort of sex-biased competition for mates that drives all sexual selection. In particular, males are hypothesized, by extension of the animal literature, (1) to have larger ranges (2) *in order* that they may increase their access to potential mates.

The anecdotal and quantitative evidence unanimously support the idea that men do have larger ranges than women. Probably if pressed, ethnographers would 'explain' such differences in economic or division-of-labor terms. Betzig (pers. comm.) in a spirit of healthy scepticism, suggested that males may be more mobile on Ifaluk because in a matrilocal system, they would have to travel farther to keep in contact with kin. She tested this hypothesis by examining the degree of relatedness between male channel-crossers and all their observed associates on the one hand, and female channel-crossers and all their associates on the other. The results were counter to her 'matrilocal model.' The relatedness (f) between males and their associates was 0.11, while for females the equivalent measure was 0.21.

The above exercise serves to emphasize two important points. First, although sex differences in ranging among humans may not be primarily a consequence of divergent reproductive strategies, the non-human literature suggests that they are. Thus, any alternative explanation is relatively unparsimonious and must bear the burden of proof. Second, even if, for example, economic factors were established as important in shaping male mobility, the present model would not necessarily be invalidated; if economic and reproductive success were positively correlated, economic competition could be viewed as a proximate factor compatible with our evolutionary analysis.

All sex differences, indeed all traits, have a developmental history as well as an evolutionary one. A full understanding of any biological phenomenon requires an explanation of both sorts of processes. Sex hormones orchestrate and integrate much of development, insuring a coherent set of traits in both females and males. It thus seems reasonable to expect that, as androgens provide males with the larger body size and stronger aggressive tendencies that form one part of their reproductive strategy, these same hormones might also condition their ability to process spatial data, thereby facilitating more extensive searching for mates. The evidence that androgens have precisely that effect, both laying down basic predispositions *in utero* and fostering their further development at puberty, is strong and growing. It is less clear at the moment, but suggested by a number of studies, that these hormones operate through their effects on brain lateralization.

Since the navigational demands on both sexes vary with the environment, we might expect selection to have provided an additional proximate pathway to adjust spatial ability to 'local' conditions. There is evidence that spatial ability is responsive to at least some sorts of experience, particularly ranging experience. Such experience seems to have somewhat stronger effects on females. This would not be surprising if, as we have argued, high spatial ability is a more critical component of male reproductive strategy. In that case, selection should have favored its emergence in response to relatively slight environmental stimulation in males, but programmed a higher threshold in females. As a result typical levels of environmental experience would produce high spatial ability only in males, but additional stimulation could elevate females to similar ability levels.

None of the foregoing analysis should be taken to suggest that sex differences in spatial ability are genetically programmed or immutable. The strong ontogenetic influences on spatial ability should be apparent from numerous clinical and field studies showing the effects of particular hormone imbalances and particular ranging experiences, respectively, on the development of spatial skills. The possibility of interaction among these sets of influences is yet to be adequately investigated. Thus, sex differences in spatial ability may develop (ontogenetically) in several ways, all of which could be mediated by the relatively well-documented androgen/estrogen pathway. Hormones may directly produce brain differences (e.g. lateralization), or may alter brain function indirectly through their effects on maturation rate or ranging activity. As either an alternative or additional pathway, ranging experience could foster spatial skill by altering hormone levels, perhaps as a result of increased activity levels. Socialization practices could promote or prevent such experience, and could do so differentially by sex. All of these scenarios are consistent with the evolutionary model developed in this chapter, but all predict considerable plasticity and within-sex variation in spatial skill.

Harris (1979) points out that attempts to explain sex differences in spatial ability historically have shifted between the classical poles of biology at one end and the workings of culture and socialization at the other. We have tried to show that this is a false and unproductive dichotomy, and that a much deeper understanding can be gleaned from the application of fully inter-actionist, evolutionary models.

Summary

1. A full understanding of sex differences in spatial ability requires a detailed model of both ontogenetic and evolutionary causes.
2. Spatial ability should be regarded as a navigational adaptation.
3. Sex differences in this trait should be analyzed in terms of a presumed evolutionary history of disruptive selection for navigational skills.
4. Such disruptive selection is argued to have its roots in differential competition for mates where males typically ranged more widely as a tactic to acquire either additional mates or the resources that would attract such mates.
5. The ontogeny of spatial ability appears to be orchestrated largely by androgens, acting both *in utero* and during pre-pubertal development.
6. At least some of these hormonal effects are likely to be a result of their organizational influences on brain lateralization.
7. Overlaying these endocrinological effects, some kinds of experience have a favorable effect on the development of spatial ability; notably, the most important experiential variable is the amount of ranging experience. In other words, the navigational demands placed on an organism seem to significantly affect spatial ability both over evolutionary time and over individual life histories.

Acknowledgements

We thank L. Betzig, M. Flinn, M. Borgerhoff Mulder and S. Berenbaum for generously allowing us to present unpublished data or results. The editors made extensive and very constructive comments on an earlier draft of this chapter, as did R. FitzGerald. Of course, any errors of fact or interpretation remain our own.

References

Alexander, D., Walker, H. T. and Money, J. (1964) Studies in direction sense. *Archives of General Psychiatry*, **10**, 337–9.

Alexander, R. D., Hoogland, J. L., Howard, R. D., Noonan, K. M. and Sherman, P. W. (1979) Sexual dimorphisms and breeding systems in pinnipeds, ungulates, primates and humans, In *Evolutionary Biology and Human Social Behavior*, ed. N. A. Chagnon and W. Irons, pp. 402–35. North Scituate, MA: Duxbury Press.

Baker, S. E. and Ehrhardt, A. A. (1974) Prenatal androgen, intelligence and cognitive sex differences. In *Sex Differences in Behavior*, ed. R. C. Friedman, R. M. Richart and R. L. Vande Wiele, pp. 53–76. New York: Wiley.

Barrett, R. J. and Ray, O. S. (1970) Behavior in the open field, Lashley III maze, shuttle box, and Sidman avoidance as a function of strain, sex, and age. *Developmental Psychology*, **3**, 73–7.

Barry, H., Child, I. L. and Bacon, M. K. (1959) The relation of child training to subsistence economy. *American Anthropology*, **61**, 51–63.

Baumrind, D. (1971) Current patterns of parental authority. *Developmental Psychology*, Monograph 4.

Benton, A. L., Hannay, H. J. and Varney, N. R. (1975) Visual perception of line direction in patients with unilateral brain disease. *Neurology*, **25**, 907–10.

Berenbaum, S. A. and Resnick, S. (1982) Somatic androgeny and cognitive abilities. *Developmental Psychology*, **18**, 418–23.

Berry, J. W. (1966) Temne and Eskimo perceptual skills. *International Journal of Psychology*, **1**, 207–29.

Berry, J. W. (1971) Ecological and cultural factors in spatial perceptual development. *Canadian Journal of Behavioral Science*, **3**(4), 129–40.

Berry, J. W. (1973) Ecology, cultural adaptation, and psychological differentiation: traditional patterning and acculturative stress. Paper presented at the Cross-Cultural Conference, East–West Centre, Honolulu, Hawaii.

Berry, J. W. (1976) *Human Ecology and Cognitive Style: Comparative Studies in Cultural and Psychological Adaptation*. New York: John Wiley.

Berry, J. W. and Annis, R. C. (1974) Ecology, culture and personality. *Journal of Cross-Cultural Psychology*, **5**, 382–405.

Blade, M. and Watson, W. S. (1955) Increase in spatial visualization test scores during engineer study. *Psychological Monographs*, **69**(12), 1–13.

Blair, W. F. (1951) Population structure, social behavior, and environmental relations in a natural population of the beach mouse (*Peromyscus polionotus leucocephalus*). *Contributions of the Laboratory of Vertebrate Biology, University of Michigan*, **48**, 1–47.

Bobrow, A. A., Money, J. and Lewis, V. G. (1971) Delayed puberty, eroticism, and sense of smell: a psychological study of hypogonadotropinism, osmatic and anosmatic (Kallmann's syndrome). *Archives of Sexual Behavior*, **1**, 329–44.

Bock, R. D. and Kolakowski, D. (1973) Further evidence of sex-linked major gene influence on human spatial visualizing ability. *American Journal of Human Genetics*, **25**, 1–14.

Book, H. M. (1932) A psychophysiological analysis of sex differences. *Journal of Social Psychology*, **3**, 454–61.

Boyette, J. G. (1966) A behavioral study of the pine mouse, *Pitymys pinetorum pinetorum*, Leconte. Ph.D. Dissertation, North Carolina State University at Raleigh.

Bradshaw, J. L. and Gates, A. (1978) Visual field differences in verbal tasks: Effects on task familiarity and sex of subject. *Brain and Language*, **5**, 166–87.

Bradshaw, J. L., Gates, A. and Nettleton, N. C. (1977) Bihemispheric involvement in lexical decisions: Handedness and a possible sex difference. *Neuropsychologia*, **15**, 227–86.

Brinkmann, E. H. (1966) Programmed instruction as a technique for improving spatial visualization. *Journal of Applied Psychology*, **50**, 179–84.

Brown, L. E. (1966) Home range and movement in small mammals. *Symposia of the Zoological Society of London*, **18**, 111–42.

Bryden, M. P. (1965) Tachistoscopic recognition, handedness, and cerebral dominance. *Neuropsychologia*, **3**, 1–8.

Bryden, M. P. (1982) *Laterality: Functional Asymmetry in the Intact Brain*. New York: Academic Press.

Buchsbaum, M. S. and Henkin, R. I. (1980) Perceptual abnormalities in patients with chromatin negative gonadal dysgenesis and hypogonadotropic hypogonadism. *International Journal of Neuroscience*, **11**, 201–9.

Burstein, B., Bank, L. and Jarvik, L. F. (1980) Sex differences in cognitive functioning: Evidence, determinants and implications. *Human Development*, **23**, 289–313.

Burton, R. V. and Whiting, J. W. M. (1961) The absent father and cross-sex identity. *Merrill-Palmer Quarterly*, **7**, 85–95.

Cashdan, E. (1984) G//ana territorial organization. *Human Ecology*, **4**, 443–63.

Chivers, D. J. (1974) *The Siamang in Malaya*. Basel: S. Karger.

Chodorow, N. (1971) Being and doing: a cross-cultural examination of the socialization of males and females. In *Women in Sexist Society*, ed. V. Gornick and B. Moran, pp. 173–97. New York: Basic Books.

Coates, G. and Bussard, E. (1974) Patterns of children's spatial behavior in a moderate-density housing development. In *Childhood City, Man-Environmental Interactions*, ed. R. C. Moore, pp. 131–41. Milwaukee: EDRA.

Coates, S., Lord, M. and Jakabovics, E. (1975) Field dependence–independence, social–non-social play and sex differences in pre-school children. *Perceptual and Motor Skills*, **40**, 195–202.

Connor, J. M., Serbin, L. A. and Shackman, M. (1977) Sex differences in children's response to training on a visual-spatial test. *Developmental Psychology*, **13**, 293–4.

Connor, J. M., Shackman, M. and Serbin, L. A. (1978) Sex-related differences in response to practice on a visual-spatial test and generalization to a related test. *Child Development*, **49**, 24–9.

Curry, F. K. W. and Rutherford, D. R. (1967) Recognition and recall of dichotically presented verbal stimuli by right- and left-handed persons. *Neuropsychologia*, **5**, 119–26.

Daly, M. and Wilson, M. (1983) *Sex, Evolution, and Behavior*, 2nd edition. Boston: PWS Publishers.

D'Andrade, R. G. (1966) Sex differences and cultural institutions. In *The Development of Sex Differences*, ed. E. E. Maccoby, pp. 174–204. Stanford: Stanford University Press.

Davidoff, J. (1977) Hemispheric differences in dot detection. *Cortex*, **13**, 434–44.

Dawson, J. L. M. (1967) Cultural and physiological influences upon spatial-perceptual processes in West Africa. Part II. *International Journal of Psychology*, **2**, 171–85.

Dawson, J. L. M. (1972) Effects of sex hormones on cognitive style in rats and men. *Behavior Genetics*, **2**, 21–42.

Dawson, J. L. M., Cheung, Y. M. and Lau, R. T. S. (1973) Effects of neonatal sex hormones on sex-based cognitive abilities in the white rat. *Psychologia*, **16**, 17–24.

Dawson, J. L. M., Cheung, Y. M. and Lau, R. T. S. (1975) Developmental effects of neonatal sex hormones on spatial and activity skills in the white rat. *Biological Psychology*, **3**, 213–29.

de Lacoste-Utamsing, C. and Holloway, R. L. (1982) Sexual dimorphism in the human corpus callosum. *Science*, **216**, 1431–2.

Dor-Shav, N. K. (1976) In search of pre-menstrual tension: Note on sex-differences in psychological differentiation as a function of cyclical physiological changes. *Perceptual and Motor Skills*, **42**, 1139–42.

Draper, P. (1974) Comparative studies of socialization. *Annual Review of Anthropology*, **3**, 263–77.

Farentinos, R. C. (1979) Seasonal changes in home range size in tassel-eared squirrels (*Sciurus aberti*). *Southwestern Naturalist*, **24**, 49–62.

Ferner, J. W. (1974) Home range size and overlap in *Sceloporus undulatus erythrocheilus* (Reptilia: Iguanidae). *Copeia*, **1974**, 332–7.

FitzGerald, R. W. and Madison, D. M. (1983) Social organization of a free-ranging population of pine voles, *Microtus pinetorum*. *Behavioral Ecology and Sociobiology*, **13**, 183–7.

Franco, L. and Sperry, R. W. (1977) Hemisphere lateralization for cognitive processing of geometry. *Neuropsychologia*, **15**, 107–14.

French, J. W. (1951) The description of aptitude and achievement tests in terms of rotated factors. *Psychometric Monographs*, **5**, 1–278.

Garron, D. (1977) Intelligence among persons with Turner's syndrome. *Behavior Genetics*, **7**, 105–27.

Gaulin, S. J. C. and Boster, J. S. (1985) Cross-cultural differences in sexual dimorphism: Is there any variance to be explained? *Ethology and Sociobiology*, **6**, 193–9.

Gaulin, S. J. C. and FitzGerald, R. W. (1986) Sex differences in spatial ability: An evolutionary hypotheis and test. *American Naturalist*, **127**, 74–88.

Gaulin, S. J. C. and Sailer, L. D. (1985) Are females the ecological sex? *American Anthropologist*, **87**, 111–19.

Gazzangia, M. S. (1970) *The Bisected Brain*. New York: Appleton.

Gazzaniga, M. S. and LeDoux, J. E. (1978) *The Integrated Mind*. New York: Plenum.

Geffen, G. and Caudrey, D. (1981) Reliability and validity of the dichotic monitoring test for language laterality. *Neuropsychologia*, **19**, 413–24.

Goldberg, S. and Lewis, M. (1969) Play behavior in the year-old infant: early sex differences. *Child Development*, **40**, 21–31.

Goldstein, A. G. and Chance, J. E. (1965) Effects of practice on sex-related differences in performance on embedded figures. *Psychonomic Science*, **3**, 361–2.

Gordon, H. W. and Galatzer, A. (1980) Cerebral organization in patients with gonadal dysgenesis. *Psychoneuroendocrinology*, **5**, 235–44.

Gross, F. (1959) The role of set in perception of the upright. *Journal of Personality*, **27**, 95–103.

Guilford, J. P. and Lacey, J. I. (1947) Printed Classification Tests. Army Air Forces Aviation Psychology Research Program Reports, Report 5. Washington: US Government Printing Office.

Hannay, H. J. and Malone, D. R. (1976) Visual field effects and short-term memory for verbal material. *Neuropsychologia*, **14**, 203–9.

Harris, L. J. (1978) Sex differences in spatial ability: Possible environmental, genetic, and neurological factors. In *Asymmetrical Function of the Brain*, ed. M. Kinsbourne, pp. 405–522. New York: Cambridge University Press.

Harris, L. J. (1979) Variances and anomalies. *Science*, **206**, 50–2.

Harrison, G. A., Weiner, J. S., Tanner, J. M. and Barnicot, N. A. (1977) *Human Biology*, 2nd edition. Oxford: Oxford University Press.

Hart, R. (1979) *Children's Experience of Place*. New York: Irvington.

Hartlage, L. C. (1970) Sex-linked inheritance of spatial ability. *Perceptual and Motor Skills*, **31**, 610.

Hatfield, J. S., Ferguson, L. R. and Alpert, R. (1967) Mother–child interaction and the effects of message structure on persuasion. *Journal of Personality and Social Psychology*, **7**, 365–414.

Hecaen, H. and Albert, M. L. (1978) *Human Neuropsychology*. New York: Wiley.

Hecaen, H., De Agostini, M. and Monzon-Montes, A. (1981) Cerebral organization in left-handers. *Brain and Language*, **12**, 261–84.

Hier, D. B. and Crowley, W. F. (1982) Spatial ability in androgen-deficient men. *New England Journal of Medicine*, **306**, 1202–5.

Hines, D. (1976) Recognition of verbs, abstract nouns and concrete nouns from the left and right visual half-fields. *Neuropsychologia*, **14**, 211–16.

Holtzman, W. H., Diaz-Guerrero, R., Swartz, J. D. and Lara-Tapia, L. (1975) *Personality Development in Two Cultures: A Cross-Cultural Longitudinal Study of School Children in the U.S. and Mexico*. Austin: University of Texas Press.

Hubbert, H. B. (1915) The effect of age on habit formation in the albino rat. *Behavior Monographs*, **2**, 1–55.

Inglis, J. and Lawson, J. S. (1981) Sex differences in the effects of unilateral brain damage on intelligence. *Science*, **212**, 693–5.

Joseph, R., Hess, S. and Birecree, E. (1978) Effects of hormone manipulations and exploration on sex differences in maze learning. *Behavioral Biology*, **24**, 364–77.

Kail, R. V. and Siegel, A. W. (1978) Sex and hemispheric differences in the recall of verbal and spatial information. *Cortex*, **14**, 557–63.

Kato, N. A. (1965) A fundamental study of the rod-and-frame test. *Japanese Psychological Research*, **7**, 61–8.

Kershner, J. R. and Jeng, A. G. (1972) Dual functional hemispheric asymmetry in visual perception: Effects of ocular dominance and postexposural processes. *Neuropsychologia*, **10**, 437–45.

Kimura, D. (1961a) Some effects of temporal lobe damage on auditory perception. *Canadian Journal of Psychology*, **15**, 156–65.

Kimura, D. (1961b) Cerebral dominance and the perception of verbal stimuli. *Canadian Journal of Psychology*, **15**, 166–71.

Kimura, D. (1966) Dual functional asymmetry of the brain in visual perception. *Neuropsychologia*, **4**, 275–85.

Kimura, D. (1969) Spatial localization in left and right visual fields. *Canadian Journal of Psychology*, **23**, 445–8.

Kitagawa, E. M. and Hauser, P. M. (1973) *Differential Mortality in the United States: A Study in Socioeconomic Epidemiology*. Cambridge, MA: Harvard University Press.

Klaiber, E. L., Broverman, D. M., Vogel, W. and Kobayashi, Y. (1974) Rhythms in plasma MOA activity, EEG, and behavior during the menstrual cycle. In *Biorhythms and Human Reproduction*, ed. M. Ferein, F. Halberg, R. M. Richart and R. L. Vande Wiele, pp. 353–67. New York: Wiley.

Kleiman, D. (1977) Monogamy in mammals. *Quarterly Review of Biology*, **52**, 39–69.

Komnenich, P., Lane, D. M., Dickey, R. P. and Stone, S. C. (1978) Gonadal hormones and cognitive performance. *Physiological Psychology*, **6**, 115–20.

Kurland, J. A. and Gaulin, S. J. C. (1984) The evolution of male parental investment: Effects of genetic relatedness and feeding ecology on the allocation of reproductive effort. In *Primate Paternalism*, ed. D. Taub, pp. 259–308. New York: Van Nostrand Reinhold.

Lake, D. A. and Bryden, M. P. (1976) Handedness and sex differences in hemispheric asymmetry. *Brain and Language*, 3, 266–82.

Landy, D. (1965) *Tropical Childhood*. New York: Harper and Row.

Lansdell, H. (1961) The effect of neurosurgery on a test of proverbs. *American Psychologist*, 16, 448.

Lansdell, H. (1969) Verbal and non-verbal factors in right-hemisphere speech: Relation to early neurological history. *Journal of Comparative and Physiological Psychology*, 69, 734–8.

Lansdell, H. and Davie, J. C. (1972) Massa intermedia: Possible relation to intelligence. *Neuropsychologia*, 10, 207–10.

Levy, J. (1969) Possible basis for the evolution of lateral specialization of the human brain. *Nature*, 224, 614–15.

Levy, J. and Reid, M. (1978) Variations in cerebral organization as a function of handedness, hand posture in writing, and sex. *Journal of Experimental Psychology: General*, 107, 119–44.

Lewis, M. (1972) State as an infant environmental interaction: an analysis of mother–infant behavior as a function of sex. *Merrill-Palmer Quarterly*, 18, 95–121.

Linn, M. C. and Pulos, S. (1983) Male–female differences in predicting displaced volume: Strategy usage, aptitude relationships, and experience influences. *Journal of Educational Psychology*, 75, 86–96.

Maccoby, E. E. and Jacklin, C. N. (1974) *The Psychology of Sex Differences*. Stanford, CA: Stanford University Press.

Mackavey, W., Curcio, F. and Rosen, J. (1975) Tachistoscopic word recognition performance under conditions of simultaneous bilateral presentation. *Neuropsychologia*, 13, 27–33.

MacLusky, N. J. and Naftolin, F. (1981) Sexual differentiation of the central nervous system. *Science*, 211, 1294–1303.

Madison, D. M. (1980) An integrated view of the social biology of *Microtus pennsylvanicus*. *The Biologist*, 62, 20–32.

Masica, D. N., Money, J., Ehrhardt, A. A. and Lewis, V. G. (1969) IQ, fetal sex hormones and cognitive patterns: Studies in the testicular feminizing syndrome of androgen insensitivity. *Johns Hopkins Medical Journal*, 123, 105–14.

Masica, D. N., Money, J. and Ehrhardt, A. A. (1971) Fetal feminization and female gender identity in the testicular feminizing syndrome of androgen insensitivity. *Archives of Sexual Behavior*, 1, 131–42.

Matthews, M. H. (1984) Cognitive mapping abilities of young boys and girls. *Geography*, 69, 327–36.

Mattson, M. L. (1933) The relation between the habit to be acquired and the form of the learning curve in young children. *Genetic Psychology Monographs*, 13, 299–398.

McGee, M. G. (1979) Human spatial abilities: psycho-metric studies and environmental, genetic, hormonal and neurological influences. *Psychological Bulletin*, 80, 889–918.

McGee, M. G. (1982) Spatial abilities: The influence of genetic factors. In *Spatial Abilities: Developmental and Physiological Foundations*, ed. M. Potegal, pp. 199–222. New York: Academic Press.

McGinnis, E. (1929) The acquisition and interference of motor habits in young children. *Genetic Psychology Monographs*, 6, 209–311.

McGlone, J. (1978) Sex differences in functional brain asymmetry. *Cortex*, 14, 122–8.

McGlone, J. and Davidson, W. (1973) The relation between cerebral speech laterality and spatial ability with special reference to sex and hand preference. *Neuropsychologia*, 11, 105–13.

McGlone, J. and Kertesz, A. (1973) Sex differences in cerebral processing of visuospatial tasks. *Cortex*, 9, 313–20.

McKeever, W. F. (1971) Lateral word recognition: Effects of unilateral and bilateral presentation, asynchrony of bilateral presentation, and forced order of report. *Quarterly Journal of Experimental Psychology*, 23, 410–6.

McKeever, W. F. and Gill, K. M. (1972) Interhemispheric transfer time for visual stimulus information varies as a function of retinal locus of stimulation. *Psychonomic Science*, 26, 308–10.

McKeever, W. F. and Huling, M. D. (1970) Lateral dominance in tachistoscopic word recognition at two levels of ability. *Quarterly Journal of Experimental Psychology*, 22, 600–4.

McNemar, Q. and Stone, C. P. (1932) The sex difference in rats on three learning tasks. *Journal of Comparative Psychology*, 14, 171–80.

Mebane, D. and Johnson, D. L. (1970) A comparison of the performance of Mexican boys and girls on Witkin's cognitive tasks. *Interamerican Journal of Psychology*, 4, 227–39.

Meizlik, F. (1973) *Study of the effect of sex and culture variables on field dependence/independence in a Jewish subculture*. Master's thesis, City University of New York.

Michael, W. B., Guilford, J. P., Fruchter, B. and Zimmerman, W. S. (1957) The description of spatial-visualization abilities. *Educational and Psychological Measurement*, 17, 185–99.

Miller, E. (1971) Handedness and the pattern of human ability. *British Journal of Psychology*, 62, 111–12.

Milner, B., Taylor, L. and Sperry, R. W. (1968) Lateralized suppression of dichotically presented digits after commissural section in man. *Science*, 161, 184–5.

Mitchelmore, M. C. (1975) The spatial ability of Jamaican and American students: a cross-cultural study. Paper presented at the Higher Degree Seminar, School of Eduction, University of the West Indies, Kingston, Jamaica.

Money, J. (1963) Cytogenetic and psychosexual incongruities with a note on space-form blindness. *American Journal of Psychiatry,*, **119**, 820–7.

Money, J., Alexander, D. and Walker, H. T. (1965) *A Standardized Test of Direction Sense*. Baltimore: Johns Hopkins University Press.

Munroe, R. L. and Munroe, R. H. (1971) Effect of environmental experience on spatial ability in an East African society. *Journal of Social Psychology*, **83**, 15–22.

Murdock, G. P. (1967) *Ethnographic Atlas*. Pittsburgh: University of Pittsburgh Press.

Nebes, R. (1971) Handedness and the perception of wholepart relationship. *Cortex*, **7**, 350–6.

Nebes, R. (1972) Dominance of the minor hemisphere in commisurotomized man in a test of figural unification. *Brain*, **95**, 633–38.

Nerlove, S. B., Munroe, R. H. and Munroe, R. L. (1971) Effects of environmental experience on spatial ability: a replication. *Journal of Social Psychology*, **84**, 3–10.

Newcombe, N., Bandura, M. M. and Taylor, D. G. (1983) Sex differences in spatial ability and spatial activities. *Sex Roles*, **9**, 377–86.

Nyborg, H. and Nielsen, J. (1981) Spatial ability of men with karyotype 47,XXY, 47XYY, or normal controls. In *Human Behavior and Genetics*, ed. W. Schmid and J. Nielsen, pp. 85–106. Amsterdam: Elsevier/North Holland Biomedical Press.

Oetzel, R. M. (1966) Classified summary of research in sex differences. In *The Development of Sex Differences*, ed. E. Maccoby, pp. 323–51. Stanford: Stanford University Press.

Payne, R. J. and Jones, D. R. W. (1977) Children's urban landscapes in Huntington Hills, Calgary. In *The Behaviorial Basis of Design*, Book 2, ed. R. Suedfield and J. A. Russell, Stroudsburg, Pennsylvania: Dowden, Hutchinson and Ross.

Penfield, W. and Roberts, L. (1959) *Speech and Brain Mechanisms*. Princeton, NJ: Princeton University Press.

Perlman, S. M. (1973) Cognitive abilities of children with hormone abnormalities: screening by psychoeducational tests. *Journal of Learning Disabilities*, **6**, 21–9.

Petersen, A. C. (1976) Physical androgeny and cognitive functioning in adolescence. *Developmental Psychology*, **12**, 524–33.

Porteus, S. D. (1965) *Porteus Maze Test: Fifty Years' Application*. Palo Alto, CA: Pacific Books.

Ramirez, M. III and Price-Williams, D. R. (1974) Cognitive styles of children of three ethnic groups in the U.S. *Journal of Cross-Cultural Psychology*, **5**, 212–19.

Ramirez, M. III, Costenada, A. and Herold, C. P. (1974) The relationship of acculturation to cognitive style among Mexican-Americans. *Journal of Cross-Cultural Psychology*, **5**, 424–33.

Ratcliffe, S. G., Bancroft, J., Axworthy, D. and McLaren, W. (1982) Klinefelter's syndrome in adolescence. *Archives of Disease in Childhood*, **57**, 6–12.

Resnick, S. M., Berenbaum, S. A., Gottesman, I. I. and Bouchard, T. J. (1986) Early hormonal influences on cognitive functioning in congenital adrenal hyperplasia. *Developmental Psychology*, **22**(2), 191–8.

Rosenthal, R. and Rubin, D. B. (1982) Further meta-analytic procedures for assessing cognitive gender differences. *Journal of Educational Psychology*, **74**, 708–12.

Rovet, J. and Netley, C. (1982) Processing deficits in Turner's syndrome. *Developmental Psychology*, **18**, 77–94.

Sadownikova-Koltzova, M. P. (1926) Genetic analysis of temperament in rats. *Journal of Experimental Zoology*, **45**, 301–18.

Saegert, S. and Hart, R. (1978) The development of environmental competence in boys and girls. In *Play: Anthropological Perspectives*, ed. M. Salter, pp. 157–75. Cornwall, New York: Leisure Press.

Satz, P., Achenbach, K. and Fennel, E. (1967) Correlations between assessed manual laterality and predicted speech laterality in a normal population. *Neuropsychologia*, **5**, 295–310.

Sears, R. R., Maccoby, E. E. and Levin, H. (1957) *Patterns of Child Rearing*. Evanston, Illinois: Row, Peterson.

Shapiro, S., Schlesinger, E. R. and Nesbitt, R. E. L. (1968) *Infant, Perinatal, Maternal and Childhood Mortality in the United States*. Cambridge, MA: Harvard University Press.

Sherman, J. A. (1967) Problems of sex differences in space perception and aspects of intellectual functioning. *Psychological Review*, **74**, 290–9.

Sherman, R. C., Croxton, J. and Smith, M. (1979) Movement and structure as determinants of spatial representations. *Journal of Nonverbal Behavior*, **4**, 27–39.

Shute, V. J., Pellegrino, J. W., Hubert, L. and Reynolds, R. W. (1983) The relationship between androgen levels and human spatial abilities. *Bulletin of the Psychonomic Society*, **21**, 465–8.

Smole, W. J. (1976) *The Yanoama Indians*. Austin, Texas: University of Texas Press.

Sperry, R. W. (1968) Hemisphere deconnection and unity in conscious awareness. *American Psychologist*, **23**, 723–33.

Springer, S. P. and Deutsch, G. (1981) *Left Brain, Right Brain*. New York: W. H. Freeman.

Springer, S. P. and Gazzaniga, M. S. (1975) Dichotic listening in partial and complete split brain patients. *Neuropsychologia*, **13**, 341–6.

Stamps, J. A. (1977) The relationship between resource competition, risk and aggression in a tropical territorial lizard. *Ecology*, **58**, 349–58.

Stewart, J., Skvarenina, A. and Pottier, J. (1975) Effects of neonatal androgens on open-field behavior and maze learning in the prepubescent and adult rat. *Physiology and Behavior*, **14**, 291–5.

Studdert-Kennedy, M. and Shankweiler, D. (1970) Hemispheric specialization for speech perception.

Journal of the Acoustical Society of America, **48**, 579–594.

Subirana, A. (1958) The prognosis in aphasia in relation to cerebral dominance and handedness. *Brain*, **81**, 415–25.

Tanner, J. M. (1962) *Growth at Adolescence*, 2nd edition. Oxford: Blackwell Scientific.

Tindal, M. (1971) *Home-range of black elementary school children*. Place Perception Reports, No. 5, Clarke University.

Tobin-Richards, M. H. (1980) The influences of experience and sex-role identity on cognitive performance. In *Proceedings, American Psychological Association*, Montreal.

Trivers, R. L. (1972) Parental investment and sexual selection. In *Sexual Selection and the Descent of Man: 1871–1971*, ed. B. G. Campbell, pp. 136–79. Chicago: Aldine.

Vandenberg, S. G. (1975) Sources of variance in performance of spatial tests. In *Children's Spatia Development*, ed. J. Elliot and N. Salkind, pp. 57–66. Springfield: Chas. C. Thomas.

Vandenberg, S. G. and Kuse, A. R. (1979) Spatial ability: a critical review of the sex-linked major gene hypothesis. In *Sex Related Differences in Cognitive Functioning*, ed. M. A. Wittig and A. C. Petersen, pp. 67–95. New York: Academic Press.

Vandenberg, S. G., Stafford, R. E. and Brown, A. M. (1968) The Louisville twin study. In *Progress in Human Behavior Genetics*, ed. S. G. Vandenberg, pp. 153–204. Baltimore: Johns Hopkins Press.

Van Leeuwen, M. S. (1978) A cross-cultural examination of psychological differentiation in males and females. *International Journal of Psychology*, **13**, 87–122.

Van Voorhis, W. P. (1941) *The Improvement of Space Perception Ability by Training*. Ph.D. Dissertation, University Park, Pennsylvania: Penn State University.

Waber, D. P. (1976) Sex differences in cognition: A function of maturation rate. *Science*, **192**, 572–4.

Waber, D. P. (1977a) Sex differences in mental activities, hemispheric lateralization, and rate of physical growth at adolescence. *Developmental Psychology*, **13**, 29–38.

Waber, D. P. (1977b) Biological substrates of field dependence: Implications of the sex difference. *Psychological Bulletin*, **84**, 1076–87.

Wada, J. A., Clark, R. and Hamm, A. (1975) Cerebral hemispheric asymmetry in humans. *Archives of Neurology*, **32**, 239–46.

Washburn, S. L. and Lancaster, C. S. (1968) The evolution of hunting. In *Man the Hunter*, ed. R. Lee & I. DeVore, pp. 293–303. Chicago: Aldine.

Webster, A. B. and Brooks, R. J. (1981) Social Behavior of *Microtus pennsylvanicus* in relation to seasonal changes in demography. *Journal of Mammalogy*, **62**, 738–51.

Weisenberg, T. and McBride, K. E. (1935) *Aphasia: A Clinical and Psychological Study*. New York: Commonwealth Fund.

Whiting, J. W. M. (1961) Socialization process and personality. In *Psychological Anthropology*, ed. F. K. Hsu, pp. 355–80. Homewood, Illinois: Dorsey Press.

Whiting, J. W. M. (1968) Methods and problems in cross-cultural research. In *Handbook of Social Psychology*. 2nd edition, vol. 2, ed. G. Lindzey and E. Aronson, pp. 693–798. Reading: Addison-Wesley.

Wickham, M. (1958) The effects of the menstrual cycle on test performance. *British Journal of Psychology*, **49**, 34–41.

Williams, G. C. (1966) *Adaptation and Natural Selection*. Princeton, NJ: Princeton University Press.

Wilson, J. R. and Vandenberg, S. G. (1978) Sex differences in cognition: Evidence from the Hawaii family study. In *Sex and Behavior: Status and Prospectus*, ed. T. E. McGill, D. A. Dewsbury and B. D. Sachs, pp. 317–35. New York: Plenum Press.

Wit, O. C. (1955) *Sex Differences in Perception*. Master's Thesis, Utrecht: University of Utrecht.

Witelson, S. F. (1976) Sex and the single hemisphere: Specialization of the right hemisphere for spatial processing. *Science*, **193**, 425–7.

Witkin, H. A. (1950) Individual differences in ease of perception of embedded figures. *Journal of Personality*, **19**, 1–15.

Witkin, H. A. and Berry, J. W. (1975) Psychological differentiation in cross-cultural perspective. *Journal of Cross-Cultural Psychology*, **6**, 4–87.

Witkin, H. A., Dyk, R. B., Paterson, H. F., Goodenough, D. R. and Karp, S. A. (1962) *Psychological Differentiation*, New York: Wiley.

Witkin, H. A., Goodenough, D. R. and Karp, S. A. (1967) Stability of cognitive style from childhood to young adulthood. *Journal of Personality and Social Psychology*, **7**, 291–300.

Witkin, H. A., Price-Williams, D., Bertini, M., Christiansen, B., Oltman, P. K., Ramirez, M. and Van Meel, J. (1974) Social conformity and psychological differentiation. *International Journal of Psychology*, **9**, 11–29.

Wittig, M. A. and Peterson, A. C. (1979) *Sex-Related Differences in Cognitive Functioning*. New York: Academic Press.

Wittig, M. A., Sasse, S. H. and Jicomi, J. (1984) Predictive validity of five cognitive skills tests among women receiving engineering training. *Journal of Research in Science Teaching*, **21**, 537–46.

Wrangham, R. W. (1980) An ecological model of female-bonded primate groups. *Behaviour*, **75**, 262–300.

Yalom, I. D., Green, R. and Fisk, N. (1973) Prenatal exposure to female hormones: Effect on psychosexual development in boys. *Archives of General Psychiatry*, 28, 554–61.

Young, A. W. and Bion, P. J. (1979) Hemispheric laterality effects in the enumeration of visually presented collections of dots by children. *Neuropsychologia*, 17, 99–102.

Donald E. Brown[1]
Dana Hotra[1]

Are prescriptively monogamous societies effectively monogamous?

Introduction

The human species uniquely forces a distinction between what Alexander *et al.* (1979:420) call 'socially imposed' and 'ecologically imposed' monogamy. Due to the environmental and technological conditions under which they live, the members of many societies can rarely achieve polygamy, even though their customs or laws allow it. In other societies – the North American is an example – environmental and technological conditions do not prohibit polygamy, but customs and laws do. The former illustrates ecologically imposed monogamy, the latter is socially imposed. The question we try to answer in this paper concerns the effect of socially imposed monogamy: does it result in what Daly and Wilson (1983) call 'effective' monogamy?

The concept of effective monogamy (or polygamy) allows a distinction between the (socially imposed) marital pattern and the actual breeding pattern (which, for various reasons, need not be the same). Daly and Wilson (1983:152) employed the ratio of male to female variances in reproductive success to measure 'the degree of effective polygamy': at 1.0 it indicates effective monogamy, while at figures above or below 1.0 it indicates, respectively, effective polygyny and polyandry. We will call this ratio the breeding system ratio, BSR.

[1] Department of Anthropology, University of California, Santa Barbara, CA 93106, USA

Daly and Wilson (1983) calculated the BSRs for two relatively simple societies for which the relevant data are available – the Xavante and the !Kung Bushmen. The Xavante variances in reproductive success, calculated only for persons aged 40 or more (Salzano et al. 1967), were 3.6 for females and 12.1 for males. The corresponding !Kung variances, calculated from expected lifetime fertilities of cohorts of 100 females and 100 males (Howell 1979), were 6.52 and 9.27, respectively. The ratio of male to female Xavante variances is 3.1, for !Kung it is 1.42. Being determined in different ways, these figures are not strictly comparable, but both indicate a degree of effective polygyny. Neither the Xavante nor !Kung have socially imposed monogamy.

To our knowledge no one has yet determined the BSR for any society with socially imposed monogamy, largely because male fertility is rarely studied, but also because sufficiently exhaustive and accurate genealogies – collected for whatever purpose – are much less common than the anthropological interest in kinship would suggest (Daly and Wilson 1983:89). Alexander et al. (1979:420) felt that socially imposed monogamy 'almost certainly' would depress male variance in reproductive success in stratified societies, but that various practices – they mention 'extramarital liaisons, and promiscuity of various sorts,' but remarriage is a relevant practice too – would temper the social imposition. For a variety of reasons, we hypothesized – as have Daly and Wilson (1983:88) – that societies with socially imposed monogamy would actually show a pattern of effective polygyny.

Among the general reasons for expecting effective polygyny among humans are the following. Societies allowing polygyny are by far the commonest, those allowing polyandry by far the rarest; this suggests that conditions favoring polygyny have been widespread. Human sexual dimorphism – in both mind and body – suggests an evolutionary history in which polygyny preponderated (Symons 1979). Even if the conditions in which humans evolved have largely disappeared, male and female psyches may still be predisposed to patterns of behavior that result in effective polygyny (Symons 1979). Hence, our primary question is:

1. Does the BSR in societies with socially imposed monogamy (which, from now on, we will simply call monogamous societies) indicate effective polygyny?

Underlying this question are a series of further questions concerning the specific interrelated factors that are likely to contribute to greater male than female reproductive variation in monogamous societies. Most of these questions emerge from the literature on sexual selection particularly the literature following Bateman's (1948) pioneering study of sexual selection in Drosophila.

2. Are there non-reciprocal simultaneous unions? Wholly marital simultaneous unions (polygamy) are ruled out by definition. This leaves wholly extramarital simultaneous unions and adulterous unions. Reciprocal unions, in which, say, two couples committed adultery with each other, promote no tendency to sex differences in reproductive variation. Non-reciprocal unions, however, have distinct effects: in most forms male reproductive variance is increased, since an extra mate enhances the fertility of one man at the expense of another. But no form increases the female variance in reproductive success, since extra mates do not normally make a woman more fertile. (The male quest for sexual variety, and contrasting female choosiness, are expectable consequences of this reproductive contrast.)

3. Do males show more variation in sequential relationships, such as remarriage? Remarriage, which can enhance the fertility of either sex, can generate sex differences in reproductive variation in monogamous societies (Mackey 1980, Lockard and Adams 1981). Historical European societies have shown a persistent tendency for men to remarry more than women (Dupâquier et al. 1981). The tendency is very widespread in modern societies (Charmie and Nsuly 1981). And if some men remarry more than women do, then more men than women must never marry – which appears long to have been the case in the United States, where there are always more single men than women (US Bureau of the Census 1968:32; 1978:40).

4. Is male fertility more sensitive to the age of spouses? Other things being equal, a woman's reproductive potential is greatest when she is near the beginning of her repro-

ductive career. A man, by contrast, has a reproductive potential that is spread more evenly over his adult life, and he typically reaches the peak of his ability to support a wife and children at an age somewhat later than the beginning of his adulthood. Consequently, males who marry or mate with younger females should be more fertile, but female fertility should be little affected by age of spouse or mate.

5. Do males show more variation in age at marriage/mating? Considerations given in 3 suggest that male age should be more variable. To the extent that male fertility is sensitive to own age, variation in age at marriage/mating may contribute to variation in male reproductive success.

6. Are males more likely to be childless? Since females have fewer incentives to choose a younger spouse/mate, males have a higher likelihood of dying before marriage or mating.

7. Is mortality higher for males? As a result of our history of sexual selection, human males typically have higher mortality than females (for reasons explored in Trivers 1972), with the result that death curtails male fertility more than female fertility.

8. Do males marry/mate later than females? If males marry or mate later, they increase their chances of dying childless or with lowered fertility.

9. Are there more males than females? All other things being equal, sex ratios above 100 promote effective polygyny, those below 100 promote effective polyandry.

Previously collected genealogical data on the Pitcairn Islanders allow some answers to these questions.

(Note that we use the term 'mate' to refer to extramarital sexual relationships that resulted in offspring; in this usage a mate is a co-parent who is not a spouse. We did not attempt to detect extramarital affairs that did not result in offspring. We use the terms 'union' or 'relationship' to refer both to marriage and mating.)

The Pitcairn data

On Pitcairn Island (Figure 8.1), settled by the mutineers of the *Bounty*, unique circumstances

provided reasonably accurate genealogies in a monogamous and essentially Western society.

Late in the 18th century, nine mutineers from the *Bounty*, along with six male and 13 female Polynesians, marooned themselves on uninhabited Pitcairn Island. By the time the colony was discovered, 18 years later, only one of the adult males still lived: 12 had been murdered, one committed suicide and one had died. Only three of the women had died. The mutiny was motivated by the desire of the men not to give up the pleasures of their Polynesian mates (Nicholson 1965:70). Most of the murders were motivated by male sexual jealousy (Nicholson 1965).

The man who survived underwent a sort of conversion, and taught the children of the island a strict Christianity. The Pitcairn community was subsequently hailed as a Christian model. Monogamy was socially imposed. The Pitcairners spoke English (but were bilingual), and the European elements in their culture were substantial (Shapiro 1936). Visitors to the island for long periods were relatively rare; even when they were more common the visitors apparently found little or no opportunity to form sexual liaisons with the Pitcairners (Shapiro 1936:107–8). Eventually the island became so crowded that the inhabitants were moved, with British assistance, to Norfolk Island (a deserted former penal colony). After a few years, however, some returned to Pitcairn. Until this century, when genealogies were collected from them, the inhabitants of Norfolk and Pitcairn Islands were very largely composed of descendants of the original mutineers and the Polynesians who accompanied them to Pitcairn.

Figure 8.1 The South Pacific showing the location of Pitcairn Island.

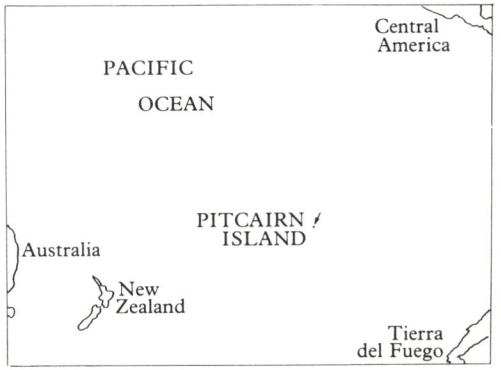

Fairly careful records of births and deaths had been kept on Pitcairn from quite early on, and it was possible – in response to the great interest Pitcairners inspired when they were found – to reconstruct the births and deaths from the years preceding careful records. In the 1920s and 1930s an anthropologist, Shapiro (1929, 1936), visited the islands with the specific goal of gathering accurate genealogies. Shapiro's work – supplemented for the period up to 1856 by the exhaustive inquiries of the historian Nicholson (1965) – provide information on births, deaths, marriages, and parentage (including illegitimacy) for all the persons descended from and including the original Pitcairners (and the few persons who joined them) up to the 1920s.

It is doubtful that many existing genealogies have been collected from monogamous peoples under such favorable conditions for the following reasons:

1. The entire populace is accounted for.
2. The smallness and remoteness of the islands – particularly Pitcairn – minimized conditions that lead to spurious genealogical data. On the one hand, the small size of the islands increased the chances that an illicit sexual relationship would be detected (note that under somewhat comparable conditions for detecting illegitimacy, !Kung determine paternity as successfully as maternity (Marshall 1976:280, Howell 1979:231–2), and note Shapiro's confidence in having detected almost all cases of illegitimacy among the Pitcairners [1936:219–20]). On the other hand, remoteness meant that it was not easy to leave the island to prevent detection of illicit pregnancies or to escape their consequences.
3. The ideological commitment to monogamy was strong, because the Christian indoctrination of the inhabitants went unchallenged (as by the media, advertising, persons of other subcultures, etc. – all factors that might divert behavior from the monogamous ideal).

Item three sets particularly difficult conditions in which to expect greater reproductive variation among males. Assuming that the very condition that fostered the monogamous ideal on Pitcairn – i.e. their desire to be good Christians – did not also foster more determination in preventing outsiders from discovering such indiscretions as did occur (an assumption that cannot now be

tested against firmer data such as blood typing), the Pitcairners thus provide desirable controls for a natural experiment to detect sex differences in reproductive variation in a monogamous society.

Combining Nicholson's information with Shapiro's, the reproductive and marital careers of 285 persons (145 males, 140 females) and their several hundred children could be established. Note, however, that for almost all analyses sample sizes are reduced from these figures due to insufficient information of one kind or another. For example, in Table 8.1 the number of females is reduced by 13 due to uncertain maternity assignments of children whose fathers remarried. For other purposes most of the excluded women can be put back. For example, in the analysis of childlessness ten of the excluded women can be counted, because it is known that each had at least one child. In a few cases uncertainty of the data necessitates a least figure or a range. Note also that many of our subjects' offspring lack death dates, so that only rarely could we measure reproductive success in terms of offspring who reach reproductive age. Consequently, we speak of fertility and reproductive success synonymously, and measure them in terms of live births.

Results

The results are presented below in the order the questions were posed earlier in the paper.

1. The BSR does not indicate effective polygyny. Table 8.1 shows the differential fertility of males and females. Three features stand out: (a) the distributions are quite similar, (b) a substantial number of subjects had no children (i.e. live births), males more so than females, and (c) the single most fertile person was not a man, but rather a woman who bore 20 children. The female variance is 23.17; the male variance is 23.64. The BSR is 1.02. This degree of deviation from perfect monogamy is highly likely to occur by chance.

2. and 3. Males showed insignificantly greater variation in simultaneous and sequential relationships as shown in Table 8.2. Males preponderated in both never marrying or mating and in forming multiple unions. Males remarried or mated adulterously 43 times (34% of

156

Table 8.1 *Differential fertility of males and females*

Live births	Female subjects	%	Male subjects	%
0	47	37.0[a]	60	41.4
1	4	3.1	3	2.1
2	6	4.7	5	3.4
3	7	5.5	6	4.1
4	4	3.1	5	3.4
5	5	3.9	1	0.7
6	6	4.7	8	5.5
7	6	4.7	10	6.9
8	11	8.7	14	9.6
9	7	5.5	5	3.4
10	4	3.1	6	4.1
11	9	7.1	7	4.8
12	5	3.9	5	3.4
13	2	1.6	3	2.1
14	0	0	3	2.1
15	1	0.8	2	1.4
16	2	1.6	1	0.7
17	0	0	1	0.7
18	0	0	0	0
19	0	0	0	0
20	1	0.8	0	0
Totals	127	100%	145	100%

[a] Actual percentage is 34 (see discussion of childlessness on p. 156)

Table 8.2 *Frequencies of marriage/mating*

	Females	Males
Never married/mated	26 (19%)	39 (28%)
Married/mated once	94 (69%)	82 (58%)
Married/mated twice	13 (9%)	18 (13%)
Married/mated 3 times	4 (3%)	1 (1%)
Married/mated 4 times	0	1 (1%)
SD	0.63	0.70

the latter is ($p < 0.001$).

5. Males did not show more variation in age at marriage/mating. Table 8.3 shows ages at first union. Although females peaked sharply between ages 16 and 20, as is expected, their remaining unions were widely spread. Males lacked the sharp peak in a single half-decade, but 76% of all who were to marry married between ages 16 and 25. The standard deviation of female age at first marriage is 6.26; the corresponding male figure is 5.2. This difference is significant ($F = 1.44, p < 0.05$).

6. Male childlessness (41%) was insignificantly greater than female childlessness (34%).

7. Male mortality was not quite significantly higher. The mean longevity of males was 44.4, of females 49.6 ($t = 1.49$, df $= 218$, $p < 0.10 > 0.05$). Proportionately more males than females died in each decade up to age 40; proportionately more females died in all but one (the 90s) decade thereafter.

8. Males married/mated significantly later than females. The average age at first union for females was 20.9, for males 22.6 ($t = 1.84$, df $= 167$, $p < 0.05$). A further perspective is provided by data on the relative ages of spouses/mates (at first union): it was between two and three times more common for the male to be older – a difference that is significant beyond the 0.001 level. Moreover, males who formed such first unions were significantly more fertile (averaging 8.27 offspring) than those forming first unions in which the female was older (averaging 6.27 offspring) ($t = 1.80$, df $= 62$, $p < 0.05$). Females in male-older first unions approached significantly greater fertility (average offspring 8.45) than those in male-younger first unions (average offspring 5.94) ($t = 1.65$, df $= 56$, $P < 0.10 > 0.05$). The male-older pattern persisted in remarriages, particularly in the remarriages of males (who almost always took

their 126 unions), while the corresponding figure for women is 38 (29% of their 132 unions). There were only two definite cases of women involved with more than one man at a time. But there were at least six cases of men involved simultaneously with more than one woman, and five of these were of a form – married man with single woman – likely to increase the gap between male and female variances in fertility. The rest of the multiple unions were sequential. Forming multiple unions had little or no effect on female fertility, but did (insignificantly) enhance the fertility of males: females who married/mated only once averaged between 5.99 and 6.30 live births; those who married/mated more than once averaged 6.23; the corresponding figures for males were 6.35 and 7.15.

4. Male fertility was more sensitive to the age of spouses. A random sample of 46 unions shows a coefficient of correlation (r) between fertility of the union and age of husband (all the sample unions were marriages) of -0.17; between fertility of the union and age of wife it is -0.49. The former is not significant;

Table 8.3 *Ages at first union*

Ages	11–15	16–20	21–25	26–30	31–35	36–40	41–45	51–55
Females	11	43	19	12	1		1	1
Males	2	30	32	10	4	2	1	

a new spouse younger than the previous one).

9. The sex ratio at birth was 104.

Discussion

Since our principal result is contrary to expectation, we wondered if our methods might have biased the results. Specifically, did we merge two populations into one, and did measuring reproductive success in terms of live births unduly inflate female reproductive variance?

In some senses the data above are drawn from two different populaces. On one hand are the original settlers of Pitcairn, whose bloody male–male competition for females left a single 'bull' as winner. On the other hand are the subsequent inhabitants, whose behavior was quite different. But for most purposes, excluding the original settlers has little effect on the results. For example, the BSR merely drops from 1.02 to 1.01, and the standard deviations given in Table 8.2 to 0.59 and 0.64.

Two subsets of the data are, however, closely connected to the distinction between the original settlers and the remainder. (1) Almost half the females who formed more than one union were in the founding generation, in which two of the women came to Pitcairn in polyandrous (and infertile) relationships with native men. Male multiple unions, by contrast, were spread evenly over the generations. Thus, after the founding generation, only 8 unions were a second or third for a woman, while for men at least 15 were. (2) Adultery was disproportionate in the founding generation. There were at least 6 fertile adulterous unions (resulting in at least 17 illegitimate children); four of these unions were in the founding generation. In all six cases the man was married to another woman at the time; in only one case was the woman married at the time. Since adultery was more of a male phenomenon, eliminating the four adulterous cases of the founding generation partially cancels out the effect of removing the female multiple unions of that generation.

To examine the effect of defining reproductive success by live births we compared male ($n = 54$) and female ($n = 39$) reproductive variances for persons (original settlers excluded) born before 1834 (the death dates for offspring of those born later are too rarely known). The result was a BSR ranging from 1.02 to 1.05. If the original settlers are included it drops to a range from 0.94 to 0.97. None of these results is significantly different from effective monogamy, nor from the results yielded by using live births.

If, therefore, the results may be accepted, what conclusions may be drawn from them? First, it must be concluded that monogamous societies, contrary to expectation, can be effectively monogamous. On the other hand, it is notable that almost every factor that was thought to promote effective polygyny was present, in the right direction, even if usually to an insignificant degree. This suggests that the reasons for thinking male variance in reproductivity would continue to be greater than the female variance were largely correct, but that the extent to which these factors would contribute to male variance was overestimated.

What cannot be concluded is that effective monogamy among the Pitcairn Islanders indicates an absence of intra-sexual competition among them or even balanced rates of intra-sexual competition. When the BSR is large, as among the Xavante, it seems safe to conclude that male–male competition is substantially greater than female–female competition, but this is a rough inference, for the precise amount that sexual competition contributes to the variances is not actually known. Many other factors, such as sterility, also account for variance in reproduction. When the BSR is low, it is a moot point as to where intra-sexual competition leaves off and the other factors begin in contributing to either sex's variances in reproductive success. Whatever the boundary between these factors, the Pitcairn case shows that prescriptive monogamy can result in a comparatively low rate of sexual competition in males, but does not show that sexual competition can be eliminated.

Finally, if we grant that the Pitcairn case

shows that a monogamous society can be effectively monogamous, can we also assume that the same is true for *modern* monogamous societies? There are reasons to doubt this: (1) The opportunities for adultery may be better. (2) Divorce and remarriage are commoner. (3) Medical and contraceptive technology limit female reproductive variance at both ends: infertility is successfully treated; deaths in childbearing reduced; excess fertility is limited.

Summary

The following points have been made in this paper:

1. It was found that the Pitcairn Islanders were effectively monogamous, and hence quite dissimilar from societies such as the Xavante.
2. It was pointed out that balanced variances in reproduction do not indicate an absence of reproductive competition.
3. It was suggested that the Pitcairn Islanders may be more effectively monogamous than would be expected in most modern societies.

Acknowledgements

We are grateful for comments and suggestions from Napoleon Chagnon, Martin Daly, Barry Hewlett, Keith Kintigh, Margo Wilson, the editors and readers for this volume, and especially from Donald Symons, whose ideas originally inspired this paper, and who patiently read its various drafts.

References

Alexander, R. D., Hoogland, J. L., Howard, R. D., Noonan, K. M., and Sherman, P. W. (1979) Sexual dimorphisms and breeding systems in pinnipeds, ungulates, primates, and humans. In *Evolutionary Biology and Human Social Behavior: An Anthropological Perspective*, ed. N. A. Chagnon and W. Irons, pp. 402–35. North Scituate, MA: Duxbury Press.

Bateman, A. J. (1948) Intra-sexual selection in *Drosophila. Heredity*, 2, 349–68.

Chamie, J. and Nsuly, S. (1981) Sex differences in remarriage and spouse selection. *Demography*, 18, 335–48.

Daly, M. and Wilson, M. (1983) *Sex, Evolution and Behavior*, 2nd edition. Boston: Willard Grant Press.

Dupâquier, J., Helin, E., Laslett, P., Livi-Bacci, M., and Sogner, S. (eds.) (1981) *Marriage and Remarriage in Populations of the Past*. New York: Academic Press.

Howell, N. (1979) *Demography of the Dobe !Kung*. New York: Academic Press.

Lockard, J. S. and Adams, R. M. (1981) Human serial polygyny: demographic, reproductive, marital, and divorce data. *Ethology and Sociobiology*, 2, 177–86.

Mackey, W. C. (1980) A sociobiological perspective on divorce patterns of men in the United States. *Journal of Anthropological Research*, 36, 419–30.

Marshall, L. (1976) *The !Kung of Nyae Nyae*. Cambridge: Harvard University Press.

Nicholson, R. B. (1965) *The Pitcairners*. Sydney: Angus and Robertson.

Salzano, F. M., Neel, J. V., and Maybury-Lewis, D. (1967) Further studies on the Xavante Indians. I. Demographic data on two additional villages: genetic structure of the tribe. *American Journal of Human Genetics*, 19, 463–89.

Shapiro, H. L. (1929) *Descendants of the Mutineers of the Bounty. Memoirs of the Bernice P. Bishop Museum*. Vol. XI, No. 1. Honolulu.

Shapiro, H. L. (1936) *The Heritage of the Bounty: The Story of Pitcairn through Six Generations*. New York: Simon and Schuster.

Symons, D. (1979) *The Evolution of Human Sexuality*. New York: Oxford University Press.

Trivers, R. L. (1972) Parental investment and sexual selection. In *Sexual Selection and the Descent of Man 1871–1971*, ed. B. Campbell, pp. 136–79. Chicago: Aldine.

US Bureau of the Census (1968, 1978) *Statistical Abstract of the United States* (89th and 99th editions). Washington, DC.

Robin I. M. Dunbar[1]

Darwinizing
man:
a commentary

The significance of Darwinian theory lies not so much in whether it is right or wrong as in its power. It provides us with a theoretical structure that has important implications in two crucial respects. First, it allows us to integrate within a single unified framework all aspects of biology and behaviour. This means that we can now translate the costs and benefits of different activities or characters into a common currency so as to be able to make direct comparisons of their relative evolutionary values. Second, the theory allows us to make very precise predictions about behaviour and morphology that can be tested in the field.

Hitherto, most theories in the social and behavioural sciences have tended to emphasize proximate mechanisms for the phenomena they have sought to explain. Chayanov's (1966) theory of peasant economies, for example, concentrated exclusively on the implications of family composition for food production and consumption. This makes it difficult to compare the predictions of his theory with theories that suggest that relationships within a community have more to do, say, with power politics. As Berté stresses in her chapter (this volume, Chapter 4),

[1] Department of Zoology, University of Liverpool, Brownlow Street, PO Box 147, Liverpool, L69 3BX, UK

Darwinian evolutionary theory provides us with an ultimate arbiter, a unique currency into which everything can be converted with the result that their respective consequences can then be compared directly in quantitative form.

The implications of these two points are profound, for they make it possible to carry out very fine-grained tests between competing theories. This has the effect of greatly speeding up the rate at which incorrect hypotheses can be discarded, so making it easier to find the correct explanation for the phenomenon under study. We need only to look to the success of physics and, more recently, molecular biology to appreciate just how effective such a research strategy can be. These two disciplines have advanced as rapidly and as far as they have not because they advocate reductionist theories but because they are able to bring very precise predictions to bear on the data available to them (see Platt 1964).

Social scientists have tended to shy away from such an approach, usually on the grounds that they study ideas in people's minds and that ideas are not susceptible to quantitative study in the way that physical phenomena are. But this is really just an obscurantist tactic, for physics itself provides us with two perfectly good examples of how to study what you cannot see directly and what you cannot put to direct experimental test. One of these is particle physics, the study of the fundamental bases of matter – a discipline that involves studying what even in principle can never be touched or manipulated, for the elementary particles of matter are in fact insubstantial forces analogous to gravity. What makes it possible for physicists to delve so deeply at this level is the fact that they can use powerful theories to make very precise quantitative predictions about what ought to happen if a given state of affairs exists at the quantum level. This allows them to develop extended causal chains that begin with unobservable particles or forces and ultimately end with observable consequences in the everyday world, be these consequences traces in a bubble chamber, marks on X-ray film or numbers on a particle 'counter'. The other discipline to which social scientists might look is cosmology, the study of the evolution of the universe. Cosmology deals with events that occurred so far in the past that we can never have any hope of observing them. Nonetheless, because everything that happens necessarily has

consequences, we can work through the relevant causal chains and identify states or events in the observable universe today that would be direct consequences of states of affairs that might have pertained in the remote past. This has allowed cosmologists to determine with some confidence the initial state of the universe and its subsequent history. Indeed, so sophisticated have these analyses become that it is now possible for cosmologists to devote entire conferences to the first three *seconds* of the universe's existence. They can do this only because the theories that they rely on (essentially those of physics) are so detailed and precise that very exact predictions are possible, thereby once again making quantitative tests a practical proposition.

A sceptical social scientist might, nonetheless, insist that while such an approach works well with physical systems, applying it to a phenomenon as complex as a human society is quite another matter. While physical systems simply follow through the inevitable consequences of a definable set of principles, human beings (like all higher vertebrates) are capable of assessing the implications of a very wide range of options and then choosing whichever strategy seems to be the most profitable under the circumstances. And one of those strategies may well be to leave the system altogether by emigrating (as the *Bounty* mutineers did, for example). The problem is, if you like, the subtlety that human beings are often able to inject into their evaluation of social situations and the consequent cunning with which they devise strategies to solve the problems thrown at them by Nature or their fellow humans. A particularly nice example of this is provided by the French nobility in the 19th century. When the *Code Civil* was promulgated in 1804 by the then imperial government, inheritance by primogeniture was abrogated. The intention was, in part, to break the stranglehold of the landed aristocracy of the *ancien régime* by forcing the dispersal of their large estates. But the nobility were able to circumvent this threat to their power base by radically reducing the size of their families while encouraging marriages within extended families (Eversley 1959). The result was certainly a regular reshuffling of estates, but without dramatically reducing the land holdings of individual families.

This kind of complexity should not deter us from tackling the problems of social behaviour on Darwinian lines, any more than physicists and astronomers were deterred by the seeming complexity of their subject matter during the early days of these disciplines. An indication of what can be done is given by Borgerhoff Mulder's study of Kipsigis marriage conventions (Chapter 3). She was able to identify three radically different factors that influenced the bride price that families were able to demand for their daughters: these were the girl's reproductive potential (essentially a function of her age), her reproductive status at the time of marriage and the future value of her labour services to her parents. All three factors had a significant effect on bride price, although between them they in fact accounted for only about 15% of the variance in the bride prices agreed between contracting parties. While obviously a long step away from providing a deterministic explanation of the variance in bride price, these analyses do imply that the calculations made by prospective in-laws when negotiating a marriage contract are immensely complex – perhaps even more complex than anthropologists have traditionally supposed.

In one sense, Darwinism's main problem has lain in its power as an explanatory framework for behaviour. This has undoubtedly tempted some researchers to generate simple unitary explanations for natural phenomena. The most pervasive of these has been that involving kin selection. For reasons which I completely fail to understand, kin selection seems to have developed into a kind of general panacea. Indeed, in some circles, it seems to have become synonymous with sociobiology as though the approach had nothing more to offer. Thus, Gray (1985), in an otherwise perceptive review of primate sociobiology, observes that 'the widespread acceptance and use of sociobiology in the social sciences ultimately depends on convincing demonstrations of [kin selection] theory's power to explain the evolution and current operation . . . social systems'. Even if the social insects are an exception, it is a fair bet that a substantial proportion of the social systems of most vertebrates can be understood without having to breathe a word about kin selection. This is certainly the case for non-human primates (see e.g. Dunbar 1987), so it would be rather surprising if humans were so exceptional. What really counts, as many of the studies in this section

of the book show, is the need to acquire mates, allies and helpers. While it may ease the wheels of negotiation if relatives are chosen, it is by no means necessarily always going to be the case that relatives make the best allies. Kinship is but one factor among many that needs to be evaluated by the individual in choosing allies and mates, and often the interests of kin selection (in the formal sense of the fitness of collateral relatives) will give way to the overriding concerns of personal reproduction (see Dunbar 1983).

The most serious methodological problem that has bedevilled Darwinism is undoubtedly the tendency to test a particular prediction and then, on finding a close fit between observed and predicted values, to conclude that the underlying mechanism must be that of the hypothesis under test. That individuals tend to form alliances with relatives in the way predicted by kin selection, for example, is taken as evidence that kin selection must be the operative factor (i.e. that alliance formation is altruistic in that the only expectation of gain is through the increased fitness of the relative concerned). But this is at best a weak inference, for, as the editors point out in their introductory chapter, many other equally valid evolutionary principles may yield the same prediction. It may well be that decisions made about alliances in the here and now are a consequence of the way in which the individual views future alliance options. For any number of reasons, relatives may prove to be more reliable allies, so that alliances formed now may enhance the probability of reciprocation in the future (for a primate example of this see Dunbar 1984).

Simple-minded unitary explanations of this kind are not, however, an intrinsic characteristic of Darwinism (*qua* a body of theory), even if they are typical of some Darwinists (*qua* practitioners of the theory), and the blame ought to be allocated correctly. This is not to say that any such arguments are necessarily wrong, but merely that they are based on weak inferential processes. They would gain immeasurably in power if they were put to the test along with other competing explanations (including possible confounding variables). This not only increases confidence in the conclusions drawn, but also has the added advantage of undermining the counter-arguments of critics before they even surface in print.

The value of this approach is emphasized by several of the papers in this part. Borgerhoff Mulder (Chapter 3), for example, used multiple regression analysis to explore the extent to which a number of factors influenced bride price in the Kipsigis. While several factors did turn out to be important, others (e.g. wealth differences between contracting families) turned out to be unimportant despite their initial plausibility. Both Betzig (Chapter 2) and Berté (Chapter 4) compared the predictions of several different theories with their observed data, thereby making it possible to exclude those hypotheses that were irrelevant. As a result, the confirmed hypothesis in each case is greatly strengthened. Similarly, in her analysis of the relationship between polygyny and pathogen stress, Low (Chapter 6) checked and rechecked her analyses by erecting and then trying to eliminate alternative confounding variables that might have accounted for the observed relationships among the data. An equally powerful alternative to multiple-hypothesis-testing is the generation of inferential chains that lead to further predictions. Crook and Crook (Chapter 5) used this technique to advantage in their study of Tibetan polyandry in order to capitalize on certain natural experiments that had occurred in their sample families. In this way, they were able to put their hypothesized explanation for polyandry to the test by comparing the consequences of this explanation with what actually happened.

This last study raises an issue that is given considerable emphasis by Chagnon in his analysis of Yanomamö kinship naming (Chapter 1), namely the role that demography plays in social systems. Demography, as a topic, has been virtually ignored in studies of both human and nonhuman primates alike, despite the fact that the demographic structure of a population unit plays a key role in determining the freedom of movement that an individual has in selecting its social partners (for more detailed discussion, see Seyfarth 1976, Altmann and Altmann 1979, Dunbar 1979). If past demographic events (notably random variations in the birth rate, in the neonatal sex ratio and in the subsequent mortality of the two sexes) result in a shortfall in the number of females of marriageable age, then not all males seeking brides will be able to acquire one. Instead, they may have to make do with what in reproductive terms may be 'suboptimal' brides (such as cripples, individuals past their peak in fecundity, those of doubtful sexual loyalty or those from elsewhere who will in consequence lack relatives that can give support or practical help to the groom).

Hitherto, as Chagnon points out, anthropologists (and biologists) have tended to study 'ideal' (or rather *idealized*) systems. They have tried, for example, to determine the kinship categories that their informants use with a view to identifying the underlying structure of the society in which those individuals live. But the real world is rarely so ideal, mainly because, in species as long-lived and slowly reproducing as man, the vagaries of the demographic processes commonly generate anomalies in the structure of the population. The result is inevitably that reality seldom matches up to the ideal for which the members of society strive. In order to operate effectively within such a system of constraints, individuals are forced to compromise on their ideals. If this means adjusting kinship designations in order to make it possible to marry, then so be it, for in the long run it is better to marry a less than ideal mate than not to marry at all, particularly if marriage is the only means whereby you can generate the large family required to hunt or farm effectively.

This tendency to compromise on ideal objectives is a characteristic of all biological systems, but it is a particularly conspicuous feature of complex societies such as those found among primates in general and man in particular. Betzig's study of chiefs' rights to fish catches and other forms of tribute on Ifaluk (Chapter 2) can serve as an example here. If people are exploited as the commoners of Ifaluk are, Darwinian principles oblige us to ask why they should be prepared to tolerate it since, all other things being equal, they would expose themselves to less risk and less exertion if they could keep the whole of their fish catch for themselves. What is it that makes it worth an individual's while submitting to the chiefs' demands and incurring these costs? Although Betzig is unable to resolve the issue in this particular case, she is able to point to at least two possible reasons, one negative (low-ranking individuals have no choice because it is too difficult to escape from such an isolated island group) and one positive (that chiefs do redistribute some of the food and this may allow individuals who have fallen on hard times to keep going). It is worth observing, in addition, that chiefs can serve other important organizing functions in society which, in the long-term, may reflect directly back on the survival and reproductive success of individual members of the society. Where the survival of individuals depends on cooperative efforts in solving major technological problems (e.g. bush clearance for new fields or building large sea-going canoes), chiefs may provide an integrative role that allows the relevant processes to take place more smoothly. Paying someone to be chief may thus simply be a form of compensation for the additional costs incurred by chiefs in having to organize the community's affairs (an activity that is generally incompatible with the time-consuming business of subsistence farming).

My intention here is not to offer speculations on the functions of chiefs, but simply to point out that explanations that might be evolutionarily relevant need not be immediately concerned with individual acts of biological survival and reproduction: in the first instance, some of them may be closer to the purely conceptual phenomena which some social scientists regard as being of central interest. The key consideration is only that we be able to trace through the consequences of those notional phenomena to identify specific effects on the survival and reproduction of individuals. Our ability to find a way out of the tangle of arguments and counter-arguments then depends only on being able to confront these various hypotheses with data from the real world. Such tests are not always immediately possible, often because the questions only emerge from the data as they are analysed, long after field work has ended. This does not, of course, mean that such tests are impossible, but it does underscore the importance of asking questions about how and why a society functions while the field work is being done. Although there are widely recognized dangers of imposing one's own views and biases onto the societies one studies, this should not distract us from the importance of framing questions. A Darwinian framework forces us to keep asking why things are as they are and, providing we are not satisfied with glib answers and unsubstantiated hypotheses, we cannot help but be directed down the right avenues by the data themselves. We may not end up with the answers that we anticipated at the outset, but in the process we will almost

certainly have been forced to delve far more deeply into the workings of complex phenomena than we would have done by passive observation alone.

There can be no doubt that the real problem where human societies are concerned is that they are extraordinarily complex. Ultimately, if we are to make any real sense of such systems, we will need to know how each component of the system works and how it interacts with other components, how each decision on one problem affects those on others and how these, in turn, feed back on the first problem. One methodological implication of this is that studies that set out to make a detailed analysis of a single component of a social system (e.g. marriage conventions or labour organization) can never do more than tinker with reality because the way a group of individuals solves a particular problem cannot be divorced from all the many other facets of behaviour and circumstance that bear on survival and reproduction. In a word, *everything* an individual is and does is part of an integrated co-evolved reproductive strategy. And this, I should stress, includes not only features like labour organization, kinship structures, alliances, child-rearing practices and religious beliefs, but also the more overtly biological factors like demographic processes and environmental conditions. Unless and until we attempt to study entire societies as integrated units, it will never be possible to generate predictive statements about the future behaviour of their members that have more than a random chance of being correct. This kind of hypothesis-testing is actually little better than the kinds of 'fishing' exercises indulged in by computer addicts in which every variable in a data-set is cross-correlated with every other variable in the hopes of finding some significant relationships.

This is not to say that we cannot make some progress on a piecemeal basis. The point is that by relying exclusively on such a research strategy we risk arriving at the wrong explanation for a phenomenon (or, at the very least, rejecting the right one) precisely because we are looking for optimal solutions to a particular problem while ignoring the fact that any optimal solution in an integrated system is necessarily constrained by other features of the system. What may, in an ideal world, be the optimum solution to a given problem will, in the real world, often be unachievable simply because it conflicts with the need to solve other problems that are equally crucial to the individual's survival and successful reproduction. In a nutshell, you cannot both eat and procreate at the same time and since, biologically speaking, we need to do both, the only possible solution is to apportion your time in such a way as to make the best of your particular circumstances.

This raises another issue that several contributors to this section have touched on, namely the fact that societies are dynamic not static systems. They can and do change over time as circumstances dictate a need. There has been a long-standing tendency for biologists in particular to view social systems as static entities and hence to study a particular population of a species as in some meaningful sense 'representative' of the species at large. It was not uncommon, for example, to go into the field to study The Baboon. But social systems are not static in this sense: they consist of individuals, each of whom is striving to maximize his or her contribution to the species' gene pool. If we have learned anything from studies of primates during the last decade or so, it has been that their social systems are interactive systems that are highly responsive to fine changes in both ecological and demographic contexts. In some respects, what we see as societies are no more than moment-by-moment solutions to problems that are particularly pressing in biological terms. The variety of social systems and social strategies that we see even within a given species is simply the consequence of the same deep structure rule (say 'Maximize the number of offspring you rear to maturity') finding expression in a variety of different forms depending on the particular demographic and environmental context.

There has, of course, been a tradition within anthropology emphasizing the fact that societies and cultures evolve (in a non-biological sense) and that cultural institutions do change when they come into contact with more powerful cultures. Nonetheless, I suspect that there has still been an implicit tendency to assume that particular societies are internally coherent and formally structured such that, in the absence of contacts with alien cultures, they will continue as they are through time. This view seems to underlie many of the more traditional theories of human social systems in which societies are viewed as having in some very real sense a life of their own such that they impose on their members certain forms or norms of behaviour: individuals simply slot into pre-existing roles whose existence is created or defined by the form of the society.

While it is certainly true that individuals within a society are not generally free to do as they wish but are often constrained to behave in certain ways, in the final analysis it is the *members* of society and not the social system that impose those constraints. And such constraints will only be tolerated so long as they are seen to be in the best long-term interests of individual members – or at least so long as those individuals feel that they lack the power to do anything about it or that actively doing so would have even worse consequences. This suggests that the mere fact of living together in a group creates internal tensions that will tend to lead towards the break-up or dissolution of the group. Such a tendency will always have to be held in check by a series of balances designed to counteract their influence. Presumably, such tensions are likely to become increasingly severe as the form of society develops to a point where some individuals are able to exploit other individuals.

This being so, we must, I think, expect that individuals will be constantly aware of their situation and will make every effort to capitalize on whatever opportunities present themselves. Several studies in this section of the book point to just such subtle shifts in behaviour. In some cases, decisions at the individual level can have a far-reaching and dramatic effect on the structure of the society as a whole, a point that perhaps emphasizes the fact that, in reality, societies are no more than the emergent properties of the set of economic, social and reproductive strategies being pursued by their individual members (see also Hinde 1976). Thus, Crook and Crook (Chapter 5) point to the changes that can occur within a traditional polyandrous Tibetan society as an individual's context and status alter. The younger brother in a polyandrous marriage will seek his own monogamous marriage whenever he can, but he can do so only providing he has access to some form of income that makes him economically independent of the traditional family farm. In recent times, such opportunities have occurred as a result of new forms of salaried employment created either by the need for a local government bureaucracy (imposed and financed by the national government) or by the expedition industry fostered by the international mountaineering fraternity. The result has been a gradual break-up of the traditional polyandrous society in those areas most affected by outside economics. This has involved not only a greater frequency of monogamous marriages, but also a tendency for the post-reproductive grandparental generation to retain control over the family farm rather than surrendering it to the reproductive filial generation when the eldest son marries. Similarly, Borgerhoff Mulder (Chapter 3) reviewed several instances in which the nature of bride-price conventions have changed over time as a result of the changing socioeconomic status of women.

But the most fascinating example of how cultural institutions can be subtly changed by the dictates of circumstance is surely provided by Chagnon's data on kinship naming by the Yąnomamö (Chapter 1). What is quite extraordinary here is the way in which individuals were willing to alter the kinship categories of genetic relatives in order to make them available as marriage and alliance partners when biologically more appropriate individuals were in short supply. Note that since it is *individuals*, not the society, who stand to gain or lose by these judgements, conflicts of interest occasionally arise between individuals who would prefer to classify the same person in different kinship categories.

What makes this a particularly interesting case is the fact that the Yąnomamö made every effort to preserve their traditional cultural names for kinship groups and instead sought to bend the rules by which the names were applied. Presumably, doing so placed less strain on the general network of relationships within the village community than the alternative strategy of overtly attempting to alter the cultural conventions themselves. In most cases, the latter course is likely to call into question the whole structure of their cultural institutions and might well generate so much strife as to lead to the complete breakdown of society, with all the adverse consequences that this would have for each individual's continued survival. Ideally, what we would like to know at this point is how successful individuals in this village were in reproductive terms compared to those in other villages who failed to make such an adjustment. One of the

conveniences of working on the social systems of higher vertebrates is that individuals often do pursue different strategies and this nearly always makes it possible to find examples of alternative strategies that can be used to compare the relative success of different solutions to the same problem.

This inherent flexibility in the social systems of higher vertebrates in general (and human beings in particular) raises one last point that needs to be stressed precisely because it has been a stumbling-block to the wider acceptance of Darwinism among social scientists. Naive interpretations of Darwinism have taken its preoccupation with genes to imply a belief in genetic determinism. The confusion has, I think, arisen because the word 'gene' happens to appear at two different points in the evolutionary process, namely at both the beginning and the end as cause and consequence of biological reproduction. Sociobiology is concerned centrally with the *consequences* of behaviour in terms of gene propagation and it is a serious mistake to assume that this necessarily implies anything about the genetic control of ontogeny or, more importantly, of behaviour itself (see also Dunbar 1986). It is one thing to assert that behaviour is geared to maximizing an individual's genetic contribution to future generations; it is quite another to infer from this that behaviour is itself genetically determined. This may be true of invertebrates, but it is manifestly not true of most vertebrates – and I take it as axiomatic that man is to be included among the vertebrates.

This said, however, I do recognize that the fault does not lie entirely with sociobiology's critics. Although a minority of the more obscure sociobiologists probably do seem to be convinced that behaviour is genetically determined (whatever that means), most of us simply use a genic metaphor without any such implications. We do so essentially for reasons of convenience: it just makes it a great deal easier to work through the implications and mathematics of a causal chain if you assume a one-to-one relationship between genes and behaviour. This usage is not, of course, without its problems, as Oyama (1985) has pointed out. Not only may the implications be misunderstood by uninitiated readers, but over-familiarity sometimes leads even the initiated to forget that the usage is metaphorical: as a result, they come to confuse the metaphor with reality. Hints of this slippage can be detected even among some of the papers in this part. In their analysis of the development of sex differences in cognitive traits, for example, Gaulin and Hoffman (Chapter 7) correctly stress the interactionist nature of development: differences in inherited genetic components can and do have important developmental implications, but these may be modified by environmental circumstances or by socialization processes. Yet, at times, even they seem to be looking for genetically determined characters that are universally valid for all humans – or at least that is the impression they are likely to create on a superficial reading.

In my view, those who concentrate on a search for species-wide universals in behaviour or morphological traits are likely to be disappointed. The number of genuinely universal traits are, I suspect, likely to run to single figures at most and probably correspond to the handful of biological 'needs' like warmth, food and procreation (see also Dunbar 1986). Beyond that, everything else is essentially a context-specific attempt to put those few universal principles into practice. It is surely in the subtlety of how individuals operating within complex sociobiological systems achieve the all-encompassing aim of reproducing effectively that the real challenge of Darwinism lies. Nonetheless, such is the elegance of the Darwinian approach that we can bring the same analytical principles to bear on the strategies of species whose behaviour is as different in its ontogeny as that of the honey bee and man.

Looking back over the chapters in this section, we have, I think, every reason to look towards the future with a sense of excitement and anticipation. While none of the chapters can perhaps lay claim to having unequivocally solved all the problems it raises, taken together they do show just what can be done to advance our understanding of complex societies when powerful theories like those of sociobiology are used to explore the workings of human societies. Taking my cue once again from the physical sciences, I would suggest that the next decade or so will see major developments in our understanding. This is not to suggest that we will end up with classical Darwinian explanations for human behaviour: that would be to misconstrue the nature of the scientific method. Rather, our

explanations will be the product of an interaction between predictive theories and the data of the real world. What we will gain is a forcing of the pace of advance because less time will be wasted pursuing irrelevant side-issues. I have no doubt that biological considerations will play an important part in whatever explanations we do finally arrive at – if only because it is inconceivable that any biological organism can rise so completely above its organismic roots as to divest itself of all trace of those roots. When all is said and done, we live and breathe and it is the very need to do so that generates most of the problems that social systems are designed to solve.

My own personal view is that we shall come to see social systems as collections of strategies aimed at generating cooperative solutions both to key environmental and reproductive problems and to a host of stresses and strains, both psychological and physiological, that are generated whenever individuals live together in close proximity. Darwinian theory will come to play a pivotal role in this not so much because it provides us with a key to understanding social systems (though I happen to believe this to be at least partially true), but because it forces us to formulate hypotheses more precisely so as to permit them to be tested against the real world.

References

Altmann, S. A. and Altmann, J. (1979) Demographic constraints on behaviour and social organisation. In *Primate Ecology and Human Origins*, ed. I. Bernstein and E. O. Smith, pp. 47–64. New York: Garland STPM.

Chayanov, A. V. (1966) *The Theory of Peasant Economy*, ed. D. Thorner, R. E. F. Smith and B. Kerblay. Homewood, IL. Richard D. Irwin, American Economic Association.

Dunbar, R. I. M. (1979) Population demography, social organisation and mating strategies. In *Primate Ecology and Human Origins*, ed. I. Bernstein and E. O. Smith, pp. 65–88. New York: Garland STPM.

Dunbar, R. I. M. (1983) Life-history tactics and alternative strategies of reproduction. In *Mate Choice*, ed. P. P. G. Bateson, pp. 423–33. Cambridge: Cambridge University Press.

Dunbar, R. I. M. (1984) *Reproductive Decisions: An Economic Analysis of Gelada Baboon Social Strategies*. Princeton, NJ: Princeton University Press.

Dunbar, R. I. M. (1986) Sociobiological explanations and the evolution of ethnocentrism. In *The Sociobiology of Ethnocentrism*, ed. V. Reynolds, I. Vine and

V. Falger, pp. 48–59. Beckenham, Kent: Croom Helm.

Dunbar, R. I. M. (1987) *Primate Social Systems*. Beckenham, Kent: Croom Helm (in press).

Eversley, D. E. C. (1959) *Social Theories of Fertility and the Malthusian Debate*. Oxford: Oxford University Press.

Gray, J. P. (1985) *Primate Sociobiology*. New Haven, CT: HRAF Press.

Hinde, R. A. (1976) Interactions, relationships and social structure. *Man*, 11, 1–17.

Oyama, S. (1985) *The Ontogeny of Information*. Cambridge: Cambridge University Press.

Platt, J. R. (1964) Strong inference. *Science*, 146, 347–53.

Seyfarth, R. M. (1976) A model of social grooming among adult female monkeys. *Journal of Theoretical Biology*, 65, 671–98.

Part II

Parenting

Helpers at the nest: childcare networks on Ifaluk

Introduction

In this chapter, tests are conducted of hypotheses positing that particular, learned social interactions by residents of a Micronesian atoll (Ifaluk) reflect a history of natural selection at the level of the individual. The empirical focus is on child-rearing networks involving grandparents, parents, and siblings. The first hypothesis is that *daughters born early in their parents' reproductive careers serve, at least for a time, as 'helpers at the nest'* (e.g. see Emlen 1984). The second is that *as a parent's chance of producing new offspring declines with age, he/she should adopt an alternative reproductive strategy in which resources and services formerly used for direct reproduction are increasingly used to increase the reproductive* *success of extant children and grandchildren.* These hypotheses are then compared with two hypotheses from microeconomic theory. However, it remains first to review the concept of 'inclusive fitness' and related concepts (cf. Betzig *et al.* this volume, Introduction).

Inclusive fitness

The theoretical work of Hamilton, Williams, and a few others, and the empirical work of a generation of biologists, has led to widespread acceptance of the view that in most species indi-

[1] Evolution and Human Behavior Program and Department of Anthropology, University of Michigan, Ann Arbor, MI 48109, USA

viduals have evolved to strive to maximize reproduction, directly or indirectly through relatives (e.g. Alexander and Tinkle 1981). Such strivings lead to what Hamilton (1964) has termed 'inclusive fitness' maximization. In social interaction, inclusive fitness is maximized when $rb > c$, where r is the coefficient of genetic relationship between interactants (genes indentical by descent), b is the reproductive benefit to the recipient of the service or resource transferred in the interaction, and c is the cost in terms of reduced future reproduction the donator of the service or resource acquires as as a result of the donation. Hamilton's rule ($rb > c$) is viewed by biologists as being enormously important because it provides a basis for making precise predictions about degrees of altruistic social interaction between genetic relatives; and because, although we can usually identify many proximate explanations for altruistic social interactions (e.g. we protect our children from danger because we love them), it provides explanation for the origin and maintenance of such mechanisms.

With regard to the two hypotheses presented in this chapter, the reproductive strategy an individual is expected to adopt (rearing children or siblings, or children or grandchildren) hinges on the benefits and costs (Hamilton's b's and c's) that the behaviors involved carry as a function of age, parity, and other circumstances.

Related concepts from models of life history evolution are 'somatic' and 'reproductive effort,' the latter of which is often subdivided into 'mating,' 'parental' and 'extraparental nepotistic effort,' and 'parental investment'. Definitions are reviewed in the Introduction to this volume. The crucial difference to be noted between the two main categories of life-effort is that somatic effort has evolved to increase the future reproductive potential of the individual by increasing the availability of resources (including survival) to be expended on reproduction, whereas reproductive effort depletes resources (including survival) that can be used for future reproduction (Williams 1966a, 1966b, Trivers 1972, Hirshfield and Tinkle 1975, Low 1978, Alexander and Borgia 1979, Alexander 1985).

Methods

The site

Data relevant to the following analysis of kinship

and social behaviour were collected by the author and a co-worker (Laura Betzig) during the summer and fall of 1983 on Ifaluk Atoll. Ifaluk is located in the Western Caroline archipelago, 350 miles east of Yap proper and 400 miles south of Guam. It consists of two small inhabited and two smaller uninhabited islets, with a total land area of 0.6 square miles, and a population at the time of the study of 446 (see Betzig's Figure 2.1, this volume). Ifaluk and other atolls in the vicinity (the nearest is 35 miles away) were formerly dominated by Yap, but are now democratically represented as part of Yap State of the Federated States of Micronesia. Yap and the FSM now interfere little with Ifaluk's local government, which remains based on kinship organized into matrilineal clans headed by chiefs.

The major influence the FSM government has had on Ifaluk affairs has been to make modern medical care and schooling available. Ifaluk's medical connection is through the *Microspirit*, a ship which, during a circuit of the archipelago that occurs roughly once every six weeks, ferries passengers to the hospital on Yap and antibiotics to the hospital-trained health-care worker (an Ifaluk native) who resides on Ifaluk. The result is a much reduced mortality rate at all ages, especially infancy (mortality rates are not too different from the US and much lower than in many Third World countries; Yap Statistical Yearbook 1980, Turke 1985).

School is taught locally by ten Ifaluk natives to boys and girls through grade eight. Boys (but not girls) are able to go on to high school at a neighboring atoll (Ulithi), but only four were in attendance during the time of our study. The local teachers receive salaries from the FSM, and therefore have much more money than members of the general population. However, the outlet for their Western currency generally is limited to those goods brought by the *Microspirit*: vodka, cigarettes, and coffee, and a limited selection of overpriced canned fish, meat, rice, and babyfood.

As far as the general population is concerned, cash, and therefore access to the aforementioned Western products, is available only through the sale of copra. Households on average sell between 10 and 20 US dollars' worth of copra (about 100–200 pounds) per visit of the *Microspirit*, i.e. about 100–200 dollars annually. Given these low incomes and the great expense of the limited goods brought by the *Microspirit*, subsistence is accomplished much as it was prior to contact with Westerners, even in the case of school teachers' families (see early descriptions in Burrows and Spiro 1957).

Taro, which is cultivated, harvested, and prepared by women, is the primary carbohydrate source of the population. Fish, which are generally caught by groups of men and redistributed by chiefs (see Betzig, this volume (Chapter 2)), provide the primary protein source; chickens, dogs, and pigs also are occasionally eaten. Besides cultivation and food preparation, women's productive time is mostly spent caring for children, weaving skirts from banana fiber or thread imported from Yap, and gathering and preparing textile materials such as coconut fiber for rope, or palm leaves to be woven into mats for roofs, walls, and floors. Besides fishing, men's productive time is spent constructing the accoutrements to fishing (nets, traps, and canoes), building and maintaining houses, caring for children, and gathering palm sap. Teenagers contribute to most of the above activities, but to a lesser extent than adults; pre-teenage children rarely work, and usually can be found playing or resting (quantitative evidence and further discussion are presented in the hypotheses and results section).

In short, Ifaluk is a traditional society, and the above description is intended to make clear that traditional subsistence practices and social organization remain largely intact. More detailed site and ethnographic description can be found in Burrows and Spiro (1957), Lutz (1980), Turke (1985), and Betzig (this volume).

Quantitative data

Interviews were the means used to gather genealogical data, from which demographic parameters were later calculated. With the help of one of four English-speaking natives, genealogies were elicited from at least one adult from each of the 56 households on Ifaluk. (Note that 'household,' as it is used here, refers to a sleeping house. Lutz (1980) counts fewer 'households,' but she is referring to '*bugots*,' which are plots of land owned by the matriline on which exists 1–4 sleeping houses of close matrilineal relatives.) We elicited only ascendant and descendant genealogical links, that is, we did not ask people to remember lateral links, such as cousin relationships. We discovered who are brothers and sisters, aunts and uncles, cousins, and so on, from whether or not individuals shared parents, grandparents, and great-grandparents. We believe that this is the simplest, most error-free way of determining extended genealogies because individuals are not required to recall, or explain to the anthropologist, complicated lateral links (e.g. ego is not required to recall whether her father's sister's children had the same or different fathers).

We have confidence in the accuracy of our genealogies, in part, because of the simplicity of our method of eliciting them, but also because reported ascending genealogical links could usually be checked to see that they complemented reported descending links. Moreover, on Ifaluk almost everyone has both genetic and 'adoptive' parents, which gives an additional basis for cross-checking genealogies. (Note that 'adoption' on Ifaluk usually does not lead to children changing residence, and in many respects is more akin to what we in the West refer to as godparenting. Analyses in progress suggest that patterns of adoption on Ifaluk are adaptive (cf. Silk 1980).)

Behavioral data were gathered by the standard anthropoligical technique of participant observation, and quantitatively through the use of instantaneous behavioral scans (Altmann 1974, Johnson 1975). Behavioral scans are well-suited to quantifying the amount of time individuals devote to particular activities, as well as frequencies of interaction between particular individuals (Johnson 1975, Hames 1979). For the present study, observations from scans were lumped into 13 categories (resting, eating–drinking, grooming–bathing, walking–running, playing, food quest, transporting, textile work, construction, child-care, copra-making, clean-up, and miscellaneous); and then lumped again according to whether the behaviors are non-productive or productive (the first five and the last eight in the above list, respectively). Details of our scanning technique are spelled out elsewhere (Turke 1985, Betzig and Turke 1986, and Betzig, this volume (Chapter 2); see also, Hames (Chapter 14) and Flinn (Chapter 11), this volume). Owing to its small size, isolation, and a climate ensuring that most daytime activities occur outdoors, Ifaluk is an ideal location for conducting instantaneous behavioral scans (Betzig and Turke 1986).

Hypotheses and results

Hypothesis 1

Among diploid, sexually reproducing organisms, including humans, the production of a full sibling increases an individual's inclusive fitness as much as the production of an offspring. This is because the probability that ego and a full sibling share any given gene is equal to that between ego and his offspring (i.e. 0.5). The question thus raised is, why in some organisms, such as termites, do most offspring forgo direct reproduction and expend all their reproductive effort helping to rear siblings; whereas in many other organisms expenditures of reproductive effort are concentrated solely on the production of offspring; and in still others reproductive effort is expended both to produce offspring and to help parents produce siblings? Alexander and Noonan (1986) argue that forgoing direct reproduction in order to help parents reproduce is likely to have the greatest net beneficial effect (high b/c, in terms of Hamilton's rule), and thus is most likely to occur, when (1) 'helper offspring' are able to provide efficient and valuable help (usually implying that new offspring require substantial care); (2) parents continue to have high, direct reproductive potential at the time when potential helpers reach an age at which they are capable of helping; and (3) not helping does little to increase an offspring's chance of direct reproduction. All these criteria are more or less satisfied in various social insects, and those that have permanently sterile castes are especially strong in satisfying criterion (2), since parents have evolved longer maximum lifespans than their helper offspring (Alexander and Noonan 1986).

Alexander and Noonan also point out that criteria 1–3 are satisfied, although probably to a lesser extent, among naked mole-rats, some birds, and social carnivores. For example, a one-year-old Florida scrub jay who leaves his natal nest and thus forgoes helping to rear siblings is usually unlikely, at that age, to win the territory he needs to begin his own direct reproduction; however, by staying to help his parents he usually substantially increases their production of his siblings (e.g. Woolfendon 1981).

Alexander and Noonan stress, though, that among birds and social carnivores, and in contrast to social insects, helpers ('workers') and reproductives ('queens' and 'kings') have apparently not evolved different maximum life lengths, and therefore the relatively inflexible, sterile, worker castes of some social insects are not expected to have evolved. In other words, in birds and mammals help given by particular offspring is expected to be easily adjusted to changes in parents and offsprings' relative reproductive opportunities. Parents are youngest and generally still have plenty of opportunities for continued direct reproduction when their first-born offspring reach an age at which they can function as helpers, and therefore first-borns more than second-borns, second-borns more than third-borns, and so on, are expected to expend reproductive effort as extraparental nepostic effort (i.e. helping parents) rather than as mating effort or direct parental effort. However, even among first-borns the tendency to give or withhold help should be reversible, because a first-born who specializes only in sibling production should find him or herself with less and less of a reproductive outlet as his/her parents senesce.

Note that parents and offspring should be in conflict over the precise point in time at which helpers should switch from being mainly helpers to mainly direct reproductives (Alexander 1974, Trivers 1974). Also, to the extent that an offspring is intended by the parent to be a helper rather than a direct reproductive, the offspring is a product of parental somatic effort rather than reproductive effort (West Eberhard 1975), which has consequences for other life history parameters such as the age of onset of senescence (Alexander and Noonan 1986).

I suggest that criteria 1–3 (above) often will be satisfied among human groups, and, in particular, at least criteria (1) and (2) seem to be satisfied on Ifaluk. Regarding criterion (1), human children obviously need plenty of care, and teenagers should be able to provide much of it, especially in societies such as Ifaluk's where subsistence is largely independent of wage labor (cf. Nag et al. 1978, Caldwell 1982). Regarding

Table 10.1 *Time spent productively according to age and sex*

Age (years)		Males				Females	
	n	% Prod.	NP/P[a]		*n*	% Prod.	NP/P[a]
0–5	24	5	283/16		27	3	243/8
6–10	13	7	131/10		14	15	110/20
11–15	4	37	43/25		12	34	98/50
16–20	6	37	74/43		11	53	70/77
21–25	8	44	75/58		4	53	42/48
26–30	10	49	38/37		17	60	70/106
31–60	17	58	142/194		13	65	72/134
61+	7	56	70/90		9	61	33/52

[a] NP/P is the ratio of non-productive to productive activity observed for a particular age group

(2), there are many instances in which offspring born early in a couple's reproductive career have reached their teenage years – and thus are capable of helping – and yet the couple is still near the height of its (direct) reproductive value. Regarding (3), offspring on Ifaluk who appear to help their parents most (oldest daughters) tend to have slightly reduced direct reproduction (Turke 1985, and below), and therefore, depending on the reaction of parents, not helping might increase their direct reproductive success. Nevertheless, to the extent that direct reproduction by helpers is compensated by inclusive fitness effects (as it appears to be for oldest daughters on Ifaluk, see below), criterion (3) need not be satisfied for the evolution of helping.

On Ifaluk, daughters are expected to be of more significant help to their parents for a number of reasons. First, they spend more time in productive activity than sons at most ages (Table 10.1). For example, over the period during which offspring are most likely to be helpers (age 11–30), daughters are more productive than sons ($p = 0.0086$; maximum likelihood ratio test of proportions; $p = 0.0043$, one-tailed *t*-test). Second, Ifaluk is matrilocal, and therefore daughters usually live in their parents' home throughout life, whereas married sons live with their wive's parents and unmarried, post-pubescent sons live in canoe houses with other unmarried male relatives. Third, the contribution daughters make to subsistence is expected to be more crucial to their parents' household than that of sons. This is because the food produced by daughters goes mainly to their own household or household compound (which is usually also their parents' household), whereas the major

food produced by sons – fish – is usually redistributed equally throughout the atoll (except that chiefs take more (see Betzig, this volume (Chapter 2)). Similarly, clothing, and most other items constructed by women and teenage girls generally remain in their household compound, whereas things constructed by men and teenage boys (sailing canoes, seines, fish traps, canoe houses) are usually more widely shared. This means that not having a daughter is more costly, in terms of lost food and other goods, than not having a son. In short, then, if Ifaluk parents use the resources and services of their offspring to produce additional offspring, effects should be most apparent among parents who produced daughters early in their reproductive careers.

Predictions

The first prediction, then, is that individuals who produced daughters early should have larger completed broods than those who produced sons early. Out of Ifaluk's population of 446, 30 females had completed their fertility (i.e. were older than age 44) and had at least one child surviving at the time of the study. In 15 cases, a surviving son was born first; and in 15 cases a surviving daughter was born first. The mean number of living offspring these women had at the time of the census was, as predicted, 4.87 (SD = 2.63) for those who bore a son first and 6.93 (SD = 3.92) for those who bore a daughter first; 4.87 is significantly less than 6.93 ($p = 0.0510$; one-tailed *t*-test, different variances, df = 28).

A stronger prediction can be made for women who bore either two sons or two daughters first.

Those who bore two sons first ($n = 11$) had on average 5.09 (SD = 2.02) offspring surviving at the time of the census; and those who bore two daughters first ($n = 7$) had on average 8.86 (SD = 4.02) offspring surviving at the time of the census; again, as predicted, 5.09 is significantly less than 8.86 ($p = 0.0295$; one-tailed t-test, different variances, df = 16). Finally, a Scheffe multiple comparison test was conducted in which the average reproductive success of women who bore two sons first (5.09) is compared to the average of women who bore two daughters first (8.86), taking into account the averages for women who bore a daughter and then a son (6.67, $n = 6$, SD = 2.07) and a son and then a daughter (5.00, $n = 4$, SD = 2.58). The statistic calculated is highly significant ($f = 8.1311$; $p = 0.0088$) (see Figure 10.1).

However, it remains to demonstrate that the hypothesis is consistent with the above findings at a proximate level. For example, it would be *in*consistent to find that the greater overall reproductive success of women who produced daughters early derives mostly from their having had greater reproductive success early in their lives. This is because very young daughters are

Figure 10.1 Completed reproductive success according to sex of first two children. Scheffe multiple comparison test of differences in mean, completed reproductive success of women who bore two daughters first (DD) and those who bore two sons first (SS), taking into account the means and variances for women who first bore a daughter and a son (DS) or a son and a daughter (SD); $p = 0.0088$.

not likely to be effective helpers. However, the above women began reproducing at age 22.9, on average, if they had a son first, and 22.6, on average, if they had a daughter first. These ages are not statistically different ($p = 0.7766$; two-tailed t-test, df = 25; age at first birth was not available for 3 of the 30 women in the sample). Moreover, reproductive success up to age 30 was nearly identical for both groups: women who bore a son first had 2.57 living offspring by the time they finished their 29th year, whereas women who bore a daughter first had 2.69; differences are *not* significant ($p = 0.8387$, two-tailed t-test, df = 25). However, women who bore a son first (i.e. back in their twenties or before) had on average only 2.64 living offspring from age 30 through 44, whereas women who bore a daughter first had 4.77 living offspring during the same 15-year period; 2.64 is, as predicted, significantly less than 4.77 ($p = 0.0325$, one-tailed t-test, different variances, df = 25). Thus nothing in the above analyses suggest that it is *im*plausible to claim that help by daughters accounts for the higher reproductive success of women who bore daughters early in life, i.e. the hypothesis appears to be internally consistent.

Females who bore a daughter first bear more children after age 29 than their counterparts who bore a son first primarily because they continue reproducing to an older age: age at birth of last child is 40.5 for women whose first child is a daughter compared to 33.8 for women whose first child is a son ($p = 0.0184$, one-tailed t-test). Birth intervals (i.e. closed intervals) after age

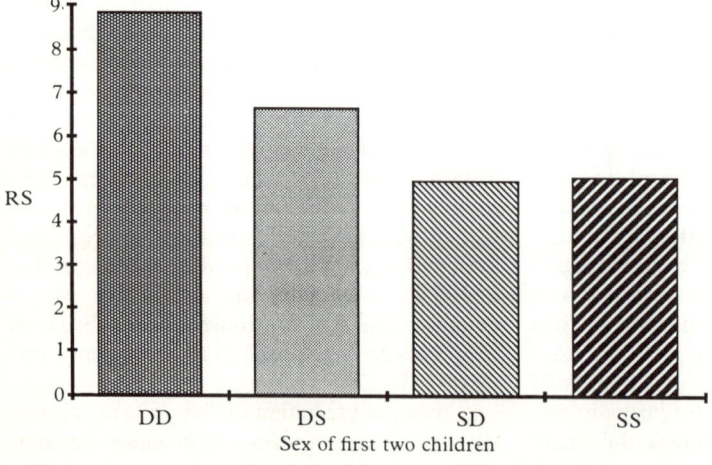

29 are about equal for the two groups of women (daughter first = 3.9 years, son first = 4.2 years, $p = 0.8464$, two-tailed t-test). Note, though, that the method of analysis in calculating birth intervals (closed intervals) for the two groups is biased such that the difference should actually be larger than that found, because birth intervals are likely to increase purely as a function of a mother's age (cf. the !Kung, Howell 1979), and mothers who bore daughters first remain reproductive until older ages than women who bore sons first.

Daughters who help parents may have less remaining effort to devote to direct reproductive success (cf. social insects). This proposition was tested in two ways. First it was assumed that a daughter can help to rear both her older and younger siblings (e.g. a 14-year-old girl may do work that helps to provide for her 11- and 17-year-old brothers). Thus, the dependent variable, 'daughter's reproductive success,' was regressed on the variables, 'her number of siblings,' and, 'her age' (the latter controls for effects of age on reproduction). The coefficient for the relevant variable, 'her number of siblings,' is negative as predicted (-0.1426; $n = 72$) and significant ($p = 0.0204$).

Next it was assumed that daughters only help to rear their younger siblings. Thus, in this case the dependent variable, 'daughter's reproductive success,' was regressed on the independent variables, 'her number of younger siblings,' and, 'her age' (again, the latter controls for the effects of age on reproduction). Once more, the coefficient for the variable, 'her number of younger siblings,' is negative as predicted (-0.1004; $n = 72$); but in this case the result is not significant ($p = 0.1359$).

Having many older siblings has no negative effects on daughters' fertility (coefficient = -0.003; $p = 0.9816$). And siblings have no detectable detrimental effects on the fertility of sons (coefficient = -0.0912; $p = 0.3350$).

Proximate mechanisms

These are at least two ways in which helpers may contribute to their parents' reproductive success on Ifaluk. First, by providing extra resources and services, daughters may reduce their mother's energetic burden thereby reducing her birth intervals (cf. Frisch and McArthur 1974); however, as noted, the Ifaluk data at best

are equivocal in this regard. Second, the human psyche, being a product of natural selection, is expected to have characteristics which, at least in the environments of evolutionary history, lead to inclusive fitness maximization. That is, the psyche should serve to assess environmental conditions that are important in reproduction and prompt the individual, via thoughts and emotions, to adopt an adaptive reproductive strategy. Thus, individuals with extra services and resources provided by helpers are expected rationally to decide that further reproduction is appropriate (i.e. foresee being able to afford another child), and they are expected to feel that it is appropriate (i.e. feel happy about further reproduction, not distressed by the thought of an additional burden).

Finally, differential childhood mortality may be (but apparently is not) the proximate mechanism underlying the finding that parents who bore daughters first have greater reproductive success than parents who bore sons first. However, this expectation is not met: 7 cases of infant or juvenile mortality were recalled by the 15 women whose first child was a son, and 8 cases for the 15 whose first child was a daughter.

Alternatives

One alternative that can be raised to account for the major result supporting the hypothesis is that mothers may sometimes claim the illegitimate offspring of their daughters as their own. This would elevate the reported reproductive success of women who bore daughters first, relative to women who bore sons first, so long as the latter don't claim the illegitimate offspring of their sons. However, doubt is cast on this alternative by the fact that during our census many young, never-married girls confidently and without hesitation stated that they have children. That is, neither they nor their parents seemed ashamed of this, and it therefore seems unlikely that other girls would be so ashamed as to attempt to deceive us. Furthermore, in a small society such as Ifaluk in which all children are nursed openly by their mothers for up to three years, it would have been difficult, in many cases, to hide maternity from us during our entire stay on the atoll; and even if we could have been fooled, other Ifalukese could not have been, and thus our cross-checking of genealogies (see methods) is likely to have revealed some inconsistencies. None were revealed. Birth intervals should provide still another clue for determining whether women sometimes claim their daughters' illegitimate offspring; that is, if it happens with any regularity, cases should arise in which a woman claims to have borne two different children (her own and a daughter's, or two by different daughters) whose birth dates are so close as to preclude the possibility. No such incidents were detected; moreover, the reader should recall that the average birth interval from ages 30–44 for women who bore daughters first is a believable 3.9 years.

A second alternative is that a preference for sons may exist on Ifaluk. Therefore, women who have sons early should fulfill this preference sooner than women who have daughters early, and thus should stop reproducing at an earlier age. However, if there is such a preference, it is a subtle one: no one was heard to voice a preference for sons, though many volunteered their view that having children (sex unspecified) was extremely desirable. More solid evidence against this alternative is that, of the women in the above sample who bore a daughter as their first child, the model position at which a son was born is child number two, and the median is position number three. Furthermore, every woman who both bore a daughter first and had greater than average reproductive success, also had at least three sons. It thus seems unlikely that a desire only for more sons is what spurs women (or their mates) on to produce, in some cases, more than a dozen children. Finally, note that in China, which is patrilineal and in which a preference for sons is well publicized, a stated basis of the preference is to continue the family name (e.g. Greenhalgh 1986); Ifaluk, however, is matrilineal, and thus lineages are traced through females.

A third alternative is that gestation and lactation costs may be greater for sons than daughters (cf. Alexander et al. 1979; for similar findings among red deer see Clutton-Brock et al. 1982). Therefore, the more sons a woman has early, the more she should lag behind in further reproduction. However, the above analyses suggest that women who bore a son first do not begin to lag behind women who bore a daughter first until almost ten years after their first birth.

If the original hypothesis is accepted over the foregoing alternatives, an interesting and potentially problematic question arises: why do not more women bear daughters first? One answer may be that prior to pacification of the region by the Germans about a century ago, the increased offensive and defensive potential sons gave the family may have balanced or even exceeded the value of services and resources provided by daughters. Thus, selection for the means to alter the sex ratio before birth may have been absent in this population until recently. Furthermore, killing a first-born son at birth in hopes of more quickly bearing a daughter would not be adaptive, since, although bearing a daughter on one's next try is likely to add almost two offspring, on average, to one's completed reproduction, one has only a 50% chance that the next child will be a daughter.

Finally, note that the above discussion does not imply that sons of today never contribute services and resources to their parents; data published elsewhere suggest they do (Turke 1985). It is implied, though, that daughters now, and in the recent past, contribute more than sons.

Hypothesis 2

This hypothesis concerns whether the elderly on Ifaluk, because of their low probability of producing additional offspring of their own, use a substantial portion of their remaining life-effort to promote successful reproduction by their extant offspring. This effort could take two forms: parental, or extraparental nepotistic. Parental effort would include care and assistance going to extant offspring; extraparental nepotistic effort would include care and assistance going to one's children's children (i.e. grandchildren). Both forms of effort should result in increased numbers of grandchildren. (In cases where the elderly lack children and grandchildren, extraparental nepotistic effort should be devoted to other close, needy relatives; this point is taken up elsewhere.) The Darwinian theoretical basis of hypotheses 2 is as follows.

Senescence

To understand the behavior of individuals who have lived past the age at which the possibility of direct reproduction begins to decline, it is necessary to understand why, in the first place, senescence occurs (Turke 1985). There are, after all, organisms that do not senesce (Williams 1957, Charlesworth 1980, Walford 1983). Early attempted explanations of why senescence occurs ignore evolutionary theory and are based on analogy to machines: machines wear out, and, thus it was argued, so do individual somas. However, two crucial problems with wear-out theories are that they fail to account for why organisms capable of morphogenesis are not capable of mere maintenance (Williams 1957); and they do not account for the tremendous variation in senescence between species – mice senesce and die in months even under ideal laboratory conditions, yet bats, built with similar 'mammalian machinery,' may live over a decade (compare the maximum longevities of a large number of species described in Comfort (1979)).

Based on ideas set forth by Medawar (1952, 1955), and as an alternative to wear-out theories, Williams (1957) developed a theory of senescence which states: (1) pleiotropic genes – genes with different effects at different time, or more accurately in different somatic environments – are common; (2) genetic effects expressed after the age of first reproduction are less heavily weighted by natural selection than are earlier effects (because, for example, due to the omnipresent possibility of accidental death, an individual is always more likely to reproduce the first time than subsequent times); and therefore (3) pleiotropic genes with even small positive effects on fitness expressed early and large negative effects expressed late can be favored by natural selection (see Hamilton (1966), for slight refinements of Williams' argument). In other words, senescence is expected to evolve as a side-effect of selection for earlier increases in reproductive value.

The genetics of Williams' theory have been formally modelled (Hamilton 1966, Emlen 1970, Charlesworth 1980), and numerous predictions from the theory have been tested, and account both for why senescence is inevitable for most types of organisms, and for variations in patterns of senescence between and within species. These predictions, of which each has empirical support, include: organisms in which soma and germ plasm are indistinct should not senesce (Williams 1957, Charlesworth 1980); artificial

selection of late breeders within a propulation should also select for later, less rapid senescence (Rose and Charlesworth 1980, Luckinbill et al. 1984); species whose adult members suffer high rates of predation (or other 'accidents') should senesce more rapidly than members of similar species with low rates of predation (Williams 1957); senescence in social insect queens should begin later and progress more slowly than in workers because workers protect queens from exogenous sources of mortality by taking extra risks unto themselves (Alexander and Noonan 1986); and effects of senescence should be detectable in wild populations (Williams 1957, Nesse 1986). Alternatively, no other published theory of senescence, including those fashionable in the medical literature, can account for all the above phenomena (Nesse 1986, Alexander 1987).

The relevance of Williams' theory of senescence to this study is that it predicts that the life span evolves as a function of the proportion of the remaining reproduction that individuals of a given age typically have before them (recall, though, that reproduction may be direct, or indirect via nepotism). More specifically, the theory predicts that maximum life span will be set at about the point at which the remaining probability of reproduction approaches zero. For *Homo sapiens*, indirect evidence suggests that for over 100 000 years the maximum life span has been set at about 100 years (Cutler 1975, Walford 1983, Hofman 1984); and direct evidence suggests that this, or a little older, was the maximum by at least a few thousand years ago (Comfort 1979, Mayer 1981, Walford 1983). In contrast, our earliest hominid ancestors, like extant apes, had maximum life spans of only about 50 years (e.g. Hofman 1984). It follows that, prior to 100 000 years ago, the reproductive potential of hominids older than age 50 was increasing – enough so that selection molded life expectancy such that it since has remained above zero until about age 100.

However, the key here is that increases in the reproductive potential of the elderly are likely to primarily have been through nepotism, not direct reproduction: with regard to our female ancestors, it is probable that menopause is an ancient hominid trait (see below), and therefore reproduction after age 45 is likely to have been indirect; and if our male ancestors were to continue to produce new offspring after age 45–55, it would have been necessary to replace post-menopausal mates with younger women, which, I believe, generally would have required combat with younger males (although once significant social stratification evolved, some older males may have controlled younger males who would do combat for them). Analogously, aged extant primates fare poorly in this regard (De Waal 1982), and there is, I believe, little reason to expect otherwise of aged, ancestral, hominid males.

Menopause
Although birth intervals may substantially increase as female non-human primates age, there is no documented evidence of their under-going menopause (Hrdy 1981). It has been hypothesized that, due to the increased duration of dependency by hominid offspring (relative to prehominids and their ancestors), menopause is a uniquely hominid adaptation. It presumably was favored by natural selection because the total number of children (and grandchildren) reared was increased by removing the possibility of further conceptions at about age 45, so that investment could be concentrated on children and grandchildren who already had been con-ceived (Williams 1957, Alexander 1974, Daw-kins 1976, Mayer 1981). Thus, if menopause evolved for the reason just suggested, it is likely also to be true (at least in environments typical of our evolutionary history) that post-menopau-sal women generally give their children and grandchildren more resources and services than they take from them.

Note that because of the certainty with which menopause curtails direct female reproduction, hypothesis 2 should in most cases apply more strongly to females than to males, since males retain some possibility of direct reproduction even at very advanced ages. This suggests that grandmaternal and grandpaternal reproductive strategies should diverge most in societies in which the possibility for direct reproduction is highest for old males, for example, among the Tiwi (Hart and Pilling 1960), and among the upper strata of highly stratified societies (Betzig 1986). On Ifaluk, no male in our census over age 50 has directly reproduced, and this is likely to have been typical of the population at least since the demise of polygyny at the turn of the century (Turke and Betzig 1985). Thus, since

the turn of the century, the reproductive striv-ings of elderly Ifaluk males should have been adjusted to more closely resemble those of elderly Ifaluk women (I am speaking here of a facultative adaptation).

In terms of Hamilton's rule, and given the prior evolution of senescence and menopause a low benefit-to-cost ratio (b/c) is expected from effort the elderly might expend to produce new offspring. For example, a post-menopausal widow who behaves like her teenage daughters by giving gifts and attention to young males (mating effort) is expected to leave fewer descen-dants than if she devoted such effort to caring for grandchildren. In contrast, care given to grandchildren generally should have a high b/c ratio, and it is for this reason that it is expected to have evolved.

Predictions
The central prediction that may be derived from the above hypothesis is that, controlling for age, individuals on Ifaluk whose parents have died should have lower reproductive success than individuals whose parents are available to pro-vide nepotism. To test this prediction, ego's reproductive success ($n = 140$) was regressed on the independent variables 'ego's year of birth' and 'ego's number of living parents.' The predic-tion is supported: individuals with more living parents generally have higher reproductive suc-cess; the coefficient (slope) for the independent variable 'number of living parents' is 0.5233, when age is controlled for, and the relationship is significant ($p = 0.0304$, $R^2 = 0.39$). Note further that in testing a different but related hypothesis, Betzig and Turke (unpublished data) have demonstrated that, among married Ifalukese couples, it is the mother's mother, rela-tive to the mother's father or either of the father's parents, who has the greatest positive effect on the couple's reproductive success. However, in all cases, except father's father which was weakly negative and statistically *in*significant, the effect of parents on their adult offsprings' reproductive success was positive.

Proximate mechanisms
Direct physical contributions to the rearing of grandchildren may be one proximate mechanism by which the elderly contribute to their extant offsprings' reproductive success. In support of

Table 10.2 *Activity budgets, in percent, by age and sex*

Age	Clean-up	Food quest	Trans-port	Textile work	Con-struction	Child care[a]	Copra prod.	Misc.	NP[b]
Males									
0–15	0	4	1	2	2	0	0	0	90
16–25	0	3	4	9	22	1	1	0	60
26–60	1	7	6	12	24	3	2	1	45
61+	1	4	2	16	33	1	1	0	44
0–15	0	5	4	2	0	2	1	0	86
16–25	1	18	12	12	3	3	3	0	48
26–60	3	25	11	11	2	9	2	0	37
61+	0	35	5	14	0	4	4	0	39

[a] This refers to direct care (feeding, holding, bathing, etc.), but does not include indirect care via association without contact.
[b] NP refers to non-productive activities; see text.

this proposition, grandmothers subjected to daily behavioral scans could have been observed as many as 384 times (once per scan circuit per grandmother). They were actually observed interacting with granchildren 13% of those times. In comparison, females over age 60 were observed eating on only 3% of possible observations, suggesting that the 13% figure attained for grandmother–grandchild interaction is not a trivial amount. Indicative of the direction of the flow of altruism in grandmother–grandchild interactions, 80% involved grandchildren less than age three; the remainder, except for one interaction with a 12-year-old, were with individuals age eight or younger.

Out of possible scan observations on grandfathers, 6% were in interaction with grandchildren. Of these 79% were with grandchildren age three or less; the other interactions were with grandchildren age five or less, again, with the exception of a single interaction with a 12-year-old. What, in particular, grandparents are likely to have been doing in the above interactions includes keeping the children from danger – especially, keeping them from the water – and teaching them social and technical skills.

The data also suggest that grandparents provide indirect services and resources that contribute to their offsprings' reproductive success. As noted, on Ifaluk most food and drink and most of the tools used in its acquisition come from the labor of adults. Behavioral scans demonstrate that elderly adults (e.g. greater than age 60) spend as much time productively engaged as younger adults (Table 10.1). Of course, a skeptic might argue that the labor of

the elderly is not very valuable, either because it is directed at useless tasks or it is inefficient. However, it can be seen from Table 10.2 that the productive activities of the elderly are not in any obvious way inferior to the productive activities of younger adults. Moreover, the *a priori* assumption that the labor of the elderly must be very less efficient than the labor of younger adults seems to me to be a cultural bias that out-of-shape Americans and Europeans find easy to adopt. Daily sightings of 70-year-old men at the tops of coconut palms tends to alleviate this bias.

Demonstrating that the elderly are productive does not, however, demonstrate that their productivity flows to their children and grandchildren. But regression analyses reported elsewhere do lend credence to this prediction, since, at all ages, including after age 60, the more offspring one has, the harder one works (Turke 1985:83–6). In contrast, having elderly parents does not increase young adult work-loads, as might be expected if resources and services flow from young adults to old (Turke 1985:88).

In addition to physical contributions of labor, elderly adults may, so long as they remain alive, contribute to the reproductive success of their offspring simply by holding kin groups together and thereby maintaining larger cooperative networks (Alexander, pers. comm.). Belonging to a large kinship network has been shown to be reproductively advantageous in other cultures (see Chagnon 1979, 1982, Irons 1981). I suspect this is or once was true of Ifaluk, since clan size generally has correlated with rank, which today (and more strongly in the past, due to polygyny) correlates positively with perquisites and reproductive success (Betzig this volume (Chapter 2); Turke and Betzig 1985; and cf. Betzig 1986).

In terms of the psychology and physiology of reproduction, the above analyses make it plausible to suggest that the care and assistance elderly parents give to adult children and grandchildren may contribute to reproduction by relieving energetic burdens of young parents, thereby (1) making parenting easier, and thus high rates of reproduction desirable, and (2) reducing physiological constraints on birth intervals. Also, grandparents may, through their efforts, help to lower the mortality of adult children and grandchildren. However, at least in recent times this effect may be trivial, since mortality is quite low on Ifaluk, due to the availability of modern medical care (Yap Statistical Yearbook 1980).

An alternative

The central result affirming the above hypothesis is that adults with living parents have greater reproductive success than adults without. This, in turn, has been backed with evidence suggesting a plausible underlying mechanism: elderly adults provide their adult children and grandchildren with services and resources. The primary alternative to this interpretation is that the services and resources alluded to are trivial, and contribute only slightly or not at all to the positive relationship between having living parents and higher than average reproductive success. Two possibilities not discussed are that parents may help their adult offspring to marry early and/or wisely, and their influence may add to the stability of these marriages (cf. Flinn this volume (Chapter 11)).

Still other hypotheses on the flow of resources between the generations and the effect of this flow on fertility are reviewed in the discussion section. These derive from microeconomic theories of motivation, and in some respects are not consistent with the hypothesis developed here.

Discussion

Both of the above hypotheses are argued in terms of reproductive benefits and costs accruing to individuals as a result of particular behaviors.

Reproductive benefits and costs sometimes parallel benefits and costs calculated in the the currencies of economic theory, and it therefore is not surprising that Darwinian and economic theory often overlap in their predictions (e.g. Hirshleifer 1977, Becker 1981, Turke 1985). However, since reproductive benefits and costs do not always equal benefits and costs as calculated by economists, there are also areas in which predictions generated from the two theories contradict each other (Turke 1985).

Economists, and demographers and anthropologists who borrow from economic theory, have developed a number of models purporting to explain variation in reproduction within and between societies (see Bulatao and Lee 1983 for a review). Two such models, which are highly regarded, and which have an economic theme at their core, are the 'wealth flows hypothesis' (e.g. Caldwell 1976, 1978, 1982, 1983) and the 'old age security hypothesis' (Leibenstein 1975, Cain 1981, Nugent 1985; also, informal models embodying the old age security rationale for high fertility are common in ethnographies, e.g. Service 1971). Both hypotheses suggest that within bounds set by the cultural environment, individuals make reproductive decisions that tend to maximize their 'utility.' The wealth flows hypothesis avers that in traditional and Third World societies the net flow of services and resources is from children to their parents. Thus, children increase parents' utility, and being utility maximizers, parents therefore strive to produce as many children as possible (e.g. Caldwell 1978:553). The old age security hypothesis states the same rationale for high fertility in traditional and Third World societies, except in specifying that children may not add to parents utility until the parents grow quite old (i.e. over a lifetime the net flow of services and resources may be from parents to offspring, but offspring are the best source of supplemental utility when parents need it most) (Figure 10.2).

Utility, however, is not well defined in these or most other economic models of goal-directed behavior (Hirshleifer 1977, Leibenstein 1981). Usually, it is loosely defined as the means to do as one pleases, but, as Hirshleifer notes, economists leave to social scientists the task of explaining variation in what it is that pleases individuals (i.e. variation in what constitutes individual utility). In turn, many concerned with the issue agree that social science theory has not derived a widely accepted predictive model for what it is that pleases people (e.g. Murdock 1972, Hirshleifer 1977, Alexander 1979, Irons 1979, Symons 1979, Mason 1983). However, Darwinian theory, through appeal to natural selection, provides a potentially acceptable solution: individuals should have evolved to be pleased by fulfilling proximate goals that maximize (or at least recently maximized) inclusive fitness (Hirshleifer 1977, Alexander 1979, 1987, Turke 1985). Thus, the utility that economists argue that we strive to maximize should be defined in terms of means for maximizing inclusive fitness. For example, wealth and power are obvious components of utility, and traditionally have given men the means to vastly out-reproduce others (as power does in other species, e.g. chimpanzees, De Waal 1982). The point is that therein possibly lies the ultimate explanation for why men everywhere strive for wealth and/or power (Betzig 1986).

I believe the utility maximization concept at the core of Caldwell's wealth flows model of fertility puts his argument on the right track through

Figure 10.2 Direction of net flow of resources between generations according to two models. In model I, parents invest heavily in children until they reach about age 15, at which time children begin to return more services and resources than they receive. The model assumes that individuals strive to mazimize utility, and that the power to do so is positively correlated with age (e.g. Caldwell 1982:69). In model II, services and resources are used to produce subsequent generations. In cases where resources flow upwards (dashed line), they are recycled to produce more offspring. The model assumes that a history of natural selection molded the capacities and propensities of individuals such that they evolved to behave in a manner that maximizes their genetic representation in future generations (adapted from Turke 1985:107).

recognizing that power, wealth, and the cost of producing children are key variables in determining levels of fertility (also Handwerker 1986). However, I also believe that, through not recognizing that utility maximization is a proximate mechanism that evolved for inclusive fitness maximization (the characteristics of which are products of a history of natural selection), the wealth flows model is likely to be universally wrong in an important detail: the net flow of resources and services in traditional societies should not be from offspring to parents. Rather, as argued in hypothesis 1 (above), parents should (and do on Ifaluk) use the services and resources offspring return to them to produce additional offspring, thus not allowing a net flow of services and resources to accumulate in the parental generation. And, as argued in hypothesis 2, parents should not have evolved post (direct) reproductive life spans if throughout human evolutionary history elderly parents generally have been net service and resource drains on their offspring. Rather, elderly parents should be strongly predisposed to invest in their offspring throughout life (see below). Evidence from Ifaluk suggests that they do, and that it results in increased reproductive success for themselves and their children.

Similarly, the hypotheses developed and supported above, in particular hypothesis 2, contradict predictions from the old age security hypothesis. They do not suggest, though, that parents and their children should not, or do not, form networks that provide mutual assistance. Humans of all ages, given their long life spans and memories, should benefit by paying short-term expenses that can yield long-term gains (e.g. a son who helps his father through a crisis can expect, if my second hypothesis is correct, many years of high return for his help). In short, however, if security networks between close kin are biased by age, the bias should be in favor of the young. Demographers should test for such an age bias not as they have (e.g. Cain 1981) by determining whether young adults sometimes assist their parents, but by determining who assists whom most when elderly couples and their adult children both are threatened by a crisis. Hypothesis 2 and the results supporting it suggest that in such cases it is the elderly who will most often act altruistically.

In terms of proximate mechanisms, parents

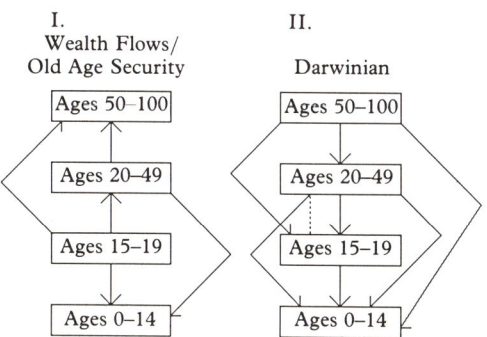

I.
Wealth Flows/
Old Age Security

Ages 50–100

Ages 20–49

Ages 15–19

Ages 0–14

II.

Darwinian

Ages 50–100

Ages 20–49

Ages 15–19

Ages 0–14

alive today are expected to resist learning to exploit their offspring in the manner suggested by the wealth flows and old age security hypotheses; in other words, given our evolution by natural selection, the use of returned resources for commodities such as excessive leisure (as explicitly suggested by Caldwell 1982:38) should not please the elderly if such use is to the detriment of their children and grandchildren. The proximate mechanisms underlying the hypothesis that altruism should flow from old to young are not known in detail, but I suggest they involve biases in the development of brain centers pertaining to love, guilt, and a sense of responsibility, such that parents feel more strongly committed to offspring than vice versa.

Summary

1. It has been hypothesized that, relative to sons, daughters on Ifaluk who are borne early in their parents' reproductive careers assist their parents in future reproduction. Supporting evidence is that, of women who have completed their fertility, those who bore a daughter first have greater reproductive success than those who bore a son first; those who bore a daughter first and second have greater reproductive success than those who bore a son first and second; the reproductive success of women who bore a son first is equal to that of women who bore a daughter first through age 29 (i.e. before helpers become functional), but thereafter those who bore a daughter first move significantly ahead; for daughters, there is a negative relationship between the dependent variable 'number of offspring produced by ego' and the independent variable 'number of siblings ego has'; for sons, there is no relationship between 'number of offspring ego has produced' and 'number of siblings ego has'; and the tendency is for younger siblings to have a greater negative effect on female ego's direct reproductive success than older siblings.

2. Elderly parents are hypothesized to adopt an alternative reproductive strategy in which resources and services formerly used for direct reproduction are increasingly used to increase the reproductive success of their extant children and grandchildren. Evidence is that, controlling for age, there is a significant positive relationship between the variables 'number of offspring ego has produced' and 'number of living parents ego has'; and the elderly are shown to produce extensive services and resources that can serve as appropriate proximate mechanisms for enhancing the reproductive success of their extant children and grandchildren.

3. It has been suggested that the foregoing hypotheses and results dispute some of the details of two widely exposed hypotheses of human fertility determinants proposed by Caldwell (1976, 1982), Leibenstein (1975), Cain (1981), and in many ethnographies.

Acknowledgements

I thank R. D. Alexander for help at many stages in the writing of this paper, as well as for developing much of the theory on which the hypotheses are based. For helpful comments, I also thank L. Betzig, M. Borgerhoff Mulder, T. Caro, M. Flinn, W. Holmes, W. Irons, and D. Symons. Financial support was privided by NSF and The Population Council.

References

Alexander, R. D. (1974) The evolution of social behavior. *Annual Review of Ecology and Systematics*, 5, 325–83.

Alexander, R. D. (1979) *Darwinism and Human Affairs*. Seattle: University of Washington.

Alexander, R. D. (1985) Evolution and human moral systems. *Zygon*, 1, 27–42.

Alexander, R. D. (1987) *The Biology of Moral Systems*. Hawthorne, NY: Aldine.

Alexander, R. D. and Borgia, G. (1979) On the origin and basis of the male–female phenomenon. In *Sexual Selection and Reproductive Competition in Insects*, ed. B. Blum and N. Blum, pp. 417–40. New York: Academic Press.

Alexander, R. D. and Noonan, K. (1986) The evolution of eusociality. Paper presented at The University of Michigan.

Alexander, R. D. and Tinkle, D. W. (1981) *Natural Selection and Social Behavior*. New York: Chiron.

Alexander, R. D., Hoogland, J., Howard, R., Noonan, K., and Sherman, P. (1979) Sexual dimorphisms and breeding systems in pinnipeds, ungulates, primates, and humans. In *Evolutionary Biology and Human Social Behavior: An Anthropological perspective*, ed. N. A. Chagnon and W. Irons, pp. 436–53. North Scituate, MA: Duxbury Press.

Altmann, J. (1974) Observational study of behavior: sampling methods. *Behaviour*, 49, 227–67.

Becker, G. (1981) *A Treatise on the Family*. Academic Press.

Betzig, L. L. (1986) *Despotism and Differential Reproduction: A Darwinian View of History*. Hawthorne, NY: Aldine.

Betzig, L. L. and Turke, P. W. (1986) Measuring time allocation: observation and intention *Current Anthropology*, 26, 647–50.

Bulatao, R. A. and Lee, R. D. (eds.) (1983) *Determinants of Fertility in Developing Countries*, vols 1 and 2. NY: Academic Press.

Burrows, E. G. and Spiro, M. E. (1957) *An Atoll Culture*. Westwood, CN: Greenwood Press.

Cain, M. (1981) Risk and insurance: perspective on fertility and agarian change in India and Bangladesh. *Population and Development Review*, 2, 321–66.

Caldwell, J. L. (1976) Toward a restatement of demographic transition theory. *Population and Development Review*, 2, 321–66.

Caldwell, J. L. (1978) A theory of fertility: from high plateau to destabilization. *Population and Development Review*, 4, 553–7.

Caldwell, J. L. (1982) *The Theory of Fertility Decline*. New York: Academic Press.

Caldwell, J. L. (1983) Direct economic costs and benefits of children. In *Determinants of Fertility in Developing Countries*, ed. R. Bulatao and R. Lee. New York: Academic Press.

Chagnon, N. A. (1979) Is reproductive success equal in egalitarian societies? In *Evolutionary Biology and Human Social Behavior: An Anthropological Perspective*, ed. N. A. Chagnon and W. Irons. North Scituate, MA: Duxbury Press.

Chagnon, N. A. (1982) Sociodemographic attributes of nepotism in tribal societies: man the rule breaker. In *Current Problems in Sociobiology*, ed. King's College Sociobiology Group, pp. 291–318. London: Cambridge University Press.

Charlesworth, B. (1980) *Evolution in Age Structured Populations*. Princeton: University Press.

Clutton-Brock, T., Guiness, F. and Albon, S. (1982) *The Red Deer*. Chicago: University of Chicago Press.

Comfort, A. (1979) *The Biology of Senescence*, 3rd edition. New York: Elsevier.

Cutler, R. (1975) Evolution of human longevity and the general complexity governing aging rate. *Proceedings of the National Academy of Sciences, USA*, 72 (11), 4664–8.

Dawkins, R. (1976) *The Selfish Gene*. Oxford University Press.

De Waal, F. (1982) *Chimpanzee Politics*. New York: Harper and Row.

Emlen, J. (1970) Age specificity and ecological theory. *Ecology*, 51 (4), 588–601.

Emlen, S. (1984) Cooperative breeding in birds and mammals. In *Behavioural Ecology: An Evolutionary Approach*, ed. J. R. Krebs and N. B. Davies. Sunderland, MA: Sinauer.

Fisher, R. A. (1958) *The Genetical Theory of Natural Selection*. New York: Dover Press (originally published in 1930).

Frisch, R. and McArthur, J. (1974) Menstrual cycles: fatness as a determinant of minimum weight for their maintenance or onset. *Science*, 185, 949–51.

Greenhalgh, S. (1986) Shifts in China's population policy. *Population Notes: Center for Policy Studies, The Population Council*, No. 56.

Hames, R. (1979) Relatedness and interaction among the Ye'kwana: a preliminary analysis. In *Evolutionary Biology and Human Social Behavior: An Anthropological Perspective*, ed. N. A. Chagnon and W. Irons, pp. 238–49. North Scituate, MA: Duxbury Press.

Hamilton, W. D. (1964) The genetical evolution of social behavior, I and II. *Journal of Theoretical Biology*, 7, 1–52.

Hamilton, W. D. (1966) The molding of senescence by natural selection. *Journal of Theoretical Biology*, 9, 12–45.

Handwerker, P. (1986) The causes of fertility decline. *American Anthropologist*, 2, 211–34.

Hart, C. and Pilling, A. (1960) *The Tiwi of North Australia*. New York: Holt, Rinehart, and Winston.

Hirshfield, M. and Tinkle, D. W. (1975) Natural selection and the evolution of reproductive effort. In *Proceedings of the National Academy of Sciences, USA*, 72, 2227–31.

Hirshleifer, J. (1977) Economics from a biological viewpoint. *Journal of Law and Economics*, 20, 1–54.

Hofman, M. (1984) On the presumed coevolution of brain size and longevity in humans. *Journal of Human Evolution*, 13, 371–6.

Howell, N. (1979) *Demography of the Dobe area !Kung*. New York: Academic Press.

Hrdy, S. B. (1981) *The Woman That Never Evolved*. Cambridge: Harvard University Press.

Irons, W. (1979) Natural selection, adaptation, and human social behavior. In *Evolutionary Biology and Human Social Behavior: An Anthropological Perspective*, ed. N. A. Chagnon and W. Irons, pp. 4–39. North Scituate, MA: Duxbury Press.

Irons, W. (1981) Why lineage exogamy? In *Natural Selection and Social Behavior*, ed. R. D. Alexander and D. W. Tinkle. New York: Chiron Press.

Johnson, A. (1975) Time allocation in a Machiguenga Community. *Ethnology*, 14, 301–10.

Leibenstein, H. (1975) The economic theory of fertility decline. *Quarterly Journal of Economics*, 89, 1–31.

Leibenstein, H. (1981) Economic decision theory and human fertility behavior. *Population and Development Review*, 7, 381–400.

Low, B. (1978) Environmental uncertainty and parental strategies of marsupials and placentals. *American Naturalist*, 112, 197–213.

Luckinbill, L., Arking, R., Clare, M., Cirocco, N.,

and Buck, S. (1984) Selection for delayed senescence in *Drosophila Melanogastor Evolution*, pp. 906–1003.

Lutz, C. (1980) The expression of emotion on Ifaluk Atoll. Ph.D. Dissertation, Harvard University.

Mason, K. (1983) Norms relating to the desire for children. In *Determinants of Fertility in Developing Countries*, vol. 1, ed. R. A. Bulatao and R. D. Lee, pp. 388–428. New York: Academic Press.

Mayer, P. (1981) Biocultural evolution of human longevity. Ph.D. Dissertation, University of Colorado.

Medawar, P. (1952) *An Unsolved Problem in Biology*. London: Lewis.

Medawar, P. (1955) The definition and measurement of senescence. *Ciba Foundation Colloquium on Ageing*, **1**, 4–15.

Murdock, G. (1972) Anthropology's mythology. *Proceedings of the Royal Anthropological Institute of Great Britain and Ireland*, pp. 17–24.

Nag, M., White, B., and Peet, R. (1978). An anthropological approach to the study of the economic value of children in Java and Nepal *Current Anthropology*, **19**, 293–306.

Nesse, R. (1986) Paper presented at The Evolution and Human Behavior Symposium (April), at the University of Michigan.

Nugent, J. (1985) The old age security motive for fertility. *Population and Development Review*, **2**, 300–9.

Rose, M. and Charlesworth, B. (1980) A test of evolutionary theories of senescence. *Nature*, **287**, 141–2.

Service, E. (1971) *Primitive Social Organization*. New York: Random House.

Silk, J. (1980) Kinship and Adoption in Oceania. *American Anthropologist*, **82**, 799–820.

Symons, D. (1979) *The Evolution of Human Sexuality*. New York: Oxford.

Trivers, R. L. (1971) The evolution of reciprocal altruism. *Quarterly Review of Biology*, **46**, 35–57.

Trivers, R. L. (1972) Parental investment and sexual selection. In *Sexual Selection and the Descent of Man*, ed. B. Campbell, pp. 136–79. Chicago: Aldine.

Trivers, R. L. (1974) Parent–offspring conflict. *American Zoologist*, **45**, 249–64.

Turke, P. W. (1985) Fertility determinants on Ifaluk and Yap: tests of economic and Darwinian hypotheses. Ph.D. Dissertation, Northwestern University.

Turke P. W. and Betzig, L. L. (1985) Those who can do: wealth, status, and reproductive success on Ifaluk. *Ethology and Sociobiology*, **6**, 79–87.

UN Demographic Yearbook (1984).

Walford, R. (1983) *Maximum Lifespan*. New York: Norton and Co.

West Eberhard, M. J. (1975) The evolution of social behavior by kin selection. *The Quarterly Review of Biology*, **50**, 1–33.

Williams, G. C. (1957) Pleitropy, natural selection, and the evolution of senescence. *Evolution*, **11**, 32–9.

Williams, G. C. (1966a) *Adaptation and Natural Selection: A Critique of Some Current Evolutionary Thought*. Princeton: University Press.

Williams, G. C. (1966b) Natural selection, the costs of reproduction, and a refinement of Lack's principle. *American Naturalist*, **100**, 687–90.

Woolfendon, G. E. (1981) Selfish behavior by Florida scrub jay helpers. In *Natural Selection and Social Behavior*, ed. R. D. Alexander and D. W. Tinkle. New York: Chiron Press.

Yap Statistical Yearbook. (1980) Published by Yap State.

Parent–offspring interactions in a Caribbean village: daughter guarding

Human kin groups may take over the competitive searching and courtship roles of the mating pair: they *breed* their members as they breed their cows and camels. It should not surprise us to find that this ready made organization would also assume responsibility for the control of paternal probability for members in whom they have nepotistic interest. These transfers of function are, I would guess, unique attributes of the human species and seem to me to be striking testimonials to the significance of inclusive fitness in our species.

(Mildred Dickemann 1981:424)

Human parents commonly exert considerable control over the mating relationships of their offspring. In some societies (e.g. The Tiwi: Hart and Pilling 1960), parents arrange the marriages of infants, or even of unborn offspring. In other societies (e.g. the Dobu: Fortune 1963), parental influence over an offspring's mating/marriage relationships is limited to friendly advice.

A variety of devices have been developed to control female sexuality. Examples include chastity belts, genital mutilations (e.g. clitorectomy and infibulation), and claustration (Dickemann 1981). A possible purpose of these devices is to enforce pre-marital and marital fidelity and hence maintain parental marriage arrangements. Other more simple day-to-day behaviors may have a similar function.

During 1978 and 1979–1980 I spent nine months conducting ethnographic field research in rural Trinidad, mostly in the village of 'Grande Anse.' In Grande Anse I frequently observed behaviors that had the apparent purpose of controlling (with or without conscious intent) the mating activities of offspring. All observed cases involved daughters. The means by which villagers attempted to 'guard' offspring included physical violence directed toward a daughter or her potential suitor(s), restricting the daughter's movements (keeping her at

[1] Department of Anthropology, University of Missouri, Columbia, MO 65201, USA

home), chaperoning (keeping her under surveillance by a family member), economic sanctions, and verbal threats of the above behaviors.

The objective of this paper is to test predictions based on the hypothesis that attempts to control the mating activities of daughters, i.e. 'daughter guarding,' are behavioral strategies that increase a father's inclusive fitness. Behavioral scan data, genealogical data, and economic data are analyzed to test the hypothesis against alternative explanations. Before presenting the results I will first briefly describe the study site and field techniques so as to provide a background for understanding the data base.

The study site

The village of 'Grande Anse' is located on the northern coast of Trinidad (Figure 11.1). It is isolated from the more heavily populated and economically developed central and western areas of the country by the steep and densely vegetated slopes of the Northern Range, which rise directly from the sea. Most of the 342 inhabitants live in the small pocket of relatively level alluvial deposits from the Grande Anse river. The surrounding hillsides are cultivated with cocoa, coffee, bananas and citrus as cash crops, and cassava, corn, dasheen, and vine tubers as subsistence items. Further inland the topography is too severe for efficient cultivation. Most of this land is undeveloped government forest reserve.

The village founders arrived about 1860 from Venezuela in small sailing canoes (Harrison 1979). Later, immigrants rowed or sailed from the nearby (40 kilometers) island of Tobago. By 1900 the community was thriving, with most villagers owning or squatting on plots of land, cultivating cocoa and subsistence crops. During the cocoa boom of the early 1900s outside interests purchased tracts of land and employed village labor. However, the cocoa market crashed during the 1920s and never recovered. Workers were laid off, and the smaller cocoa plots abandoned. Diversification into other crops such as coffee, citrus, and bananas helped to maintain the agricultural base of the village, but it never returned to the prosperity of the early cocoa days. Census data indicate that the village population has slowly declined, largely due to emigration to more developed areas (Harrison 1979).

There are a variety of ways to make a living in Grande Anse. Some are more lucrative than others. Most villagers have several part-time occupations, such as cocoa cultivation, fishing, carpentry, road work (government job), and shopkeeping. A majority of adult villagers have rights to cultivated land and spend some effort growing cash crops (e.g. cocoa, coffee) and subsistence crops. But the profits are slim and the work is hard so cultivation is the primary occupation of very few villagers today (about 13% of adult males, 8% of adult females).

At the time of the fieldwork, there were 28 co-residential father–daughter dyads, 6 part-time co-residential father–daughter dyads, and 21 non-residential father–daughter dyads in the village. About half (14 of 27) of the females between the ages of 18 and 28 did not have fathers resident in the village, but almost all had co-residential mothers (24 of 27). These figures jibe with other ethnographic studies of Caribbean populations (e.g. Clarke 1957, Smith 1962), and reflect the instability of paternal relationships.

Figure 11.1 Location of Trinidad in Caribbean Basin.

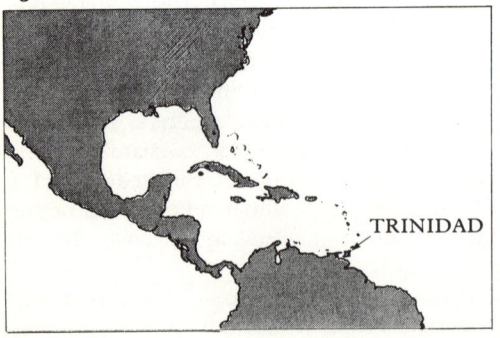

Methods and field techniques

During July and August 1978, and October 1979 through April 1980, I conducted field research in the village of 'Grande Anse' and surrounding areas. The methods and field techniques utilized in this study were designed to gather and analyze data that most reliably and objectively described: (1) day-to-day behavior, (2) genealogical relatedness, (3) economic assets and occupations, (4) past and current mating and marriage relationships, (5) residence, (6) the productivity of certain horticultural and subsistence activities, and (7) the flow of material resources among individuals (i.e. gifts and inheritances). This paper is concerned with analysis of the first five types of information, hence description of methods will be limited to them (for a more complete discussion see Flinn 1983).

To gather behavioral information useful for testing hypotheses about daughter guarding, I collected data detailing the day-to-day behavior of the villagers with an 'instantaneous scan sample' procedure (cf. Munroe and Munroe 1971, Altmann 1974, Johnson 1975, Denham 1978, Hames 1979, Munroe *et al.* 1983, Rogoff 1985, Betzig and Turke 1986).

The procedure was as follows: I travelled a set 4.7 km route through the study site once or twice daily, starting at a randomly determined time and place on the route. The route went through the entire village, passing within 20 meters of each inhabited house and each community structure (e.g. church, cricket field, water outlets). Because village houses are quite open, and because the route passed close by each house, observability was excellent. Each time an individual was observed, I recorded (with a notebook and/or tape recorder) the time, location, individual, and behavior. This information was coded within 48 hours onto computer format sheets. For each 'observation,' the date, time, one of 1375 location codes, one of 480 individual identification numbers, and one or more of 475 behavior codes were numerically recorded for computer analysis. For example, on 11 February 1980 at 6.12 a.m. I observed Hilario Ruiz throwing grain to chickens in the backyard of house No. 001. This observation was coded:

date   time   location   individual   behavior
110280   0612   0017   0012   293

I recorded about 33 000 observations in this fashion over a period of six months (173 scan routes on 152 days). Of these observations, 24 577 form the data base used in this paper. I have excluded observations recorded during the first two weeks of the procedure, observations recorded during scan routes in which less than 50% of the villagers were observed, observations of visitors to the village and observations of unidentified individuals.

During each scan I attempted to account for each individual in the village. However, Grande

Anse is not a small place, and some individuals travelled out of the village daily for school or work, resulting in incomplete scan samples. On average the scans accounted for 73% of all individuals. An additional 8% were accounted for by questioning family members about the whereabouts of the unobserved individual; most of these cases were teenagers attending a school in a neighboring village, adults away on shopping or business trips to 'town,' adults working on distant cocoa plots, and adults working in road repair crews away from the village. This information was often verified by walking out to the individual's location (e.g. cocoa plot), observing children returning from school, and so forth. The scan data accounted for a total observability rate of 81% of all individuals (cf. Hames 1979). Because the sample is incomplete, there may be some biases (Flinn 1983). However, it is unlikely that such biases would significantly affect the tests of the hypotheses presented in this paper.

A substantial number of the observations (16 541, or 66%) involved interactions between two or more individuals. Objectively defining 'interaction' was not a simple task. In general, if individuals were (1) communicating to one another, (2) touching or in close proximity (less than one meter) to each other, or (3) engaged in tasks that required mutual cooperation (e.g. hauling in a fish net), then I recorded the observation as an interaction. Most interactions were between dyads, although some multiple party interactions were recorded (e.g. three men rolling a log).

The advantages of the behavioral scan data are that they allow numerical description of the frequencies and types of behavior for specific individuals. For example, these data can be analyzed by computer to provide an objective, quantitative description of the interactions that parent–offspring relationships entail. The disadvantage is that much information is omitted in the rather crude numerical coding of behaviors.

Collecting accurate genealogies was a primary objective of the field study. Genealogies are an important source of information about parental relationships. Initially I interviewed informants from each household, usually adult females, obtaining the names, genealogical relationships, ages, and current residences of all the relatives (blood and affinal) that they could remember.

These interviews were well received, most villagers seeming pleased that someone was interested in their 'roots.' Upon returning from the interview, I assigned unique ID numbers to each individual collected in the genealogies and put all of the above information on 3 × 5 inch index cards for each individual. This information was analyzed by computer (after returning to the US) for cross reference with the behavioral scan data.

The parental relationships analyzed in this paper were widely recognized by the villagers and were readily observable. I do not believe that whatever incompleteness exists in the genealogical data is likely to have resulted in a bias that favors any of the hypotheses tested in this paper.

To test for associations between daughter guarding and resource control, information about economic assets and occupations was collected by interview (What land do you own, rent, cultivate? What major possessions do you own – e.g. house, mule, radio? What jobs do you have, and how much money do you make?). This

survey was conducted directly with informants at their place of residence, and in some cases, was corroborated by interviews with other villagers. Government land ownership maps were useful for corroborating information about land ownership (especially the precise size of landholdings, or at least the government's measurement of the acreage) and for establishing patterns of 'legal' inheritance.

In this paper land ownership is used as the indicator of individual economic status, because land was the most stable resource over time, and because land was measured more accurately and reliably than other economic assets. Land ownership is associated with mating success (Flinn 1983, 1986). I use household land as a measure of individual land ownership because land is worked jointly by household family members, the benefits are distributed among household family members, and land is not always 'owned' by individuals (see e.g. Besson 1979 for discussion of land tenure in Caribbean societies). No adjustment for the number of household members was made because this was difficult to do appropriately, and because there seemed no reason why not adjusting for house-

Figure 11.2 The frequency of parent–offspring interactions at different ages. Note the peak in father–daughter interactions at ages 11–15. These data suggest that there may be something unique about the father–daughter relationship during these ages.

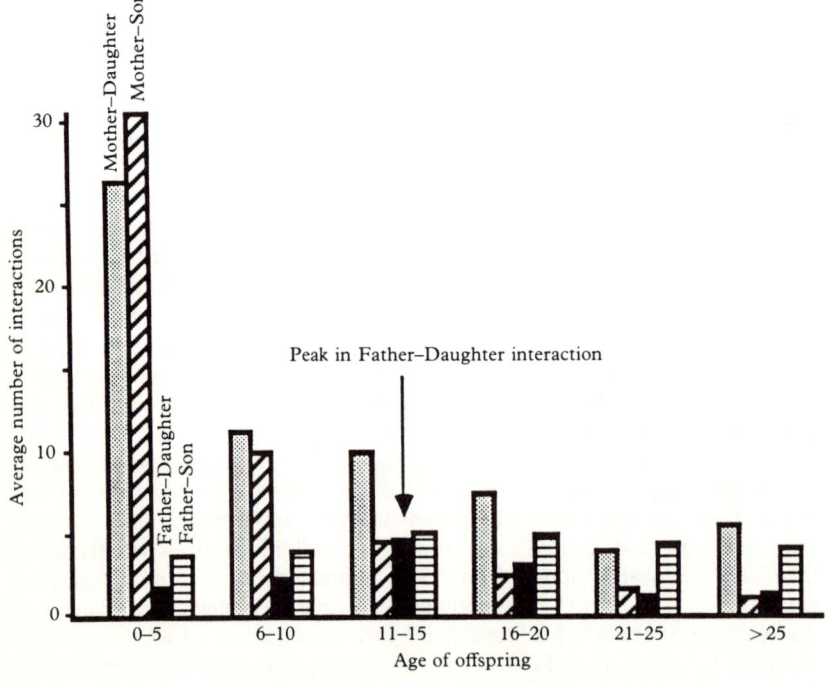

hold size would bias the results for or against any of the hypotheses tested.

The data analyzed in this paper are complete for each villager. That is, behavior (scan sample), genealogies of at least two generations in depth, current mating relationships, and land ownership are known for each of the 342 individuals in the sample population.

Results

First let us examine whether daughter guarding occurs in this population. Figure 11.2 shows the frequency of parent–offspring interactions by the age and sex of the offspring.

These behavioral scan data indicate several interesting patterns in parent–offspring interactions (Flinn 1983). Here I should like to focus on the peak in the frequency of father–daughter interactions during the ages 11–15. This peak may partially represent the efforts by fathers to control the mating activities of their daughters. There are, however, a number of other possible reasons for the peak in father–daughter interaction frequency. For instance, 11–15 year-old daughters might be doing more horticultural work with their fathers. To test this possibility I examined the scan data to see if there was an increase in the frequency of horticultural work interactions. There was no significant trend (in fact there was a slight decrease in horticultural

work interactions between fathers and older daughters, in contrast to a significant increase between fathers and older sons).

Another aspect of parent–offspring relations illustrated by Figure 11.2 is the absence of significant change in mother–daughter interaction frequences. Although informants suggested to me that mothers (and other female relatives) were at least equally as important as fathers in 'preserving their daughter's honor,' the role of the mother in daughter guarding was very difficult to analyze. There were several reasons for this. First, because the frequency of cooperative behavior with older daughters was quite high (Flinn 1983), the 'guarding' role of the mother was obscured in the scan data. Second, mothers appeared to use more subtle, less observable means of influencing their daughter's mating activities than did fathers. Third, almost all young women (aged 18–28) had mothers resident in the village (24 out of 27), whereas slightly less than half (13 out of 27) had fathers resident (see below and Flinn 1986), so the effects of mother's absence were much more difficult to evaluate than the effects of father's absence. And fourth, mothers were less likely to confront young males. For these reasons the analysis is limited to daughter guarding by fathers.

Figure 11.4 Histogram showing that males with daughters aged 10–25 have higher rates of agonistic interactions with unrelated males than do males of equivalent ages without daughters aged 10–25. $\bar{x}$ = 5.3% and SE = 0.94 for males with daughters aged 10–25. $\bar{x}$ = 1.8% and SE = 0.56 for males without daughters aged 10–25. One-tailed *t*-test is significant at $p = 0.002$. Vertical bars represent 95% confidence intervals.

Figure 11.3 The proportion of father–daughter interactions that are agonistic at different ages. The number of father–daughter dyads in each age category are: 14, 12, 10, 7, 6, and 6. The vertical bars represent 95% confidence intervals (1.96 × SE). The frequency of agnostic interactions during the 11–15 age category is significantly higher than all other age categories except 16–20 (χ^2 tests, $p < 0.05$).

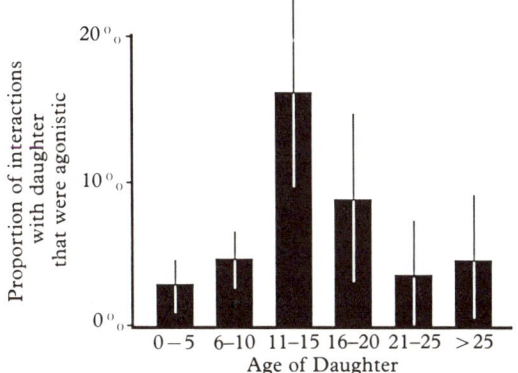

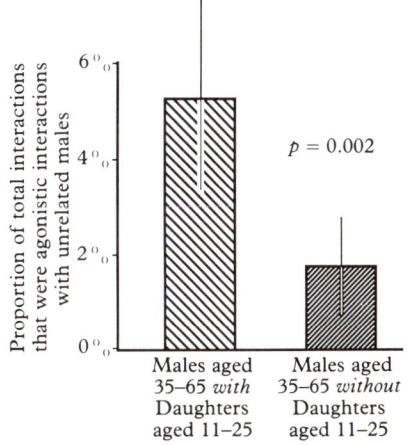

If the peak in the frequency of father–daughter interactions during ages 11–15 is at least partially due to an increase in 'daughter guarding' behaviors, then we might expect an increase in agonistic interactions (e.g. arguing and fighting; see Appendix) between fathers and their daughters that are at or approaching reproductive age. The seclusion or claustration of young women prior to marriage is common in many cultures (e.g. Dickemann 1981), and often is a period of considerable family turmoil (e.g. Daly and Wilson 1981, Wilson *et al.* 1982). Figure 11.3 indicates that the proportion of agonistic interactions between fathers and daughters peaks during the ages 11–15. Evidently there are important conflicts of interests at this time. These conflicts may arise from the relatedness asymmetry (parent–offspring conflict – Trivers 1973) or from differential experience (i.e. older, more experienced fathers know what is best for their daughters).

If the mating activities (realized or potential) of the daughter are a significant source of con-flict, then we might expect fathers to be interacting agonistically with the daughter's potential suitors as well. This hypothesis suggests the prediction that males with daughters of reproductive age (11–25) have a higher frequency of agonistic interactions with unrelated males than do daughter-less males of similar ages.

The data in Figure 11.4 support the hypothesis that fathers were guarding their daughters. I once observed the father of a 16-year-old daughter waving a machete in the face of a young man, threatening to 'cut him up' if he did not cease courting his daughter. The threat evidently was effective, as I did not observe the young couple together again, although they might have been meeting clandestinely. Not all fathers were this forceful, and they probably attempted to break up only courtships they did not approve of.

The amount of time spent at home or under supervison by a family member provides an indirect measure of the extent to which females are guarded. Figures 11.5 and 11.6 indicate a high frequency of observations of teenage (11–20) females 'at home' (defined as the parental household where the offspring resided), in contrast to teenage males, who were observed 'at home' with decreasing frequency during these ages (because older males are more likely to con-

Figure 11.5 Histogram showing that the proportion of times that offspring are observed at home (no. of observations of an individual with their household locality code/total no. of observations of that individual) according to the age and sex of the offspring. Younger offspring are observed at home more often than older offspring. Males are indicated by triangles. Females with fathers resident in the village are indicated by black circles. Females without resident fathers are indicated by open circles.

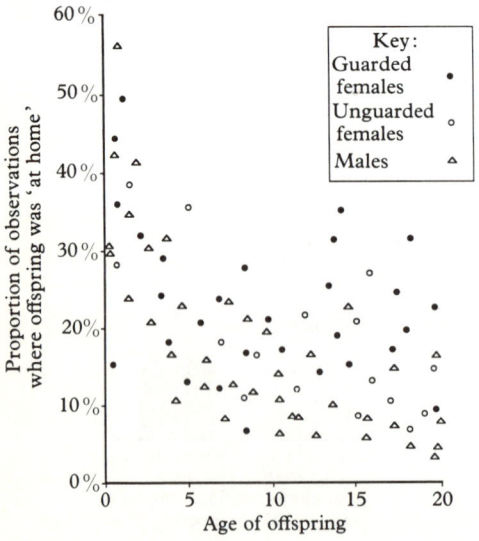

Figure 11.6 Histogram showing that older females (11–15 and 16–20) are more likely to be observed at home than are older males. For 11–15-year-old females $\bar{x} = 20.5$, SE = 2.8 vs. 11–15-year-old males $\bar{x} = 12.4$, SE = 1.8, $p = 0.24$, t-test; for 16–20-year-old females $\bar{x} = 17.6$, SE = 2.2 vs. 16–20-year-old males $\bar{x} = 8.2$, SE = 1.7, $p = 0.008$, t-test. Vertical bars represent 95% confidence intervals.

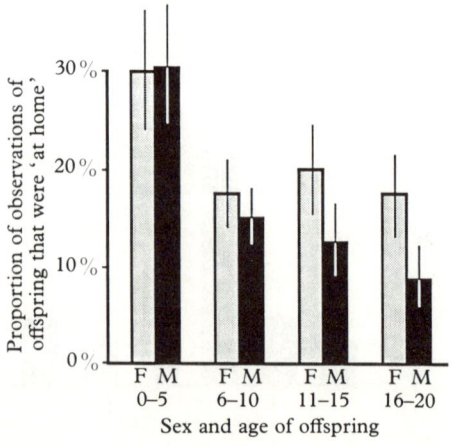

tinue their schooling at a school in a neighboring village, observations involving school attendance or transportation back from school were excluded). It is possible, however, that the difference between the sexes during these ages in the frequency of 'at home' observations is due to economic or other social factors besides guarding. Conversely, the economic roles adopted by teenage females may be influenced by parental constraints on their activities.

If fathers have a significant effect on their daughter's behavior, then we might expect that females with fathers resident in the village will have different patterns of behavior than females without resident fathers (see also Draper and Harpending 1982). Figures 11.5 and 11.7 indicate that teenage females without fathers resident in the village were observed 'at home' less frequently than teenage females with fathers resident in the village. Figure 11.8 indicates that females with fathers resident in the village were observed less frequently away from home 'unchaperoned' (i.e. no family member in the same location) than were females without resident fathers.

Villagers suggested that a primary reason why fathers guarded their daughters in Grande Anse was to increase the chances of a daughter achieving a stable mating relationship with a prosper-

ous male. Stability (i.e. permanence) of a daughter's mating relationship reportedly was important because 'divorced' females with offspring were generally less attractive as mates, and more likely to be dependent upon their families (including fathers) for the financial support and child care that might otherwise have been provided by a mate (husband). Prosperity (i.e. land ownership and income) reportedly was an important criterion for a daughter's mate because prosperous males could better support their mates and offspring. Because prosperous males have higher reproductive success in this population (Flinn 1986; see also Irons 1979b, Essock-Vitale 1984, Hill 1984, Turke and Betzig 1985, Betzig 1986), daughter guarding leading to a mating relationship with a prosperous male would increase a guarding father's inclusive fitness via an increase in the reproductive success of his grandsons (assuming that the prosperity is inherited).

If guarding by fathers has a significant effect on young females' mating relationships, then we might expect 'guarded' females to have different mating relationships from 'unguarded' females. The comparison of females with and without resident fathers again provides a useful basis for

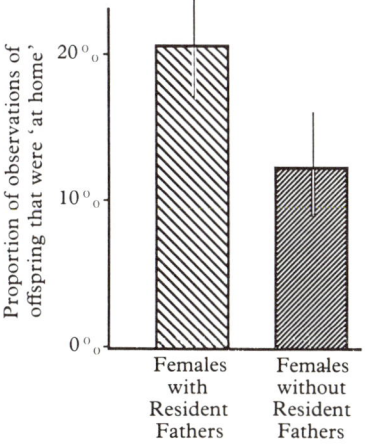

Figure 11.7 Histogram showing that older females (11–20) with resident fathers are more likely to be observed at home than are older females without resident fathers. For females with resident fathers $\bar{x} = 21.6$, SE = 2.2, vs. $\bar{x} = 14.3$, SE = 2.2 for females without resident fathers; $p = 0.027$, t-test. Vertical bars represent 95% confidence intervals.

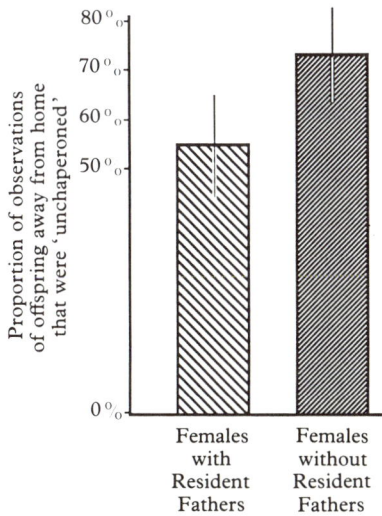

Figure 11.8 Histogram showing that older females (11–20) with resident fathers are less likely to be observed without a 'chaperone' (family member) when they are away from home than are older females without resident fathers. $\bar{x} = 52.0$, SE = 5.7. $\bar{x} = 76.3$, SE = 7.1; $p = 0.033$, t-test. Vertical bars represent 95% confidence intervals.

evaluating the effect of fathers on their daughter's mating relationships. If fathers were guarding their daughters in order to increase the likelihood of a stable mating relationship with a properous male, then we can predict that (1) young females with fathers resident in the village have more stable mating relationships, and (2) young females with fathers resident in the village have mating relationships with more prosperous males. Both predictions are supported.

The data in Figures 11.9 and 11.10 indicate that the residence of father is associated with the stability of daughter's mating relationships, and the prosperity of her mate consistent with the hypothesis that fathers guard their daughters in order to increase the chances of a 'successful' mating relationship. An alternative explanation for this result is that fathers, through their social ties, are important for arranging mating relationships with prosperous males for their daughters. Thus, it might not be the guarding *per se* (and choice by prosperous males of chaste females) that increases the likelihood of a 'successful' marriage for guarded females, but rather it is the father's efforts at arranging such marriages. This explanation is consistent with the fact that the reproductive success of young adult males is much higher if they have a resident father (Flinn 1986), suggesting that the residence of father is an important social (and economic) asset

Figure 11.9 Histogram showing that females with fathers resident in the village (or father was resident in the village until the daughter was at least 20 years old) have offspring by fewer mates than do females without fathers resident in the village. Sample includes all females under 50 years old who have had at least two offspring. These data suggest that residence of father increases the stability of daughter's mating relationships. $\bar{x} = 1.192$ and SE $= 0.096$ for females with resident fathers. $\bar{x} = 1.786$ and SE $= 0.208$ for females without fathers resident in the village. One-tailed *t*-test is significant at 0.007. Vertical bars represent 95% confidence intervals.

in mating competition. This explanation, however, does not account for the differences in behavior indicative of 'guarding' of daughters compared to sons (Figures 11.2–11.8). It is likely that both guarding and social ties provided by resident fathers contribute to the success of a daughter's mating relationships. The data do not allow for precise distinction between these two factors.

Discussion

Although parents and kin do not directly arrange marriages in Grande Anse, their influence nonetheless has significant reproductive consequences in this population. What initially piqued my interest in sex differences in parent–offspring interactions were the results of a study of the associations between parental residence and offspring reproductive success (Flinn 1986). In brief, demographic and residence data indicated that young adult males in the village with resident (living in the village) fathers had much higher reproductive success than young adult males without resident fathers. The reproductive rates of young adult females, however, were unaffected by the residence of father.

The issue raised by these data on paternal residence and reproductive success of offspring is, why are fathers bothering to be parental (e.g. guard) towards their daughters if there is no reproductive benefit? The answer suggested by the data presented in this paper is that there is a reproductive benefit realized in the grandoffspring generation. Daughter guarding ensures, or at least deceives others into believing, that

Figure 11.10 Women aged 18–28 with father resident in the village (or father was resident in the village until the daughter was at least 20 years old) are more likely to establish mating relationships and reside with prosperous males. $\chi^2 = 10.9$, $p = 0.01$.

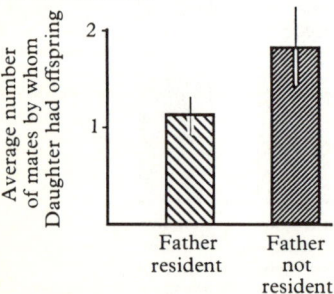

	Is father resident in village?	
	Yes	No
Mate owns >8 acres	11	2
Mate owns <8 acres	5	3
Did not move in with mate	2	9

Average number of mates by whom Daughter had offspring

Father resident / Father not resident

Mating relationship

the daughter is chaste. Fathers increase the likelihood that their daughters will marry a wealthy male by guarding because prosperous males prefer chaste females. The reasons why prosperous males prefer virgin or chaste-appearing females include (1) males do not want to care for a woman's children from previous relationships, and (2) prosperous males have more to leave to their heirs, hence desire high confidence of paternity (Dickemann 1981, Flinn 1981). Marriage to a prosperous male may not increase a woman's reproductive success, but it is likely to increase the reproductive success of her sons, if they inherit their father's prosperity (because prosperous males have higher reproductive success in this population – Flinn 1983, 1986).

Thus, although guarding by a father does not increase his inclusive fitness by increasing daughter's reproductive success, it may increase his inclusive fitness by increasing the reproductive success of his grandsons, who will have higher fitness because of being more prosperous and having a resident father. Psychological factors underlying this strategy might include pleasure derived from seeing a daughter 'happily' married, and maintaining the family 'honor.'

Another possible benefit from daughter guarding could be that males gain power or material benefits by controlling who can mate with their daughters, which could allow a father to gain additional mates for himself or for his sons (see e.g. Strauss 1949, Bourdieu 1977, Chagnon 1979, 1980, 1981, 1982, Irons 1979a). This hypothesis is consistent with ethnographic accounts of mating arrangements in a number of societies that have cross-cousin marriage rules (Flinn and Low 1986). For example, consider Hart and Pilling's (1960:15) description of mating arrangements among the Tiwi, a Australian Aboriginal society:

> Put bluntly, in Tiwi culture daughters were an asset to their father, and he invested those assets in his own welfare. He therefore bestowed his newly born daughter on a friend or an ally . . . or, the father might bestow an infant daughter on a man – or some close relative of a man – who had already bestowed an infant daughter on him, thus in effect swapping infant daughters.

Fathers in Grande Anse, however, did not have such a decisive role in arranging marriages,

and did not 'bestow' their daughters. It is not clear from the data what the conflicts of interests were between fathers and daughters concerning mate choice. It would appear that fathers were acting in their daughters' best (inclusive fitness) interests, although a relationship with a 'good provider' may be more in the father's interest than the daughter's. It was quite common for daughters to leave their children from terminated mating relationships with their parents. By ensuring that the daughter establishes a stable relationship, parents may avoid having to care for grandchildren. Fathers also seemed more approving of their daughters establishing relationships with their (the father's) friend's sons, suggesting that the enhancement of reciprocal networks may be a factor in the manipulation of daughters' mating relationships (see also Bordieu 1977).

Summary

The data indicate that:

1. Fathers have high rates of interaction with their teenage daughters.
2. Fathers have high rates of agonistic interactions with their teenage daughters.
3. Fathers with teenage daughters have high rates of agonistic interactions with unrelated males (potential suitors of their daughters).
4. Teenage females are more likely to be observed at home than are teenage males.
5. Teenage females without a father resident in the village are more likely to be observed away from home unchaperoned than are teenage females with a resident father (potential guardian).
6. Young women with a father resident in the village are more likely to establish a stable mating relationship with a prosperous male than are young women without resident fathers.

These results suggest that parental control of offspring mating is a significant aspect of reproductive competition in this human population. Many of the more subtle aspects of parental control of offspring mating relationships, such as the influence of the mother, and offspring counter-strategies, await further field research.

Flinn

Acknowledgements

I would like to thank Richard Alexander, Duncan Anderson, Laura Betzig, Robbins Burling, Martin Daly, Paul Sherman, Carol Ward, Margo Wilson and Richard Wrangham for helpful comments on the manuscript and Arinthia, Junior, Andre, Rampy and Susan for assistance with the fieldwork.

Appendix

The frequencies of interaction with different types of kin are presented in Figure 11.11.

The frequencies of the different categories of behaviors are presented in Figure 11.12.

The specific behavior codes and frequencies included in the category 'agonistic interactions' are listed below. Note that only 92 out of 1218 (7.5%) observations involved actual physical agonism, although in some cases physical agonism occurred before or after observed threats or verbal agonism.

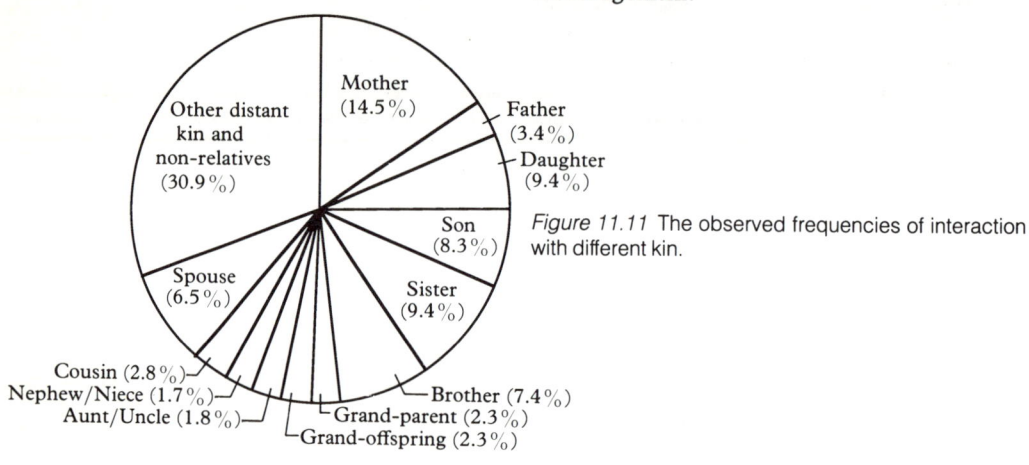

Figure 11.11 The observed frequencies of interaction with different kin.

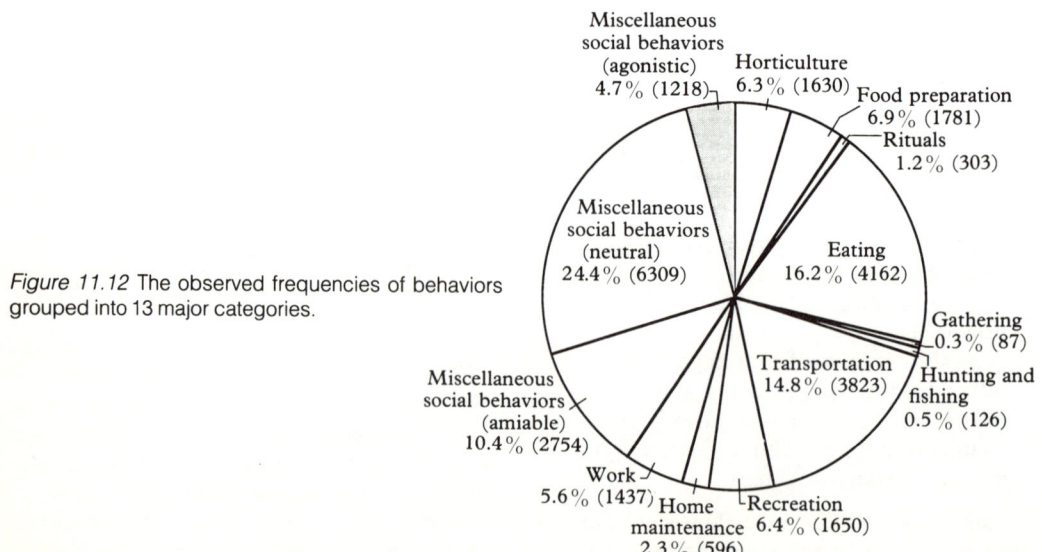

Figure 11.12 The observed frequencies of behaviors grouped into 13 major categories.

198

804 Fighting–serious (involving physical contact with the potential for substantial injury) with weapons (e.g. bottle, cutlass) (number of observations = 2, 0.2% of all agonistic interactions)

805 Fighting–serious, but no weapons (e.g. fist fighting) (5, 0.4%)

806 Fighting–moderate (few substantial blows) (7, 0.6%)

807 Fighting–'play', but with some substantial blows or tumbles (cf. #515) (23, 1.8%)

808 Fighting by throwing stones (or using slingshot) (12, 1.0%)

809 Fighting using sticks (4, 0.3%)

813 Threatening to fight an individual (I.D.#) using weapons (verbal threats and gesturing with weapon) – in the presence of the threatened individual (3, 0.2%)

814 Threatening to fight an individual (I.D.#) using weapons (verbal threats and gesturing with weapon) – not in the presence of the threatened individual (5, 0.4%)

815 Threatening to fight an individual (I.D.#) in a non-serious way, e.g. just the threat of a slap – in the presence of the threatened individual (38, 3.1%)

816 Threatening to fight an individual (I.D.#) in a non-serious way – not in the presence of the threatened individual, e.g. 'I'm going to beat that girl when she gets home' (23, 1.8%)

817 Threatening to punish an individual (I.D.#) – not serious (e.g. a mother stating that she will not give 'candy money' to her child if . . .) (127, 10.4%)

818 Threatening to punish an individual (I.D.#) – serious (e.g. a father stating that he is going to physically punish a child if . . .) (52, 4.3%)

829 Glaring at someone (I.D.#) (14, 1.1%)

847 Arguing – insubstantial, but 'unfriendly', e.g. raised voices (251, 20.6%)

848 Arguing – substantial (e.g. concerning a debt) (44, 3.5%)

856 Insulting someone deliberately (I.D.#) (32, 2.6%)

857 Cussing someone (I.D.#) (38, 3.1%)

867 Family quarrel concerning extra-marital relations (16, 1.3%)

870 Criticizing someone (I.D.#) in their presence – trivial (132, 10.8%)

871 Criticizing someone (I.D.#) not in their presence – trivial (209, 17.2%)

872 Criticizing someone (I.D.#) in their presence – serious (e.g. accusation of theft or stinginess) (24, 1.8%)

873 Criticizing someone (I.D.#) not in their presence – serious (67, 5.5%)

875 Yelling at someone (I.D.#) (41, 3.3%)

876 Screaming with pain (17, 1.4%)

877 Crying (23, 1.8%)

990 Theft (3, 0.3%)

992 Deliberate damage to another's (I.D.#) property (6, 0.5%)

References

Alexander, R. D. (1974) The evolution of social behavior. *Annual Review of Ecology and Systematics*, 5, 325–83.

Alexander, R. D. (1979) *Darwinism and Human Affairs*. Seattle: University of Washington Press.

Altmann, J. (1974) Observational study of behavior: sampling methods. *Behaviour*, XLIX, 227–66.

Beeson, J. (1979) Symbolic aspects of land in the Caribbean: The tenure and transmission of land rights among Caribbean peasantries. In *Peasants, Plantations and Rural Communities in the Caribbean*, ed. M. Cross and A. Marks, Department of Sociology, University of Surrey, and Department of Caribbean Studies, Royal Institute of Linguistics and Anthropology, pp. 86–116.

Betzig, L. L. (1986) *Despotism and Differential Reproduction*. New York: Aldine.

Betzig, L. and Turke, P. (1986) Parental investment by sex on Ifaluk. *Ethology and Sociobiology* 7, 29–37.

Blake, J. (1961) *Family Structure in Jamaica*. New York: Free Press.

Bordieu, P. (1977) *Outline of a Theory of Practice*. Cambridge: Cambridge University Press.

Chagnon, N. A. (1974) *Studying the Yąnomamö*. New York: Holt, Rinehart and Winston.

Chagnon, N. A. (1979) Is reproductive success equal in egalitarian societies? In: *Evolutionary Biology and Human Social Behavior*, ed. N. Chagnon and W. Irons, pp. 374–401. North Scituate, MA: Duxbury Press.

Chagnon, N. A. (1980) Kin selection theory, kinship, marriage, and inclusive fitness among the Yąnomamö Indians. In: *Sociobiology: Beyond Nature–Nurture*, ed. G. W. Barlow and J. Silverberg, AAAS Special Symposium 35. Boulder, CO: Westview Press.

Chagnon, N. A. (1981) Terminological kinship, genealogical relatedness, and village fissioning among the Yąnomamö Indians. In: *Natural Selection and Social Behavior: Recent Research and New Theory*, ed. R. D. Alexander and D. W. Tinkle, pp. 490–508. New York: Chiron Press.

Chagnon, N. A. (1982) Sociodemographic attributes of neoptism in tribal populations: Man the rule breaker. In: *Current Problems in Sociobiology*, ed. King's College Sociobiology Group. Cambridge University Press.

Clarke, E. (1957) *My Mother Who Fathered Me*. London: Allen and Unwin.

Daly, M. and Wilson, M. I. (1981) Abuse and neglect of children in evolutionary perspective. In: *Natural Selection and Social Behavior: Recent Research and New Theory*, ed R. D. Alexander and D. W. Tinkle, pp. 405–16. New York: Chiron Press.

Denham, W. W. (1978) BEVRECS. In: *Alyawara Ethnographic Data Base*. New Haven: HRAF Press.

Dickemann, M. (1981) Paternal confidence and dowry competition: a biocultural analysis of purdah. In: *Natural Selection and Social Behavior: Recent Research and New Theory*, ed. R. D. Alexander and D. W. Tinkle, pp. 417–38. New York: Chiron Press.

Draper, P. and Harpending, H. (1982) Father absence and reproductive strategy: an evolutionary perspective. *Journal of Anthropological Research*, 38, 255–73.

Essock-Vitale, S. (1984) The reproductive success of wealthy Americans. *Ethology and Sociobiology*, 5, 45–9.

Flinn, M. V. (1981) Uterine vs. agnatic kinship variability and associated cousin marriage preferences. In: *Natural Selection and Social Behavior: Recent Research and New Theory*, ed. R. D. Alexander and D. W. Tinkle, pp. 439–75. New York: Chiron Press.

Flinn, M. V. (1983) Resources, mating, and kinship: The behavioral ecology of a Trinidadian village. Ph.D. Thesis, Northwestern University.

Flinn, M. V. (1986) Correlates of reproductive success in a Caribbean village. *Human Ecology*, 14, 225–43.

Flinn, M. V. (1987) Mate guarding in a Caribbean village. *Ethology and Sociobiology* (in press).

Flinn, M. V. and Low, B. S. (1986) Resource distribution, social competition and mating patterns in human societies. In: *Ecological Aspects of Social Evolution*, ed. D. I. Rubenstein and R. W. Wrangham. Princeton, NJ: Princeton University Press.

Fortune, R. F. (1963) *The Sorcerers of Dobu*. New York: Dutton.

Hames, R. (1979) Relatedness and interaction among the Ye'kwana: a preliminary analysis. In: *Evolutionary Biology and Human Social Behavior*, ed. N. Chagnon and W. Irons, pp. 238–50. North Scituate, MA: Duxbury Press.

Harrison, D. H. (1979) The changing fortunes of a Trinidad peasantry: A case study. In *Peasants, Plantations and Rural Communities in the Caribbean*, ed. M. Cross and A. Marks. Department of Sociology, University of Surrey, and Department of Caribbean Studies, Royal Institute of Linguistics and Anthropology.

Hart, C. W. M. and Pilling, A. R. (1960) *The Tiwi of North Australia*. New York: Holt, Rinehart and Winston.

Hill, J. (1984) Prestige and reproductive success in man. *Ethology and Sociobiology*, 5, 77–95.

Hrdy, S. (1981) *The Woman That Never Evolved*. Cambridge, MA: Harvard University Press.

Irons, W. (1979a) Investment and primary social dyads. In: *Evolutionary Biology and Human Social Behavior*, ed. N. Chagnon and W. Irons, pp. 181–212. North Scituate, MA: Duxbury Press.

Irons, W. (1979b) Cultural and biological success. In: *Evolutionary Biology and Human Social Behavior*, ed. N. Chagnon and W. Irons, pp. 257–72. North Scituate, MA: Duxbury Press.

Irons, W. (1981) Why lineage exogamy? In: *Natural Selection and Social Behavior: Recent Research and New Theory*, ed. R. D. Alexander and D. W. Tinkle, pp. 439–75. New York: Chiron Press.

Irons, W. (1983) Human female reproductive strategies. In: *Social Behavior of Female Vertebrates*, ed. S. Wasser and M. Waterhouse, pp. 169–213. New York: Academic Press.

Johnson, A. W. (1975) Time allocation in a Machiguenga community. *Ethnology*, 14(3), 310–12.

Johnson, A. W. (1978) *Quantification in Cultural Anthropology*. Stanford: Stanford University Press.

Levi-Strauss, C. (1949) *Les structures elementaires de la parente*. Paris: Plon.

Munroe, R. H. and Munroe, R. L. (1971) Household density and infant care in an East African Society. *Journal of Social Psychology*, 85, 3–13.

Munroe, R. L., Munroe, R. H., Michealson, C., Koel, A., Bolton, R. and Bolton C. (1983) Time allocation in four societies. *Ethnology*, 22, 355–70.

Rogoff, B. (1985) Spot observation: An introduction and examination. *Quarterly Newsletter of the Institute of Comparative Human Development, Rockefeller University*, 2, 2C, 21–6.

Smith, M. G. (1962) *West Indian Family Structure*. Seattle: University of Washington Press.

Trivers, R. L. (1972) Parental investment and sexual selection. In: *Sexual Selection and the Descent of Man 1871–1971*, ed. B. Campbell. Chicago: Aldine.

Trivers, R. L. (1985) *Social Evolution*, Menlo Park, CA: Benjamin-Cummings.

Turke, P. and Betzig, L. L. (1985) Those who can do: Wealth, status, and reproductive success on Ifaluk. *Ethology and Sociobiology* 6, 79–87.

Wilson, M., Daly, M. and Weghorst, S. J. (1981), Differential maltreatment of boys and girls. *Victimology*, 6, 49–261.

Parental investment, social subordination, and population processes among the 15th and 16th century Portuguese nobility

Introduction

This paper presents an analysis of two distinctive patterns of differential parental investment in offspring among the 15th and 16th century Portuguese high nobility. The first pattern discussed is sex-biased parental investment, in which land wealth and heritable titles and offices are transmitted almost exclusively to male offspring. This pattern of parental behavior appears to form the basis of patriliny as a reproductive strategy (Hartung 1976, 1982), and patriarchal family structure in general (Boone 1986). However, as wealth and social status decreases, there appears to be a tendency to invest more and more familial wealth in female offspring, as lower status families attempt to marry their daughters 'up.' The effects of this shifting pattern of sex-biased parental investment on the male and female reproductive rates are analyzed in detail. It is shown that among the highest status families, where wealth is concentrated in male offspring, males outreproduce females, whereas among the lower nobility, where families are more likely to invest in dowries for daughters, females tend to outreproduce males. This fits the predictions of the Trivers–Willard (1973, Dickemann 1979a and 1979b) hypothesis concerning parental manipulation of sex ratios, which posits that parental

[1] Department of Anthropology, University of New Mexico, Albuquerque, NM 87131, USA

investment will be concentrated in the sex likely to produce the most descendants in a given ecological situation.

The second pattern to be discussed is differential parental investment by birth order. Preference for investment in elder children applied to both male and female offspring. For male offspring, this preference took the form of primogeniture, or restriction of inheritance to the eldest son. For females, investment in the form of dowries was often restricted to one or two daughters, usually the eldest. Younger siblings of both sexes experienced greatly reduced reproductive rates. Younger sons also experienced greatly increased mortality in wars and colonization campaigns.

In the final section of this paper, I discuss the effects of these two patterns of parental investment among the nobility on larger sociodemographic patterns through time. The period under study, beginning around 1380 and ending in the 1580s, begins with a watershed event in the later Medieval–Early Modern history of Portugal. A war of succession with Castille resulted in the establishment of a new dynasty by João I, an illegitimate half-brother of the previous Portuguese king. Most of the established families of the old regime had supported the losing Castillian side in the war, and as a result lost their lands and titles and had to flee to Castille. Their lands were transferred to João I's supporters, who in turn founded new 'houses.' Over the next few generations, their lineages proliferated, and the number of individuals of noble status increased greatly in proportion to the availability of lands and titles within the kingdom. This pattern of increasing competition within the nobility over sources of wealth will be analyzed in detail, and data will be presented which suggest that increasing mortality and the suppression of reproduction through restriction of marriage acted as significant population regulating factors among the noble class by the mid-16th century.

Materials and methods

The primary data source for this research was the *Peditura Lusitana* (Morais 1942–48), an 11-volume transcribed manuscript containing the genealogies of several hundred Medieval and Early Modern Portuguese noble lineages, or *lignages*. A *lignage* is defined by Goody (1984:228, 295) as an 'agnatically based group of lineal kinsfolk' associated with an 'aristocratic "house" whose identity over time is assured by a landed estate, claims to offices, titles, or other relatively exclusive rights.' The Portuguese genealogies, or *nobiliários*, are organized around a series of primary *lignages* associated with ducal or other high ranking houses, along with their associated cadet lineages, each of which is tied to a lesser estate or title. The *Peditura Lusitana* was compiled by a 17th century author who used a large array of supplementary documents, including letters of legitimation, land titles, marriage contracts, and military records. The genealogies are patrilineally organized and consist of lists of marriages and offspring engendered by each male in a *lignage*. In cases where men married more than once or had children by concubines, offspring were further divided under each of the mothers, who are clearly identified as to name, father's name, and father's title or position. This permitted the measurement of female reproductive performance for women who were born into and married back into the collected sample. Figures for reproductive performance and sex ratios were obtained by compiling the lists of offspring by father, mother, status group, generation, etc.

The data collected in the 1980–81 investigations in Lisbon were coded and entered into a computerized file now consisting of over 3700 individuals from the Portuguese *alta nobreza* (high nobility). The study population consists of all the male and female patrilineal descendants of the 25 highest houses, or *lignages*, in Portugal (see Figure 12.1) who were born between roughly 1380 and 1580. The social destiny (title, warfare death, religious career, marriage, etc.) of each individual is also recorded in this file, and summary statistics on rates of marriage, warfare deaths and religious careers were calculated.

Four status groups within the Portuguese nobility were defined for this analysis:

1. The first, and highest status group, consists of the primary lines of each major lineage group including the royal family and the families of dukes, counts, marquises, viscounts and barons.

2. The second group consists of the royal bureaucracy. These cadet lineages held key managerial offices in the monarchy, and include the overseers of the royal and ducal houses, secretaries of accounts and the treasury, key judges and other officials. Most of these offices were hereditary, and their holders were closely related to the primary titled lineages or the royal family. Many of these officials also had titles to lands and labor in the hinterlands as well.
3. The third group consists of the senhorial class which was primarily the landed aristocracy. These consisted of cadet lineages who held hereditary titles to lands and associated labor, often in the form of *morgadios*, or entailed estates, but held no higher office in the monarchy.
4. The lowest status group consists of men who held no known title or who held at best a small lifetime ecclesiastical military pension. Most of the men in this category were *cavaleiros*, who often spent their careers serving in overseas campaigns, and if they married, spent long periods of time away from their wives. Many of them were members of religious military orders, which provided *comendas*, or lifelong pensions, for some of their veteran members. Otherwise, males in this

Figure 12.1 Map of Western Europe showing location of study area.

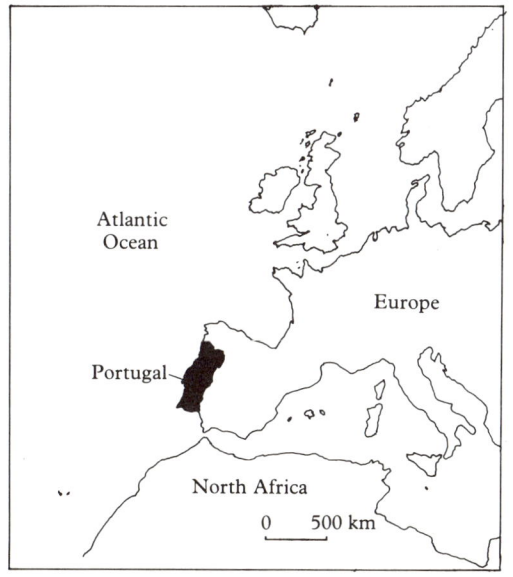

category served or were supported by the houses of more powerful noblemen. For the purposes of this analysis, all these men are grouped together because they had not acceded to any stable or substantial source of wealth.

The family listings are very complete and go far beyond the documentation of titled lineage heads. Included are male and female offspring who died in infancy and childhood, as well as men and women who never married or produced offspring and who had no direct genealogical or social significance. Subsequent analysis of data from the *Peditura Lusitana* indicate that while there is considerable under-numeration of juvenile deaths, this genealogical source contains accurate listings of virtually all individuals who lived to adulthood and entered the social arena as potential competitors for either titles or marriage partnerships. Considerable social and demographic information is supplied about each individual, including data on titles and landholdings, administrative offices, military careers (including notices of death in battle), and religious careers held by each individual who lived to enter society.

Juvenile deaths for all groups are almost certainly under-reported by a considerable degree. Table 12.1 presents frequencies and sex ratios of all reported births and of individuals who were noted as having died in childhood or were otherwise noted in such a way that it appears that they did not reach maturity (grouped by natal status). Hollingsworth (1957:12) found that among children born to British ducal families during the period 1480–1679, 31.1% died before age 15. He cites a figure of 34.1% for the Continental European ruling class from 1500 to 1699 (based on Peller 1965). Thus, juvenile deaths in the *Peditura Lusitana* may be under-reported by more than half. The sex ratios of reported juvenile deaths are also much higher than could be reasonably expected and differ significantly from the adult sex ratios.

The primary titled families have the highest level of reportage of juvenile deaths. The military/untitled group juvenile deaths are also high, suggesting that either the lower ranking families tended to report more offspring who failed to reach maturity (perhaps because they had fewer offspring to report altogether) or that some of

Table 12.1 *Sex ratios and juvenile deaths grouped by natal status (legitimate offspring only)*

	(a) All recorded births				(b) Juvenile deaths				(c) Adult ratio
	Total	M	F	Ratio	M	F	Ratio	Total (%)	
Primary titles	480	262	218	120*	48	26	185**	15.4	112
Royal bureaucracy	807	435	372	117**	49	19	258**	8.4	10
Senhorial	986	541	445	122**	68	17	400**	8.6	111
Military/untitled	1340	751	589	128**	130	50	260**	13.4	115*
Total	3613	1989	1624	123**	295	112	263**	11.3	112

(a) and (c) Asterisks denote level of difference from 50/50 ratio * < 0.05, ** < 0.01
(b) Asterisks denote significance of difference from adult ratio, showing that the sex ratios of reported juvenile deaths differ significantly from sex ratios of reporting offspring who lived to adulthood

the individuals in this group lived later into life before attaining a distinct social position. This latter effect would apply to males in particular, since they were not considered 'mature' until they had acceded to a title or social position such as a knighthood (see discussion of Georges Duby's work on noble 'youths' in the conclusion of this paper). If accession to such positions occurred at a later age among lower ranking males, numbers of juvenile deaths would be higher as well.

The adult sex ratios remain high, averaging about 112. Only the military untitled group differs significantly from a 50/50 ratio (this group has the largest sample size), but since deviations among the other groups are all in the same direction, and are quite close to each other, it is likely that they all reflect the same standard of reportage. It is tempting to suggest that the high adult sex ratios are due to differential neglect of female offspring during childhood, which has been documented for European populations of later periods (Poulain and Tabutin 1981, Wall 1981, Voland 1984), but there is no way to confirm this, and the deficit of reported female deaths in some ways argues against this interpretation. The high adult sex ratios may be due to under-reportage of women, but if they are, the standards of reportage do not appear to differ enough between status groups to account for differences in reproductive performance, nuptiality, or rates of cloistration and warfare deaths presented below.

Since birth, death, and marriage dates were unavailable for the majority of individuals in the sample, independent chronological grouping of the data was not feasible. However, since the

population is genealogically organized, it was possible to order each individual by generation within their particular lineage. To approximate the growth rate of population through time all individuals were then grouped by generation order, and each generation was treated as a 'cohort.' In the first generation, most of the individuals in the 'cohort' were born between 1380 and 1430. Individuals in the fifth generation were born roughly between 1530 and 1580.

Some further limitations of this genealogical data should be noted, particularly with reference to the measurement of reproductive performance. Male fertility is notoriously hard to measure, and I do not pretend here to offer accurate figures on the total number of offspring ever engendered by each male in the sample. The problem of enumeration of illegitimate children is particularly acute, since it is certain that many were never known, acknowledged or legitimized. Since legitimizing bastard children required a certain investment of time, money, and effort on the part of parents, one would expect men of higher social rank to have more illegitimate offspring recorded simply because they were able to have more legitimized. But there is reason to suggest they engendered altogether more illegitimate offspring in any case since they were less likely to spend long periods of time in military campaigns and were simply exposed to more women for longer periods of time. I will argue that the figures presented in the analysis below accurately represent the number of socially recognized offspring.

Measuring female reproductive performance posed a different kind of problem for this study. A considerable number of women born into the population married out of Portugal (usually into the Castillian, Burgundian, or Austrian courts) or into Portuguese lineages which were not collected. Therefore, for this analysis, reproductive performance figures are available only for women who married back into the collected sample, or approximately 32% of all ever-married women born into the population.

An additional limitation of this data source is that birth, marriage, and death dates are very seldom reported. As a result, no attempt was made to incorporate vital statistics or age at marriage data into this study.

Parental investment and elite family reproduction

The evolutionary basis for male-biased inheritance has been developed by Hartung (1976, 1982). Dickemann (1979a and 1979b) first developed the idea that the patrilineal–polygynous–hypergynous breeding structure appears to fit the predictions of an hypothesis proposed by Trivers and Willard (1973; see Hrdy 1987, for a recent review) concerning the evolution of the tendency of parents to manipulate the sex ratio of their offspring according to varying ecological conditions. Trivers and Willard argue that natural selection will favor differential parental investment in offspring of one sex or the other, depending upon which sex is likely to produce the most descendants, thereby increasing the parent's own reproductive fitness. Parental investment is defined as any investment of time or resources by the parent in an individual offspring that increases the offspring's chance of surviving and reproducing at the cost of the parent's ability to invest in other offspring (Trivers 1972). Differential investment in offspring can potentially take the form of pre-zygotic selection of gametes by the female, differential mortality *in utero*, sex-selective infanticide or neglect after birth, or the tendency to invest more in the rearing of offspring of one or the other sex.

The principal factor affecting differential parental investment is parental 'condition,' which in the Trivers–Willard model refers to the parents' health or quality of local habitat or territory. The Trivers–Willard model is based upon the fact that variation in condition affects male and female reproductive success in different ways. Simply put, 'a male in good condition is

expected to outreproduce a female in similar condition, whereas females will tend to outreproduce males if both are in poor condition' (Trivers and Willard 1973:90). Several factors contribute to this effect. The most important is that fundamental differences in male and female reproductive biology make polygamy a feasible strategy for maximizing reproductive success for males, but not females (Bateman 1948). To the extent that condition contributes to a male's ability to attract mates, males in good condition will tend to outreproduce similar females through multiple matings. Under poor conditions, the pattern is reversed since females tend to have higher resistance to environmental stress, and are more likely to survive to reproduce. And, given any within-population variation in male condition, females will choose mates in good condition, to the extent that her mate's condition can affect positively the survivability and fitness of her offspring. Thus, where polygyny is a potential mating strategy, males in good condition tend to mate with a disproportion of females in a population. This leaves males in poor condition with a shortage of mates and creates a situation of intense reproductive competition among males for mates. Where access to mates is contingent upon access to resources, resource competition among males translates directly into reproductive competition.

Among human populations, Trivers and Willard argue that socioeconomic status is the relevant variable corresponding to 'condition,' to the extent that wealth is positively correlated with reproductive success. This pattern of sex-biased parental investment should occur in any situation where the following three conditions are met:

1. Resources are unequally distributed among the population (if they were not, there would not be any differential reproduction on the basis of wealth).
2. Wealth is a stronger determinant of male reproductive performance than of female (if it were not, differential parental investment would not make any difference).
3. The socioeconomic status of parents can be conferred upon offspring and will endure into the offspring's adulthood (if it could not, differential investment would not enhance the fitness of the parent).

Table 12.2 *(a) Reproductive performance[a] of males grouped by natal status (includes legitimate and illegitimate offspring); (b) illegitimate offspring only*

	(a) All surviving offspring			(b) Illegitimate only	
	N^b	n	x̄	n	x̄
Primary titles	213	624	2.93	131	0.62
Royal bureaucracy	291	741	2.55	75	0.26
*Senhorial	414	1050	2.54	122	0.29
Military/untitled	505	768	1.52	88	0.17
Total	1423	3183	2.24	416	0.29

Kruskal–Wallis: (a) $p < 0.000$; (b) $p < 0.000$
[a] Reproductive performance is defined throughout as the number of offspring that survived to adulthood
[b] N refers to numbers of parents, n refers to number of offspring

The model can thus be applied to human populations in the following way. In stratified societies, wealth is the most decisive parameter in determining a male's ability to attract mates and to establish a stable reproductive career. Therefore, where wealth is heritable and has a positive effect on future reproductive performance of offspring, wealthy lineages that concentrate inheritance in males will outreproduce those that do not (Hartung 1976, 1982). Hence, the highest status families may gain more by concentrating investment in male offspring and curtailing or reducing investment in female offspring by eliminating them during infancy (as in the traditional Brahmin and Chinese cases), or channelling them later into non-reproductive roles (as in the Medieval European case; cf. Dickemann 1979a, 1979b).

Conversely, where the family fortune is comparatively small, lower status families may gain more by marrying daughters up than by (or in addition to) attempting to establish sons in society under poor circumstances. The inherited wealth of the daughter's higher status mate would subsequently improve the reproductive success of her future offspring. Thus, we would expect to see the level of parental investment in daughters (in the form of dowries) to be higher relative to investment in sons among lower status families than among high status families.

Systematic, quantitative data on élite family reproduction that would support the above model have been lacking. Specifically, it has not been shown that male-biased investment leads to superior male reproductive success at the top while female-biased investment leads to superior female reproductive success at the bottom. The data presented below on 15th and 16th century

Portuguese nobility support the Trivers–Willard hypothesis, particularly in terms of varying level of investment in male and female offspring and their effects on reproductive performance.

Differential reproduction by status and sex among the Portuguese nobility

Tables 12.2–12.4 show the reproductive performance of males in the sample grouped by natal (i.e. father's) and attained (i.e. actually reached as an adult) status. Table 12.2(a) shows that natal status is a significant determinant of reproductive performance among males (Kruskal–Wallis, $p < 0.001$). The Kruskal–Wallis One-Way Analysis of Variance (corrected for ties) was used to test differences in reproductive performance throughout, due to non-normal distributions of values in many cases. Table 12.2(b) presents the average numbers of reported illegitimate children only, and shows that the difference in total reproductive performance between primary titled and the lower titled males is due to the addition of illegitimate offspring. Illegitimate offspring, however, do not account for the difference between lower titled males and the military/untitled group. This suggests that other factors, including probability of marriage, number of serial marriages, and age at first marriage might better account for the difference in reproductive performance between titled and untitled males.

Figure 12.2 shows that among these elites, the effect of natal status on probability of marriage is very slight for males. However, Table 12.3 shows that if the reproductive performance of only newly-married males is considered, the difference in number of offspring due to natal status is still marked. This leaves at least two other potential determinants of the differential reproductive performance among titled and untitled males: number of serial marriages and age at marriage. Reproductive performance was found to increase with number of serial marriages (among the entire population of ever married males: Married once, $N = 788$, Average number of offspring, 3.69; Married twice, $N = 113$, Average number of offspring, 4.50; Married three or more times, $N = 15$, Average number of offspring, 6.80). Table 12.4(c) shows that the probability of marrying more than once increases considerably with attained status. Age at marriage is probably another determinant of reproductive performance, but because of the lack of consistent birth and marriage dates for this population, this factor could not be investigated. However, Levy and Henry (1960) show that marriage was earlier among the highest levels of French aristocracy than the lower nobility during approximately the same period.

We can now compare the effects of status on female reproductive performance. Table 12.5(a) shows the reproductive performance of ever-married women grouped by natal status. Within this sample, we see that female reproductive performance does not monotonically increase with

status, and that the range of variation is much smaller than among males (Kruskal–Wallis, $p < 0.618$). When the same population is grouped by conjugal status (i.e. husband's status, Table 12.5(b), differences in reproductive performance are greater (Kruskal–Wallis, $p < 0.09$) but the difference is mainly between the top three groups and the military group. Thus, marriage to higher status males appears to enhance reproductive performance for women.

Figure 12.3 summarizes the data presented in Tables 12.2–12.5 and compares male and female reproductive performance by natal and attained or conjugal status. Two main trends are apparent: (1) the range of variation in reproduction performance is less for females, and (2) low status females outreproduce low status males. Additionally, among the three higher status groups, males exhibit slightly higher reproductive rates than females. Differences between male and female reproduction among the top three status groups were not statistically significant: primary titles, $p < 0.867$; royal bureaucracy, $p < 0.650$; senhorial, $p < 0.545$ (all Kruskal–Wallis tests for differences in natal status), although the differences are all in the same direction predicted by the model. The difference between male and female reproductive performance among the military/untitled group (natal status) was significant: $p < 0.024$.

Given the higher reproductive potential of males at the top end of the scale and of females at the lower end, a corresponding pattern of differential parental investment in offspring according to sex would be expected. According to the model presented above, parental investment should be concentrated in favor of males among high status families, whereas female offspring should be favored among lower status families.

Evidence of sex-biased differential investment in the Portuguese case

In the Portuguese case, there is clear evidence that parental investment in female offspring was greater among the lower nobility than among the primary titled lineages. Figure 12.2 shows that daughters of the lower nobility were more likely to marry than their brothers, and that their probability of ever marrying exceeded those of women from the titled nobility as well. The pattern of male and female nuptiality is consistent

Figure 12.2 Proportion of men ($N = 1959$) and women ($N = 1630$) who ever married, grouped by natal status

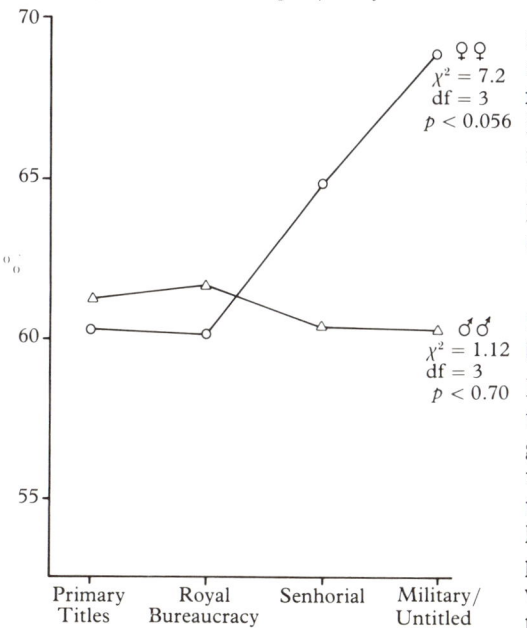

$\chi^2 = 7.2$
df $= 3$
$p < 0.056$

$\varphi \varphi$

$\delta \delta$
$\chi^2 = 1.12$
df $= 3$
$p < 0.70$

Primary Titles · Royal Bureaucracy · Senhorial · Military/ Untitled

Table 12.3 *(a) Reproductive performance of ever-married males grouped by natal status; (b) illegitimate offspring only*

Offspring of	(a) All offspring			(b) Illegitimate only	
	N	n	$\bar{x}$	n	$\bar{x}$
Primary titles	137	560	4.09	67	0.48
Royal bureaucracy	206	715	3.47	55	0.25
Senhorial	263	1016	3.86	88	0.33
Military/untitled	308	726	2.36	46	0.15
Total	914	3017	3.30	256	0.27

Kruskal–Wallis: (a) $p < 0.000$; (b) $p < 0.02$

Table 12.4 *(a) Reproductive performance of ever-married males grouped by attained status; (b) illegitimate offspring only; (c) percent married more than once*

Offspring of	(a) All offspring			(b) Illegitimate only		(c) % of N married more than once
	N	n	$\bar{x}$	n	$\bar{x}$	
Primary titles	96	456	4.75	50	0.52	22.6
Royal bureaucracy	168	776	4.62	43	0.36	18.5
Senhorial	216	981	4.54	80	0.37	13.9
Military/untitled	553	1287	2.33	127	0.23	10.3
Total	1033	3500	3.39	300	0.29	14.0

Kruskal–Wallis: (a) $p < 0.000$; (b) $p < 0.03$

Table 12.5 *Reproductive performance of ever-married women grouped by (a) natal status and (b) conjugal status*

	(a) Natal status			(b) Conjugal status		
	N	n	$\bar{x}$	N	n	$\bar{x}$
Primary titles	77	291	3.78	79	286	3.62
Royal bureaucracy	70	224	3.20	83	328	3.95
Senhorial	116	418	3.60	122	462	3.79
Military/untitled	77	256	3.32	80	209	2.61
Total	340	1189	3.50	364	1285	2.87

Kruskal–Wallis: (a) $p < 0.614$; (b) $p < 0.018$

with a hypergynous mating system: at the lower end of the scale more women marry than men; at the top, more men than women. Since marriage of female offspring involved the payment of a dowry, rates of marriage have a direct correspondence to levels of parental investment. In some cases, titles were actually transferred from the brides' father to the groom in marriage contracts. For the most part, however, dowry payments were in the form of movable goods, while titles and estates were transferred through male lines.

Further research is needed on the actual amounts and contents of dowries and inherited titles or estates at different levels of the nobility, but I suspect that the comparative reproductive value of dowries in the form of movable wealth and patrimonies in the form of landed estates varied greatly according to status. Among the highest nobility, patrimonies were quite extensive, encompassing large tracts of productive lands and labor and including a large guaranteed lifetime income in the form of rents. While dowries among the high nobility were certainly quite large, they would have to be very large indeed to equal the value of the landed estates that were passed down through male lines. However, among the lower classes of nobility, patrimonies were much less extensive, and in many cases, were incapable of supporting a noble household or of attracting a marriage partnership of suitable status (one might recall the meager patrimony of Cervantes' Don Quixote). In these cases, any movable wealth that could be invested in marrying a daughter into a higher station may actually have higher reproductive value than the estate inherited by a son.

Figure 12.4 clearly illustrates the contrasting pattern of gender bias between the upper and lower nobility. Among women, the percentage of cloistrations increases with status, a result of the fact that higher status families were less likely to invest in dowries for their daughters. Among men, the percentage of warfare deaths decreases

with status, showing that higher status males were more likely to inherit and establish themselves in Portugal rather than to spend their careers in military campaigns.

It should be pointed out that in 18th century Portugal, families paid 'dowries' to convents upon their daughters entrance into the religious profession (José Mattoso, pers. comm.). While I am not aware of evidence that this was done in the 15th and 16th centuries, it is possible that such a practice existed then as well. For the purpose of this argument, it will have to be assumed that such 'dowries' (in effect, paid to cover living expenses in a rather austere social setting) amounted to less than those which were invested in arranging a suitable marriage.

Figure 12.3 Reproductive performance of men and women grouped by status (compiled from Tables 12.2–12.5).

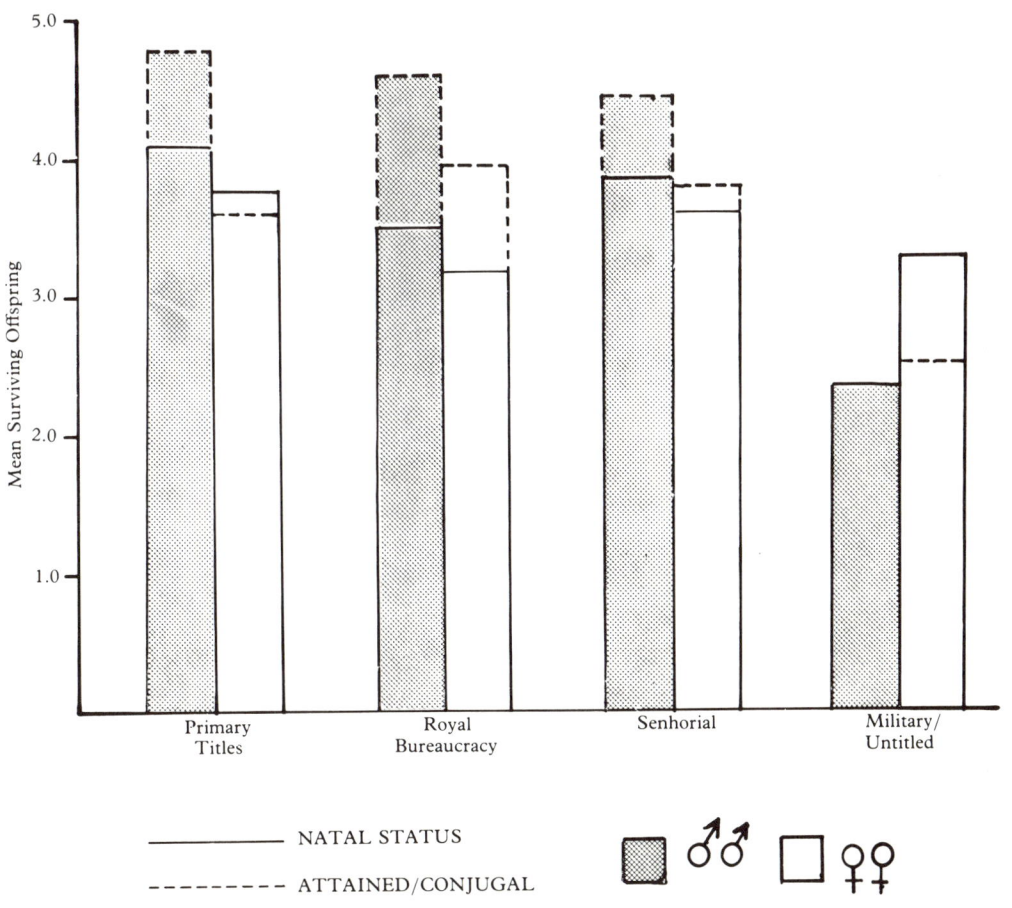

NATAL STATUS

ATTAINED/CONJUGAL

♂♂   ♀♀

209

'Where there are great riches, there are also many to devour them'

This verse from Ecclesiastes (5:11) was often quoted in Medieval texts in recognition of the fact that wealthy households tended to be larger than poor ones (Herlihy 1973). While reproductive success may be correlated with economic success, high rates of reproduction may, in highly competitive social contexts, almost paradoxically lead to downward social mobility (Herlihy 1973). Noble families faced two problems in this respect: (1) allowing too many sons to marry resulted in the proliferation of lateral branches of the family and the dissipation of the 'house,' particularly if (2) the patrimony continued to be divided between the offspring through several generations. An emergent characteristic of élite family structure in stratified societies is the restriction of familial wealth to one line (Herlihy 1973, Cooper 1976:238). Primogeniture is likely to develop as a reproductive strategy where wealth is a strong determinant of reproductive performance and where high mortality makes large family size a necessity in ensuring lineage posterity. In other words, primogeniture can be interpreted as a kind of hedging that occurs when restriction of family size *per se* is too risky due to high mortality.

Figure 12.4 Proportion of women who became nuns and men who died in warfare, grouped by natal status. From a sample of 1959 men and 1630 women.

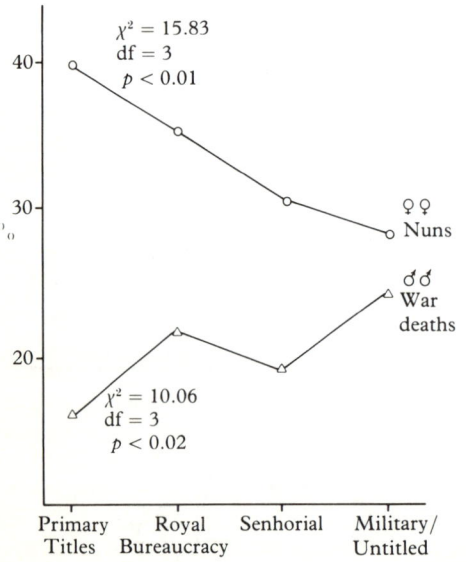

As we have seen, restriction of inheritance at the top of the hierarchical social system initially takes the form of a shift to patriliny. As competition intensifies, even more restrictive measures, such as primogeniture, typically appear.

Primogeniture should develop where the source of wealth is stable, predictable, and dependable (i.e. controllable through time), where this wealth is unequally distributed among the population, and where specific personal abilities or attributes are not overly important to the maintenance of the source of wealth. Such would be the case where wealth is in the form of rights to the surplus produced by a subject agrarian infrastructure already in place, and where these rights are a matter of inheritance of a title.

The importance of the stability and predictability of resources as determinants of inheritance patterns can be illustrated by comparing the lands-and-labor based aristocracy of Western Europe with the élites of the Italian city-states during the same period (example based on Herlihy 1977). In the Italian case, the primary source of wealth was speculative enterprise, in which financial success was dependent upon personal expertise and a good deal of chance. Family wealth required constant tending and could rise and fall in the space of a generation. Here, wealth was customarily divided up more or less equally among males, often in their early teens. The young men would go to work in counting houses, receive training in finance, and wait for their 'main chance' at financial success, which might not come until middle age, if at all. The strategy here was clearly a different sort of 'hedging of bets' on the part of wealthy parents. Among the landed aristocracy of Western Europe, this kind of hedging was unnecessary, since although yearly fluctuations in production were to be expected, lands and labor constituted a stable source of wealth from generation to generation.

Figure 12.5 shows that primogeniture was a strong determinant of male dispersion and mortality among the 15th and 16th century Portuguese nobility. This histogram shows that warfare deaths increase with birth order, reflecting the fact that younger sons were more likely to spend their entire careers at risk. Furthermore, younger sons who were killed were more likely to be killed much farther away, in India, than their elder brothers, who as youths participated in the nearby Moroccan campaigns, but soon returned to Portugal to take their place in society.

Birth order affected not only dispersion and mortality rates, but, as a critical determinant of status, determined as well who would reproduce and how much. Table 12.6(a) clearly illustrates the effects of birth order and restricted inheritance on male reproduction in the Portuguese case. Figure 12.6 shows that the general effect of birth order on reproduction is linked to probability of marriage. This is confirmed by Table 12.6(b), which shows the same data for ever-married males only: reproductive performance no longer increases monotonically with birth order, and between-group differences are much less.

Birth order had a catastrophic effect on probability of marriage among women as well (Figure 12.6), and hence, upon reproduction (see Table 12.7). Interestingly, eldest daughters were favored in the same way as sons. This appears to indicate that, as in the case of male offspring, plans for investment in daughters were highly systematized and made well ahead of time, and that specific personal attributes, such as appearance, health, or personality were less important than birth order in affecting decisions as to which

Figure 12.5 Proportion of males who lived to adulthood, who subsequently died in warfare, grouped by birth order. Each bar is further divided by place of warfare death. Statistics on birth order/death: $\chi^2 = 10.8$, df = 3, $p < 0.02$; birth order/place: $\chi^2 = 28.36$, df = 3, $p < 0.001$.

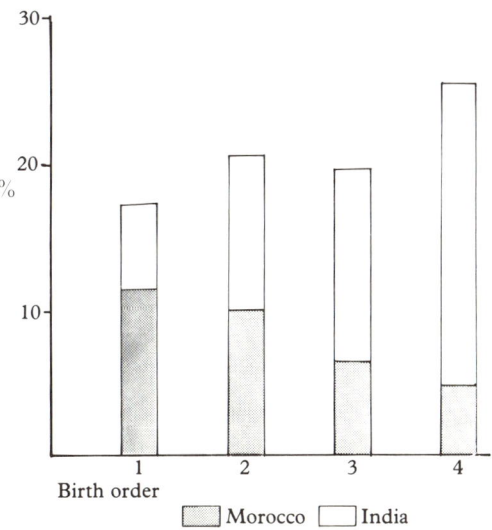

Birth order

☐ Morocco ☐ India

daughters to invest dowries in. Dowry competition and the resulting restriction of marriages among female offspring was itself closely tied to the effects of primogeniture, since primogeniture limited drastically the number of marriageable males throughout the system.

Effects of differential parental investment on larger population processes

In the sections above, I have discussed several sociodemographic processes that have a direct effect on patterns of resource/status competition among elites in preindustrial states. Figure 12.7 illustrates how these factors are interrelated, and how they lead to a situation of intensifying competition among élites for lands to titles.

In the first place, intense male–male competition is likely to develop where resources are unevenly distributed within the population, and where such resources are stable and predictable sources of status (control of agricultural surplus would be a prime example). As competition for sources of wealth increases, differences in wealth become increasingly important determinants of a male's ability to establish a stable reproductive career and to insure the survival of his lineage. As control over resources shifts to male lines, competition among élites is intensified by two factors (Figure 12.7). First, through differential investment in male offspring, the sex ratio of the élite population becomes increasingly biased in favor of males. Second, patriliny and restricted inheritance become more widespread with increasing status competition among élites, which tends to generate increasing numbers of excluded males of élite rank. Thus, family strategies aimed at insuring lineage survival and posterity generate competition among élites at the societal level, which is typically manifested in political instability warfare and territorial expansion.

In Figure 12.8, males who came of age are grouped by generational cohort, and the changing proportions of each of the defined social status categories is traced through time. This method of grouping oversimplifies the real situation in the sense that it treats each new generation as if it were a clearly demarcated event and as if all lineage generations were perfectly synchronous. In actuality, there is generational

Table 12.6 *Reproductive performance of men grouped by birth order*

Birth order	(a) All men in sample			(b) Ever-married men only		
	N	n	x̄	N	n	x̄
1	504	1561	3.10	376	1547	4.11
2	366	843	2.30	223	785	3.52
3	240	447	1.86	111	422	3.80
4+	261	434	1.66	102	386	3.78
Total	1371	3285	2.40	812	3140	3.87

Kruskal–Wallis: (a) $p < 0.000$; (b) $p < 0.09$

overlap and the accession to and vacation of titles is a continuous process.

Figure 12.8 shows that the proportion of military and untitled males increases from about 40% to about 75% during the period. The increase in the military/untitled portion of the population (as well as in the clerics, i.e. monks) is due to the fact that the number of males who are noble by birth increases with each generation, while the number of discreet titles remains the same, or increases at a much slower rate. Thus, we can say that the intensity of competition for titles among the nobility, measured in terms of number of males in relation to the number of individual titles, nearly doubled over

Table 12.7 *Reproductive performance of ever-married women grouped by birth order*

Birth order	N	n	x̄
1	143	528	3.69
2	61	238	3.90
3	30	94	3.13
4+	21	43	2.05
Total	255	903	3.54

Kruskal–Wallis: $p < 0.050$

the course of 200 years. This 200-year period was precisely the time period during which Portuguese expansion reached its zenith and in which warfare deaths among the nobility reached as high as 25% (Figure 12.9). For women, this was the age of convents. Figure 12.9 gives the

Figure 12.6 Proportion of ever-married men and women grouped by birth order.

Figure 12.7 Sociodemographic processes leading to intensifying resource competition among élites.

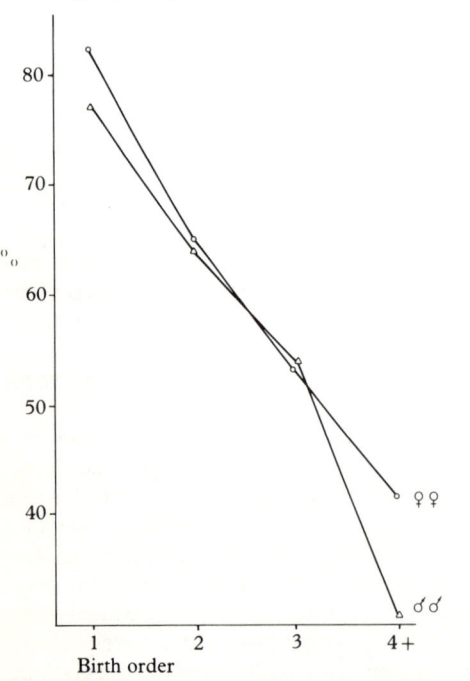

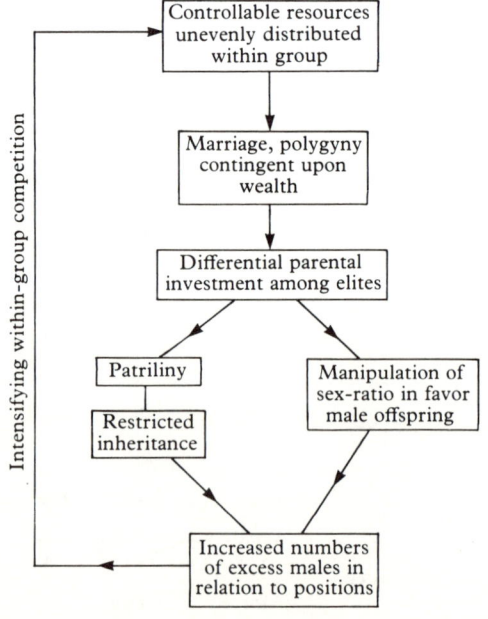

proportion of women who entered cloisters, again grouped by generational cohort. The drastic increase in the proportion of warfare deaths and cloistrations clearly parallels the pattern of increasing competition among males over titles revealed in Figure 12.8.

We are now in a position to investigate the effects of this pattern of intensifying competition on reproductive performance of men grouped by generational cohort. In Table 12.8(a) we see that the average reproductive performance among the entire male population drops by half. The proportion of males who produced no surviving offspring doubles. Even among ever-married men (Table 8(c)), reproductive performance drops by nearly 40%. This decrease among married men is probably due to increasing age at marriage although, as pointed out above, this could not be directly investigated. However, increasing age at marriage during this period has been documented in other studies. Hollingsworth (1957:14), for example, has shown that average age at marriage among British ducal families increased from 22.4 to 30.5 for males

and 17.1 to 24.7 for females from the 14th to the 18th centuries (see also Hajnal 1965:114–15).

By grouping the offspring of each generation by sex, we can gain a rough idea of what is happening to the sex ratio in response to increasing competition. The model above predicts that with increasing variance in male reproduction, the sex ratio at the top of the social hierarchy should increase in favor of males. Table 12.9 shows the sex ratio of the offspring who lived to adulthood of each succeeding generation. If the ratio is taken simply in terms of the number of living males and females who reached adulthood, there does not appear to be any distinct pattern other than a distinct general bias in favor of males. However, if the women who were channeled into celibate religious roles are removed (since they are no longer a part of the breeding population), there is a definite increase in the sex ratio as it is defined in those terms. More women are entering convents with each succeeding generation. Thus, with increased competition over titles during this 200-year period, there is an

Figure 12.8 The changing proportional representation of each of the defined status groups within the population (males only, N = 2059). Grouped by generational cohort.

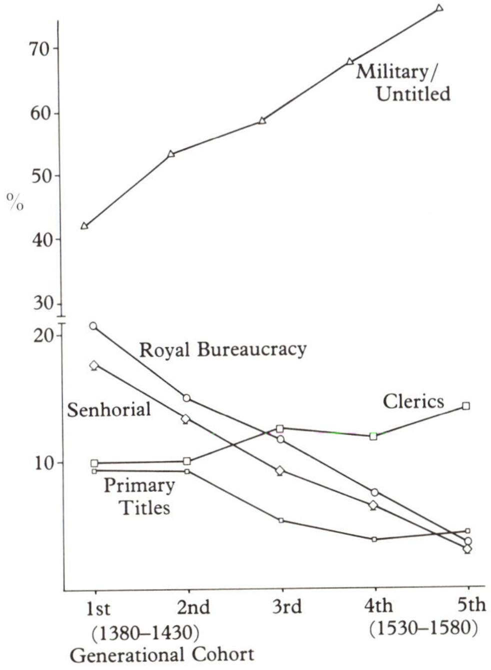

Figure 12.9 Proportion of women who became nuns and men who died in warfare, grouped by generational cohort. Cloistrations and warfare deaths increased with the intensity of competition over titles during the period 1380–1580 (compare with Figure 12.8).

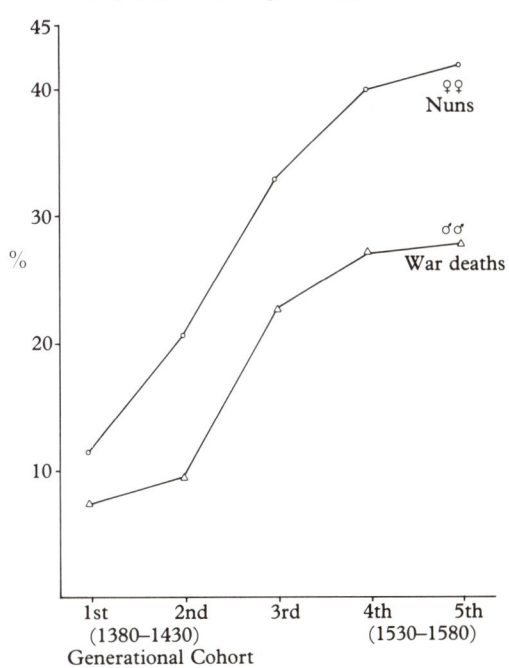

Table 12.8 *Reproductive performance of men grouped by generational cohort*

Generational cohort	(a) All men in sample				(b) % ever married	(c) Ever-married only			
	N	n	x̄	% < 1		N	n	x̄	% < 1
First	102	331	3.25	27.5	75.5	77	316	4.10	9.1
Second	169	568	3.36	28.4	79.9	135	551	4.08	14.8
Third	326	1034	3.17	34.4	70.6	230	951	4.13	15.7
Fourth	536	1087	2.03	46.5	60.4	324	1009	3.11	20.7
Fifth	475	748	1.57	60.6	56.7	269	685	2.55	34.9
Total	1608	3738	2.32	45.1	64.4	1035	3512	3.39	21.6

Kruskal–Wallis: (a) $p < 000$; (c) $p < 0.000$; '% < 1' denotes proportion producing no surviving offspring

Table 12.9 *Adult sex ratio of offspring grouped by parents' generational cohort (legitimate offspring only)*

Generational cohort	Males	Females	Ratio	Females (excluding nuns)	Ratio[a]
First	139	140	99.3	129	107.8
Second	265	225	117.8	188	141.5
Third	438	387	113.2	276	158.5
Fourth	464	378	122.7	248	187.1
Fifth	282	275	102.6	163	173.0
Total	1588	1405	113.0	1004	158.2

[a] i.e. of marriageable men and women only

increasing tendency to invest less in female offspring relative to male offspring.

Conclusion

Behavioral ecologists have noted that social hierarchical organization is a significant force for population dispersion (Christian 1970, Brown 1975, Lomicki 1982). In the sense that dominance behavior is the social analog of territoriality (Wilson 1971:196), individuals in hierarchical social groups who disperse as a result of subordination effects are analogous to 'floaters' produced by exclusion effects in single individual territorial systems. Like 'floaters,' individuals dispersing as a result of subordination effects are characterized by higher mortality rates and lower reproductive rates (Brown 1975:98). I have argued here and elsewhere (Boone 1983) that among hierarchical human groups, dispersion resulting from subordination effects can take the form of warfare against neighboring groups, territorial expansion, and colonization. In fact, controlling élites may encourage and underwrite these activities, especially when the alternative is having the competitive tendencies of their social subordinants

directed at themselves. Clearly, the landless younger sons, subordinated at the family level by the rules of restrictive inheritance, fit the floater profile in terms of mortality and reproductive rates and dispersing tendencies.

Primogeniture is often interpreted as a social means of institutionalizing succession and stabilizing competition in a society where there are always more 'applicants' than positions (Goody 1966, Service 1973, Johnson 1978). This functional interpretation is partially correct in the sense that primogeniture has this *effect*. By subordinating and dispersing excess personnel at the family level, the existing hierarchy is stabilized and preserved at the societal level. Furthermore, the dispersal effect of territorial expansion has the effect of regulating competition at the top of the social hierarchy through the higher mortality and lowered reproductive rates of males subordinated by primogeniture (see data in Table 12.7 and Figure 12.4). Additionally, where primogeniture is practiced among élites, there may be found a recurring pattern of dominant–subordinate relations between elder and younger sons, and generationally, between primary and secondary lineages (cf. Fox 1971). This dominant–subordinate pattern forms the basis of the stratification of élites into land or office-holding primary lineages and the bureaucratic and military cadet lineages. Thus the process of stratification is principally the result of genealogical decay. A portion of the younger sons subordinated by primogeniture are taken care of through appointment to somewhat lesser political offices. In fact, such offices are often created to accommodate them. In this sense, the functional organization of the state crystallizes around the process of downward social mobility, and, from an ontogenetic point of view, the unfolding functional differentiation of hierarchical social systems is a political process of creating positions for excess personnel. But while primogeniture may constitute an effective strategy for the maintenance of individual family fortunes and for stabilizing succession, it ultimately creates a highly competitive, volatile situation at the societal level with respect to the problem of excess cadet males. Rulers must choose between dispersing these individuals, for example in expansionist campaigns, or facing disorder and overthrow on the home front.

In a detailed and closely documented series of articles on noble family structure and the origin of knighthood, Duby (1977) has traced the shift to patriliny and restricted inheritance in France during the 10th through the 12th centuries, particularly in the region of Macon. Here, *de facto* primogeniture took the form of restriction of marriage to the oldest son: 'all brothers had the same rights of inheritance on their father's death. Only one of them married and begot legitimate sons. The latter, thanks to the practices of prolonged joint ownership, would collect without difficulty the rights of their uncles' (Duby 1977:74). Outright primogeniture may have been more commonly associated with entailed lands (this was clearly true in the case of the Iberian Peninsula, see discussion below), where the rule was connected with feudal law which prevented the subdivision of *fiefs*. Younger brothers may have received small inheritances (particularly new lands acquired by the father, in contrast to the patrimony itself), but possession in such cases 'was precarious, and fragments such as these bred discord between brothers and encouraged cupidity and sharpened the temptation of other brothers or nephews to seize whatever they could by force' (Duby 1977:117–18).

Duby further explores the ramifications of the problem of succession in a chapter devoted to aristocratic 'youths.' Here, the term 'youth' (*juvenis*), rather than having a strict chronological connotation, referred instead to noble males who had not yet married and established an estate. Following adolescence, a period of vagabondage was considered a necessary element in an aristocratic male's development. Vagabondage was not usually solitary, and often bands of 'youths' lived and travelled together: a newly dubbed 'youth' might arm and take with him the sons of his father's vassals who were his own age. Arms and money were provided by the house to which the young nobles and vassals were attached. The period of vagabondage was *de rigueur* for the eldest sons as well and apparently functioned to delay the young heir's marriage and accession to his patrimony: 'The eldest son who as a "youth" was surrounded by "young" companions ... began to struggle openly against the old lord .... His father would give him leave to depart with some relief, and he would not recall his son until his own powers waned' (1977:117). This is an interesting point in itself in that it indicates considerable parent–offspring conflict and competitive interaction even in the case of the rightful heir (cf. Trivers 1974). Younger sons, were destined to remain 'youths' far into middle age or indefinitely. Their usual recourse was to enter the Church or military service. Thus, Duby argues that it was this expanding group of 'youths' who constituted the 'spearhead of feudal aggression' (1977:15). As such, these bands of armed 'youths,' whose class expectations and military expertise where quite high, represented a significant disruptive potential within the noble families themselves, within the organization of the state or principality as a whole, and for the system of alliances that developed between states. And, with primogeniture spreading lower into the ranks of the nobility, these landless 'youths' were increasing in numbers. According to Duby, it is within the context of this growing problem that the Church began to take an increasing role in the affairs of the Christian states, particularly through the role it played in territorial integration and in rechanneling aggression. Early manifestations of this role in France are exemplified in the peace of God movement of the 10th and 11th centuries. Duby outlines a variety of complex features of this movement and I will recount only a few of them here.

With the strengthening of the power of regional lords and the virtual collapse of monarchial power, the peace of God movement was a response to 'conditions in an enclosed agrarian society, no longer nourished by the profits of war which had formerly been put into circulation by the sovereign' (Duby 1977:86). Warfare up until and during that time was not simply a pastime for 'youths,' it could and often did lead to palpable gain on the part of young men who had been denied inheritance through their families. (The Norman conquest of Sicily is a case in point.) It also provided a means by which the ruling élite could relieve themselves of the demands of these landless nobles, and, as the above quotation suggests, for fathers to provide directly for their own younger sons through acquisitions. The *paix de Dieu* shifted the emphasis on warfare as an institution for personal gain (at least within Christendom) to an institution for the glorification of Christianity. As such it paved the way for the segregation of 'youths' into religious military orders under the control of the Church and to their deployment in Crusades outside the Continent. Duby (1977:12) writes: 'It is obvious that it was the band of "youths" excluded by so many social prohibitions from the main body of settled men, fathers of families and heads of houses, with their prolonged spells of turbulent behavior making them an unstable fringe of society, who created and sustained the crusades.'

While the Crusades against Palestine and Syria ended by the end of the 13th century, a similar pattern of warfare continued on the Iberian Peninsula with the *Reconquista*. The availability of 'new' lands for conquests to the south of Portugal's own borders explains why we do not see the development of subinfeudation or institutionalized primogeniture associated with entailed estates until after the middle of the 13th century, when the *Reconquista* was 'completed' in the Algarve region of the Iberian Peninsula (in 1249). With this source of territory used up, intensifying competition within the state led to the institution of *morgados*, or entailed estates which carried the stipulation of primogeniture (Gama Barros 1945: vol. 8, pp. 227–53, Oliveira Marques 1975:386–7; these were similar to *mayorazgos* in Spain, cf. Cooper 1978).

The existence of a class of *cavalaria*, composed of males of noble origin, who were considered lower in status than the *fidalguia* or nobility (Gama Barros 1945: vol. 3, 345–491, Oliveira Marques 1975, 386–7, Mattoso 1985: vol. 1, 134) is the principal evidence that some system of restricted marriage/inheritance, perhaps similar to the French example cited above, existed even before the end of the *Reconquista*. This *cavalaria* appears to have consisted of nobility who, being poorer in land, sought homage to the king or other powerful houses. In any case, the institution of primogeniture in the 13th and 14th centuries hastened the appearance of landless younger sons whose only recourse was to join the Church, military service, or the ranks of the rising *burguesas* or commercial class (Oliveira Marques 1975:387, Mattoso 1975). With the development of gunpowder warfare and transoceanic sailing vessels, this pattern of dispersal of social subordinates would result in the spread of European populations over much of the planet (Wallerstein 1974:41, Boone 1983).

What is somewhat unusual about this case study, at least from a population ecological standpoint, is the appearance of large numbers of non-reproductive females – in effect, female 'floaters.' This is due, at least proximally, to the monogamous marriage system that prevailed among the nobility (as well as the rest of Europe). Monogamy, in turn, is tied to the historical development of the patriarchal lineage system of the nobility from a system of bilateral inheritance (diverging devolution, Goody 1976:3–4, 1984:11, 20, 238 and passim) which still prevailed among lower classes. Under bilateral inheritance, which is associated with plough agricultural systems (Goody 1976), land is divided equally among male and female offspring and is combined into larger units again in marriage. Thus, the families of the bride and groom have an equal stake in the marriage and in the resulting issue of the marriage. Under such an arrangement, the bride and the bride's family could be expected to have both the desire and the political leverage to discourage institutional polygyny, or in any case, the investment by the groom in any offspring other than those he had with her.

Under conditions of increasing social stratification, the female's inheritance becomes a dowry whose content has (usually) shifted in form from land to movable wealth. Hence, this kind of dowry system remains in some sense a form of bilateral inheritance, wherein land was transmitted through males, while other forms of wealth were transmitted through females when they married out of the family.

Mildred Dickemann (pers. comm.) has posed the question of why the removal of excess females takes the form of cloistration in Medieval Europe, and outright female infanticide in Rajput India. I cannot answer the question of 'why infanticide' (i.e. as opposed to some other means of removal or suppression) in India, but I would suggest that the practice of cloistration of excess female offspring in preindustrial Europe must be tied to the historical tradition of bilateral inheritance. Under such a system, daughters must have been viewed, at least officially, as equal partners in the family legacy. Further credence is lent to the idea by the fact that families are known, at least in some periods, to have paid 'dowries' to the convents – daughters were 'married' to the Church.

Summary

1. This paper presents an analysis of differential parental investment among four status groups of the 15th and 16th century Portuguese nobility.
2. Among the higher status nobility, male offspring show slightly higher reproductive rates than female offspring. Among the lower nobility, female offspring significantly outreproduce male offspring.
3. There is a corresponding pattern of parental investment biased in favor of males among the high nobility, and investment favoring females among the lower nobility, as indicated by differing rates of nuptiality by sex and by differing rates of cloistrations among women and warfare deaths among men.
4. Parental investment is also biased by birth order, favoring the eldest offspring of both sexes. This results in higher rates of mortality in warfare among younger male siblings and higher rates of cloistration among younger female siblings, as well as lower reproductive rates among younger siblings of both sexes.
5. Patterns of differential parental investment are monitored over a 200-year period between

1380 and 1580, during which time the élite population quickly outnumbers the relatively finite number of estates and titles available within the kingdom of Portugal. The effects of this intensifying competition within the population is that rates of male warfare deaths and female cloistrations increase drastically with time, and reproductive rates within the population as a whole become increasingly depressed. There is also an overall decrease in investment in female offspring relative to male offspring.

Acknowledgements

The research for this paper was funded by the Scientific Personnel Improvement Division of the National Science Foundation (1980–81) and by the Harry Frank Guggenheim Foundation (1983–84). Many thanks to Professors José Mattoso, António H. de Oliveira Marques, and António M. Dias Farinha of the Universidade Nova de Lisboa for their advice during my work in Lisbon in 1980–81. I thank the faculty and staff at the Population Research Center, particularly Dudley L. Poston, Jr, Director, for their support in 1983–84. I thank Laura Betzig, Monique Borgerhoff Mulder, and Paul Turke for their comments during the preparation of this paper. Many thanks to Mildred Dickemann and Sarah Blaffer Hrdy for their comments and encouragement during earlier stages of my research.

References

Alexander, R. D. (1974) The evolution of social behavior. *Annual Review of Ecology and Systematics*, **5**, 324–83.
Alexander, R. D. (1981) Evolution, culture and human behavior: some general considerations. In *Natural Selection and Human Behavior*, ed. R. D. Alexander and D. W. Tinkle, pp. 509–20. New York: Chiron Press.
Bateman, A. J. (1948) Intra-sexual selection in *Drosophila*. *Heredity*, **2**, 349–68.
Boone, J. L. (1983) Noble family structure and expansionist warfare in the late Middle Ages. In *Rethinking Human Adaptation: Biological and Cultural Models*, ed. R. Dyson-Hudson and M. A. Little. Denver: Westview Press.
Boone, J. L. (1986) Parental investment and elite family structure in preindustrial states: a case study of late Medieval – Early Modern Portuguese Genealogies. *American Anthropologist*, **88** (4), 859–78.

Brown, J. L. (1975) *The Evolution of Behavior*. New York: W. W. Norton and Co.

Christian, J. J. (1970) Social subordination, population density, and mammalian evolution. *Science*, **168**, 84–90.

Cooper, J. P. (1976) Patterns of inheritance and settlement by great landowners from the fifteenth to the eighteenth centuries. In *Family and Inheritance: Rural Society in Western Europe 1200–1800*, ed. J. Goody, J. Thirsk, and E. O. Thompson. Cambridge: Cambridge University Press.

Dickemann, M. (1979a) The ecology of mating systems in hypergynous dowry societies. *Social Science Information*, **19** (2), 163–95.

Dickemann, M. (1979b) Female infanticide, reproductive strategies, and social stratification: a preliminary model. In *Evolutionary Biology and Human Social Behavior*, ed. N. A. Chagnon and W. Irons, pp. 312–67. North Scituate, MA.: Duxbury Press.

Duby, G. (1977) '*The Chivalrous Society*. Translated by C. Poston. London: Edward Arnold.

Fox, R. G. (1971) *Kin, Clan, Raja and Rule*. Berkeley: University of California Press.

Gama Barros, H. de (1945–51) *História da Administracão Publica em Portugal nos Séculos XII á XV*, 2nd edition, 11 vols. Lisbon.

Goody, J. (1966) Introduction. In *Succession to High Office*, ed. J. Goody, pp. 1–56. Cambridge: Cambridge University Press.

Goody, J. (1976) *Production and Reproduction*. Cambridge: Cambridge University Press.

Goody, J. (1984) *The Development of the Family and Marriage in Europe*. Cambridge: Cambridge University Press.

Hajnal, J. (1965) European Marriage Patterns in Perspective. In *Population in History*, ed. D. V. Glass and D. E. C. Eversley. London: Edward Arnold.

Hartung, J. (1976) On natural selection and the inheritance of wealth. *Current Anthropology*, **17** (4), 607–22.

Hartung, J. (1982) Polygyny and the inheritance of wealth. *Current Anthropology*, **23**, 1–12.

Henry, L. (1956) Anciennes familles genevoises – Etude démographique: XVIe–XXe siècle. *Travaux et Documente de l'I.N.E.D.*, Cahier No. 26.

Henry, L. (1965) Démographie de la noblesse britannique. *Population*, **20** (4), 692–704.

Herlihy, D. (1973) Three patterns of social mobility in medieval history. *Journal of Interdisciplinary History*, **3**, 622–47.

Herlihy, D. (1977) Family and property in Renaissance Florence. In *The Medieval City*, ed. H. A. Miskimin, D. Herlihy, and A. L. Udovitch. Princeton: Yale University Press.

Hollingsworth, T. H. (1957) A demographic study of the British peerage. *Population Studies*, **XI** (1), 4–26.

Hollingsworth, T. H. (1964) Demography of the British peerage. *Population Studies*, **XVIII** (2).

Hollingsworth, T. H. (1969) *Historical Demography*. Ithaca: Cornell University Press.

Hrdy, S. B. (1987) Sex-biased parental investment among primates and other mammals: a critical evaluation of the Triviers–Willard hypothesis. In *Offspring Abuse and Neglect in Biosocial Perspective*, ed. R. Gelles and J. Lancaster. New York: Aldine (in press).

Johnson, G. A. (1978) Information sources and the development of decision making organizations. In *Social Archeology: Beyond Subsistence and Dating*, ed. C. L. Redman *et al.*, pp. 87–110. New York: Academic Press.

Levy, C. and Henry, L. (1960) Ducs et pairs sous l'ancien régime. *Population*, **15** (5), 807–830.

Livi-Bacci, M. (1983) The nutrition–mortality link in past times: a comment. *Journal of Interdisciplinary History*, **XIV** (2), 293–8.

Lomicki, A. (1982) Population regulation. In *Current Problems in Sociobiology*, ed. King's College Sociobiology Group. Cambridge: Cambridge University Press.

Mattoso, J. (1975) Clero. In *Dicionário de História de Portugal*, vol. I: 590–4, Joel Serrao, ed. Lisbon.

Mattoso, J. (1980) *A Nobreza Medieval Portuguesa: A Família e o Poder*. Imprensa Universitaria, No. 19. Lisbon: Editorial Estampa.

Mattoso, J. (1985) *Identificação de um País: ensaio sobre as origens de Portugal, 1096–1325*, 2 vols. Lisbon: Editorial Estampa.

Morais, C. A. (1942–48) *Peditura Lusitana: Nobiliário de Famílias de Portugal* (11 vols). Porto.

Oliveira Marques, A. H. (1972) *History of Portugal*. New York: Columbia University Press.

Oliveira Marques, A. H. (1975) Nobreza. In *Dicionário de História de Portugal*, vol. IV: 386–7, Joel Serrao, ed. Lisbon.

Peller, S. (1965) Births and deaths among European ruling families since 1500. In *Population and History*. ed. D. V. Glass and D. E. C. Eversley, pp. 87–100. London.

Peronnet, M. (1968) Genealogies et histoire: approaches méthodiques. *Revue Historique*, **92**, 111–22.

Poulain, M. and Tabutin, D. (1981) La Surmortalité du Petites Filles en Belgique au XIXe et Debut de XXe Siècle. *Annales de Démographie Historique*, **1981**, 121–48.

Service, E. R. (1973) *Origins of the State and Civilization: The Process of Cultural Evolution*. New York: W. W. Norton and Company.

Trivers, R. (1972) Parental investment and sexual selection. In *Sexual Selection and the Descent of Man*, 1871–1971, ed. D. Campbell, pp. 136–79. Chicago: Aldine.

Trivers, R. (1974) Parent–offspring conflict. *American Zoologist*, **14**, 249–64.

Trivers, R. and Willard, D. (1973) Natural selection

of parental ability to vary the sex-ratio of offspring. *Science*, **179**, 90–2.

Voland, E. (1984) Human sex ratio manipulation: historical data from a German parish. *Journal of Human Evolution*, **13**, 99–107.

Wall, R. (1981) Inferring differential neglect of females from mortality data. *Annales de Démographie Historique*, **1091**, 19–140.

Wallerstein, I. (1974) *The Modern World System*. New York: Academic Press.

Watkins, S. C. and E. Van der Walle (1983) Nutrition, mortality and population size: Malthus' Court of Last Resort. *Journal of Interdisciplinary History*, **XIV** (2), 205–26.

Susan M. Essock-Vitale[1]
Michael T. McGuire[1,2]

13

What 70 million years hath wrought: sexual histories and reproductive success of a random sample of American women

Introduction

For 70 million years, primate sexuality has been evolving. The products of this evolution are biases to our behavior which help insure that we act, whether consciously or unconsciously, to reproduce ourselves. What are the results in terms of our behavior? What are the most successful reproductive strategies for women living in the United States today? According to evolutionary theory, natural selection favors those who reproductively outcompete their peers and contribute a larger share of their genes to future generations. Behaviors with heritable components which contribute toward this end by improving a female's fecundity or the survival chances of her offspring will find expression. We are a social species: which social situations and strategies will help and which will hinder the probability of having one's genes represented in future generations?

It was our interest in exploring some of the issues raised by these questions that prompted

[1] Department of Psychiatry, School of Medicine, University of California at Los Angeles, Los Angeles, CA 90024, USA
[2] Psychiatry Service, Sepulveda Veterans Administration Medical Centre, Sepuveda, CA 91343, USA

(Note: Much of the information in this chapter originally appeared in *Ethology and Sociobiology*, **6**, 137–73 (1985).)

us to conduct a study of a targeted sample of American women. Specifically, we were interested in discovering differences in the lives of these women which might be important in determining high and low reproductive success and in determining whether there were identifiable behavioral styles which were likely to be predictive of this success.

A major line of evolutionary theory predicts that it will be the predisposition of each member of a species to act to maximize reproductive success (Williams 1966). For women, as for all female primates, this predisposition will have a social as well as a biological connotation. In order to breed and rear children successfully, a woman must not only be physically fit – capable both of conceiving and growing an infant *in utero* – but must successfully meet the challenges posed by her social environment before, during, and after her pregnancy. Though these challenges may vary from culture to culture, there exist certain basic hurdles in any competition for genetic perpetuation: a female must compete for resources for herself and her offspring; she must protect her progeny from harm; and she must compete with other females for males – for use first as inseminators, and second as potential providers of help to, and resources for, herself and her children. As regards the latter, because American society is organized around an elaborate division of labor by sex and a strong reliance upon resource exchange, there exists a particularly large payoff for retaining a male as a provider of resources for, and care-giver to, mutually conceived offspring. All of these challenges must be met within the social environment. Thus it is clear that an individual's social situation will influence how her biology expresses itself. A woman with high physiologic ability may be able to conceive children with ease but if she does not have an equally high 'social' ability which allows her to maintain the social support network of relationships and resources that facilitates raising them, it is likely that her reproductive success will be diminished.

Because human sociability appears to have evolved components which express themselves differentially in particular environments (see, for example, Daly and Wilson 1983), for any given environment behavioral styles will emerge which confer a biological advantage in relation to other behavioral styles. In meeting the basic challenges

outlined above, some women are obviously more successful than others. Are there identifiable behaviors which can be said to affect differential reproductive outcome?

Given that predispositions to behave in ways which maximize reproductive success are evolved components of human behavior, it would be expected that the following exist:

1. In the competition for males, the ability to bond with and retain a male for support after copulation will influence reproductive success. In this regard, marriage, as a proxy for this ability, should be positively associated with fecundity, while being never-married should be negatively associated.

2. Because a male who is confident of his paternity would be more likely to contribute to the support of children born to his sexual partner, promiscuity, as a behavior which could decrease that confidence, should be associated with decreased reproductive success in societies which promote serial monogamy.

3. Degree of wealth, as a proxy for access to resources, will influence fecundity. Specifically, greater wealth should be associated with higher fecundity.

4. Neurosis, as a condition which is linked to a diminished ability to conduct social relationships should be related to reduced fecundity.

In evolutionary terms, then, important questions for reproductive success are what factors influence the likelihood of a woman's marrying? Of staying married? How will her reproductive success be affected by her marital status? Are differences in reproductive potential predictive of the variations in ability to maintain the support of a male partner? How will her sexual behavior (number of partners, etc.) influence her marital status? Her reproductive success? How do such socioeconomic factors as wealth, religion, and employment influence marital status and fecundity? Is a woman's mental health related to her ability to marry and have children?

The following pages attempt to elucidate these questions. While extensive data were collected on numerous aspects of the women's lives, only data relevant to sexual behavior, and to exploring which aspects of the subjects' lives contribute to enhancing and diminishing reproductive success, are presented here in detail (for fuller discussions see Essock-Vitale and McGuire 1985a, 1985b).

There are two results sections. The first, which describes sample characteristics, organizes data in three parts: (1) demographic characteristics; (2) sex and reproduction; and (3) a comparison of the survey data with sexual data from Kinsey and his colleagues. The second section interprets the data and evaluates whether the sexual and reproductive patterns typifing a subgroup of American women are consistent with predictions derived from evolutionary theory.

Though evolutionary biology supplied the theoretical framework for this research, genetic differences between subjects with high and low reproductive success are not being posited. Rather, it is being suggested, because it is the genetic predisposition of each species member to act to maximize reproductive success, that there might be differences in the demographic and environmental characteristics of these women which might work against this predisposition. It must also be said that we are not attempting to assign causality when discussing factors predictive of diminished reproductive success. Because of the retrospective nature of this study, we are concerned only with pinpointing relationships between variables. Finally, when speaking of reproductive success, 'success' is being used only with the biological connotation. A woman who does not marry or have children is certainly not presumed to be 'unsuccessful' by any other measure.

Methods

The study was designed to meet several methodological criteria.

1. A group of 300 participants from the greater Los Angeles area was selected as optimal (Figure 13.1). This was large enough to permit considerable statistical manipulation, and small enough to be affordable and permit face-to-face interviewing.
2. Data were needed from as near a random sample as possible so that incidence figures would be representative of the larger population. To achieve this, subjects were contacted by telephone using a modified random-digit dialing procedure.
3. To avoid having to control for age, sex, race,

ethnicity, and socioeconomic status, a culturally homogenous group was selected which was readily accessible: white (which herein is used to mean Caucasians not of Hispanic origin), middle-class women living in greater Los Angeles. 'Middle class' was intentionally defined broadly. The goal was to obtain subjects who were in the broad middle socioeconomic range. The criterion that the subject be 'middle class' could be met in any of several ways, because occupation alone would be a poor guide for women. A subject could qualify as middle class on the basis of her occupation, her husband's occupation, her education, or her family's income (with cutoffs adjusted according to size of family). When qualifying as a potential subject on the basis of the family's income, we used US Census data to exclude individuals from families with incomes in the lower 25% or the upper 10% of white families of the potential subject's size of family. (For details on selection procedure for determining whether subjects met these criteria, see Essock-Vitale and McGuire 1985a).

4. An age range for subjects of 35–45 years old was selected because women in this age range were likely to have had at least one child if they were going to have children, yet were young enough so that it was likely that at least some of their children would still be at home.

Figure 13.1 Study site: Los Angeles, California, USA

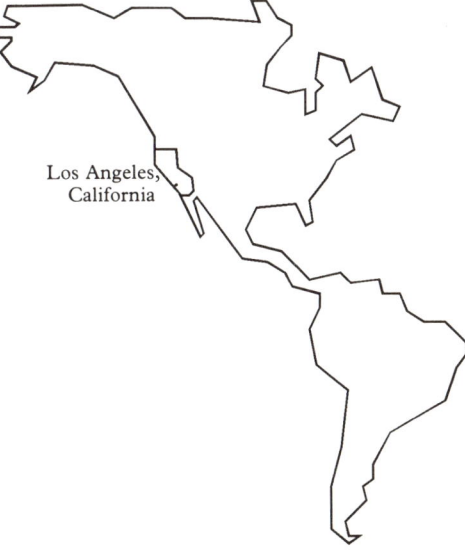

Los Angeles, California

5. Finally, the sample was limited to women born in the United States and raised by at least one of their natural parents.

Telephone interviewers averaged 4.7 hours of dialing (mean number of calls per subject = 166) to locate a subject who met the selection criteria and agreed to participate. Once a qualified subject was located, it was likely that she would agree to participate, i.e. 66% agreed. This high acceptance rate is credited to the women's interest in the topic of social relationships.

After the 300 participants were located, each was interviewed face-to-face by an interviewer who was blind to the purpose of the study. The interviewer used a standardized questionnaire which consisted entirely of questions which elicited brief, easily coded answers. Pretesting and later modifications prior to the start of the study ensured that the questions were easily understood and that administration would typically take about 5 hours, including rest periods. (For topic areas of the questionnaire and the types of data collected, see Essock-Vitale and McGuire 1985a.)

Two methods were used to assess the reliability of the information collected. The first involved requestioning subjects over the telephone, and the second involved questioning a sample of the subjects' full sibs (Essock-Vitale and McGuire 1985a).

Results: sample characteristics

Demographic characteristics

Age
The subjects' mean age was 39.6 years (SD = 3.6, median = 39).

Education
Six percent of the subjects had less than a high school diploma. Twenty-one percent were high school graduates with no further schooling. Two-thirds of the subjects had attended college or university for at least one year, and one-third were graduates (Table 13.1).

Marital status
Nearly three-quarters of the subjects were currently married, which for the study was defined as living with a legally married husband. Nearly

Table 13.1 *Subjects' level of education*

	Fre-quency	Per-cent	Cumulative percentage
Less than high school graduate	18	6.0	6.0
High school graduate	62	20.7	26.7
Technical or trade school	12	6.3	33.0
1 or 2 yrs of college	79	26.3	59.3
3 or 4 yrs of college	21	7.0	66.3
College degree	50	16.7	83.0
1 or 2 yrs post-college	24	8.0	91.0
Masters degree	23	7.6	98.6
3 or 4 yrs post-college	2	0.7	99.3
Law degree	2	0.7	100.0

Table 13.2 *Subjects' marital status*
(a) Current marital status

Status	Frequency	Percent
Never-married	17	5.7
Married	216	72.0
Separated	12	4.0
Divorced	53	17.7
Widowed	2	0.7
Total	300	100.0[a]

(b) Number of marriages

Number	Frequency	Percent
0	17	5.7
1	211	70.3
2	61	20.3
3	10	3.3
4	1	0.3
Total	300	100.0[a]

[a] Rounded to the nearest whole number

6% had never been married (Table 13.2(a)). Twenty-four percent had been married more than once (Table 13.2(b)). US Census figures are available to compare the rates of never-married and currently-married white American women of this age to the subjects (US Bureau of the Census 1982). These figures show that in 1981 approximately 5.5% of white women aged 35–44 years had never married, while 75% of white women of this age were currently married and not separated from their husbands.

Income
The subjects' income ranged from less than $10 000 per year to over $79 000 per year (Table

Table 13.3 *Family's income during the year prior to the interview*

(a) Family's income for all subjects

Income ($)	Frequency	Percent	Cumulative percent
<10 000	6	2.1	2.1
10–19 000	38	13.4	15.5
20–29 000	68	23.9	39.4
30–39 000	67	23.6	63.0
40–49 000	45	15.8	78.9
50–59 000	28	9.9	88.7
60–69 000	9	3.2	91.9
70–79 000	12	4.2	96.1
79 000	11	3.9	100.0
Total[a]	284	100.0	100.0

(b) Family's income by marital status (highest to lowest); a horizontal line separates groups which differed significantly

Marital status[b]	Frequency	Mean family income ($)
Married	203	43 127
Separated	12	35 783
Divorced	52	21 333
Never-married	15	21 167

(c) Family's income by employment status of subject; a horizontal line separates groups which differed significantly

Employment status	Frequency	Family income ($)
Not employed	74	42 432
Employed (part or full-time)	210	35 880

[a] 16 subjects declined to state their income
[b] Widowed subjects were excluded from this analysis because of the small sample size ($n = 2$)

Table 13.4 *Employment*

	Frequency	Percent
High-level professional (e.g. doctor, college professor, lawyer, engineer, business executive)	3	1.0
Other professional and technical (e.g. teacher, nurse, lab. technician)	50	16.7
Self-employed	10	3.3
Managerial and administrative	26	8.7
Sales	15	5.0
Clerical or secretarial	62	20.7
Skilled labor (electrician, plumber)	2	0.7
Labor (assembly line)	3	1.0
Service (cook, hairdresser, waitress)	5	1.7
Artistic (performance)	1	0.3
Subtotal (Full-time employment outside of home)	177	59.0
Homemaker, employed part-time	41	13.7
Homemaker, not employed	69	23.0
Full-time student	13	4.3
Total	300	100.0

Table 13.5 *Subjects' religion*

	Raised as		Currently	
	Frequency	Percent	Frequency	Percent
Protestant	177	59.0	133	44.3
Catholic	73	24.3	53	17.7
Jewish	30	10.0	29	9.7
Other	8	2.7	10	3.3
None	12	4.0	75	25.0
Total	300	100.0	300	100.0

13.3(a)). The mean family income was $37 588 (SD = $25 919, median = $34 000). Recall that subjects could be classified as 'middle class' on the basis of occupation, education, husband's occupation, or family income. Hence a wider income range was possible than if income alone had been the sole selection criterion. The subjects' family income varied with marital status (Table 13.3(b), $f_{3275} = 13.5$, $p < 0.01$) and employment status (Table 13.3(c), $f_{1275} = 3.9$, $p < 0.05$). The subjects' perception of their rela-tive wealth correlated significantly with their family income ($r_s = 0.51$, $n = 284$, $p < 0.01$).

Employment
Nearly 60% of the subjects were employed full-time outside their homes. Their job classifications are given in Table 13.4. An additional 14% were employed part-time. Twenty-three percent of the subjects were not employed outside the home.

Religion
Table 13.5 gives the religious classification of the subjects, both for how they were raised and for their current religious preference, if any. The subjects differed widely in the average number

Table 13.6 *Mean number of living close kin*

Relationship	All subjects $n = 300$	Ever married subjects $n = 283$	Never married subjects $n = 17$
Mother	0.85	0.86	0.82
Father	0.58	0.58	0.53
Full-sibs	1.74	1.75	1.59
Half-sibs	0.28	0.28	0.17
Grandmothers	0.19	0.19	0.06
Grandfathers	0.05	0.06	0.00
Children	2.13	2.25	0.18
Aunts	2.43	2.45	2.06
Uncles	2.01	2.00	2.12
Nieces and nephews	3.76	3.86	2.12
Grandchildren	0.08	0.09	0.00
Total	14.10	14.37	9.65

Table 13.7 *Type of counselors consulted by subjects*

Counselor's occupation	No. of subjects using	Percent[a]
Psychologist	94	31.3
Clergy	76	25.3
Psychiatrist	64	21.3
Family doctor	55	18.3
Social worker	22	7.3
School counselor	12	4.0

[a] Percentages do not add to 100% because subjects may have consulted none or several different types of counselors

of hours per month they spent attending religious services or engaging in activities sponsored by religious organizations: mean = 5.4 hours, SD = 9.4, median = 1, mode ($n = 134$) = 0.

Living kin

The subjects averaged 14.1 close kin (Table 13.6), where 'close' equals a coefficient of relatedness $r \frac{1}{4}$ (i.e. grandparents, parents, aunts and uncles, sibs, half-sibs, children, nieces and nephews, grandchildren).

Counseling history

A total of 211 of the subjects (70.3%) reported seeking professional help for psychiatric counseling at some point during their life. Table 13.7 shows the frequency with which various types of counselor were used. Subjects who received counseling received it for a mean of 2.6 years (SD = 4.4, range = 1 day – 32 years). Fifteen of the subjects (5%) were psychiatric inpatients at least once. For comparative purposes each

subject was assigned a mental health severity score based upon the extent of the use of professional psychological counseling, sleeping medications, and medications for 'nerves' during her life. The scores ranged from 1 (no counseling, no medications) to 7 (at least one episode of inpatient psychiatric treatment). The average severity score was 2.9. Low perceived self importance, more sexual partners, dissatisfaction with recreational activities, and less wealth were each variables significantly correlated with poorer mental health. Seven variables, when taken together, accounted for 21% of the variance of severity: ever-divorced, most help to subject from friend rather than kin, chronic health problem, number of sexual partners, number of major life events in past year, ever raped or molested (all positively associated with severity), and perceived self importance (negatively associated with severity) (Essock-Vitale and McGuire, unpublished data).

Sex and reproduction

Aspects of the subjects' sexual and reproductive histories are summarized in Tables 13.8 and 13.9. Whereas the mean age at first intercourse was 19.6 years and most subjects fell near the mean (SD = 3.1), the number of sexual partners reported varied widely. The modal score, representing 34.6% of the subjects, was 1 sexual partner, the median was 3 sexual partners, and the mean was 8.8 (SD = 23.9). Contributing to this strong positive skew were the 10% of the subjects who reported 20 or more sexual partners. Four subjects reported over 100 sexual partners. The number reporting at least one extramarital affair (which was defined as a sexual relationship with a man other than one's husband while legally married) was 23% (Table 13.8). This figure is twice that cited by Johnson (1970) as an estimate for American women, but does not differ significantly from the incidence reported by Kinsey and his colleagues (Gebhard and Johnson, 1979). For white women, the Kinsey data indicate a 17% incidence of extramarital affairs (first marriages only) for women with no college education and 21% incidence for those with at least some college. For the women of this study, the incidence of extramarital affairs also was higher among women with at least some college education (27.2%) than among women with no college education (16.2%) ($\chi^2 = 4.37$,

Table 13.8 *Sexual and reproductive history*

	n	Mean	SD	Median
Age at first intercourse	295	19.6	3.1	19
Number of sexual partners	296	8.8	23.9	3
Number of pregnancies	300	2.8	1.7	3
Number of children born	300	2.2	1.3	2
Number of living children	300	2.1	1.3	2
Number of children considered ideal	298	2.8	1.7	2

268 of 300 subjects (89%) have ever been pregnant
68 of 300 subjects (23%) have ever miscarried
35 of 300 subjects (12%) reported at least one voluntary abortion
66 of 283 ever-married subjects (23%) reported at least one extramarital affair
11 of 298 (4%) subjects at least one homosexual affair
2 of 299 subjects (1%) reported no heterosexual intercourse
166 of 282 ever-married subjects (59%) reported intercourse while not married
67 of 299 subjects (22%) reported being raped or molested
12 of 298 (4%) subjects said that it was likely or very likely that they would have a or another child, an additional 18 (6%) said it was possible, 20 (7%) said it was unlikely, and the remaining 248 (83%) said it was very unlikely
255 of 300 subjects (85%) reported at least one live birth
32 of 300 subjects (11%) reported at least one pregnancy while unmarried
11 of 254 subjects (4%) reported some doubt that the husband at the time they became pregnant was the father of the child

Table 13.9 *Pregnancies and voluntary abortions*
(a) Number of pregnancies per subject

No. of pregnancies	Frequency	Percent	Cumulative percentage
0	22	7.3	7.3
1	31	10.3	17.6
2	96	32.0	49.6
3	72	24.0	73.6
4	41	13.7	87.3
5	20	6.7	94.0
6	9	3.0	97.0
7	5	1.7	98.7
8	1	0.3	99.0
9	2	0.7	99.7
12	1	0.3	100.0
Total	300	100.0	100.0

(b) Number of voluntary abortions per subject

No. of abortions	Frequency	Percent	Cumulative percentage
0	265	88.3	88.3
1	23	7.7	96.0
2	8	2.7	98.7
3	3	1.0	99.7
4	1	0.3	100.0
Total	300	100.0	100.0

df = 1, $p < 0.05$; all marriages included in this analysis). The incidence of extramarital affairs for women married only once was 20.1% for women with some college education and 11.4% for women without any college education. Four percent of the subjects reported having had at least one homosexual relationship.

When comparing data from this study to reported norms, recall that such 'norms' have often not been derived from random samples. Certainly the Kinsey sample was non-random. Hence, we would caution that, because the reporting bias for sensitive questions is generally assumed to be one of under-reporting, it may be that the subjects of this study were unusually open in answering this question. Questions on sex and reproduction came at the end of a long interview during which topics of great emotional import (e.g. life crises, refusals of help, marriage breakups) were discussed. By this point the rapport between subject and interviewer was well established and may have been such that under-reporting was minimal. In many other repects the sexual and reproductive histories of the subjects were what would be expected on the basis of US population reports (e.g. Gebhard *et al.* 1958; US Bureau of the Census 1978, 1982), suggesting that it is unlikely that we were investigating an atypical sample. For example, 28 (9.9%) out of 283 ever-married subjects were childless, close to the roughly 8% reported by the US Census in 1979 (see Figure 12.6 in Daly and Wilson 1983, for a graph of the decline in childlessness of American women).

The average age at the first pregnancy was 22.7 years (n = 267, SD = 4.3, median = 22 years). Subjects averaged 2.8 pregnancies. The outcomes of pregnancy were classified as live births (77% of all pregnancies), still births (1%), voluntary abortions (7%), and miscarriages (15%).

With regard to the possibility of additional children, 83.2% of the subjects said that it was 'very unlikely' that they would give birth in the future, with an additional 6.7% saying an additional birth was 'unlikely.' Ever-married and

Table 13.10 *Sexual assaults: Breakdown of 67 subjects who reported being raped or molested, by age of assault and relationship to perpetrator*

	Assaulted by blood relative	Assaulted by other than blood relative	Total
Assaulted as a child (aged 17 years or under)	16	36	52
Assaulted as an adult	0	24	24
Total	16	60	76[a]

[a] Nine subjects reported being assaulted both as children and as adults

never-married individuals did not differ with respect to their perceived likelihood of having additional children ($t = 0.53$, df $= 296$, $p = 0.60$). Hence, the reproductive careers of these women were largely complete. The subjects were also unlikely to be mothers of pre-school children. Among subjects with children, the mean age of the youngest child was 11.8 (SD $= 5.5$, $n = 258$) and of the oldest child was 15.9 (SD $= 5.5$, $n = 258$).

Nearly one-quarter of the subjects answered yes to the question, 'Have you ever been raped or molested?' Table 13.10 shows these instances of sexual assault broken down by age of subject and relationship to perpetrator. For these subjects, most of the assaults occurred when they were under 17 years of age. Of the childhood sexual assaults, 30.1% were by kin. In contrast, none of the adult assaults was. Subjects who reported being raped or molested were equally likely to marry and to have as many children as those who reported no sexual assaults ($\chi^2 = 1.74$, df $= 1$, $p = 0.19$; $t = 0.83$, df $= 298$, $p = 0.41$). They reported more sexual partners than did those who reported no sexual assaults (mean 14.2 versus 7.2, $t = 2.13$, df $= 296$, $p < 0.05$).

Further comparisons to the Kinsey data

The importance of the data provided by Kinsey and his colleagues continues. Table 13.11 contrasts data from the subjects of this study to the subjects of Kinsey and his colleagues (hereafter called Kinsey subjects) using data from the Institute for Sex Research compiled by colleagues of Kinsey after his death (Gebbhard *et al.* 1958, Gebbhard and Johnston 1979). Because the data

on Kinsey subjects typically was divided into subjects with and without college education, Table 13.11 follows that format when necessary. In brief, compared to the subjects of this study, (1) the Kinsey subjects were much more likely to terminate a pregnancy with a voluntary abortion (recall that birth control pills and other recent, more reliable contraceptives were not available to Kinsey subjects), (2) the Kinsey subjects were older at their first marriage (many of the Kinsey subjects likely delayed marriage until the end of World War II), (3) the Kinsey subjects were equally as likely to report an extramarital affair, (4) the Kinsey subjects were older at the time of first sexual intercourse, (5) the Kinsey subjects were more likely to report a homosexual experience, (6) the Kinsey subjects' ideal number of children was larger. The differences between the Kinsey distributions and those found in this study doubtlessly stem from cultural differences as well as sampling differences, hence any conclusions regarding changes in the relative incidence of the behaviors under study must be guarded.

Results: reproductive success

Data from non-human primates as well as from preindustrial human societies indicate a large variance in the reproductive success of females (see, for instance, Hrdy 1981). The paragraphs below present an analysis of data collected from females living in a modern metropolis. The results, which examine the relationships between different variables and reproductive success, also show great variety.

Marital status and fecundity

A prime factor predicting reproductive success is a subject's marital status. Though many factors – for example, poverty or a demanding career – might influence a woman's ability to bear and invest time in rearing children, in American society, because of its strong reliance upon resource exchange, retaining male support after insemination has a particularly large impact. Not only do social sanctions function negatively upon children born out of wedlock and upon the mothers who bear them, an unmarried or

Table 13.11 *Comparisons to data of Kinsey and his colleagues at the Institute for Sex Research. (Sample sizes are given for this study only, because Kinsey sample sizes can only be approximated (see Gebbhard and Johnson 1979). Statistics reported are for χ^2 goodness-of-fit tests using the Kinsey values as the expected distribution.* $\star = p < 0.01$, ns $= p > 0.05$ *(no p values fell between 0.01 and 0.05)*

Topic	This study (n)	Kinsey
Probability of an abortion given a pregnancy[a]		
unmarried women★	0.64 (26)	0.82
married women★	0.03 (758)	0.19

Topic	This study (n)		Kinsey	
	Some college	No college	Some college	No college
Age at first marriage★	(184)	(99)		
less than 21 years	41%	68%	22%	35%
21–25 years	49%	25%	52%	44%
26+ years	10%	7%	26%	21%
Extramarital sex during 1st marriage (ns)	21% (141)	11% (70)	21%	17%
Under 20 years old at first intercourse★	45% (197)	69% (68)	31%	41%
Homosexual experience★	4.5% (200)	2.0% (98)	14.8%	10.9%
Number of children desired★	(200)	(98)		
0	6%	8%	8%	10%
1–2	52%	36%	12%	17%
3	20%	23%	26%	20%
4+	22%	33%	54%	53%

[a] Pregnancies are the unit of observation. Elsewhere in the table subjects are the unit of observation

divorced woman who fails to keep the father working as a provider of resources for, and caregiver to, mutually conceived offspring is likely to be at a disadvantage in terms of her ability to raise both present and future children.

According to evolutionary theory, what behaviors can women utilize to increase the likelihood that the fathers of mutual children remain to help with their rearing? While the answer to that question is both controversial and complex, with explanations ranging from continuous female receptivity to concealed ovulation (for a general discussion see Konner 1982) one conclusion seems fairly certain: the more secure a male is in his paternity, the more likely he is to contribute to the care and support of offspring belonging to a woman with whom he has mated (see Dickemann 1981, Hrdy 1981, Hartung 1985). In American society the institution of marriage, with its premise of sexual fidelity works toward this end. Hence, women who marry and who remain married may be acting to maximize their reproductive potential. Likewise, women who, for example, are promiscuous, might be working

to diminish reproductive potential because a man who has been, or believes himself to have been, cuckolded is more likely to desert a woman and her children than one who is more confident of his genetic investment (see Daly and Wilson 1985). In evolutionary terms, then, important issues for reproductive success are who marries vs. who does not; of the women who marry, who is likely to remain married; and, among married women, who is likely to have and rear children.

What factors will influence a woman's likelihood of marrying and staying married? How, in turn, will her fecundity be affected by her marital status?

Factors influencing marriage

In attempting to determine if differences in background might predict the likelihood of a subject's ever marrying, the variables age at first intercourse, number of sexual partners, ever had a homosexual relationship, ever raped or molested, raped or molested as a child, physically punished as a child, severely physically punished as a child, education, and number of childhood friends were entered into a stepwise logistic regression equation. The results indicated that being younger at first intercourse and never having had a homosexual relationship were significantly associated with ever marrying. Together, however, these two variables accounted for only 0.07% of the variance.

When discussing tactics of fitness-promoting strategies, Daly and Wilson (1983) suggest that the ideal bride has many sibs; that is, that a man's fitness-promoting strategy would be to marry into families where his children will have many aunts and uncles looking for ways to maximize their inclusive fitness. In this study, ever and never-married subjects did not differ in their number of sibs (means of 1.7 and 1.6, respectively), but never-married subjects had significantly fewer close kin than did ever-married subjects (means 9.7 and 14.4, respectively; $t(298) = 2.5$, $p < 0.05$). This effect is still suggested although no longer statistically significant when children and grandchildren are excluded from the close kin totals (means 9.5 and 12.0, respectively). Hence, the data presented here suggest that individuals who marry may come from more fecund families than those who do not marry. Analysis also shows that subjects with fewer kin produced fewer children.

As predicted, the presence of chronic incapacitating neurosis is correlated with decreased probability of marriage and few children. Women with poorer mental health, as measured by their high mental health severity scores, were significantly less likely to marry and have children. While not attributing cause, the findings do suggest that poor mental health goes hand-in-hand with atypical social relationships and diminished reproductive success. It is left to future studies to determine if the subject was depressed and therefore at a disadvantage in competing for a mate and increasing the likelihood of having children, if she failed to marry and have children and became depressed, or if her depression and failure in these regards were the product of some third variable (see Henderson 1981 for elaboration of possibilities).

Factors influencing divorce

Women who reported having extramarital affairs (sex with men other than their husbands while they were married) were married and divorced significantly more often than those who did not

$(1.5$ versus 1.2 spouses, $t(281) = 3.0$, $p < 0.01$; 0.8 versus 0.4 divorces, $t(281) = 4.9$, $p < 0.01$). The data do not imply that extramarital sex causes divorce, but suggest a relationship between the two variables. It is possible that the same women who prefer a number of sexual partners before they marry do not have their preferences for multiple sexual partners altered by marriage. In this case, they might be likely to continue to seek additional partners, both for marriage and extramarital sex. Another factor influencing the relationship between extramarital sex and divorce might be that separated (yet still legally married) women have sexual relationships with men other than their husbands and then go on to divorce.

Women with poorer mental health were also significantly less likely to remain married as were women who did not bear children. For first marriages, the probability of divorce given that no children had been born was 76.5%, whereas the probability of divorce given that at least one child had been produced was significantly less, 30.1% $(\chi^2 = 26.8, df = 1, p < 0.01)$.

Fecundity as a function of marital status

As one might expect, having a spouse was the most potent predictor of having other than zero children. Moreover, as indicated, for the subjects of this study, a marriage was significantly more likely to end in divorce if no children had been produced.

Marital status also is highly predictive of the probability of voluntary abortions. Reproduction occurs at a significant physical cost. It is likely to have negative social consequences influencing future reproductive success if a woman's ability to provide for the growing child or for her other children is compromised. Pregnancies which occur when support from a mate is unlikely thus should be more likely to end in abortion compared with those occurring when support from a mate is likely. Such support would be unlikely if an on-going marriage or other cohabitation were absent or if the spouse had reason to doubt paternity (for discussions see Alexander 1974, Dickemann 1981, Daly and Wilson 1982).

For subjects of this study, pregnancies were significantly more likely to end in a voluntary abortion if the woman was unmarried or, if married, was not certain that the husband was the father of the child. Considering all pregnancies, the probability of a voluntary abortion given a pregnancy was only 0.07. However, if the subject was not married at the time of the pregnancy, or if the subject was not certain that her husband was the father, the probabilities of abortion rose to 0.64 and 0.57, respectively ($\chi^2 = 257$ and 116, respectively, df $= 1$, $p < 0.01$), suggesting that the subjects acted to maximize their partners' confidence of paternity or that they preferred not to rear a child without the presence of a male partner.

The occurrence of a voluntary abortion could be predicted very accurately when two other variables – age at the pregnancy, and the frequency of birth control usage at the time of the pregnancy (i.e. never, sometimes, most of the time, always) – were entered with the subject's marital status into a stepwise logistic regression (Dixon and Jennrich 1981). Each of the three variables significantly improved the accuracy of predicting the probability of an abortion. Together, they correctly predicted 79% of the abortions and 87% of the non-abortions when the prior probability of an abortion (58 abortions/834 total pregnancies $= 0.07$) was known. The probability of an abortion was positively associated with being unmarried, being older, and practicing birth control at the time of the pregnancy.

Sexual activity and reproductive success

The age at first intercourse and number of sexual partners may be influenced by social strategies which ensure increased reproductive success for females and increased confidence of paternity for males. One's optimal strategy may depend on one's social environment. For example, Dickemann (1981) has reviewed environmental situations which would favor or discourage virginity and fidelity. (She describes, for instance, the increase in the degree of cloistering of women as socioeconomic status increases. Crudely put, this means it pays a woman's family members (both male and female) to guarantee the confidence of paternity of a woman's husband. The more valuable the prospective husband, the greater confidence he can demand, and the greater the cloistering efforts.) Data from the subjects of this study generally support the proposition that both homosexuality and promiscuity on the part of American, middle-class females diminishes reproductive success. Women who reported having had at least one homosexual relationship had fewer children (1.2 versus 2.2) and were less likely to ever have been married. Both the number of sexual partners and the age at first intercourse – proxies for promiscuity – were negatively correlated with number of children ($r = -0.19$, -0.23, respectively, $p < 0.01$). Age at first intercourse and number of sexual partners were themselves negatively correlated ($r = -0.17$, $p < 0.01$), i.e. women who were younger at first intercourse typically reported more sexual partners. Subjects reporting sex with men other than their husbands while they were married (who were 23% of the ever-married subjects) were significantly younger at first intercourse (17.7 versus 20.0 years, $t(279) = 5.6$, $p < 0.01$) and reported significantly more sexual partners (24.5 versus 3.9, $t(280) = 6.5$, $p < 0.01$) than did ever-married women who reported no extramarital affairs, but women who did and did not report extramarital affairs did not differ in the number of children they had (means 2.2 versus 2.3, respectively). However, because, as already stated, women who reported affairs were married and divorced significantly more often than those who did not, they were less likely to maintain the support of a spouse for their children, and thus their children, because of less provisioning, may be placed at a reproductive disadvantage.

Further analysis was done to determine which variables might predict number of sexual partners. As noted in the results section, the number of sexual partners reported by the subjects varied widely (Table 13.8). A stepwise regression was used to determine whether the number of sexual partners could be predicted by some combination of the following variables typically thought to vary with fecundity (for reviews see Kinsey et al. 1953, Symons 1979, Daly and Wilson 1983): subject's age at first intercourse, number of live births, number of children desired, rating of family's financial situation at age 13, rating of family's financial situation during young adulthood (age 18–21), rating of current financial situation, current household income, age, education level, current religion, and childhood religion. (The variable age was entered as a precaution to control for possible confoundings; the procedures used to select subjects limited the dispersion of these variables to a 10-year span, hence, the impact of age is not assessed by this analysis). The following variables made significant contributions to the predictive power of the regression equation, listed in the order in which they were entered (and each was negatively correlated with the number of sexual partners): number of live births, age at first intercourse, currently Protestant, rating of current financial situation, currently Catholic, and financial situation during young adulthood. While each of these variables significantly contributed to an increase in predictability ($f2.7$), the combined R^2 was only 0.15. This suggests that these variables, even in combination, are not very useful in estimating an individual's number of sexual partners, a point that previous reports (e.g. the Kinsey data) often failed to address.

Having been raped or molested as a child and/or as an adult was not significantly predictive of marriage or reproductive success. However, these variables were significant in predicting a high mental health severity score which itself was correlated with a reduced likelihood of marrying and having children.

Other socioeconomic factors and fecundity

Employment
In this study, subjects who were *not* employed outside the home, or who were married, usually had younger children than did those who were employed or who were not currently married (two-way ANOVA, factors Employ, $f_{2,254} = 8.76$, $p < 0.01$, and Married, $f_{1,254} = 5.88$, $p < 0.05$; Duncan's multiple range *post hoc* tests, alpha = 0.05). Contrary to what one might expect, married women who worked had as many children as married women who did not work. An investigation of fecundity by type of employment would be of interest because women in demanding professions might have less time to devote to child rearing.

Religion
We examined whether the number of live births per subject varied either with the religion in which subjects were raised or with their current religion. The number of births did not differ by childhood religion, but the effect of current religion approached significance (ANOVA, $f_{3,289} = 2.26$, $p < 0.08$), with Duncan's multiple range

post hoc tests indicating that Catholics had significantly more children (mean = 2.36) than did individuals with no religious preference (mean = 1.83). Protestants and Jews fell midway between these extremes and did not differ significantly from either (means of 2.21 and 2.17, respectively).

Desired children
The subjects' mean of 2.2 children is significantly less than the mean of their desired number, 2.8 children (correlated t-test, $t(297) = 6.21$, $p < 0.0001$). This difference between desired vs. actual number of children was present for never-married as well as ever-married subjects, although the magnitude of the difference was significantly greater for never-married (mean = 1.7) than for ever-married subjects (mean = 0.6) ($t(296) = 2.50$, $p < 0.05$). Despite this difference, most women had exactly the number of children they desired (the median and modal number of additional children desired were both zero; $n = 298$). These data suggest that women exercise great control over the size of their families, thereby achieving what they perceived to be an optimal number of offspring for themselves.

Wealth
Fertility patterns are commonly associated with socioeconomic factors such as education, religion, and wealth (for reviews see Kinsey *et al.* 1953, Symons 1979, Daly and Wilson 1983). For example, Essock-Vitale (1984) noted that, among wealthy women, women who had inherited their wealth had more children than those who had worked for their wealth. Along similar lines, it has been demonstrated among both human and non-human primates that being of high rank will give one a privileged access to resources which will in turn have a positive effect upon reproductive success (Irons 1979, Hrdy 1981, Fairbanks and McGuire 1984, Turke and Betzig 1985, Betzig 1986, Borgerhoff Mulder 1987, Silk 1987). While the subjects of this study were all classified as middle-class, within this broad category sexual behavior did appear to vary with wealth. Age at first intercourse was significantly positively correlated with current income ($r = 0.13$, $p < 0.02$) and with the subject's ranking of their wealth (on a poor-to-rich

scale) throughout their lives. The number of sexual partners reported was significantly negatively correlated with current or past wealth. Apparently, as noted by Dickemann (1981) and others before her, wealth is inversely associated with promiscuity.

Education

The incidence of extramarital affairs was higher among women with some college education (27.2%) than among women with no college education (16.2%). Greater education was also associated with fewer children and with a decreased likelihood of ever being married. Recall that greater wealth, according to our data and the studies by Dickemann, is predictive of decreased promiscuity. What remains to be assessed is the interaction between wealth and education (consider, for example, the effect of wealth within education categories).

Counseling history

In addition to being predictive of an increased likelihood of divorce and a decreased likelihood of marriage, the presence of poor mental health was also associated with decreased reproductive success. Women with high severity scores on the mental health scale had fewer children, and fewer women with high scores ever had children. This difference was not for lack of sexual partners, nor for inability to become pregnant. The high severity score women had more sexual partners and became pregnant as often as their low score counterparts. Hence, poor mental health suggests not a difficulty in attracting males or conceiving, but difficulty in selecting and keeping appropriate mates. A separate study of chronically depressed women found an increased incidence of abortion, thus indicating a disinclination to bear and/or raise conceived children (Essock-Vitale and McGuire, unpublished data).

Discussion

The data presented here validate the predictive power of evolutionary theory in examining reproductive success. The four hypotheses outlined in the introduction were supported by the analyses: marriage was positively associated with fecundity; paternal confidence was demonstrated to be influential in reproductive success

(promiscuity was associated with decreased reproductive success and paternal uncertainty was predictive of voluntary abortion); higher wealth was associated with greater fecundity; and neurosis was related to reduced reproductive success.

The use of variables presumed to be of evolutionary importance frequently yielded statistically significant predictive power of modest magnitude. Many measures which asked 'how many' showed great variability, often with very skewed distributions. These variables are of particular interest from the perspective of evolutionary theory because they provide an opportunity to see how variations in behavioral styles correspond to reproductive success. For example, the number of sexual partners, residences, friends, jobs, and hours spent in religious activities showed great variability across subjects. Such variability existed despite the sample having been drawn from what, on other dimensions, was a homogeneous group (white, middle-class women living in greater Los Angeles).

Several factors were identified which appear to promote reproductive success, and these findings lend support to previous findings and conjectures concerning factors responsible for variations in reproductive success. For example, subjects were more likely to have more children if they came from larger families (in which kin might be available as sources of assistance) and if they were relatively less promiscuous (perhaps promoting confidence of paternity and, hence, maintaining the support of the spouse). Having a spouse was the most potent predictor of managing to have other than zero children. Indeed, marriages which did not produce children were significantly more likely to end in divorce than those which did produce children. Overall, the women appeared to exercise great control over their reproductive careers, with most women reporting that they had exactly the number of children they desired. Yet a significant number of women had fewer children than they desired. Never-married women were the most likely to be dissatisfied with their fecundity, reporting a greater difference between actual and desired number of children than did ever-married women.

In summary, the data presented demonstrate the explanatory power of an evolutionary perspective in considering reproductive success.

While possible consequences of some behavioral styles have been suggested (e.g. factors influencing the likelihood of abortion), it will be the task of future reports to examine in detail the interdependence of the discussed variables. Such reports may elucidate further the impact of evolutionary theory upon human social behavior and suggest the long-term consequences of patterns of everyday events.

Summary

Reproductive history data from 300 Los Angeles women suggest a number of correlations. Among them:

1. Marriage is positively associated with fecundity.
2. Lower paternal confidence is associated with higher rates of voluntary abortion.
3. Higher wealth is associated with greater fecundity.
4. Neurosis is associated with reduced reproductive success.

Acknowledgements

The authors thank Barbara Hooper for her work in the conceptualization and writing of this chapter. Funding for the initial research project was generously provided by the Harry Frank Guggenheim Foundation. The computational resources of the UCLA Office of Academic Computing are gratefully acknowledged.

References

Alexander, R. D. (1974) The evolution of social behavior. *Annual Review of Ecology and Systematics*, 5, 325–83.

Betzig, L. L. (1986) *Despotism and Differential Reproduction*. Hawthorne, NY: Aldine Publishing Co.

Borgerhoff Mulder, M. (1987) Reproductive success in three Kipsigis cohorts. In *Reproductive Success: Studies of Selection and Adaptation on Contrasting Breeding Systems*, ed. T. H. Clutton-Brock. Chicago: University of Chicago Press (in press).

Daly, M. and Wilson, M. I. (1982) Whom are newborn babies said to resemble? *Ethology and Sociobiology*, 3, 69–78.

Daly, M. and Wilson, M. I. (1983) *Sex, Evolution, and Behavior*, 2nd edition. Boston: Willard Grant Press.

Daly, M. and Wilson, M. I. (1985) Child abuse and other risks of not living with both parents. *Ethology and Sociobiology*, 6, 197–210.

Dickemann, M. (1981) Paternal confidence and dowry competition: a biocultural analysis of Purdah. In *Natural Selection and Social Behavior*, eds. R. D. Alexander and D. W. Tinkle. New York: Chiron.

Dixon, W. J. and Jennrich, R. (1981) Stepwise regression. In *BMPD Statistical Software 1981*, ed. W. J. Dixon, pp. 251–63. Berkeley, CA: University of California Press.

Essock-Vitale, S. M. (1984) The reproductive success of wealthy Americans. *Ethology and Sociobiology*, 5, 45–9.

Essock-Vitale, S. M. and McGuire, M. T. (1985a) Women's lives viewed from an evolutionary perspective: I. Sexual histories, reproductive success, and demographic characteristics of a random sample of American women. *Ethology and Sociobiology*, 6, 137–54.

Essock-Vitale, S. M. and McGuire, M. T. (1985b) Women's lives viewed from an evolutionary perspective: II. Patterns of helping. *Ethology and Sociobiology*, 6, 155–73.

Fairbanks, L. A. and McGuire, M. T. (1984) Determinants of fecundity and reproductive success in captive vervet monkeys. *American Journal of Primatology*, 7, 27–8.

Gebhard, P. H. and Johnson, A. B. (1979) The Kinsey data: Marginal tabulations of the 1938–1963 interviews conducted by the Institute for Sex Research. Philadelphia: W. B. Saunders Co.

Gebhard, P. H., Pomeroy, W. B., Martin, C. E. and Christenson, C. V. (1958) *Pregnancy, Birth and Abortion*. New York: Harper and Brothers.

Hamilton, W. D. (1964) The genetical evolution of social behavior, I and II. *Journal of Theoretical Biology*, 7, 1.

Hartung, J. (1985) Matrilineal inheritance: New theory and analysis. *The Behavioral and Brain Sciences*, 8, 661–88.

Henderson, S., Byrne, D. G., Duncan-Jones, P. (1981) *Neurosis and the Social Environment*. Sydney: Academic Press.

Hrdy, S. B. (1981) *The Woman That Never Evolved*. Cambridge, MA: Harvard University Press.

Irons, W. (1979) Investment and primary social dyads. In *Evolutionary Biology and Human Social Behavior*, eds. N. A. Chagnon and W. Irons. Scituate, MA: Duxbury Press.

Johnson, R. E. (1970) Some correlates of extramarital coitus. *Journal of Marriage and the Family*, 32, 449–56.

Kinsey, A. C., Pomeroy, W. B., Martin, C. E. and Gebhard, P. H. (1953) *Sexual Behavior in the Human Female*. Philadelphia: Saunders.

Konner, M. (1982) *The Tangled Wing, Biological Constraints on the Human Spirit*. New York: Harper Colophon Books.

Silk, J. (1987) Social behavior in evolutionary perspective. In *Primate Societies*, eds. B. Smuts, D. Cheney, R. Seyfarth, R. Wrangham and T. Struhsaker. Chicago: University of Chicago Press (in press).

Symons, D. (1979) *The Evolution of Human Sexuality*. New York: Oxford University Press.

Turke, P. and Betzig, L. (1985) Those who can do. *Ethology and Sociobiology*, **6**, 79–87.

US Bureau of the Census (1978) Consumer income, *Current Population Reports* Series P-60. Washington DC: US Government Printing Office.

US Bureau of the Census (1982) Marital status and living arrangements: March 1981. *Current Population Reports* Series P-20, Number 372. Washington, DC: US Government Printing Office.

Williams, G. C. (1966) *Adaption and Natural Selection*. New Jersey: Princeton University Press.

The
allocation
of parental
care
among the
Ye'kwana

Introduction

It is well known that human children require
more care or parental investment than any other
primate species (Lancaster and Lancaster 1983).
While this dimension of human behavior is well
documented in the psychological literature for
Euroamerican populations (Babchuck *et al.*
1985), it has received scant, quantitative attention by anthropologists working among tribal
populations (for exceptions see Whiting and
Whiting 1975, Katz and Konner 1981, Hurtado
et al. 1985, Hewlett, this volume (Chapter 16),
Turke, this volume (Chapter 10)). The role of
alloparental care (care of non-offspring children)
has received even less quantitative attention by

social scientists (for a review see Weisner and
Gallimore 1977) although it has been a growing
theoretical concern of evolutionary biologists
(Skutch 1961, Brown 1978, Reidman 1982,
Emlen 1984). The primary goal of this chapter
is to describe the allocation of direct care to
infants by sub-adults and adults among the
Ye'kwana and to show that the degree to which
an individual engages in caregiving correlates
with options an individual has for enhancing his
or her inclusive fitness.

By direct care I simply mean different forms
of physical contact between a caregiver and care-

[1] Anthropology   Department,   University   of
   Nebraska, Lincoln, NE 68588, USA

receiver which enhances or maintains the well-being of the latter and the inclusive fitness of the former. Behaviors such as nursing, grooming, holding, and feeding are examples of direct care. Other forms of care, which one could label indirect care, include securing food, providing shelter, inculcating social and technical skills, and assistance in mate acquisition (Chagnon 1979). Although indirect care is just as important to an offspring's long-term reproductive success as direct care, it is much more difficult to measure. Furthermore, parents devote more time and energy to direct care when their offspring are infants and pre-adolescents than when they are juveniles and adults, and this investment is more aimed at offspring survival than offspring reproduction.

From an evolutionary perspective the allocation of care to children is viewed as a means for the caregiver to enhance his or her inclusive fitness by increasing a child's chances of survival and reproduction (Hamilton 1964, Trivers 1972). As a result, the probability of a caregiver investing greater or lesser amounts of care in a child should be determined by two major factors: (1) the degree of relatedness between the caregiver and child, and; (2) the ratio of the cost of care to a caregiver's fitness compared to the benefit of care to the receiver's fitness.

In most environments those caregivers most closely related to a child ego have the most to benefit by providing care and the most to lose in inclusive fitness terms by not providing care to a child ego. This is because close kin share a large fraction of their genes by common descent, and the likelihood of those genes spreading through the population will depend on the efforts they expend in promoting the survival and reproduction of closely related individuals. This does not mean that close kin will render care in direct linear proportion to their degree of relatedness (Altmann 1979), but simply that close kin will be expected to render more care than distant kin or non-kin. However, the probability of close kin, even those of the same degree of relatedness to a particular ego, rendering aid will be conditioned by the costs and benefits of care, a subject to which I now turn.

A caregiver's sex and age are the most important factors that determine the costs and benefits of childcare. Other factors such as caretaking ability and wide differences in infant needs for care affect an individual's allocation of care but they will not be considered here. The way in which sex affects costs and benefits has to do with male–female differences in the costs of reproduction (Trivers 1972). Essentially, human females, because of the biology of mammalian reproduction (Daly and Wilson 1983), usually invest more in reproduction than males. As a result their potential rate of reproduction is less which means that the cost of losing an infant or producing an infant less fit than average through inadequate care is greater compared to a male's cost. Although the cost of losing an offspring or rearing a less fit offspring will negatively affect a male's fitness a male can more easily absorb such a loss by allocating time to activities that lead to the acquisition of other mates or mating opportunities. As a result of the higher costs of reproduction for females, females are expected to invest more in infant care than males. Extant cross-cultural data on time allocation to infant care from a wide range of tribal and Euroamerican populations (Katz and Konner 1981, Babchuck et al. 1985) overwhelmingly indicate that mothers allocate more time to direct investment in offspring than do fathers. Nevertheless, fathers do invest in offspring and two of the questions I wish to deal with in this chapter are how much time is a father willing to invest in his offspring and does the father invest differently in offspring than a mother?

The mating system of a population will partially determine whether males will attempt to enhance their fitness by acquiring more mates (or mating opportunities) or by investing in offspring. In societies where polygyny is permitted males will be more motivated to expend effort in gaining additional mates; in societies where monogamy is ecologically or socially imposed (Alexander et al. 1979) males will be more motivated to invest in offspring. The Ye'kwana represent a transitional population since polygyny is traditionally permitted but today socially imposed monogamy is spreading through the population. In monogamous Euroamerican populations even when women are employed outside the home males do not compensate by increasing direct investment in offspring (Babchuck et al. 1985). As I will later show, relatively high female work-loads among monogamously married Ye'kwana women, high levels of direct care required by infants and low paternal participation in this activity would seem to limit female reproduction and hence male fitness. Among the Ye'kwana, seemingly, it would be in a male's inclusive fitness interest to either increase his work-load by assuming feminine tasks or to increase his effort in direct childcare.

However, even in the most rigidly monogamous societies male investment may not be equal to female investment in offspring for three reasons: (1) low confidence of paternity (Alexander 1974); (2) differences in the duration of male and female reproductive careers; and (3) the utility of extra-marital liaisons as an additional avenue for reproductive success – a phenomenon common in Amazonia (Carneiro 1958, Siskind 1973, Symons 1979, and Gregor 1985). For example, if a husband believes one or more of his wife's offspring are not also his he may instead devote his energy to courtship with the aim of impregnating and/or marrying another woman. A strong correlate of paternity certainty is the frequency of divorce (Flinn 1981). When a man marries a divorced woman with children from her previous marriage he knows with certainty that some of his wife's offspring are not his. As a result, a male may not be expected to invest in all his wife's offspring whereas the wife will. Even if paternity certainty is high, extra-marital liaisons can still have a high pay-off if the benefits to courtship are greater than the benefits to investment in offspring. Finally, a male may wish to invest in courtship as his wife's reproductive value declines as she approaches menopause, and ultimately he may abandon her by marrying another, younger woman.

Alternatively, one may wish to consider that low paternal investment may be a maladaptive result of phylogenetic inertia: men are less competent or tempermentally disinclined caretakers because of our long history as a slightly polygynous species. I think this explanation unlikely because it appears that males vary widely in the amount of parental investment they allocate (Katz and Konner 1981) which suggests that their behavior may be responsive to the above outlined environmental variables. A possible explanation not addressable by the data presented here is that male investment is made in indirect forms such as attaining high social status, in assisting offspring (especially sons) in obtaining high-quality mates, or in providing protection to the entire family via rare but important risk-taking activities.

An individual's age (as it correlates with reproductive ability) is the second factor that determines the costs and benefits of childcare. Prereproductive and post-reproductive individuals who lack young offspring of their own are more likely to engage in alloparental behavior than reproductive individuals who are actively caring for their own offspring. For these individuals the cost of alloparenting is low since it does not detract from their ability to care for their own offspring (but cf Turke, this volume (Chapter 10)): they either have none or they have older offspring who are in less need of care than younger kin. In addition, the very young and the old are less able to engage in alternative fitness enhancing activities, such as economically productive labor, that require a great deal of strength, skill, or endurance. As a result, childcare is an attractive alternative: it is not physically taxing and can be competently performed even by the very young (Weisner and Gallimore 1977, Borgerhoff Mulder and Milton 1985; Turke, this volume (Chapter 10)).

Variation in parental and alloparental behavior as it is determined by sex and relatedness will allow us to determine if individuals are pursuing their inclusive fitness interests in childcare. The variable of age (i.e. reproductive status) will not be strongly analyzed because the data set is not sufficiently large to simultaneously control for sex and relatedness effects.

Methods

Research for this chapter took place during 1975–1976 in the Ye'kwana village of Toki located on a tributary to the upper Orinoco river in the federal territory of Amazonas, Venezuela (see Figures 14.1). The 88 full-time residents of Toki are largely isolated from the mainstream of Venezuelan national society. Contact with non-Ye'kwana *criollos* (i.e. Spanish-speaking peasants) is largely made by men through their sale and trade of basketry and crops in the regional capital of Puerto Ayacucho, four to five days distant by canoe. The Ye'kwana engage in cash-cropping in order to secure steel goods, gasoline, outboard motors, shotguns, and ammunition but not food. Additional impact has been made by evangelical missionaries with the most important change in traditional culture being the disappearance of shamans and religious practices and the decline of polygyny. The initial goal of the project was to collect time-allocation data on all members of the village of Toki, with a strong focus on economic behavior and its relation to ecological variables. As a result, codes for child behavior and care of children were not

Figure 14.1 Location of Toki, field site for this study.

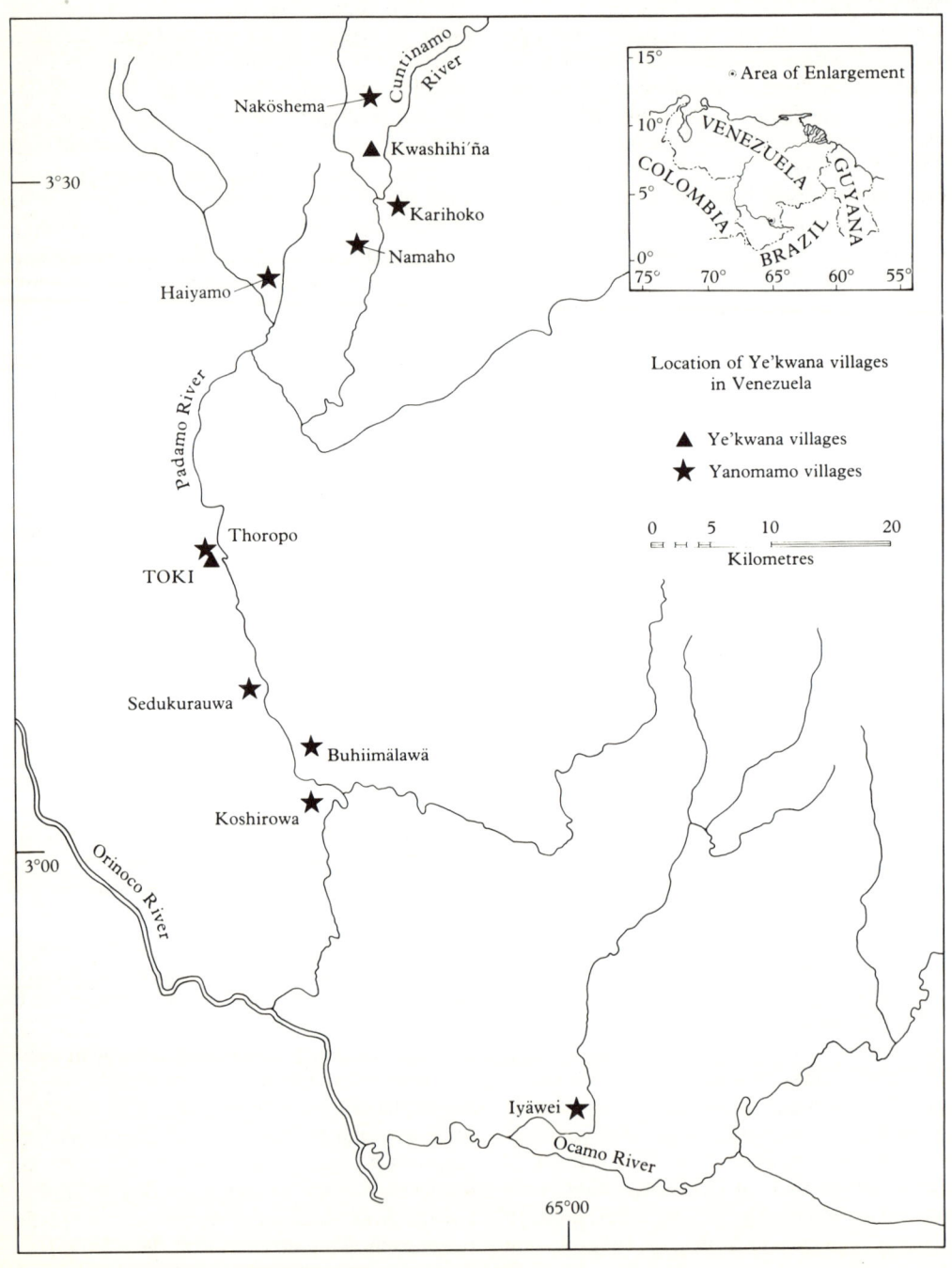

as finely resolved as would be for a study that intensively focused on parental investment.

Data on childcare and child behavior were collected using instantaneous scan sampling (Altmann 1974). Each observation represents a behavioral state as opposed to the observation of a behavioral event with a definite beginning and end (Altmann 1974: 231–2). Scan sampling is methodologically suited to give a measure of the percent of time individuals spend in various activities. Sampling occurred from 0700 hours to 1959 hours yielding a 780-minute day. Percent time in various activities are multiplied by 780 to give a measure of minutes per day (m/d) spent in various activities. It is important to note that childcare does occur at night (see Konner 1977 for information on night-time care among the !Kung). The significance of unrecorded night-time care will be discussed later in relation to underestimates of total care, especially for mothers. The procedures I used in sampling behavior have been described extensively elsewhere (e.g. Hames 1979a, 1979b, unpublished) and the reader is referred to those works for details and to Borgerhoff Mulder and Caro (1985) for broader discussion of sampling in tribal populations.

At this point it is only necessary to describe the constellation of behaviors classified by each code to allow the reader to assess the validity of the data. Instances of childcare were divided into the following categories: nursing, grooming, washing, general care, feeding, and carrying (or holding). The meaning of each is based on standard definitions but general care and carrying require comment. General care is an omnibus category that encompasses all behaviors that the others do not. It refers to such behaviors as calming, caressing, cuddling, distracting from environmental hazards, and the like. Carrying (or holding) means holding or carrying a child (usually on the hip) while moving or standing or sitting. The child is usually supported in a sling during this behavior. It is classified as a kind of care because its net effect is to protect the child from environmental hazards and allow it easy access to the breast. This is done at an energetic cost to the carrier and diminishes the efficiency at which work can be performed.

Most of the care behaviors are symmetrical interactions. That is, if a child is coded as 'being washed' then the woman doing the nursing is coded as 'washing infant'. In many instances, however, childcare was asymmetrical: a caregiver was engaged in another activity while simultaneously caring for a child. For example, caretakers frequently engage in food preparation while holding a child in a sling or nursing a child. In such cases the offspring was coded as being carried while the mother was coded as preparing food. As a result, in some of the tables on time allocation care received by offspring is much greater than the amount of care given by mothers and other caretakers.

The behavioral data I present on childcare represents an underestimate of total childcare since all behavioral observations occurred within the village during daylight hours. If an individual was absent from the village (e.g. hunting, fishing, gathering, or gardening) while I was conducting a scan I asked the nearest available family member where that individual was and what he or she was doing. During the pilot phase of this research I questioned individuals who were absent from the village during scan samples after they had returned to the village and I was able to determine that informant information on absent individuals was 94% accurate (on a sample of 48 visits to and interviews of absent individuals). The reliability of informant-generated observations was continually checked throughout research by evening visits to households to weigh resources acquired in hunting, gathering, fishing, and gardening activities. While informant-generated behavioral observations were adequate for economic activities it gives one no clear idea of whether or not an infant was being cared for while it was with its caretaker. While this is a hindrance in obtaining absolute figures on time allocation to infant care, it is not a problem in measuring differences in the amount of care allocated by caregivers if one assumes that all children were equally subject to the same bias.

It should be apparent that the above categories do not exhaust direct forms of childcare. Activities such as play, story-telling, teaching, and active and passive forms of monitoring (e.g. keeping an eye on an infant as it crawls about the floor to insure that it does not wander into the hearth) all qualify as important forms of care. A full analysis of childcare would require an analysis of patterns of social interaction and proximity which are partially completed and will be

Table 14.1 *Infant time allocation in minutes/day*

Child ID No.	Carry	Care	Nurse	Eat	Sleep	Play	Soc. Int.
0–6 months old							
1	130	111	167	0	161	6	6
2	215	158	23	0	237	45	11
3	258	174	50	3	76	25	0
4	186	160	56	0	104	72	3
5	169	200	32	32	190	11	11
Mean	192	161	65	7	153	32	4
Mean total care 418							
7–12 months old							
6	149	86	17	8	75	25	3
7	135	172	44	5	84	42	0
Mean	147	129	30	7	79	33	1
Mean total care 305							
13–26 months old							
8	74	104	31	37	31	43	6
9	170	140	35	3	75	41	3
10	23	32	18	59	82	146	14
11	42	70	5	62	31	130	13
12	28	91	0	44	51	121	12
13	25	102	10	35	55	141	22
Mean	60	90	17	40	52	104	12
Mean total care 167							
27–40 months old							
14	0	0	0	84	69	126	42
15	9	46	3	98	58	160	25
16	3	54	0	54	67	206	41
Mean	4	33	1	79	65	164	36
Mean total care 38							

presented in a companion piece to this chapter. Nevertheless, inspection of the preliminary results of these other forms of care indicates that the age/sex dimensions of care follow the same patterns as presented below.

For this analysis of childcare all village children less than 41 months of age (16 children: 9 boys and 7 girls) were selected as recipients of caregiving behavior (Table 14.1). The cutoff of 40 months was chosen empirically: children beyond 40 months receive very little direct care. All children in the sample co-resided with both biological parents throughout the study.

Results

As described above, deductions from inclusive fitness theory suggest that relatedness, sex, and age should determine the amount of care individuals allocate to childcare. The goal of this section is to present data that evaluate this hypothesis. I will begin with a discussion of the amount of care given to infants. The purpose

of presenting this data is to demonstrate that childcare is a time-consuming task which limits a caretaker's ability to engage in alternative activities (Denham 1974, Draper 1976, Hurtado *et al.* 1985). I will then turn to a description of the allocation of care by individuals according to their age, sex, and degree of relatedness to the children for whom they provided care. Finally, I will deal with the problem of low direct parental investment by fathers by hypothesizing that they may provide indirect investment in offspring.

Childcare requirements

Table 14.1 documents the time allocation of selected activities for 16 infants and children from birth to 40 months of age. The subtotal 'total care' indicates the sum of 'care', 'carrying', and 'nursing', direct forms of parental investment. Children are rank-ordered by age within the broader age categories. The obvious trend is that care diminishes with age and this trend

Table 14.2 *Proportion of time spent inside and outside the village by children less than 41 months. (Figures in parentheses indicate number of observations.)*

Age	Outside (%)	Inside (%)
0–6 months	12.9 (111)	84.8 (734)
7–12 months	24.0 (82)	75.5 (254)
13–26 months	20.6 (318)	79.3 (1219)
27–40 months	9.2 (55)	90.7 (594)

is statistically significant if age is regressed on care (Pearson $r = 0.81$, $p < 0.01$, one-tailed). But perhaps more striking is the fact that infants less than 7 months of age receive 6.96 hours of direct care per day with care diminishing sharply to 2.77 hours and 0.44 hours by the second and third years, respectively. In the first two cohorts carrying/holding rank as the highest allocation to care and its rapid diminishment thereafter coincides with a child's development of walking. It is also significant that near the mid-point of the third year nursing has all but ceased and the time allocated to eating solid foods is at its highest level.

Care outside the village

Care that a child received while outside the village is not represented in Table 14.1. While I had a clear idea of what the mother was doing in a garden (e.g. pulling weeds) I had no idea of what the child was doing. Even though there is no way of knowing what a child was doing it would be useful to determine how frequently children were outside of the village when their caretakers were engaged in economic tasks. This measure is interesting because it gives one an idea of the constraints that children place on caregivers in locations up to 6 kilometers away (i.e. forest, garden, or river) from the village where high-quality care or monitoring is necessary because of the elevated risk of environmental trauma. Table 14.2 shows the amount of time infants less than 41 months of age spend outside the village. I interpret the trends as indicating that the youngest children (0 to 6 months) are too delicate to travel outside the village and spend protracted periods of time in their mothers' slings while they labor. During the second half of the first year they are hardier and time outside the village doubles. In the second

year they are hardier than before but they are old enough to be left in the care of someone at home. This diminution of travel with mother in the third year corresponds with a radical lowering of general care as seen in Table 14.1. At this time a child is all but weaned and does not require the immediate attention of 'on demand' nursing.

Tables 14.1 and 14.2 show that young children and especially infants (children less than 1 year old) require a huge investment in time. Indeed, care given to infants is more than 90% of a mother's total labor time (see Table 14.6). If a mother were the sole caretaker of an infant and had to do her normal amount of labor she would have to put in more than a 14-hour day. In addition, as Table 14.2 suggests, she would accomplish this labor less efficiently by having to simultaneously tend to a child while she labors outside the village.

Who cares for children?

Any assistance a mother could get in childcare or labor is likely to be fitness enhancing by (1) reducing birth intervals; (2) increasing the quantity and/or quality of care (decreasing a child's probability of death) or; (3) increasing the food supply to her household to allow a mother to enhance the nutritional status of household members. Turke demonstrates this for the Ifaluk (this volume (Chapter 10)). Below I identify the kinship, age, and sex attributes of individuals who care for infants. The care a Ye'kwana child receives can be divided into two forms: passive and active. Passive care (see 'carry' Table 14.1 and 'carrying/holding' Table 14.3) occurs when the caretaker is actively engaged in some activity while he or she is in direct contact with a child. Active care occurs when the caretaker is solely providing some sort of direct care to a child.

Carrying (or holding) is a passive form of childcare; that is, by definition, a caretaker is engaged in some other activity while he or she is carrying the child. Indeed, if I determined that a caretaker had picked up a child to hold or carry it, for example, in order to calm the child then I scored the behavior as general childcare and not carrying/holding. Table 14.3 describes what the child-carrier/holder was doing when he or she was carrying a child and the

Table 14.3 *Percent time allocated to child carrying/holding by context and carrier[a]*

Carrier	Context						
	Leisure[b]	Idle	Walk	Eat	Misc. labor[c]	Food preparation	Total
Mother	37.2	8.8	11.0	8.5	9.6	2.5	77.6
	(105)	(25)	(31)	(24)	(27)	(7)	(219)
Sister	3.9	2.1	1.7	<1	<1	<1	8.9
	(11)	(6)	(5)	(1)	(1)	(1)	(25)
Female cousin	3.5	0	<1	<1	0	0	4.3
	(10)	(0)	(1)	(1)	(0)	(0)	(12)
Grandmother	1.8	0	1.1	<1	<1	<1	3.5
	(5)	(0)	(3)	(1)	(1)	1	(10)
Aunt	1.4	0	1.1	0	0	0	2.4
	(4)	(0)	(3)	(0)	(0)	(0)	(7)
Father	<1	<1	<2	0	0	0	1.4
	(1)	(2)	(1)	(0)	(0)	(0)	(4)
Brother	<1	0	0	0	0	0	0.7
	(2)	(0)	(0)	(0)	(0)	(0)	(2)
Male cousin	<1	<1	<1	<0	<0	<0	0.7
	(2)	(0)	(0)	(0)	(0)	(0)	(2)
Unrelated	<1	0	0	0	0	0	0.4
	(1)	(0)	(0)	(0)	(0)	(0)	(1)
Grandfather	0	0	0	0	0	0	0
	(0)	(0)	(0)	(0)	(0)	(0)	(0)
Total	50.0	11.7	15.6	9.6	10.3	3.2	100
	(141)	(33)	(44)	(27)	(29)	(9)	(282)

[a] Figures in parentheses indicate number of observations
[b] This activity is primarily conversation and other forms of social interaction
[c] This activity is primarily household maintenance and manufacturing

identity of the caregiver. Not surprisingly, 87% of the time a child was carried or held the carrier was not engaged in work. 'Leisure' activities (generally social interaction such as conversation) account for the majority of non-work activities with the balance more or less evenly divided between idleness, food consumption, and walking about the village. However, it should be noted that the amount of time children are carried in a work context is certainly higher than the 14% figure in Table 14.3 would indicate since these figures only measure carrying that occured within the village and not forest and garden where much of one's time is spent in labor. By focusing on caretaking by individuals other than mothers one gets a quick introduction to the role of alloparenting. One finds that if carrying in non-work versus work contexts are compared among all caregivers, mothers' proportional allocation to carrying increases while all other caregivers except for grandmothers decrease. While it is difficult to apply any statistical test to analyze this trend, it does indicate that alloparents are less willing than a mother to carry a child while they are laboring.

The results of Table 14.3 clearly show that mothers, in doing 78% of the child carrying/holding, monopolize this dimension of care. Another dimension of childcare, general childcare, is displayed in Table 14.4. The interesting result is that this trend is nearly reversed: mothers allocate but 24% of the total general care received by infants. Although the mothers' total is the highest, sisters and grandmothers are very close seconds and thirds. If carrying/holding are added to the figures on general care it turns out that mothers allocate just under half of all non-nursing care to their children (see bottom Table 14.4). This indicates that individuals other than mothers are absolutely salient to infants as sources of care.

Alloparenting, or the allocation of care to offspring other than one's own, is most likely to be a strategy of enhancing one's inclusive fitness. The benefits that accrue, which have been described above, include increasing a mother's rate of reproduction, reducing child mortality by providing more care, and allowing a mother to labor more effectively so as to enhance the nutritional and material well-being of her offspring.

Table 14.4 *Frequency of general caretaking by age class of child and identity of caretaker*

Child ID No.	Mother	Sister	Grand-mother	Aunt	Female cousin	Male cousin	Brother	Father	Grand-father	<0.125	Total
Caretaker											
0–6 months old											
1	5	6	0	0	0	0	0	0	0	0	11
2	2	9	1	0	0	1	1	0	0	0	14
3	12	0	4	23	0	6	0	2	0	0	47
4	6	21	0	0	1	5	0	0	0	0	33
5	6	0	0	0	1	0	0	1	0	0	8
Mean	12.8	7.2	1.0	4.6	0.4	2.4	0.2	0.6	0	0	22.6
7–12 months old											
6	6	0	0	0	0	0	0	3	0	6	15
7	15	0	23	0	9	4	0	0	1	1	53
Mean	10.5	0	11.5	0	4.5	2	0	1.5	0.5	3.5	34
13–26 months old											
8	7	6	0	1	0	0	0	1	0	0	15
9	6	0	1	7	13	3	6	1	0	0	37
10	0	2	1	0	0	0	0	0	0	0	3
11	5	7	0	2	0	0	0	1	0	1	16
12	5	0	25	1	1	1	0	2	0	0	35
13	5	20	2	0	0	0	1	0	0	0	28
Mean	4.6	5.8	4.8	1.8	2.3	0.7	1.2	0.8	0	0	22.2
27–40 months old											
14	0	0	0	0	0	0	0	0	0	0	0
15	1	1	1	0	3	2	0	1	1	0	10
16	2	5	1	0	0	0	2	1	0	3	14
Mean	1.0	2.0	0.7	0	1.0	0.7	0.7	0.7	0.3	1.0	8
Total	83	79	60	34	28	22	10	13	2	11	342
Percent	24	23	17.5	10	8.2	6	2.9	3.8	<1	3.2	
Total of carry and care	302	104	70	41	40	24	12	17	2	12	624
Percent	49	16.7	11.2	6.6	6.4	3.8	1.9	2.7	<1	1.9	

It should be noted that the first benefit affects the mother's fitness while the others affect the fitness of children and/or mothers. In the analysis below I assume that the main affect of alloparenting is to enhance the child's fitness. I further assume that caregivers other than parents provide care of nearly equal quality as parents. While I have no quantitative data that play on this question my year-long observations of interaction between non-parental caretakers and children lead me to believe this to be true. In fact it is my impression that young female sisters and cousins are more likely to interact intensively with children through play, conversation, and feeding than do mothers, which parallels the careful quantitative findings of Borgerhoff Mulder and Milton (1985). (Kim Hill, pers. comm., finds just the opposite to be true for the Ache.) The only occasion I found non-parental caretakers to be less competent than mothers was when girls between the ages of 4 and 7 clumsily attempted to heft a child on their hips and walk. It is also possible that young caretakers were gaining practice for future childcare, but I think this is largely a side-effect.

The simple prediction that follows is that the amount of care allocated to infants and children will be positively correlated to the degree of relatedness between the child and caretaker. To test this proposition accurately the tabular data on 'carrying/holding' and 'general care' must be normalized. Because each individual (unless two or more individuals are siblings) has a unique number of sisters, aunts, grandmothers, etc., variation in investment by different kin types may largely reflect the numbers of these kin. To control for this effect I have divided the raw scores in Tables 14.3 and 14.4 by the number

245

Table 14.5 *Childcare allocation by age–sex classification in minutes per day*

Sex	Age						
	4–6	7–11	12–16	17–23	24–37	38–50	50+
Female	24.1	34.0	20.4	51.6	48.6	50.2	96.0
	n = 6	n = 6	n = 5	n = 7	n = 3	n = 6	n = 1
Male	2.8	5.7	1.5	5.9	4.0	5.7	5.0
	n = 4	n = 7	n = 4	n = 7	n = 5	n = 3	n = 1

of kin of each type possessed by each individual. The correlation between normalized care and all nine degrees of relatedness is positive and significant ($r = 0.59$, $p < 0.05$, one-tailed). If males are removed from the sample (since their caretaking roles are insignificant) and only females are retained, the correlation is more powerful and significant ($r = 0.865$, $p < 0.025$, one-tailed).

Age and sex dimensions of care

Another way of observing the distribution of childcare is to cross-tabulate it with the age–sex class of a potential care giver. Table 14.5 shows this relationship and corresponds closely to the conclusions drawn from Table 4.14. But some new trends emerge. As expected, females allocate more time to care than males in all age-matched cohorts. While, as expected, there is variation among females corresponding to the onset of adulthood, no such differences are found among males. Male caretaking is rather constant and low throughout the male life cycle. This suggests that males and females are differentially reared in regards to their future roles as parents and alloparents.

Care and labor among husbands and wives

It has been established that females regardless of age allocate more time to direct childcare than do males. A reasonable explanation for this difference is that males have less time for direct childcare because they allocate more time to economic activities and that these labor activities are actually a form of indirect care since they are mainly designed to provide food and shelter for spouse and child. If both male and female allocation to combined labor and childcare were equal then one could assume that parental investment was equal for the sexes. For each married couple in the sample Table 14.6 compares (under the 'Wife' and 'Husband' columns) the allocation of labor, nursing (note this column does not exist for 'Husbands'), care, and the total of labor, nursing and childcare. Under the 'Wife–Husband' column it measures the difference between spouses in care (including nursing), labor, and the total of care and labor. A negative value in any of the 'Wife–Husband' columns indicates that a husband allocates more time to the activity than his wife and a positive value indicates the opposite. In 11 of the 13 comparisons wives allocate more time to labor and childcare ('Total' column) than do husbands, the average difference is 51.5 minutes/day, and this difference is statistically significant (t-test, $p = 0.006$ two-tailed). In 9 of 13 cases wives allocate more time to labor than husbands and the average difference is only 11.8 minutes/day and non-significant (t-test, $p = 0.541$, two-tailed). In 11 of 13 cases wives allocate more non-nursing care than husbands and the difference is highly significant (t-test, $p = 0.004$, two-tailed).

Given my assumptions, the data in Table 14.6 force us to reject the hypothesis that husbands compensate for lower direct investment by allocating more time to one form of indirect investment (i.e. labor). There is no statistically significant difference in labor time of husbands and wives but wives allocate significantly more time to childcare and combined labor and childcare than do husbands. However, it is clear with the addition of indirect care (labor) to husbands' direct care that husbands, contrary to the impressions in Table 14.3 and 4.4, allocate more time to care than all other of a child's relatives. Since the scan sample data does not measure all forms of investment it is possible that males (and females as well) allocate more time to parental investment. I will pursue this idea below.

Discussion

Throughout this paper the major point of departure has been on infants and their caretakers. But for purposes of discussion I want to shift focus to mothers and infants. This is because mothers are the primary caretakers of infants, and mothers, but not infants, are more able to manipulate others to provide care. I have shown that the childcare requirements of infants and very young children are perhaps beyond the

Table 14.6 *Husband–wife comparison in allocation to labor and childcare*

Couple	Wife				Husband			Wife–Husband		
	Labor	Nurse	Care	Total	Labor	Care	Total	Care	Labor	Total
1	431	37.5	34.8	503	390	16.6	407	55.7	41	93
2	368	32.5	75.8	476	376	4.8	380	103.5	−8	100
3	538	0	0	538	470	0	470	0	68	68
4	442	0	30.8	473	466	0	466	30.8	−24	11
5	534	0	15.8	550	448	4.7	453	11.1	86	97
6	434	35.0	23.3	493	499	0	499	58.3	−65	−6
7	450	22.1	4.4	477	382	0	382	26.5	68	95
8	474	31.8	36.4	542	460	7.7	468	60.5	14	74
9[a]	488	9.2	25.3	522	479	2.4	482	32.1	9	40
10[a]	319	55	27.5	403	479	2.4	482	80.1	−160	−74
11	461	13.7	10.2	485	431	15.9	446	7.6	30	38
12	502	20.6	16.0	539	476	11.3	491	25.3	28	46
13	539	5.6	17.3	561	473	5.2	479	17.7	66	88
Mean	460	20.2	24.4	505	448	5.5	454.2	39.1	11.8	51.5

[a] Polygynous marriage

work capacity of a mother if she is simultaneously expected to do a normal amount of economic labor. For example, if a mother were the sole caretaker of her infant she would have to put in a 14.5-hour day of labor and childcare. While it is conceivable a mother could work this hard, doing so would leave her little time for the care of older but still dependent offspring and the quality of infant care would undoubtedly diminish. This last point is important when one realizes that infant mortality in tribal populations ranges from 15 to 35% (Babchuck et al. 1985, Chag-non, Dow, and Cheverud, unpublished data): this suggests that a diminution in the quality or quantity of infant care would be maladaptive. To overcome this problem a mother has two alternatives: she may ask for assistance in caretaking and/or work less (i.e. ask for assistance in labor).

The data from Tables 14.3 and 14.4 indicated that infants receive care from individuals in proportion to their coefficient of relationship to the infant: close kin provide more care than distant kin or unrelated individuals. While this kin biasing in alloparenting suggests nepotistic behavior it is not clear whether reciprocity is or is not mixed with nepotism and why males compared to females of equal relatedness to infants caretake less.

To understand whether reciprocity and/or nepotism is involved in childcare one must realize that either relationship can occur over the short-term or long-term. Over the short-term it

appears that mothers with highly dependent children work less and stay at home more (see below) in order to provide intensive care for their offspring. While doing so they may also babysit the older dependent children of actively working mothers who must leave the village to garden, fish, or gather. When infants mature to ages 2 to 3, mothers may leave them in the care of formerly active workers who are now caring for recently born, highly dependent children. The data in Table 14.2 suggest that something like this is occurring but identification of caretakers is required along with evidence of role reversals through time.

The issue becomes more complex when one considers the possibility that women with dependent children are economically assisted (reciprocated) by the women for whom they babysit. Data from Table 14.6 suggests that this may be occurring. If time spent nursing is regressed on labor time the correlation is negative and highly significant (Pearson $r = -0.81$, $p = <0.001$). This means that women with highly dependent offspring (indexed by time spent nursing) work less than women with more independent children (see Hurtado et al. (1985) for similar findings). Interestingly, husband and wife labor time is uncorrelated (Pearson $r = 0.276$, $p = 0.491$). This means that a husband is not making up the difference in his wife's lowered labor allocation when she is caring for a highly dependent child. A family's food requirements should increase with each additional member, so who is making up the difference of increased productive needs and lower labor time?

The answer to that question seems to be a woman's kin. Unpublished statistical data on reciprocal garden labor exchange reveals that close kin exchanged labor more frequently than distant kin and that households tolerated greater imbalances in exchange (i.e. the difference between labor given and labor received from other households) with close kin compared to distant kin. Since women do 80% of all garden labor it is possible that women with highly dependent offspring are gaining assistance in garden labor, a woman's main economic task, from her female kin. One would predict, therefore, that households with negative exchange balances (those who received more labor than they gave) would have greater numbers of highly dependent offspring than households with positive exchange balances (those who gave more than they received). Furthermore, the very existence of garden labor exchange among women may be an adaptation to childcare constraints and not, as I have previously proposed, an adaptation to hedge against garden failure (Hames 1983:400).

Among Ye'kwana women there appears to be a long-term and a short-term pattern of reciprocal childcare. Over the short-term, women with highly dependent infants gain assistance from women without dependent infants. Later those who were assisted will reciprocate as their children become more independent. This pattern can be a result of simple reciprocal altruism or reciprocal altruism mixed with nepotism. A long-term pattern primarily occurs between mothers and daughters and is based on nepotism. When daughters are pre-pubertal they assist their mothers and when mothers are no longer able to bear children they assist their childbearing daughters. The correlation between relatedness and alloparenting supports either pattern. Whether nepotism, reciprocal altruism, or a mixture of the two will be employed will most importantly depend on the number of kinswomen a woman has in the village: when a woman has many kinswomen in the village she will more likely depend on nepotism since it is in her kin's inclusive fitness interest to assist, but when a woman has few or no kin she may have to rely on reciprocal arrangements. Resolution of these issues will require analysis of old as well as recently collected data on Yąnomanö

(see Chagnon this volume (Chapter 1)) and Ye'kwana alloparenting. The resolution promises to be complex since it apparently involves assistance in childcare and gardening through a combination of reciprocity and nepotism.

There exist two empirical studies on the allocation of childcare by kinship status that may be usefully compared to the Ye'kwana data, although neither focus intensively on the issue. Goodman et al. (1985:136: Table V) report for Agta hunter-gatherers the following rank-ordering of time allocation to childcare: mother, sister, grandmother, father, grandfather and female cousin (tie), brother, aunt, and male cousin. With the exception of father (ranked 4th among the Agta compared to 7th among the Ye'kwana) and aunt (ranked 7th for the Agta compared to 4th for the Ye'kwana) these results correspond closely to those of the Ye'kwana (Table 14.4). Denham's (1974:264) Alyawara hunter-gatherer data on child carrying by kinship relationship also correspond closely to the carrying data on the Ye'kwana (Table 14.3). All three studies show that care is more frequently done by close kin that distant kin.

Sex was found to be an important determinant of care. Table 14.5 showed that females engaged more frequently in care than males while Table 14.6 showed that husbands cared less for infants than mothers despite the fact that they are equally related to their infant offspring. In fact, as Table 14.4 indicates, in all cases when a male and female ego are equally related to an infant ego (grandmother versus grandfather, female cousin versus male cousin, brother versus sister, etc.) females invest more. These results are identical to the findings of Goodman et al. (1985) on the Agta.

To determine whether wives really invested more in offspring than husbands I hypothesized that husbands, as well as wives, provide indirect investment in offspring through household labor. Although females labor more than males the difference is not statistically significant but when labor, nursing, and care are combined as total measures of investment it was found that wives invest significantly more in offspring than husbands. There are two possible ways to resolve this question of low male investment in offspring. First, the behavioral catagories of direct and indirect care fail to capture the full range of parental investment in offspring. It is possible that husbands spend significant amounts of time in education, proximity maintenance to allow passive monitoring of young (Draper 1976), game-playing, and other forms of social interaction that enhance offspring survival and reproduction. Many of these potential forms of investment were recorded and will be reserved for a publication on Ye'kwana socialization. Also, it has been suggested to me that males may invest in their offspring by engaging in risk-taking activities such as defense against predators and enemies. However, warfare with the Yąnomamö ceased in the early 1950s (Hames 1983) and predation of offspring is more likely to be deterred by mothers than fathers since mothers are more frequently in proximity to offspring.

The second way to resolve the question of paternal (relative to maternal) parental investment is to conclude that males can make better use of their time by competing for positions of high prestige and status which will allow them to gain other mates or mating opportunities. Recent research by Kaplan and Hill (1985, this volume (Chapters 17 and 18)) indicate that Ache males who gain high status through their extraordinary economic (in this case, hunting) productivity have higher reproductive success than low status, less productive males. This is especially significant when one realizes that the Ache are monogamous and more than 90% of what a man produces is consumed by individuals outside his own family. In addition, there is a growing literature that shows a correlation between male wealth and reproductive success (Irons 1979, Turke and Betzig 1985, Betzig 1986, this volume (Chapter 2)). Therefore, a father may be allocating effort to status-enhancing activities which lead to increased mating opportunities and which have a higher pay-off than parental investment. Conversely, it is possible that high status can be traded by a father to assist his son or daughter in finding a high quality mate at an early age. If this were the case then status-seeking behavior could be seen as a form of paternal investment. Unfortunately, I do not possess data to evaluate either of these hypotheses.

I think it is clear that females or wives invest more than males or husbands in *direct* childcare and that alloparental care is, in part, determined by relatedness. However, a number of points require further clarification through research. On the issue of male–female differences in paren-

tal or alloparental childcare it is not clear to what degree there are sexual differences in *indirect* parental investment and hence total parental investment. Research should be initiated to explore those things that parents may do to enhance the fitness of their offspring outside the basics of providing food and physical care. Although alloparental care is determined by relatedness it may be blended with reciprocity (i.e. biasing exchange relationship toward kin) and mixed with exchanges of childcare for economic assistance. Finally, the local conditions (e.g. post-marital residence rules) which determine the distribution of kin and non-kin in a village setting must be understood before straightforward predictions can be made about the allocation of alloparenting.

Summary

1. Due to the nature of the Amazonia neotropical forest environment and the Ye'kwana's economic adaptations to it, infant care requirements are difficult to meet if a mother must simultaneously perform necessary subsistence tasks. Any assistance she gains in childcare or labor should positively affect infant survivorship and/or her fertility.

2. Mothers rely on close kin to assist them in childcare and garden labor. The allocation of alloparental care correlates with closeness in genetic kinship.

3. Although fathers are just as closely related to their children as mothers, fathers allocate less time to all forms of direct care measured compared to mothers. It appears that males may be following a reproductive strategy which places more emphasis on increasing mating opportunities than on parental investment in offspring; or that male care is more frequently indirect.

Acknowledgements

Funds for the preparation of this chapter were provided by the Harry Guggenheim Foundation and the National Science Foundation (BNS 84–11669). I thank P. Turke, M. Wilson, M. Daly, L. Betzig, and M. Borgerhoff Mulder for their useful comments on the manuscript.

References

Alexander, R. (1974) The evolution of social behavior. *Annual Review of Ecology and Systematics*, **5**, 325–66.

Alexander, R., Hoogland, J., Noonan, K. and Sherman, P. (1979) Sexual dimorphism and breeding systems in pinnipeds, ungulates, primates, and humans. In *Evolutionary Biology and Human Social Behavior*, ed. N. Chagnon and W. Irons, pp. 402–35. North Scituate, MA: Duxbury Press.

Altmann, J. (1974) The observational study of behavior: sampling methods. *Behavior*, **48**, 1–21.

Altmann, S. (1979) Altruistic behavior: the fallacy of kin deployment. *Animal Behavior*, **27**, 958–9.

Babchuck, W., Hames, R., and Thompson, R. (1985) Sex differences in the recognition of infant facial expression of emotion: The primary caretaker hypothesis. *Ethology and Sociobiology*, **6**, 89–101.

Betzig, L. (1986) *Despotism and Differential Reproduction*. Hawthorne, NY: Aldine.

Borgerhoff Mulder, M. and Caro, T. (1985) The use of quantitative observation techniques in anthropology. *Current Anthropology*, **26**, 232–335.

Borgerhoff Mulder, M. and Milton M. (1985) Factors affecting infant care in the Kipsigis. *Journal of Anthropological Research*, **4**(3), 231–62.

Brown, J. (1978) Avian communal breeding systems. *Annual Review of Ecology and Systematics*, **9**, 123–55.

Carneiro, R. (1958) Extra-marital sex freedom among the Kuikuru Indians of Mato Grosso. *Revista do Museu Paulista*, **10**, 134–42.

Chagnon, N. (1979) Mate competition, favoring close kin, and village fissioning close kin among the Yąnomamö. In *Evolutionary Biology and Human Social Behavior*, ed. N. Chagnon and W. Irons, pp. 221–55. North Scituate, MA: Duxbury Press.

Daly, M. and Wilson, M. (1983) *Sex, Evolution, and Behavior: Adaptations for Reproduction*. 2nd edition. North Scituate, MA: Duxbury Press.

Denham, W. (1974) Infant transport among the Alyawara tribe, Central Australia. *Oceania*, **44**, 253–77.

Draper, P. (1976) Social and economic constraints on child life among the !Kung. In *Kalahari Hunter–Gatherers*, ed. R. Lee and I. DeVore, pp. 199–217. Cambridge, MA: Harvard University Press.

Emlen, S. (1984) Cooperative breeding in birds and mammals. In *Behavioral Ecology: an Evolutionary Approach*, ed. J. Krebs and N. Davies, pp. 305–39. Sunderland, MA: Sinauer.

Flinn, M. (1981) Uterine versus agnatic kinship variability and associated cousin marriage preferences. In *Natural Selection and Social Behavior*, ed. D. Tinkle and R. Alexander, pp. 131–64. New York: Chiron Press.

Goodman, M., Griffin, P., Estioko-Griffin, A. and Grove, J. (1985) The compatability of hunting and mothering among the Agta hunter–gatherers of the Philippines. *Sex Roles*, **4**, 132–41.

Gregor, T. (1985) *Anxious Pleasures*. Chicago: University of Chicago Press.

Hames, R. (1978) A behavioral account of the division of labor among the Ye'kwana. Ph.D. Thesis, University of California, Santa Barbara.

Hames, R. (1979a) A comparison of the efficiencies of the shotgun and bow in neotropical forest hunting. *Human Ecology*, **7**, 219–52.

Hames, R. (1979b) Interaction and relatedness among the Ye'kwana: a preliminary analysis. In *Evolutionary Biology and Human Social Behavior*, ed. N. Chagnon and W. Irons, pp. 201–19. North Scituate, MA: Duxbury Press.

Hames, R. (1983) The settlement pattern of Yąnomamö population bloc: a behavioral ecological interpretation. In *Adaptive Responses of Native Amazonians*, ed. R. Hames and W. Vickers, pp. 393–427. New York: Academic Press.

Hamilton, W. (1964) The genetical evolution of social behavior. *Journal of Theoretical Biology*, **7**, 1–52.

Hurtado, M., Hill, K. and Kaplan, H. (1985) Female subsistence strategies among Ache hunter-gatherers of Eastern Paraguay. *Human Ecology*, **13**, 1–28.

Irons, W. (1979) Cultural and biological success. In *Evolutionary Biology and Human Social Behavior*, ed. N. Chagnon and W. Irons, pp. 257–72. North Sciutate, MA: Duxbury Press.

Kaplan, H. and Hill, K. (1985) Hunting ability and reproductive success among male Ache foragers. *Current Anthropology*, **26**(1), 131–3.

Katz, M. and Konner, M. (1981) The role of the father: An anthropological perspective. In *The Role of the Father in Child Development*, revised edition ed. M. Lamb, pp. 189–222. New York: Wiley.

Konner, M. (1977) Maternal care, infant behavior, and development among the !Kung. In *Kalahari Hunter–Gatherers*, ed. R. Lee and I. DeVore, pp. 219–45. Cambridge, MA: Harvard University Press.

Lancaster, J. and Lancaster, C. (1983) Parental investment: the hominid adaptation. In *How Humans Adapt*, ed. D. Ortner, pp. 33–69. Washington DC: Smithsonian Institute Press.

Reidman, M. (1982) The evolution of alloparental care and adoption in mammals. *Quarterly Review of Biology*, **57**, 405–35.

Siskind, J. (1973) Tropical forest hunters and the economy of sex. In *Peoples and Cultures of Native South America*, ed. D. Gross, pp. 226–40. New York: Natural History Press.

Skutch, A. (1961) Helpers among birds. *Condor*, **79**, 198–226.

Symons, D. (1979) *The Evolution of Human Sexuality*. Oxford: Oxford University Press.

Trivers, R. (1972) Parental investment and sexual selection. In *Sexual Selection and the Descent of Man*, ed. B. Campbell, pp. 136–79. Chicago: Aldine.

Trivers, R. (1974) Parent–offspring conflict. *American*

Zoologist, **14**, 249–64.

Turke, P. and Betzig, L. (1985) Those who can do: wealth, status, and reproductive success on Ifaluk. *Ethology and Sociobiology*, **6**, 79–89.

Weisner, T. and Gallimore, R. (1977) My brother's keeper: child and sibling caretaking. *Current Anthropology*, **18**, 169–90.

Whiting, B. and Whiting, J. (1975) *Children of Six Cultures*. Cambridge, MA: Harvard University Press.

Eckart Voland[1]

Differential infant and child mortality in evolutionary perspective: data from late 17th to 19th century Ostfriesland (Germany)

My mother has killed me,
My father is eating me,
My brothers and sisters are under the
table Eating my bones.

Taken from an English folktale recorded at the
Saunders Street Orphanage in Southport in 1915
(Gilchrist 1918–1920)

Introduction

Parental investment is based on the allocation of limited resources (Trivers 1972). Over the course of their lives, parents constantly make critical decisions concerning the use and application of their finite investment potential. In terms of evolutionary biology, this represents a problem of optimization because strategies that lead to maximization of inclusive fitness are favoured by natural selection.

Investment decisions are determined by the reproductive value of both parents and their children (Pianka and Parker 1975). Fisher (1930) defined reproductive value as the statistical probability of one's genetic contribution to the next generation, and this probability will vary over an individual's lifespan (Williams 1966).

As regards a parent's reproductive value, the decisions whether to invest in a particular offspring will depend, in part, on the further life prospects of the investor; thus, an individual will increase investment in current reproduction as his or her residual reproductive value declines with age (Pianka and Parker 1975, Pugesek 1981, Clutton-Brock 1984). As regards the reproductive value of offspring, the most adaptive parental strategy is to invest in offspring with highest variance of reproductive value, thereby

[1] Institut für Anthropologie, Universität Göttingen, D-3400 Göttingen, FRG

maximizing the effects of investment. Reproductive value of children will be influenced by such factors as age (Milinski 1978, Charlesworth and Charnov 1981), sex (Trivers and Willard 1973), demographic patterns (Fisher 1930) and the social stratification of the population (Trivers and Willard 1973, Voland 1984a).

If biologists are right in claiming that human social behaviour is optimized by selection favouring inclusive fitness maximization, then it should be possible to predict patterns of differential parental investment on the basis of parental and filial reproductive values. Empirical analyses in this direction are still very rare for human populations (cf. Daly and Wilson 1983, and Boone, this volume (Chapter 12)).

This is a surprising state of affairs, in particular because non-biological disciplines are engaged in studying the varying patterns of behaviour exhibited by parents towards their offspring; for example, some theories in the area of family sociology and social history deal with the family as an investment system having the optimal social placement of its members as its main function. There are innumerable historical examples for how the social support of children varies according to their sex and order of birth and thus contributes to family efforts directed at upward social mobility and the safeguarding of already achieved social status. Such social placement strategies have an impact on, for example, marriage, education, selection of a profession and inheritance (e.g. Bourdieu 1976, Vernier 1977, 1984, Kocka et al. 1980, Medick and Sabean 1984).

This study, some results of which have already been published elsewhere (Voland 1984b), identifies some of the determinants of differential parental investment and evaluates their influence on the reproductive behaviour of the population. In this chapter, analyses focus on patterns of investment in families characterized by the premature death of one parent, using historical data on infant and child mortality from Ostfriesland.

For whatever proximate reasons – be they primarily economic, psychological, historical or folkloristic in nature – parents develop differing attitudes towards the question of the life or death of children, and the result is differential reproduction. In cases where families experience the premature death of one parent the family invest-

ment system is drastically disturbed by the loss of one investor, and specific predictions can be made concerning the varying mortality risks of the involved children.

The following predictions can now be formulated:

1. Sex of the investee. Boys should experience a greater risk of mortality in one-parent families for two reasons. First they are constitutionally more susceptible under stress (Clutton-Brock et al. 1985, Trivers 1985); second, assuming that the early death of one parent is associated with economic difficulties for the surviving spouse and the children, daughter-biased investment may represent a more adaptive strategy for the surviving parent (Trivers and Willard 1973). This is because investment in boys only promises fitness advantages if their social environment enables them to be adequately equipped with resources for coping with male–male competition. High male mortality risks should be more pronounced in families with surviving mothers than in those with surviving fathers, because under the socioeconomic conditions prevailing among the population under study, the death of one's spouse had a much more dramatic effect, in terms of subsistence, on the women than on the men.

2. Age of the investor and birth rank of the investee. For an organism with a high residual reproductive value, i.e. at the beginning of its reproductive phase, it is assumed that it will invest less in current reproduction than an organism that is older and thus has a statistically smaller prospect of future offspring (Pianka and Parker 1975, Clutton-Brock 1984). The corresponding assumption is that infant and child mortality will decrease as the investor grows older. The same relationship should also be able to be seen as a parity effect: it is to be expected that the higher the birth rank, the lower the infant and child mortality will be.

3. Remarriage of the investor. On average, the investor's remarriage may coincide with an economic improvement in his living conditions, so that the infant and child mortality figures in these cases should remain lower than those for one-parent families. On the other hand, remarriage introduces another, genetically unrelated (potential) reproducer into the family, which can be associated with investment deficits and risks

for the respective step-children (Daly and Wilson 1985). As they have the disadvantage of having only one investor in the intra-familial resource competition, the mortality of the children of remarrying widows and widowers should be higher than that of the children from permanently one-parent families.

Furthermore, based on the well-known fact that childless widows have a better prospect of remarriage (Knodel and Lynch 1984), it is to be expected that women will utilize a reproductive strategy option, whereby they will 'give up' their first and only child in order to improve their chances for a second marriage, because this option is linked with the prospect of increased reproductive success.

Material and Methods

Demographic data from Ostfriesland, a northern German coastal region (Figure 15.1) from 1668 to 1879 were analysed. The Ostfriesland population of the 17th, 18th and 19th centuries subsisted primarily upon agriculture. The soil qualities varied greatly, from the unproductive and extremely difficult to cultivate moorlands to the sandy geest (which was poor in nutrients) and finally to the fertile marshlands. Moreover, dairy farming played an important role in the coastal marshes. Trade goods were produced almost exclusively for the local market in the villages. Social stratification was well-defined in the marshes and less well-defined in the other regions, due both to the harsh living conditions of even the farmers and to the correspondingly limited production of surplus. The population pressure of the 19th century led, on the one hand, to an increasing colonization of the moor and, on the other, to an extensive emigration to America. Inheritance traditions favoured the undivided transfer of property in the male line of descent, i.e. from testator to his youngest son.

Figure 15.1 The study site. The shaded area represents the region of Ostfriesland.

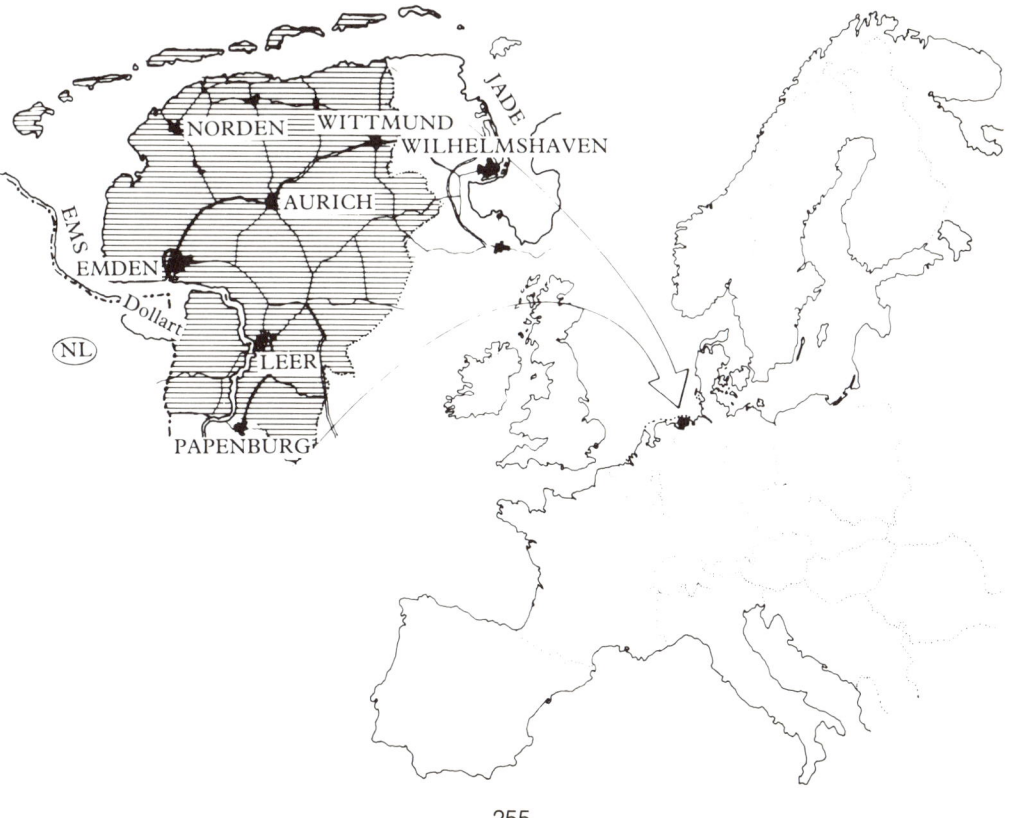

Table 15.1 *Infant and child mortality of the half-orphans according to the sex of the surviving parent*

Mortality[a]	Surviving parent								
	Mother			Father			Total		
	n	q	%	n	q	%	n	q	%
$_1q_0$	67	0.179	17.9	165	0.333	33.3	232	0.267	26.7
$_{14}q_1$	74	0.261	19.7	90	0.310	18.2	164	0.286	18.9
$_{15}q_0$	141	0.402	37.6	255	0.560	51.5	396	0.491	45.5
Unknown, but survived 1st birthday[b]	24	–	6.4	40	–	8.1	64	–	7.4
Unknown, but survived 15th birthday	210	–	56.0	200	–	40.4	410	–	47.1
Total	375	–	100.0	495	–	100.1	870	–	100.0

[a] $_xq_y$ = (number of those who died between y and $y + x$ years)/(number of the y − year olds)
[b] These cases are taken into consideration when calculating the mortality of the first year, but not for $_{15}q_0$ and $_{14}q_1$ respectively

Church records, namely baptismal, marriage and funeral registers, were collected in a familial arrangement in 'Ortssippenbücher' (local clan registers, cf. Knodel and Shorter 1976) by local historians and genealogists.

From this material, 870 families from nine parishes were selected. These families are characterized by the fact that the last-born child either survived the death of one parent during its first year of life, or was born alive after its father had died. The fate of these half-orphans form the focus of our interest, as we ask whether they survived their first or fifteenth birthday, respectively. SPSS-routines (Nie *et al.* 1975) were used to analyse the data. Further references to the data and to the techniques and methods of analysis utilized have been published elsewhere (Voland 1984b). Statistical analysis was done by comparison of the probabilities of binominal distributions (by means of the 'ẑ-test', H_0 = $\pi_1 < \pi_2$, Sachs 1972, p. 262f).

life is about twice as high when the mother dies as when the father dies, the corresponding figures tend to approach one another as the children become older.

Certainly the perinatal risk which causes a correlation of maternal and infant mortality, is partly responsible for this early disparity, but the close spatial and psychosocial relationship between mother and infant may also be responsible; for example, epidemics or subsistence crises are more likely to affect both mother and child than both father and child simultaneously because of the closer dependence of infants on their mothers. However, this unequal constellation of risks is not sufficient to explain the excessive infant mortality after maternal loss.

Indeed, the comparatively low infant mortality in the complete families of Ostfriesland (e.g. 13% in Hesel for first marriages from 1780 to 1899: Imhof 1980; also see Knodel and de Vos 1980), suggests that parents to some extent manipulate the survival chances of their half-orphaned children.

Results

Sex of investor

Table 15.1 reveals that almost half of the half-orphans die before reaching the age of 15, and one-quarter of them die within their first year of life when one of their parents has died. The death of the father or of the mother has a different effect on the children's chances of survival. While the mortality during the first month of

Sex of investee

Survivorship in one-parent families is affected by the sex of the half-orphans. Sons of mothers are significantly less likely to survive the first year than are daughters of mothers (Table 15.2). No sex differences of survivorship are observed where children are brought up by their fathers.

Table 15.2 *Infant and child mortality of the half-orphans according to the sex of the child and of the surviving parent*

Surviving parent	Child	n	Mortality[a]		
			${}_1q_0$	${}_{14}q_1$	${}_{15}q_0$
Mother	boy	201	0.204	0.262	0.421
	girl	174	0.149	0.259	0.379
	$p<$		0.05	ns	0.10
Father	boy	251	0.331	0.286	0.543
	girl	244	0.336	0.296	0.578
	$p<$		ns	ns	ns

[a] For explanation see footnotes to Table 15.1

Table 15.3 *Infant and child mortality of the half-orphans according to the sex and age of the surviving parent (excluding unidentified cases)*

Surviving parent	Age	n	Mortality[a]		
			${}_1q_0$	${}_{14}q_1$	${}_{15}q_0$
Mother	−26	48	0.104	0.341	0.413
	27–32	73	0.137	0.276	0.382
	33–38	94	0.160	0.155	0.302
	39+	66	0.106	0.268	0.349
	$p<$		ns	0.05	0.05
Father	−26	36	0.278	0.417	0.588
	27–32	110	0.309	0.324	0.543
	33–38	101	0.317	0.207	0.478
	39+	142	0.239	0.341	0.561
	$p<$		0.10	0.05	0.05

[a] For explanation see footnotes to Table 15.1

Although, drawing into consideration the consistently higher male mortality found in many avian and mammalian species (Clutton-Brock *et al.* 1985), the discrepancies in risk between mother and father-only situations again suggest that a certain degree of parental manipulation may be occurring.

The tendency of parental manipulation corresponds to the theoretical prediction (Trivers and Willard 1973). The death of one's spouse had different socioeconomic consequences for men and women, namely, a surviving husband encountered fewer economic difficulties than did a surviving wife, because men were the main subsistence providers. This may account for the differential investment behaviour observed in mother-only and father-only families. Thus, in economically stressed mother-only households, mothers were perhaps unable to raise successful sons, and were unable to pass inheritance to their sons, and therefore biased investment to their daughters. Conversely, the higher mortality of daughters in father-only households, while not statistically significant, is unexpected for physiological reasons, and may illustrate a latent preference for boys. The transfer of resources from father to son is also hardly endangered by the death of the mother, in any case it is not as massively affected as by the early death of the father.

Age of the investor and birth rank of the investee

Temporarily excluding parents who were 39 or older from the analysis, it is clear that a half-orphan's chances of survival increase with his parents' age (Table 15.3). This corresponds to the prediction that a parent's investment in current reproduction increases when his residual reproductive value decreases (Pianka and Parker 1975). Some recent evidence suggests that in other species, too, investment tends to increase with parental age (Pugesek 1981, Clutton-Brock 1984).

The curve also corresponds to the relationship between the age of the mother and the risk of parental violence towards step-children described by Daly and Wilson (1985). The authors show how the children of very young mothers run a much higher risk of becoming the victims of parental underinvestment.

An interesting point emerges from Table 15.3. While offspring mortality between the ages of 1 and 15 decreases with parental age, infant mortality, by contrast, increases with parental age; this latter finding reflects a pattern that was typical for complete families in Ostfriesland (Imhof 1980) and for other regions of Germany (Knodel and Hermalin 1984), and that seems to be an universal phenomenon of human reproductive performance (Nortman 1974). Thus the prediction regarding the negative correlation between the age of the investor and overall offspring mortality is confirmed, despite higher mortality in infancy among the offspring of old parents.

Upon reaching the age of 39, that is, the age at which the women in Ostfriesland have typically given birth to their last child (Imhof 1980), there is a partial reversal of the mortality statistics. Residual reproductive value quickly drops to zero at this age, and the reasons for the increase in offspring mortality remain unclear. Possibly they have something to do with a

Table 15.4 *Infant and child mortality of the half-orphans according to the child's birth rank and the sex of the surviving parent (excluding 9+ cases because of small sample size)*

Surviving parent	Birth rank	n	Mortality[a]		
			$_1q_0$	$_{14}q_1$	$_{15}q_0$
Mother	1	61	0.295	0.375	0.569
	2–4	199	0.141	0.290	0.399
	5–8	100	0.170	0.128	0.284
	$p<$		0.05	0.01	0.001
Father	1	144	0.340	0.313	0.574
	2–4	220	0.350	0.323	0.582
	5–8	118	0.288	0.321	0.527
	$p<$		ns	ns	ns

[a] For explanation see footnotes to Table 15.1

worsening of the economic situation of older widows and widowers due to declining productivity. This may lead to the intensified incorporation of children into the work being done to support the family, and thus to an increased and comparatively earlier exposure to the general hazards of life.

Strategic significance for parental investment decisions can also be predicted from the child's birth order. As expected, a corresponding breakdown of the data illustrates investment differentials typical for each parent (Table 15.4).

When interpreting the results, one should always remember that the variables 'birth rank' and the 'age of the mother' are highly confounded. Unfortunately, the data base does not suffice for an analytically clear separation of both of these effects.

A distinct pattern emerges: birth order has strong effects on maternal but not paternal investment. With maternal investment only, the risks of infant and child mortality are clearly much greater for a first-born child than for any later-born child. Accordingly, the child's chance of survival increases together with a higher birth rank. A widow's underinvestment in her only child and the resulting excessive mortality becomes clear, if one considers that childless women have better chances for remarriage than those with children (Knodel and Lynch, 1984). This strategy is adaptive when the reproductive success in the second marriage compensates for the loss of this one child.

Remarriage of the investor

As Table 15.5 illustrates, the relationship between the mortality of half-orphans and the remarriage of the surviving investor has various facets.

First of all, the possibility of or the motivation for a second marriage among fathers and mothers depends on parity in different ways. Women generally remarry much more rarely than do men. Even for widows with only one child the probability of a remarriage is lower than for widowers, even those with many children. These differences are marked with high parity: the probability of remarriage is twice as high for men as it is for women.

Women whose one and only first-born child dies have a prospect of remarriage that is 17% higher than that of primiparous widows whose children survive.

If one looks at the ratio of those children who die prior to the remarriage of their surviving parent with those who die subsequently, it is noticeable that the children of widows die more frequently prior to a second marriage than do those of a widower (Table 15.6). Particularly the first-born offspring of widows die at an above-average rate prior to their mother's remarriage, while half-orphans coming from father-only households die relatively more frequently during the second marriage of their surviving parent, namely subsequent to a step-mother having entered the family.

It is speculative to consider what influence the varying length of widowhood, or widowerhood, respectively, could exert on the foregoing. Is the timespan between the death of one's spouse and remarriage longer for women by an average of 7.8 months (Imhof 1981, for Hesel from 1780 to 1899) because it takes a corresponding length of time until 'impediments to marriage', namely young children from a previous marriage, no longer exist, or is it the other way around?

Even if the cause–effect relationship is not clear at the proximate level (this would require more detailed analyses based on larger samples controlling for the length of the intervals), yet the increased mortality of the half-orphans of primiparous widows (Table 15.4) can at least partly be ascribed to manipulative influences, the ultimate reason for which can be explained with the 'calculation' of a higher reproductive

Table 15.5 *The probability of remarriage (p) of the surviving parent by fate and birth rank of the half-orphans and by sex of the surviving parent (excluding 9+ and unidentified cases)*

Surviving parent	Birth rank of half-orphan							
	1		2–4		5–8		1–8	
	n	p	n	p	n	p	n	p
Mother								
Infant fate								
Died	20	0.700	57	0.491	23	0.348	100	0.500
Survived	19	0.526	97	0.557	63	0.317	179	0.469
Difference		+0.174		−0.066		+0.031		+0.031
Total	39	0.615	154	0.539	86	0.326	279	0.480
Father								
Infant fate								
Died	60	0.883	107	0.860	54	0.630	221	0.810
Survived	51	0.882	78	0.859	50	0.660	179	0.810
Difference		+0.001		+0.001		−0.030		0.000
Total	111	0.883	185	0.859	104	0.644	400	0.810

Table 15.6 *Percent infant and child deaths occurring before parental remarriage by birth rank of the half-orphans and the sex of the surviving parent (100% = all deaths, before and after parental remarriage).*

Surviving parent	Birth rank of half-orphan			
	1	2–4	5–8	1–8
Mother	85.7	71.4	87.5	78.0
Father	67.9	77.2	70.2	73.2

success by means of a second marriage. This motive cannot be demonstrated for fathers. Neither do the half-orphans having a birth rank of 1 show an increased mortality (Table 15.4) nor are there noticeably many deaths prior to the date of the remarriage (Table 15.6). On the whole, these findings lead to the overall result that a remarriage coincides with increased child mortality.

Discussion

As is well known, various physiological and social factors affect infant and child mortality, which is why the results presented here generally indicate a very high degree of variability and sometimes lower statistical significance. While one should be careful not to overinterpret individual details of the findings, I believe that the following conclusion can be derived from the general direction of the results.

From the end of the 17th to the 19th century in Ostfriesland, the mortality of infants and children was not simply a result of fate affecting all of the children equally. Christian 'respect for life' and related attitudes appear not to have provided any comprehensive or effective sanction on parental behaviour, because certain categories of children were selectively discriminated against. While evidence from historical populations of selective discrimination against children is not new (e.g. Dickemann 1979, Reynolds 1979, Wall 1981, Hammel et al. 1983, Johansson 1984, Scrimshaw 1984, Voland 1984a), these findings demonstrate that the differential psychological desirability of children accords closely with the prediction stating that individuals will manipulate investment in offspring such as to maximize their total reproductive output over their lifetimes. Parents need not of course be conscious of such goals for natural selection to favour such behavioural patterns.

While the data neither permit determination of the relative reproductive value of parents and children nor provide sufficient knowledge of the critical socioeconomic circumstances for each case, the gross pattern of these results do suggest that the reproductive values of parents and of children play a significant role in human investment decisions.

Little is known of the cognitive processes by which differences in reproductive value are actually perceived. Parents probably hold traditional norms and ideas that are little reflected upon and even less understood. The internalization of these norms and ideas leads to the contemporary opinions, attitudes and perceptions of daily life, which provide the causative context for what is done and not done. This bundle of attitudes typical for a certain region and a certain historical period towards reproductive processes in general, and towards children in particular, constitutes the proximate causes through which the ultimate causes significantly influence differential reproduction.

This process is subject to feedback. Adaptive behavioural strategies probably influence the mental climate from which they arise, and so cultural behaviour is adapted to evolutionary mechanisms by means of selective processes.

Surely it is not a coincidence that in European folktales it is the step-mother who occupies such a central role as the personification of lethal danger. This motive definitely corresponds to the fear-filled reality of half-orphans. The ambivalent role of natural parents as optimal investors on the one hand, and, on the other, as strategists having the option of underinvestment, also represented an objective threat to some children. Authentic folktales, as a mirror of contemporary mentality, have also incorporated the latent tension inherent in the parent–child relationship in the figure of the 'evil' mother, for example, in the well-known tales of 'Hänsel and Gretel' and 'Snow White'. In an early version of these tales published in 1812, it was the mother who denied her children food or who was jealous of them. Only later, probably as the result of bourgeois family ideology, was it the evil step-mother who threatened the lives of the children.

These examples indicate that the ultimate level of the reproductive strategies and their proximate psychological mechanisms are interrelated. Anthropologists can explore both aspects simultaneously, to determine the nature and course of the evolution of human social behaviour.

Summary

The allocation of parental effort is examined using data on differential infant and child mortality among half-orphans, derived from genealogical records from Ostfriesland, Germany (17th–19th centuries). Predictions concerning the effects of the sex and age of the investor and investee are tested, and the following results are found:

1. Half-orphans whose mothers have died have a 1.4 times higher risk of dying prior to their 15th birthday than do those half-orphans whose fathers have died.
2. Widows clearly favour investment in daughters, whereas widowers possibly exhibit a preference for sons.
3. Even if some of the data run contrary to the trend, investment in half-orphans generally increases in proportion with the age of the investor.
4. The children of primiparous widows have an extremely high risk of mortality.
5. For primiparous widows there is a positive interrelation between infant death and remarriage.
6. Children of remarrying mothers tend to die prior to the marriage, whereas those of remarrying fathers tend to die more frequently after the marriage.

Acknowledgements

With support of the Deutsche Forschungsgemeinschaft.

References

Bourdieu, P. (1976) Marriage strategies as strategies of social reproduction. In *Family and Society – Selections from the Annales, Économies, Sociétés, Civilisations*, ed. R. Forster and O. Ranum, pp. 117–44. Baltimore and London; Johns Hopkins University Press.

Charlesworth, B. and Charnov, E. L. (1981) Kin selection in age-structured populations. *Journal of Theoretical Biology*, **88**, 103–19.

Clutton-Brock, T. H. (1984) Reproductive effort and terminal investment in iteroparous animals. *American Naturalist*, **123**, 212–29.

Clutton-Brock, T. H., Albon, S. D. and Guinness, F. E. (1985) Parental investment and sex differences in juvenile mortality in birds and mammals. *Nature*, **313**, 131–3.

Daly, M. and Wilson, M. I. (1983) *Sex, Evolution, and Behavior*, 2nd edition. Boston: Willard Grant.

Daly, M. and Wilson, M. I. (1985) Child abuse and

other risks of not living with both parents. *Ethology and Sociobiology*, **6**, 197–210.

Dickemann, M. (1979) Female infanticide, reproductive strategies, and social stratification: A preliminary model. In *Evolutionary Biology and Human Social Behavior – An Anthropological Perspective*, ed. N. A. Chagnon and W. Irons, pp. 321–67. North Scituate, MA: Duxbury Press.

Fisher, R. A. (1930) *The Genetical Theory of Natural Selection*. Oxford: Clarendon.

Gilchrist, A. G. (1918–1920) My mother has killed me. *Journal of the Folk-Song Society*, **6**, 85–6.

Hammel, E. A., Johansson, S. R. and Ginsberg, C. A. (1983) The value of children during industrialization: Sex ratios in childhood in nineteenth-century America. *Journal of Family History*, **8**, 346–66.

Imhof, A. E. (1980) La mortalité infantile différentielle en Allemagne du 18e an 20e siècle – Resultats de recherches, certitudes et hypothèses. *Population et Famille*, **50–51**, 137–78.

Imhof, A. E. (1981) Remarriage in rural populations and in urban middle and upper strata in Germany from the sixteenth to the twentieth century. In *Marriage and Remarriage in Populations of the Past*, ed. J. Dupâquier, E. Hélin, P. Laslett, M. Livi-Bacci and S. Sogner, pp. 335–46. London: Academic Press.

Johansson, S. R. (1984) Deferred infanticide: Excess female mortality during childhood. In *Infanticide – Comparative and Evolutionary Perspectives*, ed. G. Hausfater and S. B. Hrdy, pp. 463–85. New York: Aldine.

Knodel, J. and de Vos, S. (1980) Preferences for the sex of offspring and demographic behavior in eighteenth- and nineteenth-century Germany: An examination of evidence from village genealogies. *Journal of Family History*, **5**, 145–66.

Knodel, J. and Hermalin, A. I. (1984) Effects of birth rank, maternal age, birth interval, and sibship size on infant and child mortality: Evidence from 18th and 19th century reproductive histories. *American Journal of Public Health*, **74**, 1098–1106.

Knodel, J. and Lynch, K. A. (1984) The decline of remarriage: evidence from German village populations in the eighteenth and nineteenth centuries. *Research Report 84–57 of the Population Studies Center*, University of Michigan, Ann Arbor.

Knodel, J. and Shorter, E. (1976) The reliability of family reconstitution data in German village genealogies (Ortssippenbücher). *Annales de Démographie Historique*, **1976**, 115–54.

Kocka, J., Ditt, K., Mooser, J. Reif, H. and Schüren, R. (1980) *Familien und soziale Plazierung*. Opladen: Westdeutscher Verlag.

Medick, H. and Sabean, D. W. (1984) Interest and emotion in family and kinship studies: A critique of social history and anthropology. In *Interest and Emotion – Essays on the Study of Family and Kinship*, ed. H. Medick and D. W. Sabean, pp. 9–27. Cambridge: Cambridge University Press.

Milinski, M. (1978) Kin selection and reproductive value. *Zeitschrift für Tierpsychologie*, **47**, 328–9.

Nie, N. H., Hull, C. H., Jenkins, J. G., Steinbrenner, K., and Bent, D. H. (1975) *SPSS – Statistical Package for the Social Sciences*, 2nd edition. New York: McGraw-Hill.

Nortman, D. (1974) Parental age as a factor in pregnancy outcome and child development. *Reports on Population/Family Planning*, **16**, 1–51.

Pianka, E. R. and Parker, W. S. (1975) Age-specific reproductive tactics. *American Naturalist*, **109**, 453–64.

Pugesek, B. H. (1981) Increased reproductive effort with age in the California gull (*Larus californicus*). *Science*, **212**, 822–3.

Reynolds, G. (1979) Infant mortality and sex ratios at baptism as shown by reconstruction of Willingham, a parish at the edge of the Fens in Cambridgeshire. *Local Population Studies*, **22**, 31–7.

Sachs, L. (1972) *Statistische Auswertungsmethoden*, 3rd edition. Berlin, Heidelberg, New York: Springer.

Scrimshaw, S. C. M. (1984) Infanticide in human populations: Societal and individual concerns. In *Infanticide – Comparative and Evolutionary Perspectives*, ed. G. Hausfater and S. B. Hrdy, pp. 439–62. New York: Aldine.

Trivers, R. L. (1972) Parental investment and sexual selection. In *Sexual Selection and the Descent of Man 1871–1971*, ed. B. Campbell, pp. 136–79. Chicago: Aldine.

Trivers, R. L. (1985) *Social Evolution*. Menlo Park: Benjamin Cummings.

Trivers, R. L. and Willard, D. E. (1973) Natural selection of parental ability to vary the sex ratio of offspring. *Science*, **179**, 90–2.

Vernier, B. (1977) Emigration et dérèglement du marché matrimonial. *Actes de la recherche en sciences sociales*, **3** (13), 31–58.

Vernier, B. (1984) Putting kin and kinship to good use: The circulation of goods, labor, and names on Karpathos (Greece). In *Interest and Emotion – Essays on the Study of Family and Kinship*, ed. H. Medick and D. W. Sabean, pp. 28–76. Cambridge: Cambridge University Press.

Voland, E. (1984a) Human sex-ratio manipulation: Historical data from a German parish. *Journal of Human Evolution*, **13**, 99–107.

Voland, E. (1984b) Bestimmungsgrößen für differentielles Elterninvestment in einer menschlichen Population. *Anthropologischer Anzeiger*, **42**, 197–210.

Wall, R. (1981) Inferring differential neglect of females from mortality data. *Annales de Démographie Historique*, **1981**, 119–40.

Williams, G. C. (1966) Natural selection, the costs of reproduction, and a refinement of Lack's principle. *American Naturalist*, **100**, 687–90.

Sexual selection and paternal investment among Aka pygmies

Introduction

Chagnon's extensive demographic work among the Yąnomamö (1975, 1979a, 1979b, 1980, 1981, 1982) provided much of the early empirical field evidence to demonstrate that Darwinian hypotheses were useful in explaining some human behaviors. The few other field studies of evolutionary biology among humans came from populations similar to the Yąnomamö where polygyny and accumulation of material resources existed (Gray 1985). Evolutionary predictions proposed by Darwin (1871) and Trivers (1972) (i.e. male–male competition for women) may appear to be more applicable in farming populations such as these where ritual warfare or competition for land or prestige goods are central to the cultural system. Evolutionary theory has seldom been utilized for predicting human behaviors among hunter–gatherer populations which are often characterized as peaceful or egalitarian, and where monogamy and lack of property accumulation are more common (see Hill and Kaplan, this volume (Chapters 17 and 18) for an exception). This chapter examines the applicability of evolutionary theory among a foraging population that is better known for its peacefulness rather than its fierceness – the net-hunting Aka pygmies of the Central African Republic (see Figure 16.1).

[1] Department of Sociology and Anthropology, Southern Oregon State College, Ashland, OR 97520, USA

Quantitative evidence for sexual selection among Aka pygmies is sought by re-examining published and unpublished demographic data (e.g. Hewlett *et al.* 1982, 1986a, 1986b) collected between 1974 and 1984. Once the data pertinent to sexual selection has been examined, the relationship between sexual selection and Aka paternal behaviors is considered. That is, if sexual selection is occurring, does it help us to understand the Aka paternal behaviors? Again, existing data (Hewlett, 1986) on Aka fathers are re-considered from an evolutionary perspective. The re-evaluation of the Aka data in light of evolutionary biology ends up expanding our understanding of a number of Aka behaviors, but also indicates some limitations to this theoretical perspective.

Theory

Darwin was the first to emphasize the concept of sexual selection. He pointed out that individuals who do not differ in their ability to survive may differ greatly in their mating success (sexual selection). According to Darwin, sexual selection could occur in two ways: competition within one sex for access to members of the opposite sex, called intrasexual competition by Huxley (1938), or choice by individuals of one sex for a particular member of the opposite sex, which Huxley called epigamic selection. Darwin realized that in nature it was usually males who competed with each other for access to females,

and that it was generally the females who selected particular males. The male–male competition he suggested could result in more extensive selection in males, that is, in greater variation in male reproductive success than in female reproductive success. Sexual selection is how Darwin accounted for traits that seemed unrelated to the struggle for existence (e.g. male antlers, tusks, fangs and bright plumage). But Darwin did not know why it was usually the males of most animal species which engaged in intrasexual competition and the females who did the choosing.

A. J. Batemans' (1948) experiments with *Drosophila melanogaster* provided some answers to Darwin's question. He quantitatively demonstrated that: (1) male flies had greater variation in reproductive success than did females, and (2) the frequency of copulation had no effect on female reproductive success (after the first copulation), but the more copulations a male had, the higher was his reproductive success. Bateman explained his results by suggesting that the male flies had more to gain by multiple, rather indiscriminate matings, while females did not. Females produced few and relatively costly eggs whereas males produced many and relatively inexpensive sperm. Since a male has more opportunity to increase his reproductive success by mating with many females, he may be willing to engage in intrasexual competition to gain access to females.

Darwin and Bateman's findings should be applicable to human populations (see, too, Trivers 1972). As with *Drosophila*, human males should benefit more from multiple matings than females. Human adult males invest less in reproduction than do females. Since there is a higher cost to female reproduction, females are predicted to invest more in infant care than are males. Holocultural studies have also shown that males are more likely to be the polygamous sex (van den Berghe 1979, Betzig 1986). According to Darwin and Bateman, these conditions predict greater intrasexual competition among males than among females.

Human males are expected to have greater intrasexual competition than females because males benefit more reproductively by multiple matings. The first section of this chapter examines three measurable consequences of male intrasexual competition, all of them taken from

Figure 16.1 Location of African pygmy groups mentioned in text.

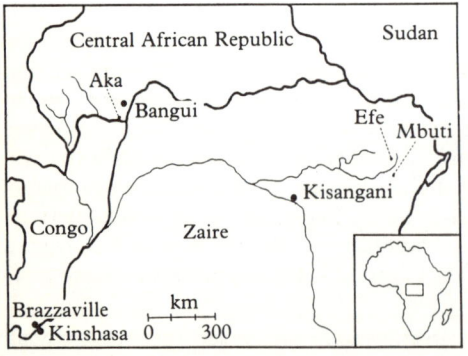

Trivers' (1972) discussion of sexual selection. First, if size of home range functions to increase matings, then one would expect larger home ranges among the more potentially polygamous sex (i.e. males). In ecological settings where females are a dispersed resource, males are predicted to have a larger home range than females because male mobility may be crucial in exposing the male to available females. Second, as a consequence of greater intrasexual competition among men, one would expect male mortality to be higher than female mortality, especially when reproductive potential is highest. Third, as a result of their higher polygamous potential, one would expect reproductive variance to be greater among men than among women.

The second section of the study considers the impact of sexual selection on human paternal investment patterns. From a cross-species perspective, human males are known for their investing – humans are one of the very few mammalian species in which males invest substantially in their offspring – while from a cross-cultural perspective, fathers are known for their lack of parental care. Cross-cultural studies have demonstrated that fathers invest very little time in the direct care of children in comparison to mothers (Whiting and Whiting 1975, Babchuck et al. 1985). Father's role also seems to vary considerably more cross-culturally than does mother's role (Barry and Paxson 1971, Katz and Konner 1981); there are the active indulgent !Kung fathers, for instance, and the Rwala Bedowin fathers who are separated from their children until they reach 7 years of age. Mother's role cross-culturally is less variable; Katz and Konnner's holocultural study (1981) found mothers to be the primary caretakers in 90% of the societies investigated. Some mothers may be indulgent in their care and others perfunctory, but they are consistently active in caregiving.

Sexual selection could affect variability in paternal investment patterns within and between cultures. Parental effort can include time and/or resources. A way men might compete for matings is by accrual or expenditure of parental resources. Some men may successfully spend time garnering resources to be used as parental investment; men who cannot may compensate for their lack of resources by spending time with their children. These predictions will be considered for explaining intracultural (the Aka) and intercultural variation in paternal investment.

The Aka

The Aka pygmies are foragers of the tropical forest regions of the southern Central African Republic and northern Congo-Brazzaville. Two groups of Aka pygmies are included in this study; about 250 Aka associated with the village of Ndele and about 800 Aka associated with the village of Bagandu. Both villages are in the Central African Republic, Ndele being about 100 kilometres west and slightly south of Bagandu.

The Aka spend about 56% of their subsistence time in hunting, 27% of their time in gathering and 17% of their time in village work (Bahuchet 1987). Although the Aka net-hunt the majority of the year and spend little or no time in the cultivation of plant foods, they are transitional foragers in the sense that a large proportion of their diet comes from domesticated village products. Seldom does a day go by without Aka consuming some manioc. In the forest they trade game meat for manioc the farmers transport into the forest, and in the village they provide labor to their village trading partner for which they receive access to his fields. The Aka reside in the village three or four months a year, in part, to assist in the clearing of the villagers' fields.

As with the Mbuti pygmies of Zaïre (Turnbull 1965, Hart 1977), most camp members, males and females, young and old participate in the net-hunt. From the time Aka leave the village and return to the forest (February–March) until caterpillar season (July–August), they often net-hunt six days a week, four to nine hours per day. Net-hunts decrease in frequency during the caterpillar season (caterpillars provide about 40% of diet at this time of year) and the major rainy season (August–October); individual and small group foraging techniques (e.g. spears, crossbows, traps) are utilized more frequently during these seasons.

The Aka are patrilineal, having shallow patri-clans, and are usually patrilocal except for a few years after marriage when the male provides bride service in the camp of his wife's family. Aka kinship terms are basically generational; *tao*, for instance, refers not only to the natural father but to all of the father's brothers as well, all grandparents are called *koko*, all offspring are called *mona* and brothers and sisters called *kadi*. As has been described for other hunting–gathering populations, the marriage and kinship rules are flexible and adaptive to situational constraints (Turnbull 1968, Woodburn 1968, Lee and Devore 1976, Chagnon, this volume (Chapter 1)).

There are four important demographic units: the nuclear family, the camp, the patriclan and the band. The camp (*lango*) consists of 1–15 nuclear families, but averages around 25–35 individuals. The core of the camp usually consists of adult males belonging to the same patriclan (*dibanda*); adult males not from the central patriclan are either temporary visitors or males providing bride service. The final demographic unit, the band, is a more elusive entity as the Aka do not have a native term for it. Essentially, it is a group of 60–100 individuals who hunt and gather in the same vicinity. Its core usually consists of two to four clans. During various seasons the band goes through periods of concentration and dispersal.

There are few Aka status positions. There is no chief in the sense of a person commanding ultimate authority, but there is the *kombeti*, who is generally an older adult male (but not aged) and who exercises his influence in subsistence and camp movement decisions in modest and subtle ways. The *nganga* is the traditional healer and provides a wide range of services to the community – e.g. divination on hunts, curing of witchcraft and herbal healing. The *ntuma* is the great elephant hunter who has often killed several elephants on his own. He leads important hunting and seasonal rituals and organizes the training of young boys in the men's secret society. If an *ntuma* exists within the camp he also often holds the position of *kombeti*.

Sharing, cooperation and autonomy are but a few of the core values of the Aka. Game captured on the net-hunt and manioc acquired through trade from farmers are shared among all camp members. Cooperation takes place each day on the net-hunt as well as in other subsistence activities. Autonomy is expressed daily as individuals in the camp decide to come and go as they wish.

Methods

The mortality data are based on interviews with 170 Aka adults from the Bagandu area and 147 Aka adults from the Ndele area (Hewlett *et al.* 1986b). Individuals were questioned about deceased parents, spouses and children, the illness that caused the death, approximate age at death and an estimated date of death. The fertility and marriage data come from 31 Aka adults over 41 years of age (13 males and 18 females) from the Ndele area and 30 Aka adults over 41 years of age (16 males, 14 females) from one section of Bagandu–Bokoka. These data come only from individuals that were known to me for some time and where cross-checking of birth histories with former spouses was possible. The data on exploration range and mating range are based on interviews with 42 adult males from the Bagandu area and 68 adult and adolescent males and females from the Ndele area (Hewlett *et al.* 1986a). The Bagandu Aka were questioned about visiting 43 places and the Ndele Aka were questioned about visiting 70 places.

Finally, the parenting data come from a sample of 15 Aka families with infants between 1 and 18 months of age associated with the Bokoka section of Bagandu (Hewlett 1986). Eight of the infants were female and 7 were male, 6 between 1 and 4 months of age (2 males, 4 females), 5 between 8 and 12 months of age (3 males and 2 females) and 4 between 13 and 18 months of age. Three types of focal sampling (Altmann 1974) were utilized: father focal all day (6 a.m. to 6 p.m.), infant focal all day and infant focal for 2 morning hours. While the infant or father was being followed some behaviors were measured continuously (e.g. holding, social interaction between caretaker and infant), while other behaviors were measured at 15-minute intervals (e.g. activity of infant/father, people touching infant/father, availability of father and mother).

Measurement of overall human parental investment is difficult. Non-human ethological studies have emphasized direct investment, such as holding, grooming, nursing and feeding of offspring. Little attention has been given to the more indirect forms of investing, such as proximity maintenance, status maintenance and inheritance of parents' resources. Although these forms of paternal investment will be considered in the analyses below, direct care will be emphasized because it was observable and, consequently, a relatively easy behavior to measure.

Results

Sexual selection among Aka

Figure 16.2 examines the fertility (number of live births) of 29 Aka men and 34 Aka women over 41 years of age. Although male variability is not as great as found in some polygynous Amazonian populations (Chagnon 1982, Daly and Wilson 1983:89), the predicted pattern of greater male variability is confirmed. For instance, male fertility ranged from no offspring to 14, whereas, female fertility ranged from 2 to 11 offspring. Aka male versus female variance fits well with the Aka pattern of 'limited polygyny' (about 15% of Aka males have more than one spouse); the variance is not as great as in more polygynous societies (Borgerhoff Mulder 1987), but is greater than in prescriptively monogamous societies (Brown and Hotra, this volume (Chapter 8)).

Aka males that are successful in intrasexual competition should have greater reproductive success. Aka leaders, such as the *kombeti*, could be considered successful competitors. One-third of the males in this position are polygynous while the average Aka polygyny rate is only 15%. Aka

Figure 16.2 Male and female reproductive success of Aka pygmies over the age of 41 years.

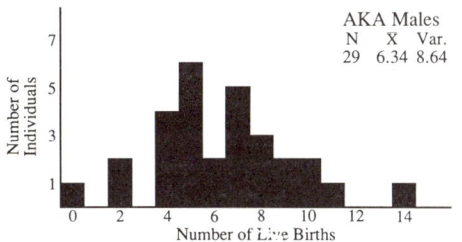

AKA Males
N   X   Var.
29 6.34 8.64

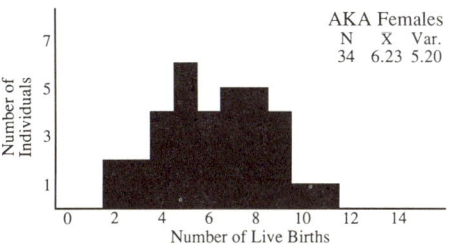

AKA Females
N   X   Var.
34 6.23 5.20

Table 16.1 *Exploration ranges of Aka males and females*

	n	M^a	SD	SE	t	df
Males	18	60.7	33.8	8.2	2.2^b	17
Females	24	41.4	13.4	2.8		

^{a} Mean distance in kilometers
$^b p < 0.025$

males that hold the position of *kombeti* do experience greater fertility than males of comparable age, although the differences are not significant (9 *kombeti* over 41 years old sired on average 7.89 children while all males over 41 sired on average 6.34 children, $t = 1.30$, df = 36).

If range affects mating increases, then males should occupy larger ranges than females to ensure that they are exposed to a number of available females (Trivers 1972:165; Gaulin and Hoffman, this volume (Chapter 7)). Since Aka live in relatively small (25–35 individuals) scattered camps where population density is less than 0.5 persons/sq km, marriageable females are dispersed. Clan exogamy also implies individuals must go some distance to locate a marriage partner. Males have a significantly larger mean 'exploration range' (see Table 16.1) than do females. Males also exhibit a greater variance in exploration range than do females. This suggests that some males have to go farther than others to find a spouse, to trade or to work for a villager.

The same males and females were also asked about their birthplace. Calculation of distances between birthplace of spouses was then possible; this measure was called the 'mating range' (Hewlett *et al.* 1986a). For females there was no relationship between exploration range and mating range ($r = -0.022$), whereas for males there was a significant correlation ($r = 0.565$), thus indicating that Aka male exploration range was a function of the distance traveled to locate a spouse.

Darwin and Bateman also predict greater male mortality due to intrasexual competition. Based on a study of Aka causes of death, Figure 16.3 clearly demonstrates the predicted pattern – Aka males run a greater risk of mortality at every age. As in other human populations (Daly and Wilson 1983), adolescent and young adult males suffer the greatest relative mortality, largely as a result of greater risk taking (Wilson and Daly 1985). A total of 30% of the Aka male deaths at this age were attributed to falling from a tree or some form of hunting and gathering accident.

In summary, Darwin's and Bateman's prediction that where one sex benefits more by multiple mating, one would expect more intrasexual competition, is supported by the Aka data: (1) Aka males ranged farther than Aka females; (2) Aka male mortality was greater than female mortality, especially in early adulthood; and, (3) Aka male reproductive variance was greater than female reproductive variance.

Aka paternal investment patterns

Aka fathers are exceptional in the fact that they provide more direct care (i.e. holding) to their infants than fathers in any other human society known to the literature (see Table 16.2 and Hames, this volume (Chapter 14)). Aka fathers are, on average, within an arm's reach or holding their infant 47% of the time in a 24-hour period. Infant holding demonstrates some of the distinctive qualities of father's versus mother's investment in young. First, fathers hold the infant less time overall, and when they do hold the infant, they hold it for a shorter period of time than the mother. Over a 12-hour period of observation during daylight hours, the father would on average hold his infant for a total of 57 minutes while the mother would hold the infant 490 minutes. The average duration of a father hold was 11.10 minutes, while an average mother hold lasted twice as long, 23.27 minutes. Second, the context of mother and father holding was also markedly different. Table 16.3 shows that fathers held their infant primarily in the camp context when not engaged in an economic activity, while mothers held their infant frequently in either setting, but especially while engaged in economic activity (e.g. on the net-hunt). When a father does help out carrying the infant on the net-hunt, it is on the walk back to camp when the mother has a heavy basket of meat and nuts. Third, Figure 16.4 demonstrates some of the different activities of mothers and fathers while holding their infant. Mothers are more likely to be the providers of nourishment and the transporters of the infant while the fathers are more likely to hug and kiss or play with the infant as they are holding. Fathers invest in relatively brief and intense episodes of activity, such as play or affection, while mothers are more inclined to invest in longer more energetically demanding activities, such as transporting and nursing.

Maintenance of proximity to the infant can also be considered a form of parental investment. It could be essential in protecting the infant from environmental factors (e.g. predators, camp fires, other aggressive children), or in transmitting cultural knowledge, such as subsistence skills. It was not uncommon, for instance, to see parents transmitting subsistence skills (e.g. use of small digging stick, knife, spear) while sitting near their 12-month old infants. Table 16.4 demonstrates that while the father is frequently available to the infant in the forest setting, he is significantly less available than the mother. Table 16.4 gives mother and father availability while they are camped in the forest; when Aka camp near the village, this disparity in mother and father availability is even greater.

The amount of father holding was not related to father availability. While camped near the village fathers were much less available to their infants than while they were camped in the forest, but there were no significant differences in overall father holding between the forest and village setting. This is a result of fathers in the village spending 52% of their day in the camp when infant holding is most likely to occur and spending only 48% of their time outside of camp. In the forest, fathers spend only 29% of their time in the camp and 71% of their time outside of camp.

Figure 16.3 Relative risk of mortality of Aka males and females.

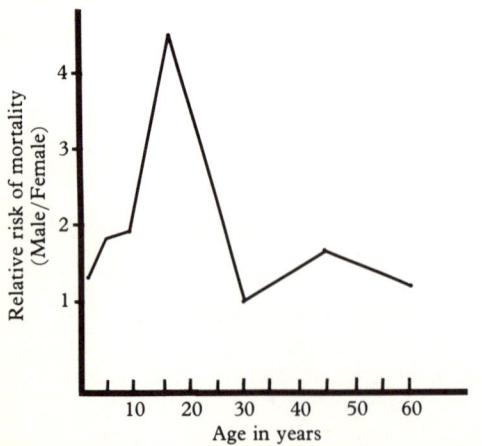

Table 16.2 *Comparison of father holding in selected foraging populations*

Population	Age of infants (months)	Father holding (% of time)	Source
!Kung	0–6	1.9	West and Konner (1976)
	6–24	4.0	
Efe pygmies	1–4	4.0	Winn, pers. comm., 1985
Aka pygmies	1–4	22.0	This chapter
	8–18	14.0	

Note: All observations were made in a camp setting

Table 16.3 *Mean percent of time mother, father and others held focal infant during daylight hours in two forest contexts: in camp and on the net-hunt*

Age of infant (months)	Forest camp				Net-hunt			
	Mother	Father	Others	Total	Mother	Father	Others	Total
1–4 (n = 6)	51.0	22.0	27.8	100.0	87.3	6.5	6.2	100.0
8–12 (n = 5)	45.3	11.2	2.3	58.8	87.8	5.9	0.0	93.7
13–18 (n = 4)	31.8	14.3	9.4	55.5	88.9	2.4	1.1	92.4

Another form of parental investment is the training of offspring in skills essential to survival. A study of Aka cultural transmission (Hewlett and Cavalli-Sforza 1986) indicated that mothers and fathers contributed equally to the subsistence training of their children, but that fathers were more likely to educate sons and mothers more likely to educate daughters. Fathers were more likely to transmit hunting, dancing and singing skills while mothers were more likely to transmit gathering and childcare skills.

The intimate nature of father–infant interactions can also be demonstrated in the kinds of infant caretaking tasks fathers perform. Aka fathers sleep in the same bed as their infant, wife and other young children. When the child wakes up at night and is not comforted by nursing, it is the father who sings to the infant and, if necessary, gets up and dances with the infant until s/he stops fussing. While fathers hold the infant, they are likely to clean mucus from the nose, pick lice from the hair and pick dirt off the body. If the infant defecates or urinates, he

Figure 16.4 Parents' activities while holding infant.

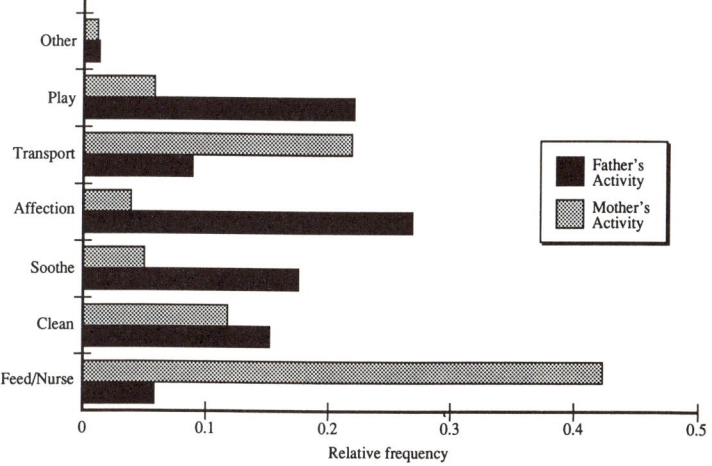

Relative frequency

269

Table 16.4 *Comparison of father and mother availability in forest setting*

Parent	Within visual range					Within hearing range (but not within visual range)					Out of area				
	n^a	M^b	SD	SE	t	n	M	SD	SE	t	n	M	SD	SE	t
Mother	6	92.7	8.0	3.6	5.3^c	6	2.0	3.9	0.9	4.5^c	6	5.2	7.4	3.3	2.2^d
Father	15	63.6	15.2	4.1		15	21.9	7.2	1.9		15	14.5	10.4	2.8	

$^a n$ = number of all-day observations
^{b} Mean scores are the average percentages of time fathers or mothers are available during daylight hours (6 a.m. to 6 p.m.)
$^c p < 0.005$ (df = 19) $^d p < 0.025$ (df = 19)

Table 16.5 *Mean numbers of minutes fathers held focal infant and some cultural and demographic variables*

Min. held	Inf. age^a	Number brothers	Number sisters	Living parents	Number wives	Status^b father	Wife from trail^c	Size^d net
40.4	1	2	2	1	1	–	Yes	L
51.2	1	2	1	2	2	K	Yes	L
106.7	1	1	1	1	1	–	No	S
117.5	1	0	1	1	1	–	No	S
45.4	1	1	1	2	1	–	No	B
41.1	1	0.5	0.5	1	1	–	Yes	M
111.8	2	0	0	0	1	–	No	S
116.1	2	0	1	0	1	–	No	M
13.0	2	2	2.5	1	2	K	Yes	L
42.5	2	0	0	0	1	–	No	S
39.7	2	0.5	1	1	1	–	No	M
25.2	3	1	2	2	1	K	Yes	L
43.3	3	1	3	1	1	–	Yes	L
13.7	3	1	1	1	2	K	Yes	L
44.7	3	2	1	2	1	K	Yes	M

^{a} 1 = 1–4 months; 2 = 8–12 months; 3 = 13–18 months ^{b} K = *kombeti*
^{c} Yes = wife came from Aka clan that resides near same forest trail to village as husband; No = wife came from Aka clan that resides some distance from primary trail
^{d} S = small (less than 30 meters long); M = medium (31–60 meters long), L = large (greater than 60 meters long); B = bride service (no net of own being used)

cleans up the mess. If the infant wants to nurse and the mother is not around, he offers his own breast to the infant. When in the village camp, fathers carry their infants with them when they go drinking *mbolu*, palm wine, often giving some of the wine to their infants.

Aka intracultural variation in paternal investment

In comparing fathers who held their infant frequently with fathers who seldom hold their infant, a generalized pattern of traits emerged. High investment fathers tended to have the following traits: no brothers, few relatives in general, wife from a distant clan, married relatively late in life, monogamous, a small hunting net, relied more on individual hunting techniques (e.g. small traps), had a close relationship with Ngandu villagers, and he and his father never held a position of status (i.e. never held the position of *kombeti*, *ntuma* or *nganga*). Aka fathers who seldom held their infant tended to have the opposite characteristics (see Table 16.5).

With the small sample size, it is difficult to determine which factor(s) is more important. Table 16.6 examines some factors that have previously been identified in predicting the level of paternal investment, and demonstrates that statistically significant differences are found

Table 16.6 *Father holding and some demographic and life-cycle variables*

Variable	n^a	M^b	SD	SE	t
Marriage type					
Monogamy	12	68.4	36.0	10.8	
Polygyny	3	26.0	21.6	15.1	2.1^c
No. of father's brothers					
None	4	97.0	36.3	21.0	
Two	4	37.3	16.8	9.7	2.6^c
One (or half-brother)	7	44.7	29.5	13.2	0.4
Infant birth order					
First-born	7	71.1	40.2	16.6	
Later-born	8	44.1	30.6	11.5	1.3
Household composition					
Parents and infant only	7	73.4	37.4	15.8	
Parents, infant and sibling(s)	8	41.8	31.0	11.5	1.6
Father's age					
Under 30	7	72.0	39.2	16.1	
Over 30	8	43.2	30.4	11.5	1.4
Sex of infant					
Female	8	58.7	33.8	13.0	
Male	7	54.7	42.5	17.3	0.08
Age of infant (months)					
1–4	6	67.0	35.3	15.8	
8–12	5	64.8	46.1	23.0	0.08
12–18	4	31.7	15.1	8.6	1.3

[a] n = number of fathers
[b] Mean scores are the average number of minutes fathers spent holding their infant during daylight hours (6 a.m. to 6 p.m.)
[c] $p < 0.01$

between fathers who have many brothers and those who have none, and fathers who are polygynous versus fathers that are monogamous. There is some indication that the number of brothers is slightly more important than polygyny. There is little difference, for instance, between the 2 monogamous fathers with 2 brothers and the 2 polygynous fathers with 2 brothers; the 2 brothers that are monogamous spent an average of 42 minutes holding their infants and the 2 brothers that are polygynous spent 38 minutes holding their infants. The number of brothers is important because the patrician forms the core of the hunting–collecting unit. If a male has a few brothers he is more likely than a male with no brothers to have a reliable economic unit. Females prefer to marry into a more economically reliable group so they seek males who have more brothers (cf.

Berté, this volume (Chapter 4)). Consequently, males with a few brothers do not have to travel as far to find a spouse and can marry earlier as more females are attracted to them. This in turn also means that the family of the wife is nearby to help support the family. Since the father who holds his infant frequently does not have a group of brothers to rely on for cooperation on the net-hunt, he relies more on individual or small-group hunting techniques and is more likely to provide labor to Ngandu farmers.

The data suggest that higher status fathers, that is those with more resources (brothers), invest less direct care in their infants. A high status male is one who has many brothers, two wives and has a father who was an *ntuma* or *kombeti*. Indirect evidence exists to suggest that fathers with more brothers are of higher status and have in fact more resources. First, of the 7 *kombeti* in the study areas for which reliable geneological data exist, all had at least two full brothers. Second, higher status Aka males (i.e. those in position of *kombeti*) had significantly fewer caries than males of the same age (Walker and Hewlett 1987), suggesting that they had a diet higher in protein and fat. The better diet may also explain why the *kombeti* are on average 3 cm taller than the average adult Aka (i.e. they have had better diets than other adult males). One might infer that their children may also have a better diet as a consequence of having a higher status father. Third, as demonstrated earlier, the *kombeti* generally has more than one wife and more children, a sign that he has more resources. Greater reproductive success of the *kombeti* would contribute to the future status and reproductive success of the child. This does not mean that the father who does not hold the infant contributes less; he provides different types of investment. For instance, much of his time may be spent talking with other males so as to maintain his status. This status maintenance 'indirectly' benefits the infant. Fathers with fewer resources (brothers) compensate by spending more time in the direct care of their infant.

Finally, cultural explanations for this variability should also be considered in future studies. The cultural transmission study mentioned above demonstrated that Aka culture is transmitted primarily from parent to child. According to a cultural transmission model developed by Cavalli-Sforza and Feldman (1981), this form of

Table 16.7 *Comparison of father presence with infants or children among selected foraging and farming populations*

Population	% of time father is present or within view during observations	Primary setting of observations	Source
Gusii	10	house/yard and garden	1
Mixteca	9	house/yard	1
Ilocano	14	house/yard	1
Okinawan	3	public places and house/yard	1
Rajput	3	house/yard	1
!Kung	30	camp	2
Aka pygmies	88	forest camp	3

Sources:
1. Whiting and Whiting 1975
2. West and Konner 1976
3. This chapter

transmission predicts great intracultural variability – precisely what we find in paternal investment patterns. Unfortunately, longitudinal data to test the model (i.e. to determine if investing fathers socially reproduce high investing fathers) do not exist.

Intercultural variation in paternal investment

Like many other foragers, the Aka have few accumulable resources that are essential for survival. Males essentially inherit a most important resource, brothers. Aka males also contribute slightly fewer calories to the diet than do females (considering that females also contribute on the net-hunt (Bahuchet 1987)). In societies unlike the Aka, where resources essential to survival can be accumulated or where males are the primary contributors to subsistence, sexual selection theory would predict that fathers in these societies would invest more time competing for these resources and consequently would spend less time with their children. In contrast, where resources are not accumulable or men are not the primary contributors to subsistence, men overall would spend more time in the direct care of their children. Holocultural and field studies tend to support this hypothesis. Katz and Konner (1981:195) found that father–infant proximity (degree of emotional warmth and physical proximity) is closest in gathering–hunting (gathered foods by females are principle resources, meat is secondary) populations and most distant in cultures where herding or advanced agriculture is practiced. In the latter, cattle, camels and land are considered the essential accumulable

resources necessary for survival. These findings are consistent with Whiting and Whiting's (1975) holocultural study of husband–wife intimacy. They found husband–wife intimacy to be greatest in cultures without accumulated resources or capital investments. While there are other factors to consider (e.g. protection of resources and polygyny rate), there is a strong tendency for fathers/husbands to devote more time to their children/wives if there are no accumulable resources.

Table 16.7 examines father availability in societies that have been investigated with systematic observations. The data support the holocultural findings that fathers in societies with accumulable resources are less likely to spend time near children than fathers in societies where there are few accumulable resources and where men contribute less to the diet than females.

Katz and Konner also found that in societies where hunting by men was the primary mode of subsistence (i.e. hunter–gatherers not gatherer–hunters), father–infant proximity was distant. This is consistent with recent field studies conducted among Ache foragers. Meat and honey collected by Ache men represent the majority of calories consumed (Hill and Kaplan, this volume (Chapter 17)), and Ache fathers hold their children on average only 10 minutes per day (Hill *et al.* 1985). This is the lowest amount of paternal holding recorded for a foraging population that has been quantitatively investigated; no other population where males contribute the majority of subsistence foods has been intensively investigated.

While the above hypothesis correctly predicts differences between intensive farmers and gathers, and between hunter–gatherers and gatherer–hunters, it is not useful in predicting intercultural variability among foraging populations where females contribute significally to the diet (i.e. gatherer–hunters, such as Efe, !Kung and Australian Aborigines, and hunter–gatherers, such as Aka and Mbuti). Table 16.2 demonstrates some of the variability in direct paternal care of infants in systematically observed populations where females contribute significantly to the diet. Among the Efe and !Kung, females contribute substantially more calories than the men (Lee 1979, Peacock 1985), and Aka men and women contribute nearly equal amounts (Bahuchet 1987). Men in all three societies are not responsible for the majority of the calories consumed and there are no accumulable resources essential for survival. Consequently, a father's reproductive success in these societies may be enhanced by contributing more time to the direct care of infants than among the Ache fathers for instance. Females in these populations would also benefit by selecting males who would be willing and capable of doing childcare because the women are less dependent on men for subsistence. But the above hypothesis would predict that Aka fathers should spend less time with infants rather than more time as indicated, since they contribute more to subsistence than Efe or !Kung fathers.

Other evolutionary factors often cited as influencing the level of paternal investment are not useful in explaining intercultural variability among foragers where females contribute the majority of the resources. Paternity certainty, sex ratio and level of polygyny, are important factors for evolutionary biologists, but none of these factors help to explain why Aka fathers do substantially more direct caretaking than Efe or !Kung fathers. Based on blood analysis, paternity certainty is known to be above 95% for both !Kung and Aka, therefore it is not helpful in explaining differences in paternal care between these two groups. The sex ratio for individuals over 15 years of age is 0.86 for !Kung (Lee 1979:48), 1.10 for Efe (Bailey and Peacock 1987), and 0.90 for Aka. According to the sex ratio hypothesis, if there are many more adult males than adult females, as is found among the Yąnomamö, then male–male competition for females is predicted to be greater and males contribute less to the direct care of infants, but the

Efe have the greatest number of males to females yet they do just as much infant holding as !Kung. Consequently, the sex-ratio hypothesis is not useful for these data.

Level of polygyny is also considered an important factor in predicting direct paternal care. In societies where levels of polygyny are high, direct care by fathers is predicted to be low because male–male competition is also expected to be higher, and if the father is polygynous he must divide his time between more children. But the Efe and !Kung levels of polygyny are much lower than the Aka (3–4% among Efe and !Kung versus 15% among the Aka); paternal infant care should be just the opposite of that which is found.

At this point, these factors do not help explain the extraordinary level of paternal investment found among the Aka. Two ecological factors unique to Aka and other pygmy net-hunters are more useful in understanding the behavior of Aka fathers. First, Aka females have to travel farther more regularly than either Efe or !Kung females. Aka females travel just as far as Aka males to participate in the net-hunt, about 8–20 kilometers per day. Efe women work for Lese farmers and !Kung females usually gather goods, in both cases usually not far from the camp. In both of these groups an older female sibling is often the preferred secondary caretaker, not the father as among the Aka. Aka fathers may be preferred over female siblings because of the greater distances traveled by Aka females. Older female siblings would not be able to carry infants for any great length of time on the net-hunt, whereas the father could.

The second unique feature of Aka culture is that male and female subsistence patterns overlap for the majority of the year. The net-hunt and caterpillar collecting are the predominant subsistence activities during the year and both are activities in which male and female subsistence activities overlap. Both Efe and !Kung have subsistence activities in which husband and wife participate together, but they are infrequent and generally involve gathering rather than hunting activities. Regular long-distance travel may explain why Aka fathers help with infant care on the net-hunt (Aka fathers do more infant caretaking on the net-hunt than Efe or !Kung fathers do in a camp setting), but male and female overlapping subsistence activity may be an important factor in understanding why Aka fathers do so much more caretaking than !Kung or Efe in the camp setting.

It is difficult to identify precisely what mechanism(s) encourages greater direct paternal investment when husband and wife subsistence activities overlap. Mammals and especially humans are known for their propensity towards emotional attachment (Bowlby 1969). Aka fathers' extensive interaction and familiarity with their children may generate greater emotional attachment, and therefore greater concern and involvement in their children's well-being. The family is the basic economic unit, family members are more intimate than in most cultures (sleeping and 'working' together), and there is a need to have an adult secondary caretaker rather than an older sibling. Consequently, Aka fathers may be willing to invest more in offspring than what is necessary to maximize reproductive success.

This overview of intercultural variation suggests a pattern similar to that found in intracultural variation: generally, men will spend more time with their children when they have fewer resources to offer. An important way in which men may compete for matings is by accrual/expenditure of parental resources. Intraculturally, Aka fathers with more brothers have more resources available to them, and consequently, spend more time in activities such as status maintenance rather than in direct childcare. Aka fathers with no brothers and few resources spend considerably more time in the direct care of children. Interculturally, societies in which men accumulate essential resources (e.g. land or cattle) or contribute the majority of calories to the diet, spend significally less time in the direct care of children than do men in societies where males contribute less to the diet than do females. Fathers in these societies have fewer resources to offer and therefore reproductive success is enhanced by contributing to the direct care of children. It is also to the female's reproductive advantage in such societies to select men that demonstrate the desire and ability to do direct childcare.

Summary

1. Darwin's (1871) and Bateman's (1948) prediction that where one sex benefits more by multiple mating, one would expect more intrasexual competition, is supported by Aka demographic data: (a) Aka males ranged farther than Aka females; (b) Aka male mortality was greater than female mortality, especially when mating began (i.e. early adulthood); and, (c) Aka male reproductive variance was greater than female reproductive variance, and males were the more polygamous sex.

2. Distinctions in intrasexual competition between the relatively peaceful Aka 'forest' people and the 'fierce' Yąnomamö are simply a matter of degree, being more pronounced among the 'fierce' people.

3. Sexual selection influences paternal investment patterns both intraculturally and interculturally. Generally, men will spend more time with their children when they have fewer resources to offer.

4. Evolutionary predictions were less useful in explaining why Aka fathers invested so much more time in the direct care of their infants in comparison to !Kung and Efe fathers. Male and female overlapping subsistence patterns and long-distance travel required by Aka females on the net-hunt appear to be critical factors.

Acknowledgements

Research for this chapter was supported by grants from the Wenner-Gren Foundation, University of California Humanities Fund, and the Swan Fund. I am indebted to the government of the Central African Republic, especially to Jean-Claude Kazagui, le Haut Commissaire de la Recherche Scientifique et Technologique, for facilitating the project. Etobe, Boseke, Samole, and Maman provided special insights into Aka parenting, and Justin Mongosso assisted tremendously with logistical advice. I also wish to acknowledge the useful comments of the editors of this volume, as well as Napoleon Chagnon, Donald Brown, Donald Symons, Jesus Cardozo, Michael Jochim, Serge Bahuchet and P. Herbert Leiderman on earlier drafts of this chapter.

References

Altmann, J. (1974) The observational study of behavior: sampling methods. *Behavior*, **48**, 1–21.

Babchuck, W., Hames, R., and Thompson, R. (1985)

Sex differences in the recognition of infant facial expression of emotion: The primary caretaker hypothesis. *Ethology and Sociobiology*, **6**, 89–101.

Bahuchet, S. (1987) Food supply and uncertainty among Aka pygmies (Loybaye, Central African Republic). In *Coping with Uncertainty in Food Supply*, ed. I. de Garine and G. A. Harrison. Oxford: Oxford University Press (in press).

Bailey, R. C. and Peacock, N. R. (1987) Efe pygmies of northeast Zaïre: subsistence strategies in the Ituri forest. In *Coping with Uncertainty in Food Supply*, ed. I. de Garine and G. A. Harrison. Oxford: Oxford University Press (in press).

Barry, H. III and Paxson, L. M. (1971) Infancy and early childhood: cross-cultural codes 2. *Ethnology*, **10**, 466–508.

Bateman, A. J. (1948) Intra-sexual selection in *Drosophila*. *Heredity*, **2**, 349–68.

Betzig, L. L. (1986) *Despotism and Differential Reproduction: A Darwinian View of History*. Hawthorne, NY: Aldine.

Borgerhoff Mulder, M. (1987) Reproductive success in three Kipsigis cohorts. In *Reproductive Success: Studies of Selection and Adaptation in Contrasting Breeding Systems*, ed. T. Clutton-Brock, Chicago: University of Chicago Press (in press).

Bowlby, J. (1969) *Attachment and Loss*, Vol. 1, *Attachment*. New York: Basic Books.

Cavalli-Sforza, L. L. and Feldman, M. (1981) *Cultural Transmission and Evolution: A Quantitative Approach*. Princeton, NJ: Princeton University Press.

Chagnon, N. A. (1975) Genealogy, solidarity and relatedness: Limits to local group size and patterns of fissioning in an expanding population. *Yearbook of Physical Anthropology*, **19**, 95–110. American Anthropological Association, Washington.

Chagnon, N. A. (1979a) Is reproductive success equal in egalitarian societies? In *Evolutionary Biology and Human Social Behavior: An Anthropological Perspective*, ed. N. A. Chagnon and W. Irons, pp. 374–401. North Scituate, MA: Duxbury Press.

Chagnon, N. A. (1979b) Anthropology and the nature of things. In *Evolutionary Biology and Human Social Behavior: An Anthropological Perspective*, ed. N. A. Chagnon and W. Irons, pp. 522–6. North Scituate, MA: Duxbury Press.

Chagnon, N. A. (1980) Kin selection theory, kinship, marriage and fitness among the Yąnomamö Indians. In *Sociobiology: Beyond Nature/Nurture?*, ed. G. W. Barlow and J. Silverberg, pp. 545–71. Special Symposium Publication No. 35, American Association for the Advancement of Science. Boulder: Westview Press.

Chagnon, N. A. (1981) Terminological kinship, genealogical relatedness and village fissioning among the Yąnomamö Indians. In *Natural Selection and Social Behavior: Recent Research and New Theory*, ed. R. D. Alexander and D. W. Tinkle, pp. 490–508. New York: Chiron Press.

Chagnon, N. A. (1982) Sociodemographic attributes of nepotism in tribal populations: Man the rule breaker. In *Current Problems in Sociobiology*, ed. B. Bertram *et al.*, pp. 291–318. Cambridge: Cambridge University Press.

Daly, M. and M. Wilson, M. (1983) *Sex, Evolution, and Behavior*. Boston: Willard Grant Press.

Darwin, C. (1871) *The Descent of Man, and Selection in Relation to Sex*. New York: Appleton.

Gray, J. P. (1985) *A Guide to Primate Sociobiological Theory and Research*. New Haven: Human Relations Area Files.

Hart, J. A. (1977) From subsistence to market: a case study of the Mbuti net hunters. *Human Ecology*, **6**, 325–53.

Hewlett, B. S. (1986) Intimate fathers: paternal patterns of holding among Aka pygmies. In *Father's Role in Cross-Cultural Perspective*, ed. M. E. Lamb. New York: Erlbaum.

Hewlett, B. S. and Cavalli-Sforza, L. L. (1986) Cultural transmission among Aka pygmies. *American Anthropologist*, **88**, 15–35.

Hewlett, B. S., van de Koppel, J. M. H. and Cavalli-Sforza, L. L. (1982) Exploration ranges of Aka pygmies of the Central African Republic. *Man(N.S.)*, **17**, 418–30.

Hewlett, B. S., van de Koppel, J. M. H. and Cavalli-Sforza, L. L. (1986a) Exploration and mating range of Aka pygmies of the Central African Republic. In *African Pygmies*, ed. L. L. Cavalli-Sforza, pp. 65–79. New York: Academic Press.

Hewlett, B. S., van de Koppel, J. M. H., and van de Koppel, M. (1986b) Causes of death among Aka pygmies of the Central African Republic. In *African Pygmies*, ed. L. L. Cavalli-Sforza, pp. 45–63. New York: Academic Press.

Hill, K., Kaplan, H., Hawkes, K., and Hurtado, A. M. (1985) Men's time allocation to subsistence work among the Ache of Eastern Paraguay. *Human Ecology*, **13**, 29–47.

Huxley, J. S. (1938) The present standing of the theory of sexual selection. In *Evolution: Essays on Aspects of Evolutionary Biology Presented to Professor E. S. Goodrich on His Seventieth Birthday*, ed. G. R. de Beer, pp. 11–42. Oxford: Clarendon Press.

Katz, M. and Konner, M. (1981) The role of the father: An anthropological perspective. In *The Role of the Father in Child Development*, ed. M. Lamb, pp. 189–222. New York: Wiley.

Lee, R. (1979) *The !Kung San: Men, Women, and Work in a Foraging Society*. Cambridge: Cambridge University Press.

Lee, R. B. and DeVore, I. (eds) (1976) *Kalhari Hunter–Gatherers*. Cambridge, MA: Harvard University Press.

Peacock, N. R. (1985) Time allocation, work and fertility among Efe pygmy women of northeast Zaire. Ph.D. Dissertation, Harvard University.

Trivers, R. (1972) Parental investment and sexual

selection. In *Sexual Selection and the Descent of Man*, ed. B. Campbell, pp. 136–179. Chicago: Aldine.

Turnbull, C. M. (1965) *Wayward Servants: The Two Worlds of the African Pygmies*. Garden City: Natural History Press.

Turnbull, C. M. (1968) The importance of flux in two hunting societies. In *Man the Hunter*, ed. R. B. Lee and I. DeVore, pp. 45–53. Chicago: Aldine.

van den Berghe, P. L. (1979) *Human Family Systems: An Evolutionary View*. New York: Elsevier.

Walker, P. L. and Hewlett, B. S. (1987) Dental health and social organization among African Pygmies and Bantu. *American Anthropologist* (in press).

West, M. M. and Konner, M. J. (1976) The role of the father: An anthropological perspective. In *The Role of Father in Child Development*, ed. M. Lamb, pp. 185–217. New York: Wiley.

Whiting, B. B. and Whiting, J. W. M. (1975) *Children of Six Cultures: A Psychocultural Analysis*. Cambridge, MA: Harvard University Press.

Wilson, M. and Daly, M. (1985) Competitiveness, risk taking, and violence: The young male syndrome. *Ethology and Sociobiology*, **6**, 59–73.

Woodburn, J. (1968) An introduction to Hadza ecology. In *Man the Hunter*, ed. R. B. Lee and I. DeVore, pp. 49–55. Chicago: Aldine.

Kim Hill[1]
Hillard Kaplan[2]

Tradeoffs in male and female reproductive strategies among the Ache: part 1

Introduction

In the following two chapters we examine reproductive decisions faced by Ache men and women. Rather than treating one specific aspect of reproduction in detail, we will explore the manner in which reproductive decisions mutually constrain one another and often involve a complex series of tradeoffs between alternative behavioral options. Although many specific reproductive behaviors in non-human organisms have been well studied by behavioral biologists, and the implications of these studies are increasingly appreciated by anthropologists, the extent to which reproductive decisions involve multiple tradeoffs and adjustments made in relation to

the strategies employed by other individuals is less well appreciated (Dunbar 1983).

Fitness tradeoffs among the Ache vary as a function of age, sex, and reproductive status. Such variation often leads to conflicts of interests between individuals who also share some common fitness goals. In these chapters, we present a series of hypotheses about the factors involved in reproductive decision-making among the Ache and, to the extent that our data allow, test them with relevant data on Ache reproduction,

[1] Department of Anthropology, Emory University, Atlanta, GA 30322, USA
[2] Department of Anthropology, University of New Mexico, Albuquerque, NM 87131, USA

mating, time allocation to activities, and resource acquisition. We begin by looking at the reproductive decisions faced by Ache males and the tradeoffs that may be involved. The next chapter considers female reproductive tradeoffs and points of common interest and conflict between spouses. Family we examine conflicts and cooperation between adults, their offspring, and other band members. Although our discussion will focus exclusively upon the Ache, we hope that the general applicability of the tradeoff approach will be clear.

The focus of our analysis is upon actual behavior and its fitness consequences. Throughout the discussion, we use words and phrases such as 'faced with a tradeoff', 'stategy', 'decisions', 'attempt to', 'deceive', and 'believe' which, in ordinary usage, imply conscious intent and knowledge of action. These phrases, however, are not employed here with any implication of conscious intent, but rather as a shorthand for describing patterns of behavior which appear to serve specific functions and which are putatively shaped directly by natural selection. The exact (proximate) mechanisms underlying the behavioral patterns we describe may vary widely: from physiologically controlled growth and fertility to unconscious associations to self-conscious logic (and even self-deception). Our purpose here is to examine the relationship between behavior and ecological variables in light of evolutionary theory. We make no specific assumptions about the character of the mechanisms which produce the behavior of interest.

The Ache

The Ache are a native population of eastern Paraguay. Until recently, they were full-time nomadic hunter–gatherers. In the 1970s, most of our study population (the Northern Ache at Chupa Pou, see Figure 17.1) came into permanent peaceful contact with the Paraguayan society and were settled in loosely organized agricultural colonies similar to the tribal horticultural villages found throughout much of lowland South America (Hill 1983). Although the Ache are now involved to some degree in both farming and wage labor, this paper will present economic and reproductive data primarily derived from either the pre-contact period (through interviews) or

from foraging trips in the forest we observed between 1980 and 1985. Thus, we are trying to describe the reproductive tradeoffs that faced Ache adults as full-time foragers. Specific reproductive data from the pre-contact and post-contact period were pooled only when no significant differences between them were found. All data on time allocation, food production and food sharing were acquired on foraging trips. Currently among our study population about 25% of adult persons days (Hawkes *et al.* 1987) are spent in the forest living in a manner similar to the pre-contact Ache life style (see Hill 1983 for discussion). On forest foraging trips the Ache live in small bands which move camp almost daily and subsist entirely from wild food products (Hill *et al.* 1984). Life on mobile foraging trips is geared to immediate subsistence needs; all food is generally eaten within two days of its acquisition and foraged foods are only rarely brought back to the settlement and in very small quantities. The band composition and daily routine of Ache on observed foraging trips has been described in detail (Hawkes *et al.* 1982, Hill and Hawkes 1983, Kaplan 1983, Hurtado 1985).

When foraging in the forest, Ache men and women generally set out from camp early in the morning in single file line. After about a half hour, the men begin to spread out and systematically search for game or honey. Male foraging effort is highly cooperative. When the men hunt, they space themselves just far enough apart so that they do not overlap in their search but close enough so that they can call to one another if game is encountered. About 60% of all game taken is captured in cooperative pursuits. The women and children walk slowly, making frequent rest stops, towards a previously agreed upon general direction or to a specific site for the night's camp. Game taken in the morning is brought to the women's group so that the men may continue hunting unencumbered. If honey is found by a man, women are called to the site, to bring an axe so that men can chop open the hive. Women wait, and carry away in pots whatever is not eaten on the spot. Early in the afternoon women establish a new camp and spend some time exploiting nearby vegetable or insect resources. Most important among these is the inner fiber of palm trees which can be sucked or squeezed for its starch. Children generally stay close to their mother or in the small camp clearing with other children and 'babysitters'. Because the Ache are so nomadic, there are no playing spaces for children that are truly safe. During rest stops, mothers simply sit on the uncleared forest floor, and even in camp, only the underbrush is cleared in a small circle. The forest floor remains covered with leaf litter and a large array of biting insects, and undisturbed primary forest is generally only an arm's reach away.

Men generally return to camp late in the day carrying game taken in the afternoon. Small (monkeys, armadillos, pacas) and medium-sized game (peccaries and deer) make up the vast majority of the meat component of the diet (Hill *et al.* 1984). Meat is widely shared after cooking, and is almost invariably distributed by a man other than the one who actually killed the animal. There appears to be no bias in distribution with respect to the relationship between the acquirer of a game item and its consumers (Kaplan *et al.* 1984). The notable exception to this is that men consume very little meat from game items that they themselves killed (ibid).

Sex differences in reproductive strategies: an overview

Recent work in biology has shown that the reproductive strategies employed by individual orga-

Figure 17.1 Ache home ranges (shaded) around 1955.

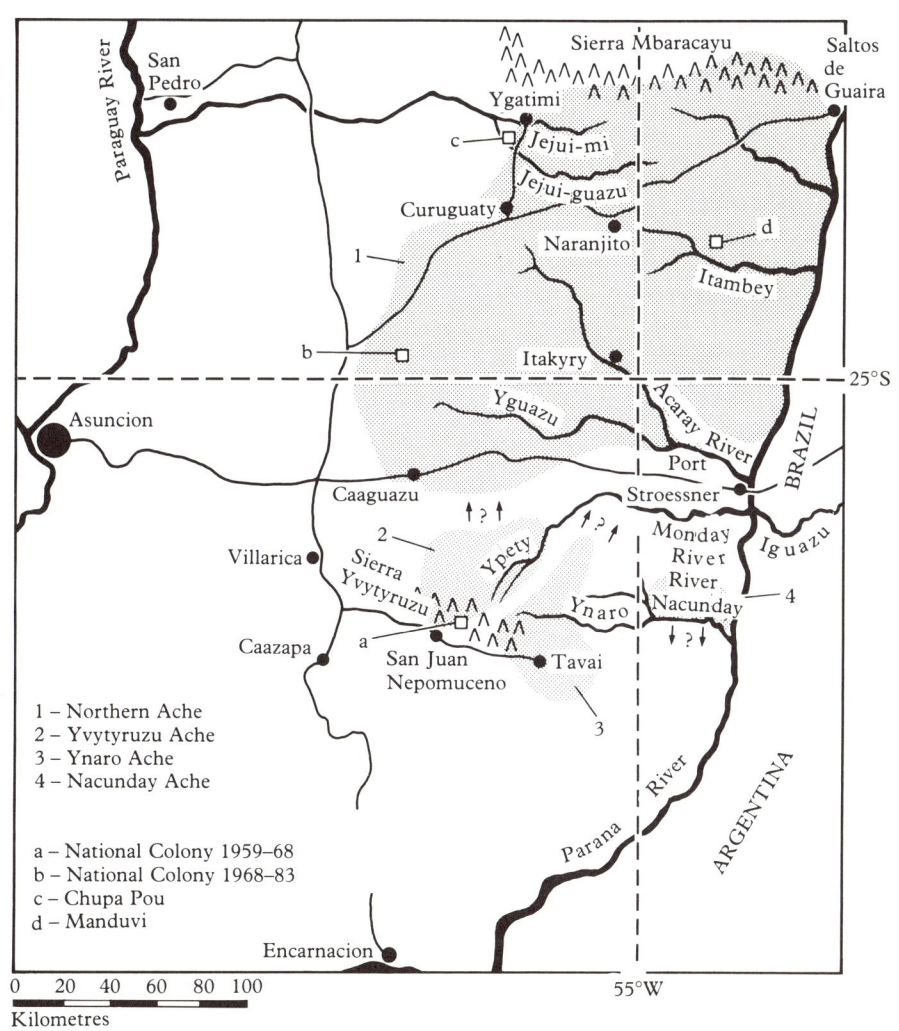

1 – Northern Ache
2 – Yvytyruzu Ache
3 – Ynaro Ache
4 – Nacunday Ache

a – National Colony 1959–68
b – National Colony 1968–83
c – Chupa Pou
d – Manduvi

0   20   40   60   80   100
Kilometres

nisms often differ dramatically with respect to age and sex of the organism, even in the same ecological circumstances (e.g. Stearns 1976, Wrangham 1979a, Clutton-Brock *et al.* 1982). In mammals, sex differences in reproductive strategy are particularly notable because females are committed to internal gestation and lactation, and generally invest a great deal more than males in the survivorship and viability of their offspring. Since time and energy are limited resources, the number of offspring that individual females can potentially produce is generally lower than that of males who often contribute no more than their sperm to their progeny. This suggests that females should be more choosy than males about when to mate and with whom to mate, and as a result, that males should compete among themselves for access to females. These observations have led to the theoretical expectation and, ultimately, to the generalization (Bateman 1948, Williams 1966, Trivers 1972, Clutton-Brock and Harvey 1977, Wrangham 1979b) that females primarily increase their fitness by increasing the amount of food they acquire (i.e. by increasing parental investment in offspring) whereas males primarily increase their fitness by acquiring more matings (i.e. by investment in mating).

The situation becomes somewhat more complex in cases such as humans and many species of monogamous birds and mammals (see Wittenberger and Tilson 1980 for a review) in which male parental investment is often crucial to offspring survival. In such cases males, like females, should be selective about the scheduling of mating, and their choice of partners. In addition, females should be particularly concerned about the quality and amount of parental care that potential mates have to offer. However, there still exist some important differences in the factors affecting male and female reproductive decisions. Among mammals, females internally gestate their young. They therefore can be sure that all offspring they produce are theirs. In contrast, males always face the possibility that their mate's offspring are actually the progeny of another male who also copulated with their mate. From the perspective of females, then, there is a potential tradeoff between 'promiscuity' and 'fidelity'. Females can mate with several males in order to increase the total amount of paternal investment they receive

(Hrdy 1981). However, this strategy carries with it the risk that males, if they lack confidence of paternity, will abandon their mate or reduce their parental investment. The fitness costs and benefits of this strategy must be weighed against those associated with fidelity and potentially higher individual investment from a single male.

From the perspective of males, there is a potential tradeoff between parental and mating investment. Once a male has obtained a mate, he can allocate the remainder of his reproductive effort into parental investment and help his mate maximize the number of viable offspring produced. Alternatively, he can allocate some proportion of his reproductive investment into acquiring additional mating opportunities with other females in whose offspring he may invest to a greater or lesser degree. One variation of this strategy is for a male to attempt 'clandestine' mating with other females and to 'deceive' that female's principal mate into investing in the offspring produced (see Trivers 1972, Dawkins 1976 for similar discussions of male and female strategies in species where both partners invest in offspring).

Sex differences among foragers

In addition to the more generalized mammalian sex differences, there appear to be some species-specific sex differences among humans. The resources which human foragers typically exploit (and have probably exploited for at least the last 100 000 years) can roughly be divided into those which are hunted and those which are collected. In general, males both hunt animals and collect vegetable foods, whereas females generally avoid the pursuit of resources which require great strength or speed (Murdock 1967). As primates who usually carry their dependent young, human females would probably pay a high price in offspring mortality if they engaged in hunting (Hurtado 1985, but see Goodman *et al.* 1985 who present data suggesting that Agta women hunt and so not show associated excessive child mortality; these women are aided by dogs, however). These sex differences in foraging strategies may have resulted in the commonly observed pattern that foods acquired by both sexes are shared in family units and human children are provisioned by both parents. Although the questions of why food sharing, high male parental investment and a sexual division of labor evolved in human societies merit careful investigation (see Kaplan 1983, Hurtado 1985, Kaplan and Hill 1985a, for some suggestions in light of Ache data), in the present discussion we treat these features of behavior among human foragers as givens, and examine male and female reproductive strategies in that light.

While living in the forest, Ache males provide 87% of the calories consumed by the entire group (Hurtado *et al.* 1985). The majority of these calories are derived from hunting which occupies most of the daylight hours for men. Time allocation studies indicate that adult Ache men spend a mean of 6.6 hours per day in the search and pursuit of game animals or honey, and butchering game (Hill *et al.* 1985). They also spend 0.7 hours in tool work or camp work, and about 4 hours per day resting, eating, or in light activity. In contrast, Ache women while in the forest spend 1.9 hours per day walking (moving camp) and only 1.9 hours per day acquiring or processing food (Hurtado *et al.* 1985). They spend an additional 1.9 hours in tool manufacture or camp work, but the remainder of their day (5.9 hours) is spent resting, light activity, and in simultaneous care of children. Women spend very little time in activities that do not allow for close proximity to, and frequent monitoring of, dependent children (Hurtado *et al.* 1985). Infants under 2 years spend virtually 100% of their time with their mothers, about 80% of which is spent in direct tactile contact with them (determined from 6 focal day observations of Ache infants). In the forest, men clearly specialize in food acquisition and provisioning while women specialize in child care.

Given the factors that affect fitness for males and females, respectively, and given their characteristic sexual division of labor, the dilemma facing both sexes is to determine the optimal amount of time and energy that should be allocated to each of several alternative forms of parental and mating investment.

Methods

Details of the methods used to collect data on food production, time allocation, and sharing have been previously published (Hawkes *et al.* 1982, Hill and Hawkes 1983, Kaplan *et al.* 1984, Hill *et al.* 1985, Hurtado *et al.* 1985, Hill *et al.* 1987). Time spent in activities was determined by following focal subjects for an entire day ($n = 63$ man days, $n = 63$ women days), or by sampling all activities for all members of a camp at ten-minute intervals ($n = 594$ man days, $n = 461$ women days). Food acquired by individuals was weighed with hanging spring scales, and time spent in various food-related activities was measured with a stopwatch. Sharing patterns were monitored by scoring consumers and acquirers of most food consumed by members of foraging bands. Acquirers of resources were identified by direct observation or by asking Ache informants 'who killed it' (in the case of meat) or 'who got it' (in the case of collected resources). Only a single acquirer was given by informants for each resource item even when lengthy cooperative effort was involved in the acquisition of a resource. Heights and weights of Ache men and women were measured using a standard tape measure mounted to a wall, and an electronic bathroom weigh scale.

Demographic data are based on interviews conducted with Ache men ($n = 32$) and women ($n = 32$) between 1980 and 1985 about their genealogical and reproductive histories. Informants were asked about their own marriages and offspring, along with those of their parents, siblings, and offspring. This allowed for some cross-checking of information, and provided information on individuals who were deceased or not present during interview periods. Since the Ache do not keep records, ages for individuals born before 1975 were determined from a relative age list of the entire population matched with population age–sex composition tables, and using dated events as a reference (similar to the procedure used by Howell 1979). We also matched old photographs of various individuals with current children of known ages in order to determine more accurately the ages of people born between 1955 and 1975. We consider age estimates to be approximate (within 5 years for adults) although this error decreases with individuals under 30 years of age. Since many of the results reported here represent preliminary analyses using a subset of a larger body of data, descriptive statistics presented are often based on small sample sizes. In addition, the sample size varies from one test or statistic to another because not all information relevant to each question was asked or accurately determined from each interview. All cases where the accuracy of a data point was suspect (e.g. the birth date of a child who died) were eliminated from statistics dependent on that information.

Male reproductive tradeoffs among the Ache

Food sharing

While men are the primary food providers among the Ache, data show that most of the food they produce does not go to their own nuclear family, nor does most of the food consumed by the nuclear family come from the male head of the household (Kaplan *et al.* 1984). Instead, all food, and especially meat, is shared among all the members of foraging bands. As mentioned above, the acquirer of game very rarely has any direct involvement in its redistribution. Typically, as each game animal becomes ready for consumption, it is passed to a man who, in turn, distributes pieces to all or most families in the band. Even monkeys weighing less than 3 kilograms are distributed to all families in the band (unless several monkeys are distributed at once, and in these cases, part of each monkey is still distributed to most families). Extent of resource sharing outside the nuclear family is shown in Table 17.1. The data indicate that 91% of the meat consumed by individuals was killed by someone outside their nuclear family, and as a corollary, more than 90% of the meat that a man acquires is consumed by individuals outside his nuclear family (Kaplan and Hill 1985a). Given that average band size was 9–10 families, the 90% figure indicates complete pooling and sharing of meat. Moreover, we found that women and children eat no more meat from that acquired by their husbands and fathers than would be expected by chance if all food were simply pooled and redistributed (Kaplan *et al.* 1984). This sharing probably benefits all families by reducing daily variation in food intake (Kaplan and Hill 1985a) and may generally be explained by models of reciprocal altruism (Trivers 1971, Axelrod and Hamilton 1981, see also Kaplan and Hill 1985a for tests of alternative hypotheses regarding Ache food sharing).

Table 17.1 *Food sharing by individual resource*

	% consumed by nuclear family of acquirer	Sex of major producer
Meat		
Collared peccary	11	m
White-lipped peccary	11	m
Armadillo	9	m
Monkey	10	m
Paca	5	m
Deer	6	m
Coati	9	m
Miscellaneous[a]	13	m
Honey		
Honey (*Apis melifera*)	15	m
Miscellaneous[a]	19	m
Collected resources		
Palm fiber	31	f
Palm heart	28	m
Oranges	32	f
Virella (*Campomanesia zanthocarpna*)	92	f
Kurilla (*Rheedia brazilense*)	77	f
Larvae	42	f
Miscellaneous[a]	36	f

Adapted from Kaplan and Hill 1985a
[a] Includes items taken in quantities too small for obtaining accurate sharing measures. Miscellaneous collected resources are mostly fruits; miscellaneous honey includes all honey produced by bees other than *Apis melifera*; miscellaneous meat includes birds, fish, and other animal species taken rarely

Nevertheless, some men, because they are better hunters (acquire more meat per hour hunting), hunt more hours, or have fewer dependants, provide much more food than they receive (Hill and Hawkes 1983, Kaplan and Hill 1985a). Even though there are consistent long-term differences between hunters in the amount of meat they acquire (some men differ more than fourfold in hunting returns even after 30 days of observation sampled over a three-year period – ibid), there is no correlation between the calories of food acquired by a family and the total number of times its members were recorded eating food during scan sampling (Pearson $r = 0.31$, $p = 0.12$, $n = 25$ families – see Kaplan and Hill 1985a: 233 for more details). Although it is possible and perhaps even likely that good hunters and their families are given slightly more meat than poorer hunters (but that our test was not sufficiently sensitive to reveal those differences) there is no doubt that the differences in food production between families are much larger than any differences in food consumption, if they exist (contrast with Betzig this volume (Chapter 2)). These differences in men's contributions are a frequent topic of conversation in Ache bands (i.e. who is a 'good giver' vs. a 'non-giver').

Despite the observed sharing pattern, we hypothesize that differences in food production *do* represent different levels of parental investment by men in their own offspring. This is because acquirers are acknowledged and known by all members of a band (spot checks asking who killed which game item confirmed this) and some types of associated 'rights to future benefits' may accrue to high food providers, their wives, and children. Specifically, we hypothesize that better hunters receive two types of benefits from the food they give away but never receive in return. The first is better treatment of their wives and children, a form of parental investment. We expected other band members to favor the children of better hunters so that those men would remain in their band and continue sharing food. Visual inspection of census data on band composition through time shows that men (and their families) frequently switch band residence. Benefits to children of a good hunter may take many forms. If, for example, a child of a good hunter becomes ill, band members might be more willing to remain in one location (campsites are generally occupied for only one night) until the child recovers. Other band members might treat children of good hunters better by grooming them, playing with them, carrying them, babysitting them while their mother acquires vegetable resources, etc. People may also be more tolerant of food begging by the children of good hunters, and give them enough extra food to make a difference to their health but not enough to produce a measurable difference with our field methods.

The second benefit likely to accrue to high producing men in a context of band-wide food sharing is an increase in mating opportunities. Since females other than the hunter's spouse also receive a share of the food that each man provides, we expected females to reward better hunters by allowing them more frequent sexual access. This would have the double effect of providing a direct (mating) incentive for a good hunter to remain with the band in which the female resides, and the indirect incentive (his possibility of paternity) for him to continue pro-

viding food for her and her children after the children he could possibly have fathered were born (see Smuts 1985 for similar situation in baboons). In other words, according to this hypothesis, food shared by good hunters with unrelated members of the band represents both parental investment through indirect effects on the survivorship of their 'legitimate' offspring and mating investment through increased access to extramarital sex. Poor hunters (those characterized by lower mean daily meat acquisition) may be willing, in turn, to accept a slightly lower probability of paternity in order to continue receiving a share of the food provided by the better hunter for themselves and their possible offspring.

Available data from 28 men (all men in the sample were observed for more than 220 hunting hours) paired by age and differentiated by hunting ability (mean kilograms meat acquired per hour spent hunting) lend some support to these two hypotheses (see Figure 17.2). Better hunters (those who acquire more meat per hour hunting) have higher survivorship (to age 15) of their reported offspring than do poor hunters (74% $n = 56$, vs. 63% $n = 36$, Wilcoxon signed ranks one-tailed $p = 0.05$). Better hunters are also more frequently reported as lovers in extramarital relationships (25 times vs. 12, χ^2 $p < 0.05$), and have more illegitimate offspring (as acknowledged by women, mean of 1.43 vs. 0.43, Wilcoxon signed ranks one-tailed $p = 0.05$, all results from Kaplan and Hill 1985b). However, some potential problems with the interpretation of these results should be mentioned. First,

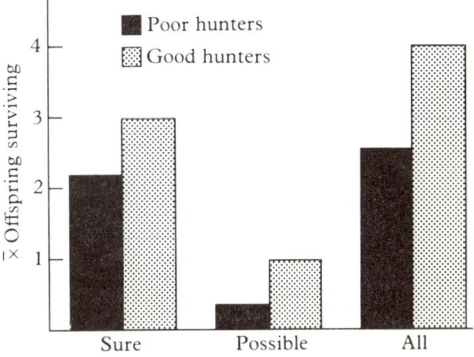

Figure 17.2 Mean number of children surviving to the present for poor and good hunters. For sure children, $p = 0.15$; for possible children and all children, $p = 0.05$. (Adapted from Kaplan and Hill 1985b.)

higher rates of hunting success and higher survivorship of children while positively correlated, may not be causally related. One could easily imagine that any heritable tendency toward better general levels or health or robustness might also result in both better hunters and children who survive at a higher rate. The data necessary to test between these two alternative explanations are difficult to obtain in a natural field setting with a small population. There is also a potential problem with the data on mating access. The numbers of lovers and illegitimate offspring used in this test are determined by women's reports, and thus present a very real possibility of reporting bias. However, we believe it likely that the same factors which would make it more likely for a woman to want to report a man as her lover, also make it more likely that he will in fact be her lover if she has any at all. In addition, possible fathers (i.e. 'illegitimate') of children are often publicly acknowledged and we have never encountered a case where a possible father reported by a woman denied that he had been involved in frequent sexual relations with the mother of a child.

Time spent in food acquisition versus childcare

The above data suggest that male hunting may be considered both mating investment (i.e. an activity leading to more frequent matings with a greater number of females) and parental investment (i.e. provisioning one's own children and the children of others to obtain better treatment of one's offspring). If some hunting time is mating investment, we should find that men with children face a different tradeoff to those without children (because men with children also have the option of direct parental investment). With this in mind, we have developed a simple tradeoff model that may allow for a *post-hoc* understanding of interesting differences in Ache male time allocation.

We propose that the relationship between fitness and cumulative time spent in an activity is of key importance here. If Ache foragers are trying (or designed) to maximize fitness, they should allocate time to those activities which give the highest fitness payoffs. However, the relationship between time investment and fitness for many activities is probably not linear but negatively accelerated (see Figure 17.3). This type of curve is likely to characterize the relationship because, at some point, additional increments of time spent in an activity are unlikely to provide the same fitness benefits as did the initial time increments spent in that activity (hence the curve that describes such a relationship is called a 'diminishing returns curve'). For example, while some amount of time spent hunting, grooming, or doing childcare each day is likely to be important to an individual's fitness, at some point, additional time spent in these activities is unlikely to produce the same fitness rewards as did earlier time increments. Additional food consumed each day beyond some point will not have the same nutritional benefit as did the food consumed earlier in the day when nothing had been eaten. The tenth hour per day spent grooming is unlikely to be as important as the first.

The fact that the fitness benefits associated with different activities are often likely to be characterized by diminishing returns curves suggests that no one activity will continually provide higher fitness rewards than all others. If fitness is to be maximized, Ache men should choose the appropriate mix of time spent in alternative activities on the basis of the relationship between time spent and fitness benefits derived for each activity. This means, however, that the precise amount of time that should be spent in each of an array of potential activities can only be predicted by knowing the shape of the fitness curve that is associated with cumulative time spent in each alternative activity. Unless one can measure the relationship between time spent in an activity and fitness, it is not possible to predict *a priori* whether more or less time should be spent in particular activities, as a function of changing conditions.

For example, since children probably benefit from some amount of direct paternal interaction (teaching, playing, grooming, etc.), men with children must tradeoff those benefits with the benefits associated with spending more time hunting and providing more meat. Men without children do not face this tradeoff and therefore may spend more time acquiring food when all else is equal. This hypothetical interpretation of the tradeoffs faced by Ache men is in agreement with (and partially derived from) Ache data. Amount of time spent hunting is inversely correlated (Pearson $r = -0.35$ $p < 0.01$, from Hill

1983) with the number of dependent children men have on a foraging trip (this is not correlated with age) when hunting ability is controlled for (this is necessary because of the relationship described below). It is important to note however that the opposite prediction could have been just as easily made: men with more children have more need to provide food and would therefore spend greater amounts of time hunting (this might be true if others determined whether to encourage a man to remain in the band on the basis of the *difference* between the amount he provides and the amount his family consumes). Also, if there are forms of mating investment other than hunting, such as returning to camp early and flirting, men without children might quit earlier. This means that the model, while possibly a useful framework for thinking about how time allocation decisions are made if men attempt to maximize fitness, is not useful in its present state for predicting time allocation changes. If, however, our model is correct and Ache men are allocating time to activities in a way which maximizes their fitness, the Ache data suggest that with band-wide food sharing, men without children continue to obtain the greatest benefits from hunting longer than men with children, who benefit most from whatever parental care is provided in camp. This would also seem to suggest that 'family men' exploit the mating investment of single men (whose daily food acquisition is, on average, more than 2000 calories higher than their consumption – Kaplan and Hill 1985a) to support their children. If the model is correct, we should find a *positive* relationship between the number of dependants and a man's hunting effort in societies where food is shared little and there are no alternative avenues for obtaining fitness benefits from the production of surplus food.

In the context of wide-scale food sharing, the tradeoff model of time spent in activities also suggests that men should vary in their relative emphasis on mating versus parental investment depending upon their hunting skill. Although the fitness benefits associated with direct childcare are perhaps equal for all males with the same number and ages of children, the fitness benefits associated with increased investment in hunting should be higher for men who acquire more meat per unit time spent hunting. The reasoning behind this prediction is illustrated in Figures

17.3(a) to (d). Fitness should continue to increase as a function of quantity of meat acquired, since hunters have never been observed to acquire more food than band members consume, and since greater food production by individual hunters is positively associated with number of matings and offspring survivorship (see above). There should be some reward for each additional increment of food provided daily within the range of daily hunting success that characterizes Ache men. On the other hand, as fatigue increases and more total food is available to band members, the value of additional food decreases and the costs of continuing to hunt increase. Thus net benefits (benefits – costs) from time spent hunting begin to diminish (Figure 17.3(a)). Higher hunting return rates result in greater fitness benefits per unit time invested in hunting because the slope of the fitness/time spent hunting curve for good hunters is steeper initially and probably drops off more slowly than would be the case for poor hunters (compare Figures 17.3(a) and (c)). This may lead to the expectation that, under these conditions, better hunters should spend more time hunting than do poor hunters. This expectation is in agreement with available data on Ache men. Time spent hunting by Ache men is positively correlated with hunting return rate (Pearson $r = 0.34$, $p < 0.01$, from Hill 1983). However, this result cannot be considered a test

Figure 17.3 Shaded areas show optimal time allocation for high return and low return hunters with 10 units of available time. Better hunters should spend more time hunting under conditions described in the text.

Optimal time allocation for low return hunter

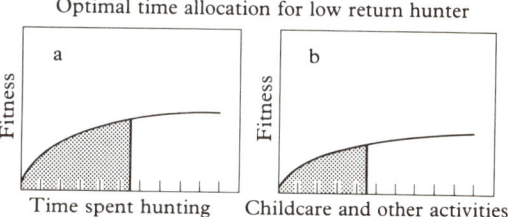

Optimal time allocation for high return hunter

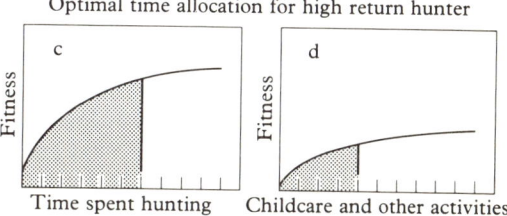

of the model, since the model was partially derived from the available data. Again, one test implication of the model is that the relationship between hunting return rate and time spent hunting should be *negative*, in societies where men can produce more food than their families can consume and sharing is minimal so that surplus food cannot be turned into additional fitness benefits.

Clearly, modelling time allocation is a difficult task because it requires translating the costs and benefits from very different activities into a single currency: effects on fitness. The challenge we face is to develop predictive models that can be tested with empirical data.

Life history strategies – when to mate

There appear to be three principal reproductive options for adolescent Ache males. First, they can attempt to find a suitable spouse and begin to produce their own offspring. Second, they can attempt to mate occasionally with any females in the population that will cooperate. Third, they can remain with their natal families and help raise their younger siblings (with whom they share on average between 25% and 50% of their genes; not all siblings are full siblings because of high rates of divorce and extramarital affairs). This situation, in many respects, appears analogous to the tradeoffs faced by territorial nesting birds (see Emlen 1984 and Brown 1978 for reviews) and some social carnivores (e.g. Moehlman 1983). When available territories for foraging and mating are in short supply, young birds and mammals often do not reproduce until they are large enough to successfully defend a territory. Instead they remain with their parents and help raise their younger siblings. They do so by provisioning them at the nest and by protecting them while their parents forage. This form of behavior, referred to as 'helping at the nest,' is associated with an increase in the number of offspring their parents raise to adulthood (see Emlen 1984 for review) and has been shown to directly result in higher parental reproductive success in one study (Brown and Brown 1982). Although it has not been demonstrated empirically, the data suggest that these young male birds achieve higher fitness by investing in their siblings than by attempting to reproduce on their

own, because establishing a territory is difficult when they must compete with larger full-adult birds. Some human data also suggest that helpers at the nest increase parental reproductive success (see Turke, this volume (Chapter 10)).

Ache males, because they provide most of the food consumed by band members, probably must be able to acquire much more food than they themselves consume before they are desirable as a mate. This is not because of the need for direct provisioning of potential mates and offspring (band-wide sharing takes care of this) but probably instead because of the other band members' treatment of a man's spouse and offspring as a function of the amount of food he produces. Couples who reproduce before they can contribute enough food to the band to compensate for their own consumption may be treated rather poorly. Minimally, men should be able to provision themselves, their spouse, and one offspring before they are considered by females as a desirable mate. Ache data partially support this hypothesis. The two men in our sample of long-term hunting returns (Kaplan and Hill 1985a, table 9) who have never had a spouse during 8 years of observation both produce a mean of over 2000 calories of meat per day *less* than the median daily caloric production of meat from the other 15 adult men on whom we have long-term hunting data and who have been married on and off throughout the observation period ($x = 4568$ cal. meat/day vs. 6970 cal. meat/day; men also produce between 1000 and 4000 cal. honey/day with the same two men probably producing considerably less based on our impressions). The data presented in the next chapter on the effects of paternal mortality on offspring survivorship also suggest that paternal investment is critical to offspring survival, even in the context of band-wide food sharing.

We calculate the daily caloric requirements of adult Ache males and females at 4640 and 2779, respectively (this calculation is a slightly modified version of that published in Hill et al. 1984, using the more accurate time allocation data from Hill et al. 1985 and Hurtado et al. 1985, and separating the costs of lactation from women's daily caloric expenditure). Nursing an infant probably adds another 1000 calories to these requirements (Taylor and Pye 1966). Since males generally provide 87% of the calories consumed by the group, they may have to be able to acquire some 7325 calories per day (4640 + 2779 + 1000 = 8419 × 0.87 = 7325) in order to meet the nuclear family's average consumption level (or more precisely, the level at which the family's contribution to the band equals their food consumption) without placing extra burden on their spouse. This figure is almost twice the amount they need in order to provision themselves. Therefore, during the time period when they can acquire more calories than they themselves consume but when they acquire less calories than are necessary to make them a desirable mate, they might be expected to help provision their parents' offspring. Available data suggest that by the time Ache adolescent males reach the age of 16–17 years of age, they acquire more calories than they themselves consume (Figure 17.4). However, they do not acquire the 7325 calories they need to fully meet the observed levels of consumption for a family of three until they are approximately 19 years of age (this measurement includes males who at this age have not yet acquired spouses, thus the acquisition of a spouse is not responsible for the increased food production). Demographic analyses show that for Ache males, the average age of first marriage is 19.8 years (SD = 1.7, $n = 13$) and of first reproduction is 21.9 years (SD = 4.5, $n = 33$). This is consistent with the expectation that males must acquire enough calories to feed a family before they are desirable mates (it might be argued that males should become desirable

Figure 17.4 Sample sizes, in person days measured, for males and females, respectively, are: 4–5 years 26, 15; 6–7 years 19, 21; 8–9 years 16, 19; 10–11 years 21, 13; 12–13 years 23, 13; 14–15 years 80, 24; 16–17 years 82, 19; 18–19 years 72, 7; 20–21 years 66, 15; 22–23 years 117, 19; 24–25 years 47, 49.

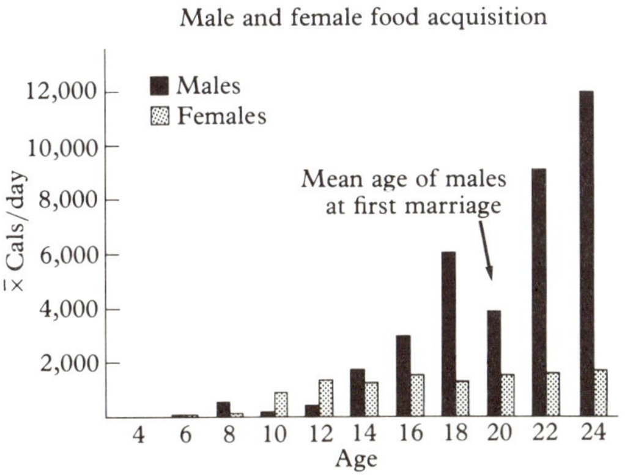

Male and female food acquisition

as mates earlier because of the lag time between marriage and the birth of the first child; however, since, as mentioned above, there are stable long-term differences between men in hunting ability, females may wish to see concrete evidence of a man's hunting ability before choosing him as a mate). It also suggests that when males between 16 and 20 years of age live with their parents, they may indirectly provide food for their siblings and obtain better treatment for their families as well. We might expect that those males who are able to acquire over 7000 calories at a younger age will marry younger than average. Although it is our impression that this is generally the case among the Ache, we do not have enough data on the food production of individual adolescent males to test this hypothesis. Of course, there is also a good chance that adolescent males are using the extra food they provide to acquire certain types of benefits for themselves (especially mating opportunities) and may therefore not be functioning as 'helpers at the nest' even during the period when they cannot acquire their own mate.

If 'helping-at-the-nest' is a behavioral option which adolescent males actively choose, we should find differences between individual males on the basis of their birth order. Those individuals who have fewer younger siblings should leave their natal families earlier in search of a mate (even if their chances of finding one are slight) and thus have higher lifetime reproductive success. In addition, women who give birth to more males or whose first offspring is a male might be expected to have higher reproductive success (in the F1 generation) than those females who produce fewer males or whose first offspring is female. Ache data however do not confirm this prediction. Women who have completed their reproductive careers and whose first surviving offspring is male have fewer offspring who survive to adulthood ($x = 4.6$, $n = 20$) than those women whose first surviving offspring is female ($x = 6.3$, $n = 8$). This difference is significant ($t = 2.27$, $p = 0.03$). However, the correlation between number of children who survive to adulthood and the sex ratio of the first half of the completed family that a woman produces is positive, and not significant (Pearson $r = 0.22$, $p = 0.31$). Although there is some possibility that adolescent males do provide food for their siblings and function as helpers-at-the-nest, the

287

data suggest that the effect on a woman's reproductive success of producing male offspring early in her reproductive career is weak if it exists at all, and may in fact be negative. If first-born female offspring truly result in higher reproductive success for parents, it remains to be determined whether this is due to their own alloparenting efforts, or to the benefits provided by a young wife's husband who may reside matrilocally for some time providing food to the family of his bride.

Summary

Ache males are faced with several tradeoffs as they attempt to pursue a reproductive strategy that will maximize their inclusive fitness. These tradeoffs are examined in this chapter, and the major points raised are:

1. As Ache males reach sexual maturity they are faced with the tradeoff between attempting to reproduce early, but often unsuccessfully, and helping their parents to raise more offspring successfully. Data do not suggest that the presence of adolescent males positively affects the reproduction of their parents relative to parents without adolescent male offspring. This leads us to suggest that adolescent Ache males may primarily expend time and effort trying to acquire matings for themselves.
2. Data suggest that better hunters are able to acquire more matings than poor hunters, and their offspring are characterized by higher survivorship. Data also indicate that better hunters spend more time hunting than do worse hunters. We suggest this is because hunting gives higher fitness payoffs than can be expected from time spent in any other activity. The fact that better hunters acquire more matings, and that their children have higher survivorship may indicate that for Ache males, important fitness benefits can be gained through increased food acquisition, even when most resources are shared evenly among band members.
3. Band-wide food sharing, while probably motivated by the fitness benefits of reduced variance in food intake, can only be fully understood when additional reproductive benefits to high producers are considered.
4. Ache males who have produced offspring are faced with a tradeoff between expending time and resources in parental or mating investment. This tradeoff is probably responsible for the negative correlation between time spent hunting and number of dependants for Ache males.

Acknowledgements

This research was supported by L. S. B. Leakey Foundation grants to Hill and Kaplan, and by NSF grant numbers BNS-8121209, BNS-8309834, and 538228, and by NIH grant number 1-RO HD16221-01A2. We would like to thank Wayne Robbins and Graciela O'Cariz for their help and hospitality in Paraguay. Kristen Hawkes, Ana Hurtado, and Kevin Jones collected some of the reported data and provided useful comments and criticisms. Extremely useful comments were also provided by L. Betzig, M. Borgerhoff Mulder, M. Daly, R. Dunbar, P. Turke, and M. Wison.

References

Axelrod, R. T. and Hamilton, W. D. (1981) The evolution of cooperation. *Science*, **211**, 1390–6.

Bateman, A. J. (1948) Intra-sexual selection in *Drosophila Heredity*, **2**, 349–68.

Brown, J. L. (1978) Avian communal breeding systems. *Annual Review of Ecology and Systematics*, **9**, 123–55.

Brown, J. L. and Brown, E. R. (1982) Helpers: effects of experimental removal on reproductive success. *Science*, **215**, 421–2.

Clutton-Brock, T. H. and Harvey, P. H. (1977) Primate ecology and social organization. *Journal of Zoology*, **183**, 1–39.

Clutton-Brock, T. H., Guinness, F. E. and Albon, S. D. (1982) *The Red Deer: The Behavior and Ecology of the Two Sexes*. Chicago: Chicago University Press.

Dawkins, R. (1976) *The Selfish Gene*. Oxford: Oxford University Press.

Dunbar, R. I. M. (1983) Life history tactics and alternative strategies of reproduction. In *Mate Choice*, ed. P. Bateson, pp. 423–34. Cambridge: Cambridge University Press.

Emlen, S. T. (1984) Cooperative breeding in birds and mammals. In *Behavioral Ecology*, ed. J. R. Krebs and N. B. Davies, pp. 305–39. Sunderland, MA: Sinauer.

Goodman, M. J., Griffin, P. B., Estioko-Griffin, A. A. and Grove, J. S. (1985) The compatibility of hunting and mothering among the Agta hunter-gatherers of the Philippines. *Sex Roles*, **12**(11), 1199–1209.

Hawkes, K., Hill. K. and O'Connell, J. (1982) Why

hunters gather: optimal foraging and the Ache of eastern Paraguay. *American Ethnologist*, 9(2), 379–98.

Hawkes, K., Kaplan, H., Hill, K. and Hurtado, A. M. (1987) Ache at the settlement: contrasts between farming and foraging. *Human Ecology* (in press).

Hill, K. (1982) Hunting and human evolution. *Journal of Human Evolution*, 11, 521–44.

Hill, K. (1983) Adult male subsistence strategies among Ache hunter-gatherers of eastern Paraguay. Ph.D. Dissertation, University of Utah.

Hill, K. and Hawkes, K. (1983) Neotropical hunting among the Ache of eastern Paraguay. In *Adaptive Responses of Native Amazonians*, ed. R. Hames and W. Vickers, pp. 139–88. New York: Academic Press.

Hill, K., Kaplan, H., Hawkes, K. and Hurtado, A. (1984) Seasonal variance in the diet of Ache hunter-gatherers in eastern Paraguay. *Human Ecology*, 12, 145–80.

Hill, K., Kaplan, H., Hawkes, K. and Hurtado, A. (1985) Men's time allocation to subsistence work among the Ache of Eastern Paraguay. *Human Ecology*, 13, 29–47.

Hill, K., Hawkes, K., Kaplan, H. and Hurtado, A. (1987) Foraging decisions among the Ache: new data and analysis. *Ethology and Sociobiology* (in press).

Howell, N. (1979) *Demography of the Dobe !Kung.* New York: Academic Press.

Hrdy, S. B. (1981) *The Woman that Never Evolved.* Cambridge: Harvard University press.

Hurtado, A. (1985) Women's subsistence strategies among Ache hunter-gatherers of eastern Paraguay. Ph.D. Dissertation, University of Utah.

Hurtado, A., Hawkes, K. and Kaplan, H. (1985) Female subsistence strategies among Ache hunter-gatherers of eastern Paraguay. *Human Ecology*, 13, 1–28.

Kaplan, H. (1983) The evolution of food sharing among adult conspecifics: research with Ache hunter-gatherers of eastern Paraguay, Ph.D. Dissertation, University of Utah.

Kaplan, H. and Hill, K. (1985a) Food sharing among Ache foragers: tests of explanatory hypotheses. *Current Anthropology*, 26(2), 223–45.

Kaplan, H. and Hill, K. (1985b) Hunting ability and reproductive success among male Ache foragers. *Current Anthropology*, 26(1), 131–3.

Kaplan, H., Hill, K. and Hurtado, A. (1984) Food sharing among the Ache hunter-gathers of eastern Paraguay. *Current Anthropology*, 25, 113–15.

Moehlman, P. D. (1983) Socioecology of silver backed and golden jackals, *Canis mesomelas* and *C. aureus.* In *Recent Advances in the Study of Mammalian Behavior*, ed. J. F. Eisenberg and D. G. Kleinman. Special Publication Number 7, American Society of Mammalogists.

Murdock, G. P. (1967) *Ethnographic Atlas.* Pittsburgh: University of Pittsburgh Press.

Smuts, B. (1985) *Sex and Friendship in Baboons.* Chicago: Aldine.

Stearns, S. C. (1976) Life history tactics: a review of ideas. *Quarterly Review of Biology*, 51, 3–47.

Taylor, C. and Pye, O. (1966) *The Foundations of Nutrition.* New York: Macmillan.

Trivers, R. L. (1971) The evolution of reciprocal altruism. *Quarterly Review of Biology*, 46, 35–57.

Trivers, R. L. (1972) Parental investment and sexual selection. In *Sexual Selection and the Descent of Man, 1871–1971*, ed. B. Campbell, pp. 136–79. Chicago: Aldine.

Williams, G. C. (1966) *Adaptation and Natural Selection.* Princeton: Princeton University Press.

Wittenberger, J. F. and Tilson, R. L. (1980) The evolution of monogamy: hypotheses and evidence. *Annual Review of Ecology and Systematics*, 11, 197–232.

Wrangham, R. W. (1979a) Sex differences in chimpanzee dispersion. In *The Great Apes: Perspectives in Human Evolution*, ed. D. A. Hamburg and E. R. McGown, pp. 481–9. Menlo Park: Benjamin/Cummings.

Wrangham, R. W. (1979b) On the evolution of ape social systems. *Social Science Information*, 18, 335–68.

Kim Hill[1]
Hillard Kaplan[2]

18

Tradeoffs in male and female reproductive strategies among the Ache: part 2

Introduction

In the previous chapter we presented background information on the types of reproductive decisions that generally face male and female mammals, and human hunter–gatherers in particular. After short sections on the background of the Ache study population and our methods of measurement and analysis we also discussed tradeoffs between parental and mating investment among Ache males. In this chapter we will focus on the reproductive tradeoffs by Ache females, and then go on to examine the areas of likely cooperation between spouses as each sex pursues an optimal reproductive strategy. Finally, we consider conflicts of interest between parents and their offspring, and some of the reproductive conflicts between band members.

Female reproductive tradeoffs among the Ache

Food sharing

Unlike food resources acquired by Ache men, much (30–40%, on average) of the food that

---
[1] Department of Anthropology, Emory University, Atlanta, GA 30322, USA
[2] Department of Anthropology, University of New Mexico, Albuquerque, NM 87131, USA

291

Ache women produce is consumed directly by their own nuclear families (Table 17.1, previous chapter) and is preferentially distributed to them (Kaplan *et al.* 1984) One possible explanation of this finding is that the benefits of reciprocal food sharing are much greater for hunted foods than for collected food resources. Because hunted foods generally come in large packages (a single white-lipped peccary, for example, can provide some 50 000 calories) and because daily hunting returns vary considerably, men, on some days, acquire much more food than their families could consume before it spoils and, on other days, acquire no food at all. Food sharing reduces this variance and the associated food waste, resulting in higher mean daily food consumption per capita (and also higher mean fitness value of the food consumed if the relationship between daily food intake and fitness is characterized by a diminishing returns curve, Kaplan and Hill 1985a). In contrast, the sharing of vegetable items which are often acquired simultaneously by all women in the band and which come in smaller packages, does not increase average available food energy per capita substantially (ibid). Consistent with these results, we also found that average package size (in calories) and daily variability between families in the acquisition of different resources are positively correlated (Pearson $r = 0.74$, $p < 0.001$ and $r = 0.51$ $p < 0.05$, respectively) with the extent to which they are shared (ibid). We suspect that the extreme elaboration of Ache meat sharing relative to other foraging peoples is due to two factors. First, because meat comprises so high a percentage of the diet (about 60%) and because the Ache pattern of meat acquisition is characterized by high day-to-day variance which is not synchronized across hunters (Kaplan and Hill 1985a), the Ache benefit more from the pooling of food resources than would other foragers such as the Dobe !Kung who rely more heavily on a stable plant food base. Second, more than 50% of the meat the capture is acquired with some degree of cooperative effort, and band-wide foraging returns increase as a result (Hill and Hawkes 1983). It seems unlikely to us that Ache men would cooperate in food pursuits if the spoils were not shared afterwards.

Another possible explanation for the difference in food sharing between resource types typically acquired by women and those acquired by men is that women do not benefit from increased access to mates when they share out the food they acquire. In other words, while men may achieve higher fitness by transforming some of the food they provide into extramarital mating through food sharing with other band members, women, whose fitness probably does not increase *directly* as a function of the number of their sexual partners and who need not provision others to find willing extramarital sex partners, benefit more from direct provisioning of their young.

Regardless of which of these (or other possible) explanations accounts for the variation in food sharing, Ache sharing data show that the foods acquired by women have a more direct impact on their own family's food consumption. This difference in food sharing appears to be related to time allocation as well.

Time spent in food acquisition vs childcare

Because men provide most food consumed by the Ache, we expect the fitness payoff curve for time spent in food production by Ache women to drop off quickly and rapidly. Unlike male food acquisition which is directed towards provisioning the entire band, a female's food acquisition probably yields diminishing returns as it approaches the point at which her own family is well fed. However, women with more children should continue to receive fitness from a greater amount of food than those with fewer children, and thus they should spend more time in food acquisition each day before switching to other activities (Hurtado 1985). As we mentioned in the section of men's time allocation, however, this is only expected if the fitness value of time spent in food acquisition increases more as a function of the number of offspring than does the fitness value of time spent in any other alternative activity.

One other important activity is direct childcare. The value of childcare also probably increases as a function of the number of children a woman has. In order to ensure high survivorship, children of all ages probably require some period of time each day which their mothers devote to taking care of their needs to the exclusion (partial or total) of other activities. Thus, women face a tradeoff between time spent caring for children and providing them with food.

The fitness value of time spent in childcare for young children is probably very high because the Ache live in a dangerous environment. Ache children during mobile foraging spend all their time in uncleared or poorly cleared small spaces of dense tropical forest. Micro-organisms cause frequent skin and gut infections, exposure to moisture and cold often results in respiratory infections, poisonous or biting insects are common, snakebites to young children are almost always fatal, and many plants have thorns or spines which when imbedded in the skin may lead to severe infections (Hurtado 1985, Kaplan and Dove 1987).

The effect of these conditions on the value of time spent in intensive childcare is probably greatest for infants. Demographic data suggest that infancy is a dangerous period for Ache children: 37% of all childhood mortality occurs before the age of two ($n = 113$ children who died before 15 years). Moreover, our sample shows 100% mortality ($n = 4$) for children whose mothers die before they reach two years of age (cf. Voland, this volume (Chapter 15)). Not surprisingly, Ache women with an infant spend almost 100% of their time in its presence (Hurtado et al. 1985). However, as children get older, the need for direct care probably diminishes, and the types of care and supervision they require probably become more compatible with simultaneous participation in other activities.

This suggests that the tradeoff between food provisioning and direct intensive supervision should change with the child's age. The presence of older children (who are not yet old enough to acquire much food for themselves) should increase women's time allocation to food acquisition but presence of infants should reduce time spent foraging in favor of direct childcare. Ache data are in agreement with this logic. Women with more weaned dependants (approximately 3 to 8 years of age) produce significantly more calories than women with fewer weaned dependants (Pearson $r = 0.33$, $p = 0.02$, from Hurtado et al. 1985). Mothers with nursing infants spend significantly less time in food acquisition than other mothers currently without nursing infants (women paired by age and number of offspring, data from some women, whose infants were weaned during the field period, were paired against themselves; paired t-test for normalized scores $p < 0.001$, from Hurtado et al. 1985).

When the number of other dependent offspring is controlled for, Ache women who are not currently nursing children ($n = 43$ women, $x = 29$ min/day) spend more than twice as much time exploiting palm products in the forest as do nursing mothers ($n = 33$ women, $x = 10$ min/day, Hurtado 1985). It should be noted again that these data cannot be used to test our predictions from the tradeoffs model because the predictions were partially derived from Ache time allocation data.

The model does, however, generate some expectations about female time allocation tradeoffs in other contexts. The value of food acquisition should be higher in cases in which men provide a lower proportion of the calories eaten by children and when food sharing is less extensive. In such cases, even nursing infants may increase rather than decrease maternal time spent in food acquisition. If a young mother could not count on other individuals to provide the extra food necessary for her to bear the energetic burden of lactation, we might expect her to work more hours with an infant or undergo rapid weight loss (e.g. Whitten 1982). Similarly, factors such as environmental hazards which affect the value of direct childcare for children should also affect time allocation to food production. In less hazardous environments, nursing mothers may be willing to entrust their infant to a less competent caretaker such as an older sibling of the child, and again, infants may increase maternal time allocation to food production. Finally, in cases in which food production is compatible with high quality childcare, the tradeoff may cease to exist.

The scheduling of reproduction and the apportionment of investment

When to reproduce

Although adolescent girls begin menstrual cycling at 14.3 years of age on average (SD = 0.6, $n = 25$), the mean age for females at first birth is 18.5 years (SD = 2.5, $n = 26$). Abstinence cannot account for this period of infertility because most adolescent girls are sexually active (and often married) by the time they reach puberty. Also, since women provide only a small percentage of the calories consumed by their families, it is unlikely that their own food production abilities seriously constrain the timing of their first reproduction. In any case, by age 16 they produce, on average, as many calories per day as do adult women (Figure 17.4, previous chapter). Because females are on average more closely related to their own offspring than to their younger siblings (because they may not share the same father) and because they can exploit their potential husbands' parental investment (Charnov 1981), they should probably begin to reproduce as early as they can do so with a reasonable chance of success, rather than function as 'helpers at the nest' for their parents.

However, since successful reproduction requires that females nourish their offspring both during gestation and then for some period following birth directly through their own energy reserves (i.e. through lactation), females face a tradeoff between early but generally less successful reproduction and later but often more successful reproduction. Other things being equal, the earlier a female reproduces the more offspring she can potentially rear in a lifetime. However, if she begins to reproduce before she has accumulated sufficient fat reserves to nourish a developing offspring, it is probable that the child will not survive and all the energy expended in its production will have been wasted. We hypothesize that Ache adolescent females reproduce as early as they can viably rear an offspring but delay reproduction (presumably, through physiological mechanisms) until they have accumulated sufficient fat reserves to do so (Frisch *et al.* 1971; see also Huss-Ashmore 1980 and Borgerhoff Mulder this volume (Chapter 3)).

Data on female growth and reproduction at the permanent mission settlement offer some preliminary support for the hypothesis that females delay reproduction until they have sufficient fat reserves to sucessfully complete pregnancy and lactation. Just prior to puberty, female weights begin to dramatically increase as does their weight to height ratio. This suggests that they are increasing in body fat during this time period. This spurt of growth continues to early adulthood and ends with first reproduction (see Figure 18.1). Interestingly, the mean age of first reproduction corresponds well to the age at which females achieve the mean weight for adult females in the population (i.e. 18.5 years).

It should be noted that the data do not address the issue of whether females could reach this weight at an earlier age and therefore begin reproduction earlier, and whether there are other factors (acquisition of knowledge, social skills, pelvic development, etc.) that are responsible for the late age of female reproduction.

Interval between births

Demographic data from births in the forest before contact indicate that Ache women living as full-time foragers had a mean interbirth interval of 3.2 years (SD = 1.4, n = 143 closed intervals). Individual intervals, however, range from 1.2 to 9.0 years, and the mean for individual women ranges from 1.9 to 5.0 years. These data raise several questions concerning women's reproductive strategies. Why is the Ache interbirth interval so long, or, alternatively, why is it not longer? What determines the variation between Ache women? Why do some other human groups have much shorter (e.g. the Hutterites, Tietze 1957) or longer (e.g. the !Kung San, Howell 1979) interbirth intervals than do the Ache, and what conditions are likely to shorten or lengthen interbirth intervals?

All organisms face tradeoff between the quantity and quality of offspring produced. More low quality offspring or fewer higher quality offspring can be raised. By shortening birth spacing (or, for other organisms, increasing clutch size)

Figure 18.1 Sample sizes, in individuals weighed, for males and females, respectively are: 0–1 years 7, 13; 2–3 years 12, 9; 4–5 years 14, 7; 6–7 years 10, 7; 8–9 years 6, 5; 10–11 years 4, 5; 12–13 years 5, 9; 14–15 years 10, 8; 16–17 years 7, 6; 18–19 years 9, 2; 20–21 years 7, 1; 22–23 years 8, 4; 24–25 years 12, 7.

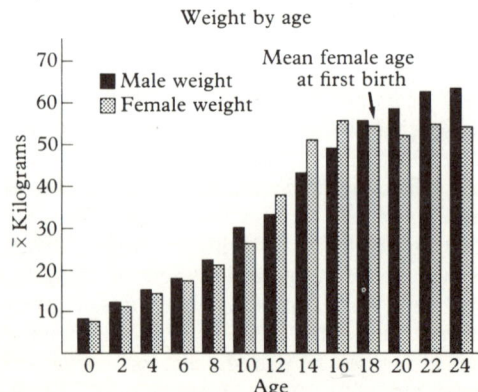

more total offspring can be produced in a lifetime. However, shortened birth spacing can also lead to higher offspring mortality, especially if the amount of food or direct care provided by parents affects survivorship. Human infants are extremely altricial and a long period of learning and growth is necessary before they will be able to successfully reproduce. Therefore, in 'deciding' when and if to produce another child, human females must determine the effects of investing time and energy in an additional offspring on the survivorship and mating success of the ones they already have. These effects should be weighed against the fitness benefits associated with increasing total offspring production (physiological mechanisms might mediate this 'decision' process). In theory, at least, there should be an optimal birth interval which maximizes the production of reproductively viable offspring. The optimal birth interval should occur at the point in which the negative effects associated with the production of an additional offspring are low enough that they are offset by the net fitness increase associated with total offspring output. Blurton Jones (1986) demonstrated that the modal interbirth interval among !Kung women foragers is in fact the one that results in the greatest number of offspring who survive to adulthood. Unfortunately, difficulties with accurately determining the interbirth interval (i.e. to the month) of Ache children who died as infants and are not easily placed in our relative age list (i.e. to determine their age and hence the interval between their birth and that of their next oldest sibling – see methods section) have hampered our attempts to replicate this result with Ache data (this problem arises even when 'replacement' intervals are excluded from the analysis).

In most animal and human contexts, food may be the principal limiter of interbirth intervals and clutch sizes. While time may often be shared between caring for newborn infants and attending to the demands of older children (teaching, grooming, protecting, etc.), food resources are finite and cannot be given to both offspring simultaneously. One offspring's consumption occurs directly at the expense of the other. This means that a female should not conceive until the food supply she can expect in the next time interval is enough to ensure high probability of survivorship for both offspring. For human for-

agers, the best possible guarantee of a sufficient energy supply for an additional offspring is, again, probably body fat reserves (Frisch and McArthur 1974).

If food supply and body fat are the critical limiters of interbirth interval, we should be able to detect a change in mean post-contact interbirth intervals, since weight data show that Ache women have significantly increased in weight over the past 3–5 years ($x = 2.3$ kg weight gain, t-paired test on 17 women, $p < 0.001$, women's weights in 1985 were paired against their weights measured previously). As expected, interbirth interval has decreased significantly since the Ache began to live at the agricultural colony (x pre-contact = 3.2 years, x post-contact = 2.9 years, $t = -1.67$, $p < 0.05$). Of course, there are many other possible interpretations of this result. However, some interpretations can be ruled out. Ache women do not use bottles to feed their children, do not generally wean their offspring until they become pregnant, and infants are carried in a front sling which allows them to suckle at will (cf. Konner and Worthman 1980). This suggests that changes in nursing frequency are probably not important here.

If body fat reserves determine when a woman is likely to successfully reproduce again, we should also expect to find that the offspring of women with low body fat should have lower survivorship than the norm (i.e. when their mothers are matched with other women of the same age and at the same stage in the reproductive cycle). This prediction is supported with Ache data. When women were paired by age, heavier women ($x = 8.9$ kg heavier for 19 randomly age-matched pairs) had significantly higher offspring survivorship (63% vs. 48% survive to 15 years or present, $n = 192$ children, Wilcoxon signed ranks two-tailed $p = 0.04$), and have more current living offspring ($x = 0.89$ more living children, Wilcoxon signed-ranks two-tailed $p = 0.05$). Heavier women were not more likely to be married to high return hunters in this sample, so the effect is not due to the quality of their spouse.

Comparative data on another independent small population of Ache provide some support for the hypotheses that women's fat levels strongly influence their fertility and the mortality of their offspring. We observed an isolated population of Ache foragers on the Ñacunday river in southern Paraguay (see Figure 17.1, previous chapter) during two weeks of 1985. This group first made contact in 1979, and had lived in an area that was diminishing rapidly in size due to hostile Paraguayan colonists. We accompanied the group on one foraging trip out from their mission base, and the production and consumption levels were the lowest we have seen on any Ache foraging trip (data not yet tabulated). In keeping with this, adult members of the population were shorter and considerably lighter than our sample from the northern Ache population. Interestingly, southern women who were shorter ($x = 144$ cm, $n = 10$ vs. $x = 147$ cm, $n = 37$) and lighter (42.8 kg, $n = 13$ vs. 51.9 kg, $n = 37$) than northern Ache women (and had a lower weight/height ratio, $x = 0.30$ vs. 0.35 kg/cm) also had fewer reported live births per post-reproductive women ($x = 4.8$, $n = 22$ vs. $x = 6.75$, $n = 37$) and higher offspring mortality (51% $n = 136$ children born vs. 38% $n = 295$) before age 15. Because the data on the southern group are currently pooled to produce population averages, we cannot test for statistical significance of the differences between the two groups, but the findings are suggestive. The fact that heavier women have significantly higher reproductive success to date both within our northern Ache sample and in the two group comparison agrees well with the generalization among non-human animals that differential nutrition is a major determinant of variation in female fitness (e.g. Wrangham 1979, Clutton-Brock *et al.* 1982, Whitten 1983).

Juvenile sex ratios, and juvenile size differences between the sexes

More than 50 years ago Fisher presented logical arguments to suggest that, in sexually reproducing organisms, parental investment should be allocated equally to both sexes such that an equivalent amount of resources are expended on producing males and females (Fisher 1930). This was later formalized mathematically (Shaw and Mohler 1953, MacArthur 1965). The implication of this theory is that, if males and females are equally costly to raise, equal numbers of both sexes should be produced. If, however, one sex is less costly to raise than the other, more of that sex should be produced (see Charnov 1982 for thorough discussion).

Data from Ache reproductive histories show an *at birth* sex ratio of 116 males to 100 females ($n = 385$ children born). The trend of Ache women to produce more male than female offspring is widespread in the population, and significant (*t*-paired test of males vs. females born to 71 women, two-tailed $p = 0.01$). In addition, Ache boys survive at a higher rate than girls (63% vs. 53% survive to 15 years or present, *t*-paired test of male vs. female survivorship on 69 women, two-tailed $p = 0.04$), and, until they are approximately 12 years of age, boys weigh more than girls of the same age (Figure 18.1). The facts that more Ache males are born, more boys survive and male children are apparently better fed suggest that parents invest more in their male than in their female offspring when they are young. However, because more males are born, the *theory* suggests that, over the *entire* period of parental investment, Ache boys must be cheaper to raise overall than are Ache girls. This means that if parental investment is higher in males than females during early years (more are produced and they survive at higher rate), male offspring must be less costly later on.

Several factors could theoretically lower the cost of males relative to females as they grow older. First, Ache males from the age of 16 onward produce substantially more food than do females (Figure 17.4, previous chapter). Second, there are important differences between males and females in the ages at which they marry and reproduce. Demographic data suggest that Ache males generally marry 6 years later than do Ache females (males $x = 19.8$ years, SD = 1.7, $n = 13$; females $x = 13.6$ years, SD = 0.5, $n = 16$) and mean age at first reproduction is 3.4 years later in males (21.9 years vs. 18.5 years, as reported above). This means that during their first few years of high food production Ache males have no dependants of their own to support. In addition, a much larger percentage of males never marry and reproduce (19% for males, $n = 72$ versus 2% for females, $n = 63$) and can be expected to contribute to their parents and siblings throughout their lifetime (this may be true even for married men because of the sharing pattern and their high levels of food production; i.e. if some sort of credit is given to the families of men for the food they contribute to the band).

The data suggest that Ache parents may generally expect resource *benefits* rather than costs from their male offspring for several years after their female offspring have begun to have children of their own. It is also important to note that a male-biased sex ratio at birth or in census data is commonly reported among mammals and birds that are characterized by high levels of alloparental investment in siblings (helping at the nest). However, the possibility of males being cheaper because of their effectiveness as helpers at the nest is not supported by the analysis presented in the previous chapter. If Ache males were providing food to their parents and siblings before starting their own families, we would expect to find an increase in reproductive success for those women whose first-born offspring were male. As reported in the previous chapter this prediction is not met.

Another factor which might decrease the cost of males over the entire investment period is high male mortality due to warfare. However, we believe this would actually increase the cost of males further because all deaths from warfare ($n = 22$) that we have analyzed took place at an age when males would have been contributing food to their parents and siblings rather than accepting food from their parents.

We have also examined one possible proximate explanation of the male-biased sex ratio at birth. It has been pointed out to us (D. Stephens, pers. comm.) that an increased interbirth interval after male offspring are born, relative to the interbirth interval after female offspring, would lead to a male-biased sex ratio at birth. This possiblity was tested with Ache data, but no difference in the interbirth interval after either sex offspring was discovered (post-male ibi $x = 3.04$ years, post-female ibi $x = 3.12$ years, $t = 0.946$, $p = 0.82$).

Regardless of the proximate mechanism behind the male-biased sex ratio at birth among the Ache, the ultimate cause of the observed sex remains obscure. The possibility of an effect due to the spatial structure of the population (Charnov 1982:67–92) should be examined, as well as the possibility that the results are due to the small sample size (despite the reported significance levels). Comparative research on at-birth sex ratios in different South American populations, testing the predictions of adaptive hypotheses and tracing patterns of genetic relatedness, would help us determine whether such differences are due to ecology, sampling error, or historical factors such as genetic drift. Sex ratios

as high or higher than the one we report here are common in the junior age grades of native South American populations (e.g. Salzano et al. 1967, INDI 1981, Melanconen 1982:82, Hurtado and Hill 1987) and another independent Ache group in southern Paraguay for which we have data also shows a male-biased sex ratio at birth (sex ratio = 120, $n = 119$ births). Particularly notable is the fact that the sex ratio of children between birth and 14 years for all of the native populations in eastern Paraguay combined is male biased (sex ratio = 112, $n = 6057$ children, INDI 1981). The possibility of adaptive sex ratio manipulation implies another reproductive tradeoff to be faced by Ache men and women; namely, how much should they invest in one sex offspring versus the other?

Cooperation and conflict between spouses

Type of parental investment, interbirth interval, and sex ratio

The previous chapter and the earlier part of this one discuss some of the constraints on male and female reproductive behaviors among the Ache and the ways that such constraints present a series of tradeoffs for individuals. The nature of the tradeoffs suggest several areas where spouses should be in agreement and disagreement about how to allocate their time and energy to reproduction. Areas of greatest agreement should be in male and female time allocation to different types of direct parental investment, decisions about interbirth interval, and the apportionment of investment between offspring of different sexes.

Spouses should be in close agreement concerning the amount and type of parental investment to allocate to each of their offspring relative to their other offspring, if the male has 100% confidence in his paternity and has fathered all of the female's offspring. To the extent that this is not the case, however, a male should favor the offspring in which he has highest paternity confidence and attempt to provide that or those offspring with more parental care relative to other offspring than would be ideal from his spouse's viewpoint. Even in the event of a perfect compromise (each spouse adjusts his/her behavior to the fitness interests of the other spouse equally), this means that children living with a father who has low confidence in paternity (especially if it is zero) should suffer higher mortality (cf. Daly and Wilson 1985). This is confirmed by demographic data on the Ache. Children whose reported biological fathers die before they are 15 years old and are raised by other men, have significantly higher mortality than those whose reported biological fathers remain alive and married to their mothers (43.3% of $n = 67$ vs. 19.3% of $n = 171$ die before the age of 15, $\chi^2 = 13.2, p < 0.001$).

Similarly, although the results are not quite statistically significant, children who are raised by women other than their mothers (because their biological mothers die before they are 15 years old) appear to suffer higher mortality than those raised in intact families (36.1% of $n = 61$ vs. 25% of $n = 184$ die before age 15, $\chi^2 = 2.8$, $p = 0.09$). More importantly, 100% ($n = 4$) of the children in our sample, whose mother died when they were under two years of age, also died vs. 33% ($n = 241$) mortality for children whose mothers do not die before they are two years old. Data from cases in which both biological parents survive, but separate from each other before the child reaches the age of 15, are somewhat more equivocal. While children over two years of age seem to suffer no greater mortality if their parents separate (18.9% of $n = 37$ vs. 19.4% of $n = 154$ die before the age of 15), there is a (non-significant) trend towards infants under two years having a higher risk of death if parents separate (27.5% of $n = 29$ vs. 15.9% of $n = 261$ die before age two, Fisher exact test $p = 0.10$). Clearly, it would be of interest here to determine whether children whose divorced parents remain in the same band have higher survivorship than those whose parents reside in different bands, but because of high rates of migration between bands (away, then back again, etc.), this analysis requires more complete data on pre-contact band composition through time than we have yet collected.

These data suggest that there are conflicts of interests between spouses in the apportionment of parental investment when their biological relationships to the children in question differ. They also suggest that, initially, female parental investment is of greater relevance of offspring survival but that, with age, male parental investment becomes increasingly important (cf. Vol-

and, this volume (Chapter 15); also see data on infanticide below).

Fidelity versus promiscuity

An important conflict in parental investment strategies is likely to arise over the use of hidden matings by females as a means to increase total parental investment in their offspring (Hrdy 1981). Our data suggest that the Ache frequently engage in extramarital sexual liaisons. In fact, the Ache recognize three types of fatherhood. One type refers to the man who is married to a woman when her child is born. Another type refers to the man or men with whom she has had extramarital sexual relations just prior to or during her pregnancy. The third type refers to the man who *she* believes actually inseminated her (he can either be her current or ex-husband, or one of her lovers – types 1 or 2). The frequency of extramarital relations is sufficiently high that Ache women report a mean of 2.1 possible fathers for each offspring ($n = 66$ offspring from 17 women).

If men provide parental investment directly in proportion to their confidence in paternity, women can increase total parental investment in their offspring by allowing the total confidence in paternity for all potential fathers to sum to greater than 100%. This is accomplished through the deception of both the legitimate mate and the additional sexual partners into thinking that the number of other potential fathers is fewer than is actually the case (thus increasing each male's confidence in his own paternity). In addition, since Ache men share all meat acquired throughout the band, a woman, by having affairs with good hunters, may convince them to remain in their band, therefore providing more food for her children. Additional 'fathers' may also be especially important to women's fitness in light of the relatively high levels of adult male mortality among the Ache. Children are frequently killed when their fathers die, presumably because other band members do not wish to provision them (see below). Thus, if other men in the band believe that they may be the father of the child in question when his mother's spouse dies, they may be less likely to kill the child.

The price to be paid if extramarital affairs are

discovered, however, can be quite high. When another candidate for the genetic father of a child is suspected, the primary male partner ('legitimate' spouse) may overcompensate in lowering his level of investment in that offspring, leading to less rather than more total parental investment for the child in question. Moreover, women who develop a reputation for engaging in extramarital sex may also have difficulty finding a new mate if they are abandoned by their spouse.

All of this suggests that there is a potential tradeoff between the increased investment in offspring provided by additional possible fathers and the possibility of reduced investment, mate desertion, or even infanticide (a relatively common phenomenon among the Ache) by the woman's legitimate spouse. If this tradeoff does constrain women's reproductive decisions, there should be a predictable pattern concerning which women decide to engage in extramarital affairs and when. First, since we have found that the children of above-average hunters have higher survivorship (presumably due to higher quality male parental investment) than those of poor hunters (Kaplan and Hill 1985b), women married to above-average hunters should be less likely to engage in extramarital affairs. On the other hand, women with low quality mates may gain much more than they lose by giving a higher quality male some confidence in paternity at the expense of their current mate's paternity confidence. Unfortunately, this prediction cannot be tested with currently available Ache data.

Extramarital mating by males is probably also an important source of conflict. The situation, however, is somewhat different. While a female can 'trick' a male into investing in another male's offspring by convincing him that he may be the 'true' father of the child, a male cannot deceive a female into investing in the offspring of another woman. If a male diverts some potential parental investment from his wife's offspring into acquiring additional mating opportunities or investing in children of another woman, this is in direct conflict with the interests of the female spouse (since she obtains no fitness benefits from those matings but pays the cost in terms of reduced investment in her offspring). Diverting parental investment may still be possible in the context of the Ache sharing pattern. If men receive some 'credit' for the food they provide to other band members and if such credit can either be used

to obtain better treatment of his 'legitimate' spouse and offspring, or to acquire mating favors, the use of such credit to obtain mating favors conflicts with the interests of his spouse. For example, other men who learn that they have been 'cuckolded' might no longer wish to motivate the offender to remain in the band, even if he is an excellent hunter, and change their treatment of the offender's spouse and children. It is also possible, however, that the extra matings that a man acquires as a good hunter sharing out more food do not actually cost his wife and offspring directly, but are primarily costly in terms of their implications for spouse switching. This is discussed below.

Male time allocation to hunting is one possible area of conflict here. If some proportion of hunting time is used to acquire additional mating opportunities, women might prefer men to abandon the hunt and to return to camp earlier than the men would wish. This conflict becomes especially likely in view of the difference between the male and female sharing pattern. When men return to camp, women often leave their children in their husband's care and acquire vegetable resources. Since hunted foods are shared throughout the band but collected foods are disproportionately consumed by the collector's family, female food acquisition represents a more direct form of parental investment. Females, then, may attempt to pressure males to return early from hunting, rather than continue to produce food which will be used to acquire additional matings. This potential conflict may be most significant when a woman has several children which she must care for and feed.

Changing spouses

Another important area of conflict between men and women concerns spouse switching. Men and women over 38 years of age report a large number of spouse changes (since the Ache practice no formal marriage rites, we define spouse as an adult partner of a relationship which includes sexual relations and cohabitation for longer than a week; this conforms closely to the Ache definition of spouse, covered by the term, 'breko') in their lifetime ($x = 11.7$ spouses for 15 women, SD = 2.9; $x = 10.8$ spouses for 11 men, SD = 6.1). Both males and females should search for a new spouse when it will result in an increase in their fitness. Again, however, there is a tradeoff involved in spouse switching. When individuals have the opportunity to acquire a higher quality mate (e.g. for males, one which is more fertile, or a better caretaker of children and, for females, a better hunter or one that will invest more in her children), they must calculate the probable losses of parental investment in their current offspring against the potential future gains in fitness with offspring produced by the new mate. In addition, they must also calculate the costs of investing in children from previous marriages if the new mate has already reproduced. This suggests that mate switching after several children are born is more costly and should be less common (however, changes in reproductive value of males and females as they age might lead to the opposite prediction, see below). Ache data are in agreement with this prediction. Men and women show a mean of 7.5 (SD = 4.1) spouse changes before their second child is born and only 3.3 (SD = 3.0) spouse changes after their second child is born (we picked the second child because any short 'fling' can produce one child, but two children generally represents a significant period of cooperative investment by spouses) despite the fact that the later period generally represents more than twice as many years of their reproductive career. This difference is significant ($n = 26$, t-paired $p < 0.01$), but we must be careful in the interpretation of this finding. As reported above, separation of parents after a child reaches the age of two does not lead to increased mortality in our sample. This means that the fitness cost to children of parents who separate may be primarily a decreased probability of finding a mate rather than increased mortality. On the other hand, the sample of children whose parents divorce after they are 2 years old but before they reach the age of 15 is quite small, and a significant effect may be discovered when more cases are coded and included in the sample. A third possibility, however, is that separation of a child's parents in Ache society has no important effect on that child's survival or reproductive success and that the finding we report above is due to another unrelated factor. For example, if time spent together correlates well with compatability between spouses, couples with more children (i.e. those who have spent more time

together would be less likely to separate because the sample represents those couples who are most compatable.

Mate switching probably often involves conflicts of interests between spouses because it is unlikely that both partners simultaneously benefit from it. Spouses who are well matched in quality when they marry may not remain so through time. Reproductive females, as they age, tend to decrease in reproductive value through time because the potential number of additional offspring they can produce decreases as they approach menopause. Ache males from puberty to old age, on the other hand, probably increase and then decrease in reproductive value (as does their food production, Hill and Hawkes 1983, and apparent political power). Also, the availability of alternative mates for both partners changes through time. This suggests that most spouse switches should be initiated by the individual whose value is increasing relative to his/her mate. In addition, if high producing males sometimes decide to switch spouses as a result of extramarital liaisons, those affairs threaten his spouse even if they involve no direct costs to her during their duration (see section on fidelity and promiscuity above). In any case, our informant data suggest that spouses are rarely in agreement about mate switching and that such changes are often actively resisted. For example, females often threaten to let children die if the father abandons them. This is an effective way to escalate the costs of desertion for a male, and frequently results in the father taking custody of the child (33% of the time, $n = 51$) or mortality of infants under two years (27.5% of the time, $n = 29$ vs. 15.9% mortality of 241 children whose parents did not separate).

Parent–child cooperation and conflict in reproduction

As mentioned earlier, it may be in the interests of juvenile males and females to delay costly attempts at reproduction even after the age at which they are physiologically capable of reproducing. During this time period, they can increase their genetic representation in subsequent generations by investing in their younger siblings and continue to acquire the skills and knowledge necessary to ensure successful reproduction. Males may do this through food acquisition and females through caretaking of children.

This form of investment in kin is generally in the interests of their parents and may also be the best strategy for a juvenile to maximize his or her own fitness. However, at some point, the interests of parents and their children should diverge. Adults, on the average, share only one-fourth of their genes with their grandchildren and if they remain capable of continued reproduction are therefore more likely to want their children to invest in siblings rather than beginning their own reproduction (Hamilton 1964). Children, on the other hand, on average share one-half of their genes with their siblings (less in the Ache case where confidence in paternity is well below 100% and divorce is frequent) and with their own offspring, so they should not favor their siblings. Children should therefore decide to invest in siblings or their own offspring based on the relatedness they believe they have to siblings, and the differences in probability of successful reproduction (reproductive potential) between themselves and their parents (ibid). This may be expected to lead to a conflict of interest (Trivers 1974) where parents attempt to discourage their children to marry, even when they are capable of finding a suitable mate. Among the Ache, this may be the case for young males. Several male informants reported that their parents strongly discouraged then from marrying or even carrying on sexual affairs when they were in their late teens and early twenties. Their parents forced them to sleep in the center of the camp where they could be observed easily, and during the day they were encouraged to hunt at the outermost periphery of the hunters in the band, most distant from the women and children. How parents could coerce their sons to cooperate is less than clear however, so it may be that both parents and children are in agreement about this delay in male reproduction (however, several informants strongly insisted otherwise). In any case, if sons decide to invest in siblings or their own offspring based on the reproductive potential of their parents and themselves, we might expect to find sons whose parents are old (and presumably have lower reproductive potential) to marry and reproduce at an earlier age than other males in the population.

It should also be mentioned that this tradeoff between investment in siblings and producing one's own children is likely to be different when both parents invest in offspring (Charnov 1981). Since a man or a woman's investment in his/her own offspring will be augmented by his/her spouse's investment, each unit of investment in one's own offspring has a greater potential fitness payoff than investment in siblings. This favors earlier reproduction in the bi-parental investment case, even from the perspective of the grandparents' interests. Nevertheless, the potential for conflict between parents and their children in the timing is not completely eliminated by this effect.

Reproductive conflict and cooperation between band members

Food sharing and infanticide

Band members who are not closely related to one another cooperate in several ways. Foraging activities are organized so that individuals often sacrifice their own food production to maximize the entire amount of food acquired by the band. Data from cooperative hunts indicate that men reduce the amount of meat they themselves capture by calling other men to the hunting site (Hill and Hawkes 1983). Men also frequently pass by honey and inform other band members of its location so that they can continue hunting and another person can acquire the honey. All of this cooperation occurs in the context of band-wide food sharing (Kaplan et al. 1984).

This pattern of cooperation and food sharing means that all band members contribute to the raising of each other's offspring. Moreover, since food is shared out in proportion to family size (unpublished data), any man with a smaller family pays a disproportionate cost in the raising of children from larger families, if he produces equivalent amounts of food as the men with larger families. The sharing of food should therefore create important conflicts of interests between band members who would prefer to have more food invested in their own offspring rather than in those of others. The existence of conflicts of interest is supported by Ache data on infanticide and child homicide.

For analytical convenience we have divided

infanticide/child homicide into two types (we consider infanticide/child homicide to be any behavior leading to immediate death of a child, such as suffocating, drowning, burying alive, hitting with a club, etc.). The first form generally occurs with children younger than two years of age (6.9% of all children born, $n = 291$). Children in this category are usually killed by their parents because they are considered non-viable. This could be because of illness, deformity, or because the birth spacing between them and their next oldest sibling is too short. In the Ache case, this category may also include infants killed by parents to adjust offspring sex ratio, and those killed by other males to bring a female back into reproductive cycling rapidly (see Hausfater and Hrdy 1984). Unfortunately our current information does not allow us to distinguish which of these various possibilities is most probable in each case. When both parents are involved in the decision however, they are presumably weighing the costs of raising these children against the benefits of raising possibly more viable children in the future. In such cases, there should be few or no conflicts of interest, either between spouses or between band members.

Another type of infanticide/child homicide is quite different, however. This form (2.8% of all children who reach two years of age, $n = 247$) almost invariably occurs after the death of the child's father or his abandonment of the child's mother. The difference in child mortality due to this factor is dramatic in children over two years of age who would normally have a good chance of survival to adulthood. If a child's father lives until the child reaches or would have reached age 15, there is only 0.6% ($n = 181$ children) chance of its being killed after the age of two. If, however, a child's father dies before it reaches or would have reached the age of fifteen, it has a 9.1% ($n = 66$ children) chance of being killed after the age of two (younger children in this category appear to be at higher risk). This difference is statistically significant (Fisher exact $p = 0.002$, $n = 247$ children). Interestingly, for most of these homicides, informants reported that the children were killed *because* their father had died. The mother of the child is never involved in the direct act of killing (unlike the cases of children under age two). However, we cannot determine the extent to which she was opposed to the action. These data suggest that band members do not want to provision the offspring of other men. They do so when those men are alive and are providing food. When those men die, there is no longer any incentive to provision their children.

Conclusions

Much of the analysis and discussion presented in these two chapters is *post hoc* and derived from descriptive data we collected on the Ache. These data, however, allow us to make a variety of explicit predictions about the character of male and female reproductive tradeoffs that can be tested in the future with data from the Ache and other human groups. Several tentative conclusions can be drawn from the available data. First, reproductive decision-making involves tradeoffs between alternative behavioral options. The allocation of time and energy towards, for example, the survivorship of one offspring means that it cannot be allocated to the production or survivorship of other offspring. Early reproduction may increase the total number of offspring an organism can produce but may entail lower survivorship for these offspring. This suggests that in order to predict which of several behavioral options will be favored by natural selection, it is necessary to determine *both* the fitness costs and benefits associated with each of those options. Fitness benefits alone cannot select between alternatives.

Second, the choice of one behavioral alternative rather than others has important implications for the costs and benefits associated with other reproductive decisions. For example, male decisions to invest heavily in offspring affect the costs and benefits associated with mate switching and promiscuity. As investment in children increases, so too do the costs of mate abandonment if one is caught in extramarital liaisons.

Third, the costs and benefits associated with alternative behavioral options can vary as a function of the options chosen by other individuals in the population. For example, the fitness costs and benefits associated with food production and childcare for women vary as a function of male strategies (and vice versa). If males allocate a great deal of time and energy to the acquisition of food resources which they will share, the value (benefits minus costs) of time spent in food production decreases for females, and therefore the relative value of childcare time increases. Similarly, the fitness value to males of time spent in childcare is much lower if females have already chosen a strategy that includes high quality childcare. This means the fitness value to males (both in terms of parental and mating investment) of time allocated in hunting and of food sharing varies as a function of female decisions to allocate time to childcare.

A fourth point which we have not yet addressed explicitly is that the fitness costs and benefits associated with alternative behavioral options are likely to vary as a function of local ecology. Cross-cultural data suggest that not all foraging peoples adopt as strict a sexual divison of labor as do the Ache. !Kung San women, for example, are reported to provide a much greater proportion of the calories their children consume than do Ache women (Lee 1979). !Kung men appear to spend less time hunting and more time in camp than do Ache men (Lee 1979; but see Yellen 1977, Hill 1983 and Draper 1987). We suspect that those differences can be accounted for in terms of the differential distribution of collected versus hunted food items in their respective environments (factors which affect the costs and benefits of time spent hunting versus gathering for men and women), the kinds of environmental hazards to which children are exposed (affecting the value of intensive childcare) and, possibly, the differential costs associated with foraging (see Blurton Jones and Sibly 1978 for a discussion of heat stress and foraging among the !Kung). The principal task faced by anthropologists is to determine the factors which account for those similarities and differences across human groups and across individuals within human populations.

Summary

In this chapter we have examined reproductive tradeoffs faced by women and then discussed the possible areas of cooperation and conflict between spouses, parents and children, and unrelated band members as they pursue their optimal reproductive strategies. Important points raised by Ache data are as follows:

1. Women share food less than men because they cannot gain a fitness advantage by using food to acquire greater numbers of matings. Data show that women adjust the amount of time they spend in food production or childcare as a function of the age and number of children they have. It was suggested that the tradeoff between these two activities favors childcare for infants, because of the danger of the Ache environment, but favors food production when the number of older dependents who must be fed increases.

2. Females face a tradeoff concerning when to first reproduce, and how to time subsequent reproduction. We suggested that both these fertility parameters represent a tradeoff between quality vs. quantity of offspring that can be produced, and we further suggested that body fat is one physiological mechanism involved in 'deciding' this tradeoff. Ache data support the hypothesis that increased body weight has a positive effect on female fertility.

3. Another tradeoff facing Ache females concerns how much and what kinds of resources to partition to producing offspring of the two sexes. It was noted that the at-birth sex ratio is male biased, and males show higher childhood survivorship. The explanation for these observations remains unclear.

4. While some areas of cooperation in the reproductive strategies of spouses may exist, potentially strong conflicts are also likely. Males are expected to be less inclined to invest in offspring who may not be their own. Despite the interests of females to successfully rear such offspring, Ache data show that children who live with step-fathers because their real fathers have died have significantly higher mortality than those children whose fathers are alive.

5. Strong conflicts between spouses are also likely over the females' use of hidden matings to acquire extra parental investment, and the male's diversion of resources to acquire increased numbers of matings.

6. Spouse changes are frequent among the Ache and probably reflect changing assessments of the reproductive value of a current mate.

7. Although both parents and their offspring may increase fitness when the offspring provide alloparental investment in siblings, the tradeoff faced by each party is not equivalent. Because parents are more related to their own children than are grandparents, and because

spouses can exploit an unrelated partner's investment, offspring are likely to want to begin their own reproductive careers before their parents would want them to do so.

8. Because of band-wide food sharing, unrelated band members are unlikely to be favorably disposed to a child whose father has died and is therefore not providing any food. This appears to lead to an increased level of infanticide/homicide on those Ache children whose father have died.

Acknowledgements

This research was supported by L. S. B. Leakey Foundation grants to Hill and Kaplan, and by NSF grant numbers BNS-8121209, BNS-8309834, and 538228, and by NIH grant number 1-RO HD16221-01A2. Wayne Robbins and Graciela O'Cariz provided assistance and hospitality in Paraguay. Kristen Hawkes, Ana Hurtado and Kevin Jones collected some of the reported data and provided useful comments and criticisms. Extremely useful comments were also provided by L. Betzig, M. Borgerhoff Mulder, M. Daly, R. Dunbar, P. Turke and M. Wilson.

References

Blurton Jones, N. (1986) Bushman birth spacing: a test for optimal interbirth interval. *Ethology and Sociobiology*, **7** (2), 91–105.

Blurton Jones, N. and Sibly, R. (1978) Testing adaptiveness of culturally determined behavior: do bushmen women maximize their reproductive success by spacing births widely and foraging seldom? In *Human Adaptation and Behavior*, eds. N. Blurton and V. Reynolds, pp. 135–58. London: Taylor & Francis.

Charnov, E. L. (1981) Kin selection and helpers at the nest: effects of paternity and biparental care. *Animal Behavior*, **29**, 631–2.

Charnov, E. L. (1982) *The Theory of Sex Allocation*. Princeton, Princeton University Press.

Clutton-Brock, T. H. Guinness, F. E. and Albon, S. D. (1982) *The Red Deer: Behavior and Ecology of the Two Sexes*. Chicago: Chicago University Press.

Daly, M. and Wilson, M. (1985) Child abuse and other risks of not living with both parents. *Ethology and Sociobiology*, **6**, 249–62.

Draper, P. (1987) !Kung work: the effects of season, sex, age and number of dependants on adult work effort. *Human Ecology* (in press).

Fisher, R. A. (1930) *The Genetical Theory of Natural Selection*. Oxford University Press.

Frisch, R. and McArthur, J. (1974) Menstrual cycles: fatness as a determinant of minimum weight for height necessary for their maintenance or onset. *Science*, **185**, 949–51.

Frisch, R. E., Revelle, R. and Cook, S. (1971) Height, weight and age at menarche and the 'critical weight' hypothesis. *Science*, **174**, 1148–9.

Hamilton, W. D. (1964) The genetical evolution of social behaviour. Parts 1 and 2. *Journal of Theoretical Biology*, **7**, 1–52.

Hausfater, G. and Hrdy, S. B. (eds.) (1984) *Infanticide: Comparative and Evolutionary Perspectives*. Chicago: Aldine.

Hill, K. (1983) Adult male subsistence strategies among Ache hunter–gatherers of eastern Paraguay. Ph.D. Dissertation, University of Utah.

Hill, K. and Hawkes, K. (1983) Neotropical hunting among the Ache of eastern Paraguay. In *Adaptive Responses of Native Amazonians*, eds. R. Hames and W. Vickers, pp. 139–88. New York: Academic Press.

Howell, N. (1979) *Demography of the Dobe !Kung*. New York: Academic Press.

Hrdy, S. B. (1981) *The Woman that Never Evolved*. Cambridge: Harvard University Press.

Hurtado, A. (1985) Women's subsistence strategies among Ache hunter–gatherers of eastern Paraguay. Ph.D. Dissertation, University of Utah.

Hurtado, A. M. and Hill, K. (1987) Early dry season subsistence ecology of the Cuiva foragers of Venezuela. *Human Ecology* (in press).

Hurtado, A., Hawkes, K., Hill, K. and Kaplan, H. (1985) Female subsistence strategies among Ache hunter–gatherers of eastern Paraguay. *Human Ecology*, **13**, 1–28.

Huss-Ashmore, R. (1980) Fat and fertility: demographic implications of differential fat storage. *Yearbook of Physical Anthropology*, **23**, 65–91.

INDI (1981) *Censo y Estudio de la Poblacion Indigena del Paraquay*. Asuncion, Paraguay: Instituto Paraguayo del Indigena.

Kaplan, H. and Dove, H. (1987) Infant development among the Ache of eastern Paraguay. *Developmental Psychology*, **23**(2); 190–8.

Kaplan, H. and Hill, K. (1985a) Food sharing among Ache foragers: test of explanatory hypotheses. *Current Anthropology*, **26**(2), 223–45.

Kaplan, H. and Hill, K. (1985b) Hunting ability and reproductive success among male Ache foragers. *Current Anthropology*, **26**(1), 131–3.

Kaplan, H., Hill, K., Hawkes, K. and Hurtado, A. (1984) Food sharing among the Ache hunter–gatherers of eastern Paraguay. *Current Anthropology*, **25**, 113–15.

Konner, M. and Worthman, C. (1980) Nursing frequency, gonadal function, and birth spacing among !Kung hunter–gatherers. *Science*, **207**, 788–91.

Lee, R. B. (1979) *The !Kung San: Men, Women and*

Work in a Foraging Society. New York: Cambridge University Press.

MacArthur, R. H. (1965) Ecological consequences of natural selection. In *Theoretical and Mathematical Biology*, eds. T. H. Waterman and H. Morowitz. Blaisdell, NY.

Melanconen, T. (1982) Marriage and reproduction among Yanomamo Indians of Venezuela. Ph.D. Dissertation, Pennsylvania State University.

Salzano, F. M., Neel, J. V. and Maybury-Lewis, D. (1967) Further studies on the Xavante Indians. *American Journal of Human Genetics*, **19**, 463–88.

Shaw, R. F. and Mohler, J. D. (1953) The selective advantage of the sex ratio. *Amererican Naturalist*, **87**, 337–42.

Smuts, B. (1985) *Sex and Friendship in Baboons*. Chicago: Aldine.

Tietze, C. (1957) Reproductive span and rate of reproduction among Hutterite women. *Fertility and Sterility*, **8**, 89–97.

Trivers, R. L. (1974) Parent–offspring conflict. *American Zoologist*, **14**, 249–64.

Whitten, P. L. (1982) Female reproductive strategies among vervet monkeys. Ph.D. Dissertation, Harvard University.

Whitten, P. L. (1983) Diet and dominance among female vervet monkeys (*Cercopithecus aethiops*). *American Journal of Primatology*, **5**, 139–59.

Wrangham, R. W. (1979) On the evolution of ape social systems. *Social Science Information*, **18**, 335–68.

Yellen, J. (1977) *Archeological approaches to the Present: Models for Reconstructing the Past*. New York: Academic Press.

Parental behavior in humans

Introduction

Human beings make numerous decisions throughout their lives which affect their own and their close relatives' reproduction. For example, in many societies, it is common for young adults to face a choice between marriage and child-bearing, on the one hand, and helping parents to raise their younger siblings, on the other hand. Later in life, these same individuals frequently must choose between having more children or devoting all of their effort toward caring for existing children. How much effort and how many resources to devote to sons versus daughters, or to first-born versus late-born children, are other comon choices.

The papers in this volume all deal with the theory that people evolved to make these decisions in ways which maximize the reproduction of their own genes. This evolutionary theory of human behavior does not assume that people consciously pursue replication of their genes. Rather, they pursue shorter-term goals such as getting enough to eat, establishing and maintaining social relations which they find rewarding, seeking sexual satisfaction, taking care of children, and so forth. Somehow, the human nervous and endocrine systems process information

[1] Department of Anthropology, Northwestern University, Evanston, IL 60201, USA

about an individual's environment and life circumstances and translate this into a set of goals, aspirations, interests, feelings, values and so forth. These goals, aspirations, and so on, in turn guide behavior. Selection has shaped human neural and hormonal mechanisms so that people want and seek what best serves the survival of their genes in the particular environments in which they find themselves. This theory can be summarized in technical language as follows: people evolve to maximize their inclusive fitness by tracking both their environment and their own condition and behaving in ways which are adaptive given the information gained.

The papers in Part II of this volume apply this theoretical perspective to parenting in a number of different social settings. They do this by presenting carefully collected and analyzed data aimed at determining how particular behavior affects either reproduction itself or some resource or condition which is conducive to reproduction. All of the papers report high quality research and as a group these papers make a significant increase in the quantity of empirical research on human parenting as a set of evolved reproductive strategies.

Earlier research on parenting as evolved strategies

Only ten or so years ago papers of the sort presented here were virtually non-existent. A recently published review of evolutionary research – Gray's *Primate Sociobiology* (1985) – provides a convenient source from which to gauge the growth of evolutionary research on human social behavior. In going through his bibliography, I count roughly 60 papers which are devoted primarily to empirical work on human behavior as evolved strategies. The present volume by itself, therefore, represents a large quantitative leap in the amount of material treating human behavior as an evolutionary strategy.

Turning more specifically to the subject of parenting, I find only 15 papers in Gray's bibliography which are devoted primarily to evaluating empirically the idea that human parenting

behaviors are inclusive fitness maximizing strategies (Hartung 1976, 1981, 1982, 1985, Dickemann 1979a, 1979b, 1981, Chagnon *et al.*. 1979, Gaulin and Schlegel 1980, Daly and Wilson 1981, 1982, Flinn 1981, Gray and Wolfe 1981, Lenington 1981, Lightcap *et al.* 1982). There are, of course, also a number of primarily theoretical papers or books and a few textbooks which discuss human parenting at some length in evolutionary terms and occasionally include some empirical data aimed at evaluating the theory. Important as these theoretical publications are, without empirical work of the sort reported by the papers reviewed in Gray (1985) and the papers in this volume, no real progress can be made toward understanding human parenting as a set of evolutionary strategies. We need both theory and empirical work as always, but, in my evaluation, at present empirical work is the item in shorter supply and hence in need of emphasis. To be complete, I should also note that several papers of the sort described above have also appeared since Gray's book went to press (Bugos and McCarthy 1984, Daly and Wilson 1984, 1985, Essock-Vitale and McGuire 1985a, 1985b, Borgerhoff Mulder and Milton 1985). Thus roughly 20 papers have appeared in the last decade. Part II of this volume increases the quantity of material by about 40%.

The papers in Part II also make a very significant contribution in at least two other ways: they vastly increase the number of topics researched and they vastly increase the extent to which hypothesis testing is combined with ethnography.

Earlier papers concentrated on a limited range of topics: the Trivers–Willard hypothesis, Alexander's (1974) hypothesis regarding paternity confidence and paternal investment, male-biased inheritance of property, child abuse, infanticide. These papers expand the list of topics researched by adding 'helping at the nest,' grandparenting as an alternative to direct reproduction, careful comparison of evolutionary and alternative microeconomic theory of demography (Turke, Chapter 10), parental manipulation of offspring mate choice (Flinn, Chapter 11), effects of parental investment strategies on social structure, warfare, and colonization (Boone, Chapter 12), effects of presence or absence of husband, and paternity confidence on female reproduction in modern societies, and effects of religion, family size and neurosis on reproduction in modern societies (Essock-Vitale and McGuire, Chapter 13), alloparenting (Hames, Chapter 14), and tradeoffs between mating and parental effort for males (Hames, Hill and Kaplan (Chapters 17 and 18), Turke, Hewlett (Chapter 16)), adjustments of parental investment strategies in response to death of mate and remarriage (Voland, Chapter 15), economic activities as reproductive strategies, body weight and birth intervals, and conflict of interest between spouses (Hill and Kaplan). At the same time, the papers continue to investigate earlier themes: the Trivers–Willard hypothesis (Boone, Voland), paternity confidence (Flinn, Hill and Kaplan), child abuse and infanticide (Voland, Hill and Kaplan) as well as celibacy as an alternative to infanticide (Boone). Thus these papers build well on the earlier literature and at the same time break new ground.

A high proportion of these papers also are products of research which incorporated ethnography in an important way. The later appearance of such research in the literature on parenting as an evolved strategy no doubt is a result of the fact that ethnography is an especially time-consuming form of research. Such research is especially valuable, however, because it allows us to explore more closely the way in which various behaviors are responses to the specific constraints and opportunities of particular local social environments and particular local ecological settings. Examples of this include the following: Turke's elucidation of how a local setting gives females more potential than males as 'helpers at the nest'; Flinn's demonstration of how men's manipulation of their daughters' mate choices is a response to local variation in male reproductive strategies; Hames' relating alloparenting to labor demands; Hewlett's elucidation of intracultural variation in male emphasis on parenting and of the effect of the similarity of male and female movements for economic purposes on male parenting, and Hill and Kaplan's explanation of how wide food sharing by good hunters serves as a mating strategy as well as a form of parental effort. It is true that some of the adjustments to local conditions are not fully demonstrated at present; nevertheless, they serve as examples of what can be done by combining ethnography and evolutionary theory.

A tentative overview of human parenting as evolved strategies

These papers cover a wide enough range of strategies to allow us to begin to sketch out a relatively complete picture of the environmental cues people evolved to be sensitive to and how they respond to these cues. Such an overall picture can be a useful guide to future research even though it is necessarily tentaive. One can summarize the picture that emerges from these papers by thinking of the choices that women and men face as they pass through a relatively typical life history.

Women, it appears, have evolved to be sensitive to opportunities to serve as the equivalent of 'helpers at the nest,' and perhaps to be sensitive to the relative costs in direct reproduction and benefits in indirect reproduction of such helping. Women seem also to be sensitive to whether they have sufficient resources to begin child-bearing and child-rearing. Among the American middle class, presence of a husband and confidence that the husband will recognize the child as his seem to be important cues that resources are available. Absence of these things make a woman much more likely to opt for abortion. Essock-Vitale and McGuire's paper makes this clear. A similar use of husband's absence as a cue to seriously contemplate infanticide has recently been reported (Bugos and McCarthy 1984).

It seems logical that if women have evolved to be sensitive to choices that can increase reproduction of their genes, they would be sensitive as well to loss of resources as a possible cue to begin weighing the advantages of either child abandonment or at least diminished parental effort. Voland's, Boone's, and Hill and Kaplan's papers all give data indicating that this also is true. Some of these data also indicate that parental investment is distributed among children with sensitivity to their reproductive value, and that resources (wealth, presence of a spouse) and status (one's place in a social hierarchy) are taken into account somehow as indicators of how much to invest in a particular child. Sex and parity are characteristics of the child itself that also appear to be taken into account in a salient way.

A similar issue that women must weigh is when to cease having children and, in effect, when to put all of their remaining reproductive efforts into rearing existing children and perhaps aiding in the rearing of grandchildren. Turke's data from Ifaluk indicate neatly that different women will make this choice at different ages and at points at which they have different numbers of children. The data indicate that those who go on bearing children longer do so in response to the presence of daughters as helpers in the task of child-rearing. Essock-Vitale and McGuire's data suggest that the final outcome of this sort of decision-making in the American middle class is a similar scaling of family size to resources in the form of income and number of relatives who might be available for aid. Their data also introduce some other interesting variables which seem to act as similar cues relating to child-bearing: neurosis and religion. That neurosis should be perceived by both a women and her husband as a form of limited resources, or at least as something equivalent to limited resources, is not surprising. Nevertheless, it is interesting to see this expectation borne out. Very little of the literature on human social behavior as evolutionary strategies has paid attention to the idea that people would evaluate their own characteristics as indicators of how to behave. It is good to see attention directed toward this type of variable as a proximate cue. My own impression is that people do evaluate their abilities and adjust their behaviors in important ways in response to what they perceive as 'internal' resources.

The effect of religion on reproduction is also something that is interesting and has not been examined empirically from an evolutionary point of view. No doubt some observers would point out that a high birth rate for Catholics can readily be explained by their church hierarchy's position on birth control and abortion. But this may not be the whole story. Catholic birth rates are not high enough to suggest that all Catholics, or even most, are following strictly the church's proscriptions of most forms of birth control. They, too, are making decisions to limit births, but have somewhat different perceptions of how many children are desirable. It would be interesting to know how much their higher birth rate reflects larger families in the previous generation and hence a perception of more sources of assistance in child-rearing, and whether or not different assumptions about how much one needs to invest in a child (how much one needs to do

in the way, for example, of providing education) are influencing these decisions.

Why Protestants and Jews have more children than secularists is also an interesting question. Could it be that membership of a religious community makes people feel that they have more resources for child-rearing, more willing helpers, in a way similar to the way family size apparently influences perceptions of resources? I am sure other suggestions can be made. Although Essock-Vitale and McGuire's work only begins to look into these issues, the work is important in that it opens questions of this sort.

It is perhaps an incidental irony that the secularists who have the lowest reproductive rate are probably those most likely to take seriously the theory explored by the papers in this book. Thus we have some data to support Alexander's (1979) view that believing in evolutionary theory is a maladaptive trait.

It should perhaps also be noted that closely related to these decisions about parenting are certain decisions concerning mating. Hill and Kaplan suggest that human beings throughout their lives evaluate their mate's appropriateness and the desirability of switching mates. Although this is logically a matter of mating-effort, it is very much tied up with and influenced by parenting. The effect of switching partners on the welfare of children would certainly be an important decision relating to parenting and one which people have probably evolved to make carefully.

The data suggest that men have evolved to make a similar sequence of choices which is somewhat different in the specifics. It is not surprising to discover that, in many societies, young men devote more effort to mating and less to parenting when compared to young women. Men are the sex which, more than women, must compete for mates, and thus must devote more time and resources to mating effort. This naturally limits the time and resources available for parenting. Several of the papers indicate that men, especially younger men, devote more effort to mating and that they must make choices regarding the tradeoffs between mating effort and parental effort. The papers by Turke, Hewlett, Voland, Hill and Kaplan, and Hames all provide data supporting this view. Hewlett's data also contain the interesting suggestion that, in at least some societies, men who are less successful at mating devote more of their time and resources to parenting. Also very fundamental is the fact that eventually most reproductively successful men do parent.

Although men must as a rule devote more effort to mating than women, especially in their younger years, they nevertheless parallel women in facing decisions about when to begin their reproductive careers. In contrast to women, however, the choice is more likely to revolve around whether to gather more resources for mating or whether to acquire a wife and begin expending those resources. For women, the choice is more frequently a choice between initiating child-bearing versus assisting parents in rearing siblings or gathering more resources for child-bearing. The papers by Boone and by Hill and Kaplan both shed light on this aspect of male reproductive strategies.

Despite the greater emphasis on mating at the expense of parenting, men – as noted above – also do parent and face decisions similar to those mentioned above for women. For example, men also appear to have evolved to decide when changing conditions indicate they should abandon a child, or at least diminish their investment in a particular child. Also, they make decisions concerning how to vary parental investment in response to a child's reproductive value as influenced by the child's age, sex, and place in the birth order. Voland and Boone both present data suggesting that men make these decisions in ways which are reproductively advantageous.

Hill and Kaplan's data also suggest that men as much as women must concern themselves throughout life with the possibility of switching mates. No doubt in many societies the choice can also be one of acquiring additional mates rather than switching mates.

Hill and Kaplan's data also explore the conflict of interest between spouses over extramarital sex. Women can use extramarital sex as a means of gaining resources for themselves and their children but must weigh the effect of this on the husband's willingness to invest in their children. Similarly, men can gain reproductive advantages by seeking extramarital liaisons, but in doing so place themselves in conflict with their wives.

The data on male parenting and mating strategies also demonstrate the ways in which the pre-cise nature of male reproductive strategies are adjusted to local conditions both cultural and ecological. For example, Hill and Kaplan demonstrate that sharing the fruits of the hunt equally among band members is a means of gaining mates. Hewlett provides another example by showing how the similarity of male and female movements for resource gathering causes Aka pygmy males to put more effort into parenting than men in societies where resource gathering takes them further away from women in their daily activities.

Flinn's data on daughter guarding begins to explore a male strategy which is probably rare among non-humans. Specifically, this is the strategy of manipulating offspring's mate choices. Judging from the ethnographic record in general, human beings – both male and female – have evolved to take a large interest in their offspring's mate choices and to attempt to have a positive influence on them. It is good to see data detailing how this evolved propensity is expressed in a specific ethnographic setting.

Of course, this overview of human parental strategies will no doubt change in some way and certainly become richer in detail as more research is reported. Nevertheless, it is reasonable to say that we know much more now than we did ten years ago. It is also interesting to note how the empirical work which has appeared since the first theoretical work has shifted the focus of attention. Much of this shift has been, as I see it, to focus more on the subtle ways in which human activities influence fitness; for example, ways in which sharing food leads to mating opportunities, or that older men fighting with younger men enhances their daughters' mate choices.

Issues not explicitly addressed

These papers also raise some issues implicitly which I would like to make more explicit. There are two such issues: quantitative measurement of fitness costs and benefits, and the relationship between social rules and individual strategies.

Inclusive fitness theory states that organisms evolve to choose from among possible courses of action those actions which yield the highest net fitness benefit over a lifetime. To test this rigorously, one needs to measure the quantitative effect of various behaviors on fertility and survivorship. A significant criticism of evolutionary research is that such quantitative measures have by and large not been made (Gray 1985). Instead, the quantitative theory is used to make qualitative predictions: more help to closer kin, etc. Although statistical data are often reported, it is more a matter of demonstrating that a trend is not likely to be a result of sampling error rather than an actual quantitative measure of the fitness costs and fitness benefits.

Some of the papers here come close to estimating actual costs and benefits, and the paper that comes closest is Turke's. In order to demonstrate that young women function as 'helpers at the nest,' he uses his data to estimate the effect on the reproductive success of first-born daughters on their mothers' reproductive success. His estimate suggests that women who enjoy the aid of a first-born daughter have roughly two children more during their later reproductive years, when the daughter is actively helping, than do those who lack such help. At another point, he estimates the effect of sibling number on a daughter's reproductive success. Here the results are ambiguous. Sibling number has a significant negative effect, but younger sibling number has only a statistically insignificant effect. It would be interesting to know whether a larger sample would yield a significant result for the effect of younger siblings. However, if we take the results at face value, daughters helping mothers makes evolutionary sense. The mother gains at no detectable cost to daughter.

Turke then asks why not infanticide. Here his estimates of parents' gain become especially relevant. If successful in having a daughter after eliminating a son, the woman will be closer to the situation of those who have a daughter first. The birth interval after an infanticide would be shorter than after a surviving birth, but nevertheless the mother would be at least a year older and thus not quite in the situation of a mother who has a daughter first. Also, she has only roughly a 50% chance that the next child will be a daughter. Given the estimates we have, she stands a 50% chance of gaining two children, or roughly stands to gain one child by dispatching one child. On the surface, it would seem that the gains and losses cancel one another. However, this is not quite the case. First, if the next child is a daughter, the mother will be a little older when her second child arrives, and

not in the same advantageous position she would have enjoyed if the first-born had been a daughter. Second, her own chance of surviving (and of remaining fertile if she survives) are less than 100%. Thus, given the numbers we have, the best guess is that infanticide would not pay. The absence of infanticide fits theoretical expectations.

Of course, if Turke had set the best possible estimates of fitness costs and benefits as his goal, he would have wanted to estimate confidence intervals for these components of fitness which he has estimated. He might also have wanted to estimate exactly what a woman's life expectancy is (or was in the recent past) at first childbirth. The point I wish to emphasize by pushing his data as far as I can is that he may be much closer to a reasonable estimate of fitness costs and benefits than he thinks. I believe it is time for those like Turke and others who have measured quantitative effects of particular behaviors or circumstances on reproductive success to begin thinking about such estimates.

Some researchers might suggest that, since many of the conditions to which people are responding are evolutionarily novel, we cannot expect adaptiveness; that is, we cannot expect that behavior will be finely tuned to optimal form in terms of quantitative costs and benefits (cf. Symons 1979). In my estimation, it is an open question exactly how capable people are of responding adaptively to the range of environments found in contemporary societies, and in the ethnographic and historical records. It is also a question which can only be answered by measuring the precise fitness costs and benefits of particular behaviors. Thus, measurements of this sort are important even if one expects that, owing to environmental novelty, they will not reveal adaptiveness (Caro and Borgerhoff Mulder 1987). All expectations should be tested empirically.

The relationship between individual strategies and conventional, moral, and jural rules is an interesting question that is not explicitly addressed in most papers. However, Boone does note that primogeniture was created as a new rule among the Portuguese nobility at the point in their history when additional resource acquisition become difficult and equal inheritance threatened to undermine the privileged position of the nobility. In effect, Boone is saying people made up a new rule because they saw it to their advantage to do so (and that the perceived advantage corresponded to their reproductive advantage). Presumably, those who made up the rule and gained by it were the parents of noble families, and those who lost, the young siblings of these families, had insufficient power to resist the establishment of this new rule.

Although Boone does not explore this issue at length, I wish to suggest that he and others with similar data do this so that we can begin to see how new rules and new social systems are generated by individuals' attempting to make the most of changing circumstances. Often this probably means more powerful individuals make the most of a new circumstance at the expense of less powerful individuals.

This is especially important as an issue for several reasons. First, anthropologists have generally not looked at rule changes empirically and have often cultivated the impression that rules somehow are created by a reified culture or society, rather than by the conscious machinations of individuals. Another reason is that some of the more serious misunderstandings of evolutionary interpretations of human behavior rest on the assumption that people are, in effect, uninclined or unable to manipulate, circumvent, and modify rules or that their motivations for doing so cannot be shaped, even in part, by evolved psychological mechanisms as opposed to symbolically transmitted culture (e.g. Sahlins 1976).

What I think is most needed to shed light on this issue is for researchers to keep in mind the issue of how self-interested individuals treat rules – whether it be to try to enforce them, break them, or change them. Attention to exactly how rules are invoked and how people react to their being invoked will, I believe, allow us to see how rules get created, manipulated, used, and modified, and how individuals do these things to achieve proximate goals that make evolutionary sense. I also believe that, although large rapid changes in rules are rare, and therefore hard to observe, the smaller-scale manipulations and modifications that are common and easy to observe will allow us to see how self-interested individuals interact with other self-interested individuals to create, maintain, bend, break, and modify rules as a part of their individual strategies, and how these processes create systems of rules.

Closing comment

Over the last ten to twelve years, a significant amount of empirical research has been reported which allows us to evaluate inclusive fitness theory as a theory of human behavior. It is too early to say, in my opinion, whether the theory in its current form will be as successful a theory of human behavior as it has been as a theory of animal behavior. Nevertheless, the results are positive enough to justify some optimistic statements. Whatever else happens, new data have been uncovered. It is now clear, for example, that variables such as genetic relatedness and reproductive value are important predictors of trends of behavior in a wide range of societies. In fact, we have yet to see a serious empirical test which shows these variables to be irrelevant. The trends in the data are predominantly in the directions predicted by the theory, especially when the predictions are derived by a small number of logical steps and do not involve a large number of problematic assumptions. More rigorous tests will need to be made. These include tests measuring precise costs and benefits, tests measuring the heritability of specific norms of reaction, and tests which carefully clarify the relationship between individual strategies on the one hand, and social rules and cultural traditions on the other hand (cf. Gray 1985). However, even if those more rigorous tests should disconfirm the precise quantitative predictions of inclusive fitness theory, we will still be left with the fact that the theory in its present form uncovered a lot of novel data, data which cannot be found in any introductory anthropology text or any other type of social science text. Thus, the worst future outcome of the sort of work presented here would be that the theory eventually fails, but much new data was uncovered. The best possible outcome would be substantial confirmation of the theory with only minor modification. It is also important to note that the actual outcome will eventually be determined by further pursuit of the lines of research reported here. Whatever happens, the work reported here is bound to be important for the future of the social sciences.

References

Alexander, R. D. (1974) The evolution of social behavior. *Annual Review of Ecology and Systematics*, 5, 325–83.

Alexander, R. D. (1979) *Darwinisn and Human Affairs*. Seattle: University of Washington Press.

Borgerhoff Mulder, M. and Milton, M. (1985) Factors affecting infant care among the Kipsigis. *Journal of Anthropological Research*, **41**, 131–262.

Bugos, P. E. and McCarthy, L. M. (1984) Ayoreo infanticide: a case study. In *Infanticide: Comparative and Evolutionary Perspectives*, ed. G. Hausfater and S. B. Hrdy, pp. 503–20. New York: Aldine.

Caro, T. M. and Borgerhoff Mulder, M. (1987) The problem of adaptation in the study of human behaviour *Ethology and Sociobiology* 8.

Chagnon, N. A., Flinn, M. V., and Melancon, T. F. (1979) Sex-ratio variation among the Yąnomamö indians. In *Evolutionary Biology and Human Social Behavior: Anthropological Perspective*, ed. N. Chagnon and W. Irons, pp. 290–320. North Scituate, MA: Duxbury Press.

Daly, M. and Wilson, M. I. (1981) Abuse and neglect of children in evolutionary perspective. In *Natural Selection and Social Behavior: Recent Research and New Theory*, ed. R. Alexander and D. Tinkle, pp. 405–16. New York: Chiron Press.

Daly, M. and Wilson, M. I. (1982) Whom are newborn babies said to resemble? *Ethology and Sociobiology*, **3**, 69–78.

Daly, M. and Wilson, M. I. (1984) A sociobiological analysis of human infanticide. In *Infanticide: Comparative and Evolutionary Perspectives*, ed. G. Hausfater and S. B. Hrdy, pp. 487–502. New York: Aldine.

Daly, M. and Wilson, M. I. (1985) Child abuse and other risks of not living with both parents. *Ethology and Sociobiology*, **3**, 197–210.

Dickemann, M. (1979a) Female infanticide, reproductive strategies, and social stratification: a preliminary model. In *Evolutionary Biology and Human Social Behavior: An Anthropological Perspective*, ed. N. Chagnon and W. Irons, pp. 321–67. North Scituate, MA: Duxbury Press.

Dickemann, M. (1979b) The ecology of mating systems in hypergynous dowry societies. *Social Science Information*, **18**, 163–95.

Dickemann, M. (1981) Paternal confidence and dowry competition: a biocultural analysis of purdah. In *Natural Selection and Social Behavior: Recent Research and New Theory*, ed. R. Alexander

and D. Tinkle, pp. 417–38. New York: Chiron Press.

Essock-Vitale, S. M. and McGuire, M. T. (1985a) Women's lives viewed from an evolutionary perspective. I. Sexual histories, reproductive success, and demographic characteristics of a random sample of American women. *Ethology and Sociobiology*, **6** (3), 137–54.

Essock-Vitale, S. M. and McGuire, M. T. (1985b) Women's lives viewed from an evolutionary perspective. II. Patterns of helping. *Ethology and Sociobiology*, **6** (3), 155–74.

Flinn, M. (1981) Uterine vs. agnatic kinship variability and associated cousin marriage preferences: an evolutionary biological analysis. In *Natural Selection and Social Behavior: Recent Research and New Theory*, ed. R. Alexander and D. Tinkle, pp. 439–75. New York: Chiron Press.

Gaulin, S. J. C. and Schlegel, A. (1980) Paternal confidence and paternal investment: a cross-cultural test of a sociobiological hypothesis. *Ethology and Sociobiology*, **1**, 301–9.

Gray, J. P. (1985) *Primate Sociobiology*. New Haven, CT: HRAF.

Gray, J. P. and Wolfe, L. D. (1981) Parental certainty, subsistence, and inheritance revisited. *Journal of Human Evolution*, **10**, 277–8.

Hartung, J. (1976) On natural selection and the inheritance of wealth. *Current Anthropology*, **17**, 607–22.

Hartung, J. (1981) Paternity and inheritance of wealth. *Nature*, **291**, 652–4.

Hartung, J. (1982) Polygyny and inheritance of wealth. *Current Anthropology*, **23**, 1–12.

Hartung, J. (1985) Matrilineal inheritance: new theory and analysis. *Behavioral and Brain Sciences*, **8**, 661–88.

Lenington, S. (1981) Child abuse: the limits of sociobiology. *Ethology and Sociobiology*, **2**, 17–29.

Lightcap, J. L., Kurland, J. A., and Burgess, R. L. (1982) Child abuse: a test of some predictions from evolutionary theory. *Ethology and Sociobiology*, **3**, 61–7.

Sahlins, M. (1976) *The Use and Abuse of Biology*. Ann Arbor: The University of Michigan Press.

Symons, D. (1979) *The Evolution of Human Sexuality*. Oxford: Oxford University Press.

Prospects

Evolutionary approaches to human behavior: What does the future hold?

The important predictions in evolutionary biology derive from a concept of adaptation based on a selfish-gene model of natural selection and take this form: given that all organisms throughout their history have been subject to this kind of genetic bookkeeping, any given organism is expected to have certain properties and not have others. The properties are expected to form a closely-optimized strategy for the maximal proliferation of the genes that directed the development of the organism. No compromise with any other goal, like the survival of the species, is expected. Inspection of the organism will disclose whether it does or does not have the predicted properties.

Williams (1985: 12)

In the natural sciences a person is remembered for his best ideas; in the social sciences he is remembered for his worst.

Unknown

Introduction

At a small conference on evolutionary approaches to human behavior, at a midwestern university in 1981, a distinguished social anthropologist addressed himself explicitly to the graduate students in the audience. He advised them not to associate themselves with this 'fad' because, among other things, the anthropology panels of national granting agencies simply would not fund studies in this arena. The same man, although listed as a discussant, acknowledged that he had not attended any of the presentations and had not read any of the manuscripts. Similarly, at a conference that followed publication of George C. Williams' 1966 book, *Adaptation and Natural Selection: A Critique of Some Current Evolutionary Thought*, a distinguished evolutionary biologist proclaimed Williams' volume to be 'a *bad book*!'

Two decades later, the biologist just mentioned would have liked to take credit himself for the basic idea in Williams' book – that natural selection is most effective at lower levels in the hierarchical organization of life. The social anthropologist, however, may not live long enough to experience a similar reversal. Not only is it easier to accept ideas about one's work that originate within one's own discipline, but biolo-

---

[1] Museum of Zoology, University of Michigan, Ann Arbor, MI 48109, USA

gists are not as fearful as are social scientists that theoretical shifts conceal ideological goals or biases, or may promote them incidentally.

The ideas of Williams, and Hamilton's (1964) development of inclusive fitness theory, appeared mainly between 1957 and 1967 (see also Fisher 1958). By 1977, they had transformed evolutionary ecology, behavioral ecology, the study of social behavior, population genetics, and most aspects of evolutionary biology. After 20 years they are so thoroughly imbedded in biology as to be virtually unnoticed aspects of nearly every biologist's basic dogmas.

It will not be the same in the social sciences. In some human-oriented disciplines – such as sociology, economics, and political science – there is still only an occasional enthusiast, viewed by most of his colleagues as a more or less harmless oddity. In psychology there has been a little more activity, and only scattered hostility, the latter possibly because psychologists never thought evolution was very important to them, and still do not.

Anthropology is different. Anthropologists do a lot of describing, and they often do broad-scale comparative studies; so do biologists. Archaeological anthropologists try to reconstruct the long-term past from fragmentary evidence; so do biologists. Biological and physical anthropologists are necessarily concerned with organic or genetic evolution, as are biologists, though organic evolution has never been seen as central theory in anthropology because its relationship to culture has always been vague, and culture is the central theme of the long-term and broad-scale comparative studies of anthropologists.

Anthropologists long ago adopted the basic tenets of organic evolution from the discipline of biology and adapted and emphasized them according to their own needs. Biological anthropologists, for example, teach population genetics, although often with an emphasis on genetic drift that is surprising to biologists – because changes via drift carry little or no implication of better versus worse. The concept of adaptation as reproductive fitness has never been prominent in anthropology.

In social and cultural anthropology the term evolution took on its own special meaning, referring to patterns of cultural change, often without reference to mechanisms, or implications of genetic change. In the last several decades there have been assiduous efforts to steer clear of suggestions that contemporary cultural variations have anything to do with genetic variations among the peoples of the world. I think everyone senses the persisting tendency to turn any such opinions or possibilities to ends deleterious to groups with less power and influence by judging or characterizing them as less 'attractive' or 'inferior.'

In summary, anthropologists have believed that they understand evolution perfectly well, and that they had incorporated it correctly, and as far as they dared, into their discipline. This attitude, and concern about the use of evolution as ideology, have caused a hostility far more powerful and persistent than in most other social sciences, and far exceeding the alarm of those biologists who 20 years ago thought that they understood evolution perfectly well without the ideas developed by Williams and Hamilton. In my opinion, this hostility is a central deterrent to progress in the use of evolutionary theory to advance human self-understanding. Without it, more people in the human-oriented disciplines would be able to incorporate the ideas and findings of evolutionary biology into their thinking in a constructive way, without feeling that they necessarily have to cross an ideological and interdisciplinary fence, or alter their fundamental approach with respect to human behavior.

To the extent that the social sciences are indeed *sciences*, biases, fears, and interdisciplinary competitiveness have the potential for affecting evolutionary approaches to human behavior only on a short-term basis. Even temporary hostility, however, can debilitate the careers of young scientists.

What about the longer term? Can we accelerate the abatement of emotional rejections and unreasoned fears and hostility? If we assume that the hostility will pass, eventually, what then can we expect of the evolutionary approach? What would be the ideal culmination of its application? What is the importance of the papers in this volume? How do they measure up, scientifically? How do they differ from those appearing in earlier, similar volumes? I want to approach these questions by discussing, first, some of the reasons for disagreements and hostility between those utilizing evolutionary approaches and others who operate in the human-oriented disciplines.

20. What does the future hold?

The problem of interdisciplinary differences in goals and methods

Considerable confusion has occurred because the arena of evolution and human behavior, as with the discipline of anthropology, overlaps both science and the humanities. These two aspects of human endeavor differ strikingly in some respects, and when their practitioners argue directly with one another there is special perplexity because each group is unfamiliar with the other's methods and goals.

Scientists typically pursue topics within which there exist cores of factual discoveries – within which statements can be made that approach undeniability. The earth is round; night follows day; three species of American cicadas emerge from the ground every 17 years; secondary sex ratios in most mammals are slightly male-biased; etc. Moreover, the undeniable or factual parts of science are its centerpiece. All scientists work in reference to this centerpiece, theorizing and testing outward from it, and seeking to expand its base by using ideas and speculations and hypotheses to locate new facts. Perhaps because of the preoccupation of science with the undeniable, its method has come to embody the principle of testability or repeatability. The vertebrate paleontologist, George Gaylord Simpson, thus called science a self-correcting method of finding out about the universe.

Scientists, then, seeking to advance their own careers and in competition with one another, engage themselves in stripping away erroneous and imprecise structures, added to the core of factual knowledge by themselves or others, and replacing them with structures that, as they see it, are more nearly correct. They do this by hypothesizing and testing and arguing and criticizing. Because science is not ideal, its practitioners often try as well to dismantle perfectly valid aspects of the perceived factual centerpiece contributed by competitors. In science, though, the requirement of repeatability in method, and the adherence to topics for which undeniability or factuality is possible, mean that such over-zealousness eventually will be exposed – by still other competitors engaged in advancing their own careers. The delay is often extensive, because of either lack of interest or the inertia of power differentials within the political structures of science; but one can be fairly sure that the next generation of scientists, competing among themselves, will locate many of the exaggerations and falsehoods of one's own generation and understand more clearly who got things straight and who did not, and who did it first.

One might say that the method of science, requiring repeatability and preoccupation with facts, amounts to an eventual *forcing* of agreement; anyone who denies established facts will lose his reputation and credibility if he cannot show *scientifically* that he is right – i.e. using means that are themselves repeatable and subject to falsification if that is possible.

Scientists who undertake evolutionary analysis of human behavior tend to suppose that those who approach the same subject from other perspectives – such as philosophy, theology, history, ethics, aesthetics, or other aspects of the humanities – have the same methods and goals as themselves. This is not the case. First, and most important, even though there are undeniable facts in the humanities, they are typically not the centerpiece. Quite the opposite, such disciplines are preoccupied with meaning, or value, and these concepts are interpreted individually – or at least not universally – and therefore lead toward diversity and disagreement rather than universality and undeniability. Practitioners of the humanities are concerned with what literature, art, music, aesthetics, religion – and even ethics and history sometimes – mean to *different* individuals or *different* groups. They are preoccupied with variations in interpretations, which arise out of differences in interests. The sciences literally avoid such topics, and so – at least until recently – have tended to stay out of the business of human behavior, particularly in realms of meaning and value, which are central to human social endeavors.

Whatever bodies of facts do underlie the activities of humanists, they are typically not regarded as the central issue. Even in history, which is often scientific, interpretations based on meanings or values specific to particular groups or individuals may be massively influential. While in science interpretations involving different meanings or values are seen as either irrelevant or as impediments to progress, in the humanities elucidating them may represent the principal goals. One of the reasons is that humans alone, among all of the objects in the universe available for study, change their behavior as a reaction to the *findings* of those analyzing them. Any human who knows this is virtually certain to alter what he says or thinks about human activities so as to cause responses in directions he himself desires; similarly, he may resist statements by others – factual or not – that he believes will alter human activities in ways contrary to his own interests. People are likely to suspect that those who analyze human activities choose their topics and adjust their methods and conclusions – consciously or not – so as to serve their own interests rather than those of others.

Controversies in science typically precede resolutions resulting from new facts or corrections of errors. This is possible because the continuing focus is on locating and establishing undeniable facts. Controversies in the humanities, on the other hand, may be endless because they concern the meaning of particular events or activities to different individuals or groups, whose interests in the matter may always differ.

The central aspect of scientific methodology is repeatability. The methodology of the humanities, on the other hand, may better be described as rhetoric (e.g. Raymond 1982). As a result, humanists who believe that scientists are entering the areas of meaning or value may be defensive, and scientists attacked by humanists may be perplexed or indignant. The humanist may believe that a scientist delving into human activities is trying wrongly to promote as universal some particular meaning, to destroy the notion of meaning or value as subject to interpretation, or to deny the meaning that particular humanist favors. Those with particular political beliefs, who also believe that scientists may be showing, or attempting to show, weaknesses in their ideology, may take up this kind of argument. The scientist attacked for such reasons, and by rhetoric as well, may in his turn see the attack as *ad hominem*, and, using the ethics of his own discipline, may regard it as reprehensible on that account.

Changes in the subject matter of the humanities are not cumulative in the way of changes in science (see also Smith 1984). They are better described as sequential changes in meaning, or in sophistication about meaning. They occur not necessarily because additional knowledge has been gained (even if it has), but because the social–cultural milieu has been altered.

Humanists typically are not chastised for out-and-out *errors* in criticism. What they write is typically not dissected into correct and incorrect aspects – into facts and errors. A competitor in the humanities is someone whose opinions, interpretations, or values differ from one's own. Attacking such a competitor – as, say, in a critique of a contribution to literature – is more likely to mean trying to destroy his credibility so that your own view will prevail. There may be no factual basis or criterion of repeatability to make one person wrong, another right. One wishes to substitute one's own interpretations, and one is also less likely to parade any core of accuracy that might exist in the other's viewpoint so as to build from it a cumulatively expanding factual structure. Humanists' careers are not so much ruined by errors, or even by evidence of deliberate misleading, as by having what they say be regarded as trivial or ridiculous, or irrelevant to most peoples' interests.

The critic or competitor, among humanists, packages the ideas of his competitors so they can be attacked as a unit, and in this and other ways personalizes his attack. Thus, he may speak of the 'programs' of particular individuals, or label endeavors headed by one or a few individuals and then set out to destroy the entire package so identified, in order to substitute his own, or just to show his devastating ability to identify triviality and explain generality in meaning. Because so much in the humanities depends on personal interpretations, the prestige that comes from this kind of demonstration is likely to be useful in the future. The method of destruction of a competitor's work or ideas, rather than including locating a core of 'truth' or correctness and building from it, is likely to involve identifying the weakest parts of the opponent's arguments and using them to argue that the entire package is useless. Leon Kamin, a social psychologist at Princeton, for example, writes in *Psychology Today* (1985) that the philosopher Philip Kitcher (1985), in his attack on Edward O. Wilson's 'early program,' 'Lumsden and Wilson's program,' 'Alexander's program,' and 'pop [read human] sociobiology' in general has shown, as Kitcher also claims, that 'the ladder of sociobiology is rotten at every rung.' Kitcher's methodology often fits the description of the humanist's approach given here as, for example, when he selects what he sees as the weakest 2 or 3 of a list of 25 predictions from Alexander's (1979) book and suggests that their weakness destroys not only all the others as well but the entire idea from which they arise. A scientist's approach would be to see, first, whether all of the predictions indeed arose from the same theory, then locate the strongest and 'riskiest' predictions and test them. As these were confirmed or rejected he might go on to test still others, but at some point in the procedure he would regard the underlying theory as provisionally either correct or incorrect. The weakest predictions would be of least, not most, interest to him. The reason is that the scientist is typically not *simply* trying to destroy the credibility of his competitor, or to use him to parade his own devastating wit or critical ability (although scientists often try to do these things along the way), but to get to the next line of investigation – to identify the next crucial hypothesis and test it (and to receive the credit due him for such accomplishments). Kitcher makes little effort to provide alternative theory, but in the spirit of the humanities simply criticizes.

One of the more interesting aspects of the current debate on the border between the sciences and the humanities, with evolutionary biologists on the 'science' side, is that a small group of scientists in acknowledged political agreement (Marxist) have adopted both the methodology and the language of the humanists. They attack the 'adaptationist's program' not by describing its strongest arguments and adjusting or building from them but by repeating its *weakest* supposed examples and tenets, always linked to the same people, whose names also label the 'programs' being attacked. Writings by others using the same theories – sometimes less assailable, and often less well publicized outside biology – are usually omitted entirely. This tactic appears as an extension of the idea of attacking the weakest arguments of a single author: Attack only the most vulnerable statements or works of the best publicized authors in a field easily represented as a package ('sociobiology') and imply by extension that everything else in the 'field' is wrong too. Let the everything elses remain unnoticed, if possible. It is ironic that Wilson's (1975) effort to promote the study of social behavior from an evolutionary viewpoint by calling it 'sociobiology,' and to promote his own views as the core of the 'discipline,' provided such critics

with the ready-made, personalized package they needed. It is also ironic that Segerstrale (1986), in what she calls an ' "in vivo" analysis of the sociobiology controversy,' becomes so embroiled in the opinions and reciprocal attacks of Wilson and Lewontin that she fails to cite a single one of the three authors (Hamilton 1964, Williams 1966, Trivers 1971) who provided the theoretical advances responsible for Wilson's (1975) book, hence the entire 'controversy.'

The problem of motivation

One of the reasons humanists and other non-biologists resent probes by evolutionary biologists into human activities may be a feeling that by seeking generalities, or universals, biologists either detract from the humanists' central topics of meaning and value, with their flavor of diversity in interpretation, or else imply that any and all variations depend on genetic variation. Additionally, to ascribe universal goals to life effort, even in historical (evolutionary) terms, may imply things about motivation and consciousness, as well as about individual differences, that seem unacceptable to a humanist (or anyone!). Thus, to speak of a tendency or propensity produced by natural selection, or a lifetime shaped by evolution, seems to many to be genetic determinism that erases notions of free will, choice, and plasticity in behavior. To some it seems to justify evil or selfish acts as genetically determined or developmentally inescapable. This kind of skepticism leads such critics to deny even the possibility of an evolved human nature.

The concept of morality, which seems always to involve a core of mystery, can be used to illustrate this problem. Because morality involves conflicts of interest, it cannot easily be generalized into a universal despite virtually continual efforts by utilitarian philosophers to do that; morality does not derive its meaning from sets of universals or undeniable facts (Alexander 1987). A second, and considerably more troublesome source of mystery involves the question of motivation, hence consciousness or deliberateness. To serve one's own interests incidentally, or thwart those of another inadvertently, may not be judged immoral; to do either deliberately is likely to be so judged.

For example, the results of Buss (1985, 1987) suggest that human females are more concerned about the resources a potential mate controls than are males, while males are more concerned about various aspects of physical appearance and health in potential mates than are females. So long as such differences seem to depend on attitudes that are more or less unconscious and unfocused we view them with interest, and perhaps amusement. A little transformation into the conscious and deliberate, however, creates the images of 'golddigger' and 'male chauvinist.' In a sense those with an evolutionary approach, attempting to determine and bring into our conscious understanding the 'ultimate' goals of human lifetimes and their social activities, are threatening to turn something regarded as moral into something immoral; they threaten by suggesting that the forces which molded humans from non-humans would have caused us to be immoral if we had understood them all along. Such a change may well be seen as justifying immorality, or at least modelling humans as immoral, thus leaving us in painful doubt and thwarting manipulations toward greater group-cooperativeness that explicitly portray us as basically moral and unselfish.

Any vagueness, then, about the concept of 'motivation' in a discussion of morality as an evolved phenomenon is likely to be used by critics to support either accusations of genetic determinism or acceptance of immoral behavior as biological law. Unfortunately, such vagueness is likely to be present for a long time in efforts to explain how lifetimes (hence, somehow, motivation, consciousness, conscience, and all the rest) have been designed by evolution, whether or not the explainers are guilty of such implications (Alexander 1985, 1987).

This excursion, contrasting science and the humanities, is particularly relevant because most of the papers in this volume were written by anthropologists who regard themselves as scientists. But the members of the American Anthropological Assocation, at least, have long debated whether to call themselves scientists or humanists; and I suspect that much of the criticism of this volume will come from those who count themselves among the latter.

Is the evolutionary approach appropriate?

A particularly interesting case of resistance to evolutionary analyses of human behavior – perhaps including some confusion over the issues just discussed – is that of the evolutionary biologist, John Maynard Smith (1983, 1984, 1985). His (1985) review of the philosopher Philip Kitcher's (1985) critique of 'pop sociobiology' is instructive, and I will discuss both publications in some detail here.

Maynard Smith begins his review by referring (as did Kitcher) to 'efforts to apply biology to human affairs ... [that] ended up as justifications for racial, sexual, and class inequalities.' He says that Kitcher's and his own experiences have '... left us cautious about proposals to use biological theory to plan human institutions.' He adds that Kitcher is '... unsympathetic to the claim that evolutionary biology can guide political judgment ...' He suspects that Kitcher was 'unsympathetic before he started work on this book.' So do I. But this introduction is chaff thrown in the eyes of the reader: None of the three 'programs' Kitcher undertakes to demolish ventures into the realms whose history supposedly leave both Maynard Smith and Kitcher filled with trepidations, and neither Maynard Smith nor Kitcher has been able to accuse them of such. As with similar dire warnings by Gould and Lewontin (1979), Lewontin (1979), Kamin (1985), Lewontin et al. (1985), and other 'anti-sociobiologists,' this is a warmup to make the reader think he is about to hear something he is in fact not going to hear. All of this misleading nonsense uses the word 'biology' to mean 'genetic' or at least 'physiological,' rather than 'the discipline which studies life,' its virtually universal meaning outside philosophy and medicine and a few other disciplines (Alexander 1987). This particular brand of anti-sociobiology begins by trying to link modern evolutionary biologists either to 19th century racism or to more recent efforts to show that IQ differences are genetic, or both. No doubt Maynard Smith is correct when he says that 'Prejudices are inevitable.' But particular ways of using them are not therefore justified.

Maynard Smith assures us that Kitcher is authoritative and on the mark (at the end he will conclude that 'This is an admirable book') by telling us that 'Unlike some other authors he has undertaken a genuine study. He does understand the ideas he is criticizing. He has the biological background ... and the mathematical ability ... [and] above all he presents sociobiology in its strongest and most coherent form …' Maynard Smith may be less convinced on the middle two points than he wishes us to believe, however, as he uses about 25% of his space to show that two of Kitcher's basic arguments are off-target: that hybrid inferiority and lowering of mean group fitness are principal reasons for the absence of optimality in evolutionary adaptation. The idea is to denigrate modern evolutionary approaches to adaptation. Maynard Smith notes that hybrid inferiority can scarcely explain absence of optimality in long and complexly-evolved traits involving many loci. He also points out that modern evolutionary biologists do not spend much time on the concept of mean group fitness. He could have mentioned that the people Kitcher attacks were in the first wave of those who adopted Williams' (1966) suggestion that adaptation is just better versus worse in the immediate situation. As Maynard Smith suggests, the investigators Kitcher attacks were also among the first to realize that mean group fitness is essentially an artifact of the arithmetic of population genetics, which for decades aided and abetted the misleading notion that selection acts primarily at the group level, despite Fisher's (1958) admonition that this was not what he was talking about in 1930.

Williams (1966) and Hamilton (1964) generated the entire approach that Kitcher criticizes, and a lack of potency in group selection was a fundamental assumption in that approach from the beginning. The idea of mean group fitness was for 30 or 40 years a source of considerable confusion to even the most astute biologists, and it is ironic that many people who think that evolutionary biology is not on solid ground until it is entirely underlaid with mathematical formulae still fail to realize that errors of this size and significance can appear and be perpetuated *because* of particular ways that mathematics may be used in biology. The mean fitness error gave rise to a misuse of the term 'genetic load' and led to what was called 'Haldane's Dilemma,' after an error of Maynard Smith's early mentor, the distinguished mathematical biologist, J. B. S. Haldane (see Brues 1964, 1969, Wallace 1968). The error arose (at least in part) because of the necessity (in mathematical equations) of assuming that the better genotype in a selective process always has a fitness of 1.0, the less fit

genotype some fraction of this number. This necessity exists because otherwise numerical indicators of fitness will climb, causing equations dealing with selection to become impractical. Thus Haldane concluded that rapid evolution was too costly to occur – that it would lead to the extinction of whole populations. This result derived because introduction of beneficial mutants, at first rare, seemed to lower the 'mean fitness' of the population. Try it: multiply the fitness of a new mutant – 1.0 if it is beneficial – times the number of its copies and the fitness of the old allele being replaced (<1.0) times the number of its copies. You will see that the more beneficial the new allele is, and the rarer it is, the lower will be the mean fitness of the population after it is introduced. Now do the exercise with *several* beneficial new mutants, and you will understand Haldane's dilemma, and why Muller's (1950) concept of the 'genetic load' of mutants became perverted to include even beneficial alleles. Alice Brues (1964) first made this error plain and noted that, in this sense, evolving can never be more costly than not evolving.

At the end of his criticisms on these points Maynard Smith insists that Kitcher 'understands very well.' One wonders how he could tell. And one is again reminded of the old system, in natural history, of first establishing the authority of the person whose anecdotes you are about to espouse as the God's truth (Schneirla 1950). Maynard Smith is about to tell us that Kitcher's criticisms of those evolutionary biologists dealing with humans are on target – because, as Maynard Smith has repeatedly suggested in earlier papers (and to me personally), he cannot see how to explain humanity using evolutionary principles.

Maynard Smith and Kitcher both strongly support the evolutionary study of non-human organisms, and have virtually no criticisms of it. This is a kind of study that Maynard Smith himself has pursued for decades – in ways that Kitcher obviously approves of as much as Maynard Smith approves of Kitcher's criticisms of others. But both draw the line at applying the same approach to humans. Maynard Smith agrees that 'Man is an animal and has evolved by the same processes as other animals.' He says that 'The debate is between those who, while accepting that man is an animal, argue that he is such a peculiar animal that evolutionary biology can have little to say about his social behavior ...' and those who think 'the study of human societies, just as of ant societies, must be rooted in biology.' The inclusion of 'just as of ant societies' in this statement is more chaff, designed to imply that anyone who thinks that humans can be analyzed using an evolutionary approach also thinks that humans are really just like ants. The use of 'biology' and 'rooted in biology' causes the reader to concentrate on 'genetic' rather than 'evolutionary.' The question is: If Kitcher and Maynard Smith think humans are exempt from an evolutionary approach because the species is so 'peculiar,' then what alternative would they suggest? Can they possibly believe that human social behavior – in all its peculiarity and uniqueness – came about as a result of forces alternative to evolution? What forces? How do any such forces *relate* to the evolution that produced humans? What approaches are permissible, and how do we decide? And since every species, not merely the human one, is unique, might not other species be so 'peculiar' as to be inaccessible via approaches that include the principles of organic evolution? If so, which ones, and how do we tell? (The British ecologist, David Lack, would have agreed with Kitcher and Maynard Smith, but as a devout Christian he had a ready alternative, and he invoked it – Lack 1965). I am particularly surprised at Maynard Smith here, because, in 1983, he reiterated (without reference) Conant's (1951) assertion that, in science, 'a theory is only overthrown by better theory, never merely by contradictory facts.' What is the theory alternative to an organic evolution guided chiefly by natural selection that might explain the peculiar human species? What theory does Kitcher (or any one else?) erect to replace an evolution guided largely by natural selection (see also Maynard Smith 1983, Williams 1985). (In the Maynard Smith article I cite here, it is his intent to demonstrate that evolution is guided chiefly by natural selection.) Is it some political prescription?

Maynard Smith agrees with Kitcher (and so do I) that there is 'no special underlying theory ... no autonomous theory of the evolution of behaviour' – no need, one assumes they are both implying, for the term 'sociobiology.' While Maynard Smith allows that he does not like Kitcher's phrase 'pop sociobiology,' he does see the need for a label 'for the application of sociobiology to human beings, and I have no better one to offer.' One wonders not only why we need a special term for using evolution to study human behavior if we do not need one for using it to study the behavior of all other organisms, but also how obvious alternatives like 'human sociobiology' slipped past Maynard Smith, especially since he came so close to saying that particular one. But this would not be a derogatory term, and Kitcher's enterprise (or, as he and other philosophers – and Lewontin and Gould now, who have adopted such language – would term it, his 'program') seems to be to find weak spots in the evolutionary approach to human behavior and from them extrapolate (or try to get the reader to extrapolate) that the whole approach is useless, and even pernicious.

Although Maynard Smith concurs with the term 'pop sociobiology,' he argues that certain of the uses to which Kitcher puts it are 'unfair.' One senses that the scientist in Maynard Smith emerged at that point, causing uneasiness with an approach he had not yet quite put into perspective. Yet, he also makes the (to me) incredibly sweeping statement that he finds Edward O. Wilson's arguments 'generally ill-formulated and empty of content.'

But Maynard Smith is not quite through yet with the human (pop) sociobiologists. He appears to question the assumption of an 'unconscious relationship-calculator and fitness-maximizer influencing our conscious actions.' He actually lays the questioning on Kitcher and says that 'If I were Alexander [and were confronted with this questioning], I would reply that, if the claim is true, then it is up to psychologists to discover the mechanism.' But Maynard Smith's apparent reluctance in regard to such mechanisms – if I am correct in reading such a reluctance out of his statements here and elsewhere – is almost beyond credibility. All of his own work – for example, on evolutionarily stable strategies – demands the assumption of just such calculators in every species right across the animal and plant kingdoms. Apparently, Maynard Smith believes either that (1) any such calculators in humans would have to be conscious (since *some* things are conscious), and thus obvious, or that (2) humans either lost the ability to act reproductively or never possessed it. He says that the claim that 'people behave so as to maximize their inclusive fitness . . . is probably false,' and that he finds it 'hard to believe' that the things that '. . . sociobiologists . . . say . . . about real societies . . . are right.'

Kitcher contends that 'folk psychology' is a better predictor of human behavior than evolutionary theories based on inclusive-fitness-maximizing. He does not take up the question why it should be so. Nor does Maynard Smith, apparently, see any connection between this exercise of Kitcher's and his own rejection of the idea of sophisticated reproductive cost–benefit assessment by humans. I suggest that Kitcher's 'folk psychology' (which Betzig, pers. comm., describes as 'Kitcher's intuition') works as well as it does *because* humans have evolved to be reproductive cost–benefit analyzers. But conscious application of evolutionary hypotheses does better most of the time. Moreover, as those with evolutionary approaches refine their knowledge and their science, their hypotheses will improve in relation to 'folk psychology.'

No one doubts that rapid and dramatic technological and social changes cause humans to make many and important 'evolutionary mistakes' – i.e. to fail to maximize their inclusive fitness because the environment is novel. But this is a far cry from assuming that they are not *evolved* to maximize fitness, as evolutionary biologists claim. All through history non-human organisms have made the kinds of mistakes that Maynard Smith implies exempt humans from the evolutionary approach.

Some of the resistance to evolutionary approaches must represent honest fear of the effects of mistakes. Fear of mistakes, however, must associate with *all imperfect* efforts, and certainly all efforts to understand humans – not just those of evolutionary biologists – involve mistakes that have to be corrected. But I cannot agree with those who assert that evolutionists are *less* scientific than their predecessors in the social sciences. We are all being exhorted (appropriately) to develop testable hypotheses and test them, but the truth is that hypotheses of any shape or form – and testable hypotheses *a fortiori* – have always been virtually absent from some of the very subdisciplines of the social sciences from which the admonitions are coming. I return to this question later.

A third source of reticence, not to be taken lightly, is conflict with an accepted ideology.

Perhaps all three sources of reservations exist in all people, one more important in some, another in others. One can only hope that they will all be diminished, dissipated, or used constructively, as our ability to incorporate evolutionary theory in the quest for self-understanding grows.

The infanticide controversy

Kitcher (1985) also criticizes Dickemann's (1979) analysis of infanticide. His argument is basically that of Harris (1979), though he does not cite Harris: 'Strictly speaking . . . daughters are an *economic* loss. How this translates into the "currency" of reproduction is a matter for investigation . . .' (p. 316). 'Whether female infanticide is a strategy that maximizes inclusive fitness for upper-class parents is an entirely open question' (p. 326). Kitcher's ultimate conclusion is the same as that of Harris '. . . the long-term interests of the genes are being sacrificed in the cause of status, influence, and perhaps money in the immediate future.' His view is that 'greed' runs the system, and that greed need not have anything to do with reproduction. (This view denies the significance of evolution but provides no workable or complete alternative theory.)

Like Dickemann and Harris, Kitcher suggests that high-ranking families use sons to consolidate and maintain their wealth and rank. No one has doubted this. In Dickemann's model this leads to more descendants, also of high rank and great wealth, via male offspring. Harris and Kitcher deny that there is any reason for expecting wealth and rank to be related to reproduction.

Kitcher discusses what he calls 'details' that cause it to be 'very difficult to discover an analysis that yields anything like Dickemann's conclusions.' Kitcher's 'details' seem to me to be entirely inadequate to the task he assigns them. First, he asserts that '*If nothing else changes* . . .' parents who kill their daughters decrease the total number of their offspring. Later he acknowledges that something does change – namely, women relieved of nursing ovulate sooner. This fact diminishes his point, but he tries to reinflate it by asking why women in Asia do not employ wet-nurses, as they did in Victorian England. By implication they were not trying to maximize reproductive success in the first place. Here he bypasses a traditional form of parsimony. Evolution of both genes and culture proceeds not from nothingness but from last year's model (some modern authors have started calling this 'phylogenetic inertia'). One cannot expect the best strategy imaginable to be in place for every organism everywhere. As Dawkins (1976) put it, no one expects pigs to have wings, even if they would be useful now and then (a main reason is that the stages required to get there may not themselves be adaptive). Moreover, wet-nurses are not likely to be free of charge, so Kitcher also cannot ignore the expense of providing them for daughters. The fact is that in these societies daughters are costly to high-ranking families in multiple ways, and they interfere with the production of sons. As far as I can see, no one had discredited this proposition.

Kitcher seems in this instance to have missed the significance of his own admonition (p. 328): 'The general moral is ... we need to trace the history of cultural institutions, recognizing how institutions affect the dispositions of those who grow up in societies dominated by them and how, in turn, those dispositions modify existing institutions. In tracing this history, we shall suppose that human beings have propensities that lead them, when they grow up in certain social and physical environments, to acquire as adults the desires and aspirations with which we are familiar.'

No one knows why wet-nurses were not employed in India, because we have not analyzed either history or the current situation well enough. Perhaps the intensity of desire for many children, well-known in India, is so great and so universal that it is difficult or impossible to get anyone to nurse another's child. Perhaps something else. Whatever the case, Kitcher's implication that admonitions such as his 'general moral' (above) are not a part of Dickemann's view of things is invidious, as this quote from Dickemann (1979: 327) shows: 'The ultimate test of the applicability of this model must depend, then, not only on a larger sample of more refined demographic data than I possess, but also on specification of the interaction between demographic structures and their ecological and historical contexts, something which is not attempted here.' If every study of human behavior by an evolutionist ended with such a caveat it would not denigrate the evolutionary approach.

Is the evolutionary approach flawed?

The evolutionary approach assumes that lifetimes evolve as reproductive events or sequences. This has been a basic tenet since Darwin (1859). Accordingly, we should consider Kitcher's (1985) admonition that 'It cannot be taken for granted that economic gains will translate into reproductive gains.' Harris' (1979) statements are similar. These statements could be revised to say: 'It cannot be taken for granted that access to resources correlates with reproductive success.' Arguments that rank or status has nothing to do with reproductive success, if correct, would render impotent the entire current evolutionary approach to human behavior. This argument (e.g. Vining 1986) is widely regarded as the strongest general attack on evolutionists' assumptions. I am interested here in how the assumption is generated and whether or not it is justified (see also the introduction to this volume, and Betzig 1986).

I will begin with the following statements, which I regard as general observations or accepted facts.

1. People do strive to control resources. That is, people seek wealth and material possessions; they seek access to the 'good things of life.' They also seek status, good reputation, and power, which they use to gain and maintain control of resources.

2. Non-humans also strive to control resources: food, waterholes, territories, nests, shelter, overwintering sites, mates.

3. Non-humans seem always to use resources in reproduction, except for failures from incomplete information (an animal didn't know that a particular food item was poisonous), miscalculations (an animal wrongly judged an opponent defeatable), or novel environments (as with moths around electric lights).

4. Humans, on the other hand, frequently do not use resources in reproduction, and moreover do not generally believe that reproduction is the sole significance of either resource control or the proximate mechanisms of resource control.

5. All organisms have evolved, including humans.
6. Because of the rapidity of change in human culture, humans have probably injected uniquely great amounts of novelty into their environments. Novelty can cause the proximate mechanisms of reproductive success (such as pleasure, resource control, or pleasure that leads to or results from resource control) to lead to activities that are not reproductive. When the proximate mechanisms of reproductive behavior are multilayered and complex, as they evidently are to a greater degree in humans than in any other species, this evolutionary 'mis-firing' can be extremely confusing and misleading.

Vining (1986) provides an extensive review of data indicating that 'fertility differentials among contemporary humans are not consistent' with the postulate that 'individuals exploit favorable environments to increase their genetic representation in the next generation.' He notes: 'That wealth, power and rank are ceaselessly and obsessively striven for, as well as monitored in others, is obvious to all observers of human behavior ... That modern humans exploit what they are able to obtain in the way of status and rank to produce, and to help relatives to produce, more offspring than those of lower rank and status seems clearly *not* to be the case. In fact, precisely the opposite appears to be true. The striving for, if not the actual possession of, status and power, seems, on average, to deter rather than to stimulate reproductive effort in humans.'

I expect that Vining is correct – at least sufficiently correct to establish the paradox he discusses – although I doubt that he or anyone else has shown that parents do not use their wealth, power, and rank (hereafter designated as WPR) to help and encourage their *children* to produce more offspring than others do (raising questions about his phrases 'helping relatives to produce' and 'in the next generation'). I would like to analyze Vining's finding with respect to background theory and intervening or proximate variables:

First, the significance of reproductive success in evolution does not depend on demonstrations of the relationship of reproductive success to any particular traits, but on irrefutable logic. A

farmer I know, asked about the possibility that a young bull he wished to sell was sterile, hesitated, and then finally commented: 'Well – he comes from a long line of fertile ancestors.' None of us – no living creature – had a single sterile ancestor, right back to the beginning of life. This logic can be taken a step further. None of us had a single ancestor who was unable or unwilling to put forth whatever minimal effort was required for success in reproduction while it was alive – and that effort would have to include securing a mate, copulating with it, and also very likely giving some parental care.

Population genetics and probabilities enter the picture when we argue that those variants which leave the greatest numbers of successful descendants in any short run of generations are most likely to be represented (genetically) after a long run of generations. (Note that this model of natural selection is not exactly the same as Vining's.) Except in cases of actual reversals of environmental influences, this effect is probably expected by all modern biologists (I stress that an important consequence involves the nature of long-term cumulative changes in traits).

Therefore, when Vining and others tell us that data on reproductive success indicate that widespread or universal traits – such as striving for WPR – correlate negatively with reproductive success (RS), biologists are not likely to abandon the postulates that (1) evolution is universal and inevitable in all forms of life, (2) natural selection is its principal guiding force, or (3) natural selection leads to the accumulation of genes that contribute to traits yielding higher reproductive success. Rather, biologists are likely to ask: (1) Have certain features of the human environment reversed, fracturing the correlation between RS and WPR? And (2) which particular combinations of human traits have interacted with features of the (especially social) environment, and how, to effect such reversals? If we are somewhat like moths flying non-reproductively or anti-reproductively around electric lights, then precisely how and why did it come about? How much must we understand about human behavior to comprehend how and why the unexpected happened? Will we be able to use this new comprehension to extend our self-understanding? Vining implies not by saying that sociobiology has little to offer sociology because of a negative association between resource acquisition and reproductive success in contemporary society and that sociobiology must, for the moment, confine itself to the study of 'constants of human nature …' I answer the last two questions affirmatively, and I disagree with Vining, as I expect do most or all of those concerned with incorporating evolutionary theory into our efforts at self-understanding. (See also, Williams 1985, who notes that we are not currently testing Darwin's theory but testing how it applies. We do not abandon the basic paradigm after one or a few tests fail, but seek reasons for the failure.)

Wealth, power, and rank are outcomes that must be striven for consciously – perhaps in ways that utilize all of our most distinctive human mental attributes (intelligence, consciousness, foresight, self-awareness, free will, memory, conscience, morality, and so forth). Indeed, socially competitive striving within and between competitive groups is likely the context in which we evolved our human attributes (Alexander 1979, 1987).

Contrarily, it is not necessary (typically) to strive (intelligently, consciously, deliberately) for children; rather, it is necessary to strive in these fashions to *avoid* them (as an aspect of spacing them optimally, toward the end of maximizing RS or any other goal). In other words, striving for pleasure typically leads automatically to the production of children *unless conscious, deliberate, and sometimes intelligent steps are taken to prevent it.*

In the course of diverging from other primates, humans evidently evolved toward increased parental investment (PI), meaning that they have benefited from spacing births increasingly widely and from giving more PI to each offspring. The basic evidence for this assumption is that human offspring seem to require and receive more PI – and to receive it across a longer period – than the offspring of other primates. As Darwin noted, each organism's resources are finite, and what a parent gives to one offspring it cannot give to another. The human kind and degree of social striving for WPR is usually seen – and I believe accurately so – as a heritage of this trend toward increased PI.

In social striving for WPR, the hostile forces – the environments of success or failure – are composed primarily of other humans. What is involved is an evolutionary unending race to see who can best use his consciousness, purpose, intelligence, etc. to secure resources. Because the major or sole competitors are conspecific – for humans in ways that may be unique – they will always be no more than a jump behind, *no matter what extremes are achieved during the race* (other species are less likely to be principal hostile forces than for non-human forms with less overall control over their environments). The same unique human attributes listed above, the striving in which they are used, and the resources gained by their use provide WPR to offspring, grand-offspring, and sometimes collateral relatives. Vining does not claim that persons with more WPR do not use them to *aid* the offspring and grandchildren that are produced – only that they are not used to *produce* more. Descendants of people with WPR typically do themselves also have WPR, and last wills and testaments tend to leave WPR to relatives in ways that closely approximate inclusive-fitness-maximizing (IFM).

Except for a small proportion of prospective parents who discover to their dismay that the usual activities of wedded bliss do not yield offspring, *production* of children, then, is typically not striven for in the conscious, deliberate, intelligent sense. What is striven for is the pleasure of sex, or wedded bliss, or orgasms, or sexual harmony, or emotional intimacy, or long-term bonds. These somewhat less intelligent, less uniquely human kinds of striving are generally sufficient not only to produce children, but, I suggest, to produce more children than, during most of history, an ordinary pair of spouses could save or make reproductively successful. Everyone may use uniquely human attributes in efforts to secure and keep desirable mates, but this process primarily contributes to PI – i.e. is part of the effort to make offspring successful, and not specifically an effort to produce them.

It is expensive to conceive babies and then lose them, either as infants or later. Where the environment has been predictably spare across millenia, then, we expect physiological traits or not-so-conscious behaviors to lead to wide spacing of babies, and some evidence supports the expectation (Konnor and Worthman 1980). But where the environment may vary dramatically, we might expect those unique attributes of intelligence, consciousness, and foresight to come into play when wider spacing is called for, and to recede in favor of letting nature take its course when times are better.

So we have a circumstance in which intelligence, consciousness, and purpose are brought into play to (1) gain WPR, (2) increase the interval between babies, so as to increase PI for each baby, and (3) provide and distribute resources in the interests of one's offspring, other descendants, and collateral relatives. The same attributes are not being stressed in *producing* babies.

Now we bring on the scene three major changes: (1) more and better resources for use in PI than were ever available before, (2) partly coincidentally, more pleasure outlets (and perhaps better ones), and (3) easier and cheaper ways to prevent babies while yet enjoying the glories of sex.

We might expect the initial result to be an increase in the birth rate because of relaxation of concern for spacing babies widely enough to ensure their survival. Whether or not this increase would persist would depend on (1) how important *relative* amounts of WPR are to descendants, (2) pleasurable uses of WPR (such as sexual access to more desirable, and perhaps more, partners), and (3) how much striving is necessary to prevent offspring while indulging in the pleasurable activities that would normally lead to babies.

If humans assessed the probability of raising babies to be successful in terms of *absolute* resources available, then, as technology and agriculture increased available resources, we would expect birth rates to rise because mated pairs relaxed their efforts to space babies widely. If, on the other hand, offspring success is largely determined by what is available to them relative to the offspring of others (for example, if success depends on WPR, which is relative and dependent on social competition), then something different might happen. Parents might assess the advisability of producing offspring by not the *absolute* amount of available resources but the *relative* amounts of those resources they control, or are likely to control in the relevant future, especially compared to others of about the same ages and stages (see also Turke, unpublished data). Thus, in a time and place of relative affluence, but in which the likelihood of securing property, jobs, and other resources comparable to the best or even most of society are diminishing, efforts to avoid children might be enhanced.

More than this, if certain kinds of pleasures come to accord with success in efforts to secure WPR – as we would expect over long terms in any species in which WPR correlate with RS – then the pleasures may be sought as their own reward so long as reproduction ensues and its success is roughly proportional to success in attaining WPR. Striving for WPR thus becomes an alternative to baby production, or comes into conflict with it, when baby production conflicts with baby success. This will be true for nearly all individuals early in sexual maturity – for varying periods depending on circumstances – so that tendencies and abilities to restrict or avoid baby production may be expected universally in humans at some times in their lives or under some circumstances. Given this circumstance dramatic increases in pleasure possibilities associated with WPR – especially when coincident with novel and easy methods of baby prevention – may be expected to reduce baby production in ways contrary to IFM, and when baby production and/or rearing conflict with maximizing pleasure from novel availability of phenotypic indulgence.

To say it again, if sufficient pleasure derives from WPR, if babies interfere with this pleasure, if we are given easy ways to prevent babies, and if judgments about optimal amounts of PI depend on how much neighbors and associates are giving to their offspring, then the effect Vining has identified may be precisely the one that would be predicted in modern affluent humans, from biological evolutionary theory.

I would not be surprised if all of the above conditions are met in contemporary society, and are largely responsible for the steps in what has been called the 'demographic transition.' Even if this is not so, generating hypotheses of this kind about variables that intervene between Darwinian predictions and reproductive or genetic survival outcomes, and figuring out ways to test them, is the appropriate route for biologists and other scientists interested in explaining the kind of paradox that Vining has reviewed and developed.

Two conclusions follow: First, investigators studying non-human species assume, with validity, that striving for resource control represents striving for reproductive success. Second, investigators studying humans can also assume, with validity, that striving for resource control by humans represents striving for reproductive success – at least in terms of the history of human environments, whether or not such striving actually correlates with reproductive success now. This second conclusion is acceptable, I believe, unless and until one or more of the following becomes true:

1. Humans are shown not to have evolved by the same rules as other organisms.
2. Evolution is shown not be guided principally by natural selection.
3. Human environments are shown not to involve massive novelty of the sort leading to disruption of the connection between resources control and reproductive success.
4. Investigations on humans repeatedly lead to results that do not make sense in light of the above reasoning or from the conclusion that striving for resource control in humans represents striving for reproductive success in confusingly novel environments.

Skeptics like Kitcher, Harris, and Vining would apparently require that every scientist who wishes to apply evolutionary theory to humans must first prove all over again that it is valid, specifically when applied to humans. If they mean, by this kind of parsimony, that failure to elucidate intervening variables can create a kind of selectionist optimism that expects pigs to fly, even without wings, then I agree completely. For example, showing that high-ranking parents exert more parental effort with sons and low-ranking parents more with daughters (e.g. Dickemann 1979, Betzig and Turke 1986) is provocative and positive support for a Trivers–Willard (1973) interpretation (i.e. that in polygynous species, high-ranking or unusually healthy parents can gain reproductively by favoring males), and for any non-human species it would probably be accepted as a satisfactory conclusion. With humans, we are more interested in how they come to do it, what they think about why they do it, and whether it is really true. Anything humans do can also become a model for future behavior, whether or not one openly subscribes to any version of the naturalistic fallacy. None of these problems makes Dickemann's or Betzig and Turke's kinds of findings any less scientific than the same results with a non-human species. They only make it less likely that the interpretation is pre-

cisely correct, and also make us more concerned that we understand the situation correctly.

Are evolutionists who study human behavior unscientific?

Skeptics of evolutionary approaches to human behavior often argue that investigators adopting this approach do not follow scientific procedures: They are said to utilize unacceptable forms of 'ad hoc' hypothesizing, and to tell 'just-so' stories.

I have diagrammed the procedures of science in Figure 20.1. To what degree do evolutionists in general, and the contributors to this volume in particular, operate outside such procedures?

The ideal sequence in the diagram in Figure 20.1 is probably (1) (2) (3) (4) (5) (3) (4) (5) etc., with publication at (4). Also ideally, each bout of hypothesizing and testing involves all reasonable hypotheses matched against one another, and explicit efforts to falsify each. Also ideally, steps (8) (9) (10) will involve some additional data-gathering after (6).

Step (10), using the old paradigm, is only valid as a test when the test (3) cannot be considered a test of the paradigm itself. If several or numerous tests within a particular paradigm fail, then step (10) becomes less reasonable and step (9) is indicated.

Many 'theoretical' papers involve publication at step (2), or, at least, publication without specific tests using data gathered for the purpose. Data gathered for other purposes can be used, if the original purpose was unlikely to bias with respect to the hypothesis being tested. Sometimes tests using 'logic' are merely tests using

Figure 20.1 The procedures of science

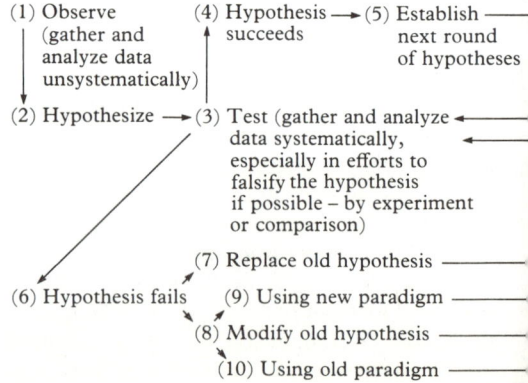

well-established facts (data gathered for other purposes and for one reason or another regarded as correct). For example, in a recent discussion about how it can be demonstrated that natural selection is the principal guiding force of evolution, a philosopher challenged the value of my statement (Alexander 1979) that in living forms changing the direction of selection seems always to change the direction of change. I regarded this apparent fact as a strong test because it seems to deny the role of principal guiding force to two of the three possible candidates (drift and mutations) while simultaneously supporting the third (selection). It is thus a 'test' based on already gathered 'data.' Once stated it can be made stronger, of course (or falsified), by checking in the future to see if it always holds true, and if not whether or not there is a pattern to the exceptions that explicitly denies the application.

'Ad hoc' hypothesizing appears to be an accusation levelled at people who employ step (8), especially going through step (10). In evolutionary studies, the aim of critics of this procedure often appears to be denigration of the entire evolutionary paradigm. As Williams (1985) put it, these critics are the kind of people who, if their car or watch stopped running, might suppose that there is something wrong with the basic laws of physics. Contrary to such critics, 'ad hoc hypothesizing' is how science has always worked. Williams (1985) notes that some critics have the 'mistaken view that predictions are tested to check on the truth of general theory, when they are rather being tested to check on the truth of a particular understanding of the phenomena involved.'

Evolution is a simple theory. Applying it to understand life, however – which is the most complicated phenomenon we have yet encountered in the universe – is one of the most difficult tasks before us. We must not be deterred by those whose skepticism or rejection rests on a refusal to school themselves in the intricacies of biological science, and who, as a result, interpret every difficulty as evidence of failure of the basic theory.

Evolutionary studies of human behavior often appear in the sequences 6 → 8 → 9 → or 6 → 8 → 10 (Figure 20.1) because investigation of human behavior is probably the most difficult procedure in the universe to make scientific. In no other scientific enterprise do we use the attributes we wish to study to do the study, and study an organism designed to deceive us. Moreover, when we study humans, we study the most extremely complex item yet known to us.

Ways of verifying (testing) hypotheses

The goal in science is to identify hypotheses and demonstrate their correctness. The manner of testing hypotheses is the crux of the matter in determining the value of conclusions. The three general methods by which one can do this amount to supporting what in the end remains as the most likely correct hypothesis. The three procedures, from least effective to most, are these:

1. Locate data that agree with the hypothesis. The weaknesses of this approach are that (a) the data may also agree with other unmentioned hypotheses and (b) no direct effort is being made to identify the Achilles heel of the hypothesis. When alternative procedures are difficult, however, supporting data can have some (even if trivial) significance: When I began a list of general statements about human kinship systems (Alexander 1977), I argued that, even if each alone is trivial, and even if some are not really predictions anymore, to discover that, say, 100 such generalizations (or principles) support an explanation from natural selection would not be trivial (e.g. Alexander 1979).

2. Attempt to list all alternative hypotheses and seek to support them, eventually choosing the one that seems best supported. This method, employed by Hoogland and Sherman, both together (1976) and separately (1977), has certain weaknesses and has been criticized by most philosophers of science, including Ghiselin (1969). First, it tends to lead to the false impression that all reasonable hypotheses have been considered, when this end may never be accomplished. Second, it leads to the use of 'straw men,' either deliberately or unconsciously, and to a less than rigorous test on this account. Indeed, almost by definition, as with the first procedure (above), it amounts to supporting one's consciously or unconsciously favorite hypothesis. Third, it fails to focus on the most

331

likely hypothesis and to explore its specific weaknesses. Finally, it is usually a tedious and expensive method of locating the best explanation for a given phenomenon, because it fails to capitalize upon what is already known about the relative merits of existing hypotheses, even sometimes including the pretense that from the start all are more or less equally acceptable. The weakness of this approach is also shown by considering the case in which there is but a single hypothesis: Presumably, all one could then do is to dream up alternatives, however weak, against which to 'test' it.

3. Explicitly seek to falsify the hypothesis. This method is the most widely used and respected in science. It is commonly called the Popperian approach (Popper 1963), but Darwin employed it repeatedly, explicitly, and generally (see Alexander 1979). Its chief virtues are that it seeks the most vulnerable requirements of the proposition and exploits them to the utmost, and it does not require the pretension that all alternative hypotheses have been erected and tested. As Popper said, the most 'risky' tests are the best. Darwin (1859) sought the worst cases known from nature and postulated situations that *if* they existed would falsify evolution by natural selection. He knew that, if his hypothesis was correct, it should explain all *observable* cases but not all *imaginable* ones (Alexander 1979).

In earlier papers (Alexander 1974, 1977, 1979) I analyzed the avunculate and the asymmetrical treatment of cross and parallel cousins to falsify the hypothesis that *these practices show* that evolution is not relevant to the patterning of human sociality. I did this by generating and supporting a reasonable hypothesis from natural selection to meet explicit and particular objections denying the role of 'biology' (i.e. relatedness, and a history of natural selection) in the structuring of kinship systems (e.g. White 1947, Schneider 1961, Sahlins 1976).

Then I supported the selection hypothesis (both the broad one and its specific subsets) by showing supportive correlations from published data for both the avunculate and the treatment of cross and parallel cousins (additional data provided by Kurland 1979, Gaulin and Schlegel 1980, and Flinn 1981). Finally I added support for the general selective hypothesis by showing that genetic asymmetries also coincide with

asymmetrical cousin treatment, predicting successfully the societies in which each kind of cousin marriage is likely to be stressed, and the frequencies and distribution of all four kinds of cousin marriages, and tying together the avunculate and cousin marriages in cases where confidence of paternity is not low. The avunculate and asymmetry in cousin marriages are outstanding complexities of human kinship systems in general, and no explanation for them with any generality of predictiveness had previously been proposed. In effect, I falsified the hypothesis that these cases show that natural selection is inconsistent with the patterns of human sociality. I did not either suggest that low confidence of paternity provides explanation for all cases of either the avunculate or cousin treatment or claim that the suggested explanations were indeed the correct ones. Others and I have continued to seek (and to find) additional factors involved in both phenomena (Alexander 1977, 1979, Kurland 1979, Hartung 1976, Gaulin and Schlegel 1980, Flinn 1981, Flinn and Low 1986).

Recently, another question involving the avunculate was posed by Laura Betzig and Paul Turke (pers. comm.). Why do chiefs on Pacific Islands, in societies with uxorilocality, and evident high confidence of paternity, pass chiefship to their sister's sons rather than to their own? The answer appears to involve the necessity of passing chiefship to a male who is not only a close relative of the chief but also a successor who will be logical and acceptable to those over whom he will be chief. Because men live in the 'clan territories' of their wives (chiefs do not live with their 'subjects'), their sons do not grow up in the region which will require a successor to the chief. Sister's sons are the closest male relatives who do (see also Flinn 1981).

The general points that (1) sister's children are a man's closest relatives in the next generation other than spouse's children and (2) as confidence of paternity diminishes sister's children are increasingly appropriate recipients of beneficence – and may become the *most* appropriate recipients (Alexander 1977, 1979, Kurland 1979) – remain the same, and one or both is involved in every hypothesis generated about the avunculate so far. (The question of why uxorilocality prevails in such regions remains unsolved – but see Ember and Ember 1971, Ember 1974.)

The continuing need for better hypotheses

Biologists using evolutionary approaches to human behavior may accept hypotheses that are too simple – because they appear to be consistent with evolutionary theory – and they often do not work hard enough to use intervening (or proximate) variables to help test and refine their hypotheses (see also Williams 1985, Symons 1987). For example, I wonder if culture has not driven the system of female-biased infanticide that Dickemann discusses even farther than she argues, in a direction positively correlated with reproductive success. Dickemann cites reports that the Jhareja subcaste of India killed *all* female infants at birth. In Indian society rank is evidently regarded as of crucial importance to everyone. Lower-ranking people sacrifice everything possible to elevate the rank of their descendants, and high-ranking people sacrifice to keep their rank.

Infanticide is evidently biased toward females not only in stratified societies but virtually everywhere it occurs. Regardless of the reasons, male offspring – probably males in general – are more highly regarded. Recent reports of a rise in female infanticide in China with efforts to restrict families to one child are an illustration. So are the controversies over using amniocentesis to sex embryos and discard some, primarily females. Even if we do not know the reasons for the phenomenon, we may ask: Where in the world has there not been a tendency to give special congratulations to the parents who produce a son?

Suppose that one's family is currently ranked at the top in a society in which rank is unusually precious, and that extreme effort is required to maintain top ranking. Might not the mere presence of female children be a negative influence? If a top-ranked family had *only* daughters surely its position would be threatened. And would it not be enhanced by the production of only sons?

I am suggesting that rank may be so precious, and so tied to maleness, that in stratified societies culture may sometimes carry efforts to bias offspring toward maleness virtually into the form of a potlatch, in which one cannot afford to lose rank even if the only way to avoid that is to kill all of one's daughters, even at seemingly great (reproductive) expense. Rather than rank and wealth resulting in female infanticide because of the low value or net costliness of females, females may be killed sometimes strictly to *preserve* rank.

Whether or not this scenario has validity I suggest that, rather than the long-term interests of genes '. . . being sacrificed in the cause of status, influence, and perhaps money in the immediate future . . .,' what *look like* the *short-term* interests of the genes are being sacrificed in favor of their *long-term* interests by the acquiring and maintenance of status, influence, and wealth. I look forward to the unravelling of the intervening variables, proximate mechanisms, and history that will explain the rest of the situation. 'Special genes' for female-biased infanticide, incidentally, are not a part of the hypothesis – only abilities to imitate success and anti-imitate failure, and their application – Flinn and Alexander 1982).

I also wonder if Daly and Wilson (1981, 1983), in their studies of child abuse, may have failed to take into account a slightly different hypothesis than the one they tested. Perhaps the effect on the *pair bond* of having a child related to one parent but not to the other is decisive in predicting abuse (by *either* the real parent or the nonparent, or by the two jointly), not the relatedness *per se* or the fact that one spouse is unrelated to the child, so that the child will not yield reproductive benefits for the unrelated adult. The pair bond is the system whereby a very great proportion of each adult's lifetime reproduction will be realized. This 'pair-bond' hypothesis accounts for Daly and Wilson's report that adopted children are not abused more than children living with two real parents; because the relationship of the adoptee with its new parents is symmetrical, adoptees are even likely to *reinforce* the pair bond. The pair-bond hypothesis also predicts that either spouse or both may be involved in the abuse when only one spouse is the parent, as newspaper accounts indicate is true; Daly and Wilson's hypothesis does not seem able to account for this fact.

Consider Figure 20.2, which diagrams a conflict of interest proposition relevant to the child care and pair-bond interpretations of child abuse. A and C each strive to create the optimal situation for themselves. A seeks to create Situation Z, drawing C into her circle of interests without losing B. C seeks to draw A into his circle of interests without B coming along. B seeks to follow his mother, thus also to insinuate himself into C's circle of interests. If C convinces A that he is more important to her than B, he may abuse B (in the extreme eliminating him from the situation by killing him); and he may seek to get A to affirm her acceptance of this situation by cooperation or tolerance in his abuse of B. If C is unsuccessful, A and B reject C and continue together.

During A's and C's efforts to shift the situation from X to Z or Y, respectively, B may be expected either to seek to retain condition X or create situation Z, since Y equals his worst outcome. But he must be exceedingly careful not

Figure 20.2 A conflict of interest proposition relevant to the child-care and pair-bond interpretations of child abuse. Interests of three individuals – A, B, and C – are represented by circles. A is the mother of B. C is a potential new spouse for A. In situation A, at the outset, the mother's interests overlap very broadly with those of her child, while those of the potential new spouse do not yet overlap the interests of the other two individuals. The optimal situation for A and B is Z, in which C has been caused to accept A and B as if both their interests broadly overlapped his own. The worst situation for B is Y, in which C has convinced A that it is in her interests to abandon B and assume that her interests broadly overlap those of C, even though he has not accepted that his interests in any way relate to those of B.

Situation (X)

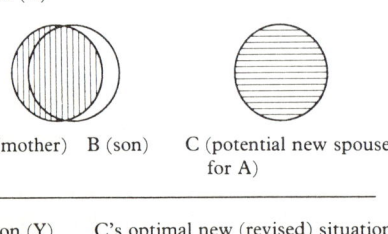

A (mother)   B (son)   C (potential new spouse for A)

Situation (Y)   C's optimal new (revised) situation (= B's worst situation)

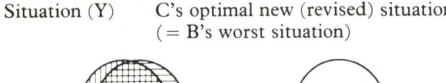

A C   B

Situation (Z)   A's optimal new (revised) situation (also may = B's optimal situation)

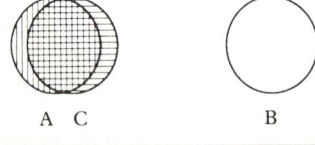

C A B

to create situation Y by promoting a close relationship between A and C which could itself lead to his own estrangement. He avoids this by both ingratiating himself to C and slowing the progress of overlap of A and C's interests so it does not get too far ahead of his relationship with C.

A, on the other hand, may be expected to 'lead' in the convergence of her interests with those of C more than B wants her to because she is somewhat less afraid of situation Y.

Are the studies reported in this volume scientific?

How would the studies reported in this volume differ if they had not incorporated an evolutionary approach?

First, and perhaps contrary to the suppositions of some, they would probably have been less scientific (less repeatable, less likely to contribute to a *cumulative* growth of knowledge). The reason is that nearly every one of these studies, whatever else its shortcomings, is quantitative, involving the systematic gathering and analyzing of data. Cultural and social anthropology have typically been based on evidence derived from interviews and expressed qualitatively and as interpretations. Such accounts are not useful unless the work is repeated more systematically; they are not reliable, or comparable to other studies. Quantitative work is not by any means restricted to those taking evolutionary approaches, but it is part of the heritage of the discipline of biology.

Second, the papers here all assume that the ultimate (evolved) function underlying all behavior is maximizing reproductive success, which means, usually in some complexly indirect way, maximizing the likelihood of survival of one's genetic materials. This assumption replaces several others in human-oriented disciplines, namely: (1) no assumption of function at all, (2) maximizing the likelihood of personal survival, (3) maximizing some particular proximate rewards (e.g. pleasure) and minimizing some particular proximate punishments (e.g. pain), (4) maximizing the likelihood of survival of some other individual (e.g. spouse, friend, leader, child), (5) maximizing the likelihood of survival, happiness, or success of one's social group (however defined), (6) maximizing moral-ity, 'goodness,' social service, or altruism, and (7) maximizing the good (or happiness) of the greatest (possible) number of humans (see Alex-ander 1987). The new assumption from recent evolutionary biology may be wrong. I suspect not, but if it is that should become apparent as studies like these – Williams' (1985) 'inspection of the organism' – multiply. In any case, the assumption of RS maximization as function is at the moment the only hypothesis consistent with the theory that virtually everyone agrees accounts for life on earth.

Third, all of the chapters that deal with social interactions make efforts to include actual genea-logical relations, and treat variations in genetic relatedness as an important variable. Spousal and other reciprocal interactions of non-kin or distant kin are distinguished from interactions among close kin. Although genealogies have always been a part of ethnographic analysis of kinship systems and patterns of social behavior, until the late 1970s they were not related to Hamilton's (1964) notion of inclusive fitness maximization. Until the middle and late 1970s, no study of the social behavior of non-human species relied upon individual identification coupled with complete genealogical histories. Biologists now realize that without such informa-tion they are blind to the significance of most social activities. Anthropologists have always known that kinship was crucial in human socia-lity, but without Hamilton's insights they could not fully understand why. There was no compre-hensive set of theoretical paradigms for inter-preting kinship systems. These papers show that those days are gone forever.

Fourth, all authors in this volume explicitly seek to test one or more hypotheses. If their tests or their hypotheses are less than ideal, critics should compare their efforts to studies of human sociality in the past. Most, I believe, are without identifiable or explicit hypotheses at all, let alone tests.

Let us review some of the procedures employed by the authors in this volume, with an eye to comparing them both with earlier work and with the ideals of scientific procedure.

Chagnon (Chapter 2) *describes* kinship pat-terns. In this sense he is in the tradition of anthropological ethnographies. He also has an enormous amount of systematically gathered data amenable to statistical analysis, and he assumes efforts to maximize inclusive fitness (IFM). In these senses he is not traditional. He found one thing that is easy to interpret as consis-tent with IFM (that adult males call more young women by kin terms indicating potential wife than is really the case). He found two things he cannot as easily explain: (1) men classify kin faster than do women and (2) men use 'vague endearing' terms less often than women. For the amount of work he carried out, these might be seen as meager results. I would say, rather, that they attest to the expense and difficulty of analyz-ing human sociality; and we can be sure that much more will be extracted from this study.

Gaulin and Hoffman (Chapter 7) review evi-dence that human males and females differ in 'spatial ability' and conclude that they do, and that androgens trigger the divergence. They argue, from both human and non-human data, that this difference has arisen in conjunction with more extensive mate-seeking by males. Cur-iously, they do not explicitly discuss effects of the largely male activities of war and hunting in this context.

Crook and Crook (Chapter 5) propose that the monomarital system of Tibetan polyandry, and its family size and structure, are imposed by par-ents on their children so as to maintain the func-tionality of the farm by never producing more children than can subsist and rear children on it. This is the model I proposed in 1974, explain-ing fraternal polyandry as a combination of par-ental manipulation and kin selection in the maintenance of control of a non-partable resource. Polyandry would then be a con-sequence of the *importance* of the farm, the labor required to extract its resources, and the fact that farms have been historically divided to a minimal size for family success.

Crook and Crook's calculation of the fitness of males in polyandrous marriages seems incom-plete in certain regards. Thus, it appears to refer to numbers of descendant and collateral relatives (offspring and nephews and nieces) rather than the results of effort exerted on behalf of such relatives. For polyandry the problem is complex for at least three reasons. First, a man may help nephews and nieces in other households, as well as in those in his own (polyandrous) household. Second, younger brothers almost certainly do not have equal access to their older brother's wife. Third, a younger brother who would have no children if he did not join his brother polyandrously would add to his fitness just by helping nieces and nephews, without having any children of his own.

Betzig (Chapter 2) found that chiefs on Ifaluk are deferred to, do less physical labor, and give their relatives disproportionate amounts of goods they redistribute. Although she reports the chiefs' constant admonitions to the whole group, and acknowledges the possibility of a 'managerial' benefit, she is reluctant to suggest that what they do is 'productive work.'

To accept this point, one would have to conclude that academics, inventors, foremen, administrators, executives, generals, and leaders and thinkers of all sorts are less 'productive' than the people they oversee or to whom they transmit their thoughts, and that what they do is mostly leisure, and exploitative. This need not be true. If an organizer or inventor causes a cooperative group to double its production, that person has been as *productive* as all other group members combined. If all who are exempt from physical labor are thereby exploitative, one would have to assume that corporations which hire executives are being altruistic. One must also consider the probable value of chiefs in developing and maintaining group unity in connection with the almost perpetual war that typified this region up to only 50 years or so ago.

In this instance Betzig, like others in this volume, has simply slammed up against one of the shortcomings of behavioral scans that are especially severe in studies of humans. Behavioral scans cannot tell what is going on in people's minds, and more goes on there, presumably, than is true for the members of any other species. Unfortunately, interviews and related methods do not necessarily inform us accurately either. For various reasons, little might be gained by asking either chiefs or others to describe the chief's value, or lack of it, to the group as a whole or to the individuals asked. (A second shortcoming of the behavioral scan method is that individual observations on different behaviors cannot be compared in quantitative terms. Effort – in terms of calories or risk – may be grossly different for behaviors that are entered as equivalents in a behavioral scan sample.) Of the studies reported here, those of Flinn (Chapter 11) and Kaplan and Hill

(Chapters 17 and 18) seem to me to be good examples of explicit and formal use of both behavioral scans and other sources of information, such as interviews.

Borgerhoff Mulder (Chapter 3) assumes that variations in bridewealth among Kipsigi reflect differences in benefits to brides and grooms and their respective parents. She tests to see if in the Kipsigis reproductive success is involved. Her suggestion that 'low price paid for older brides is not due to some unspecific undesirability which leads to their delayed marriage' leaves us wondering why these women married later.

Borgerhoff Mulder says that she predicted that a groom's father living far from a bride's father will have to pay more for a bride and that her data support the hypothesis. She made the prediction because brides living close to their natal home may give more of their labor to their parents than to their husbands (or their husbands' families?). One wonders whether other, different hypotheses – just as compatible with evolutionary theory – are equally or better supported. Borgerhoff Mulder deals with some aspects of this question, but I have reservations. It is my experience that people who sell almost anything – objects, produce, domestic animals, or any kind of goods for which the price is subject to barter – are likely to charge less when they sell to relatives or friends, including neighbors, even when the item in question has no possibility of somehow itself returning to be useful to the seller. Neighbors and friends are people with whom one tends to have continuing – even lifetime – reciprocal interactions (this is true of relatives too, but the additional variable of genetic overlap is involved there). Is the lower price part of a continuing reciprocal interaction? This is especially pertinent since Borgerhoff Mulder says (Chapter 3) that affines 'help each other with agricultural work and preparations for large ceremonies but this cooperation derives more from their common *kokwet* membership [i.e. the fact of their geographic proximity] than from affinity *per se*.'

I also wonder if Borgerhoff Mulder's finding that the distance women live from their fathers is not associated with desertion by wives or wifebeating eliminates the hypothesis that parents are better able to assist and keep track of nearby daughters and grandchildren, in ways contributing to the parents' reproductive success. (Berté

Table 20.1 *Types of scientific 'investigations*

Sequence	Kind of data	
	Subjective	Objective
Hypothesis generated first	Data must be gathered 'blind'	Data do not necessarily need to be gathered 'blind'
Data gathered first	Hypothesis must be generated independently	

(Chapter 4) found that among K'ekchi Indians the cost of securing a bride for one's son is slightly higher if the bride comes from another village; the reason here, however, is that the cost of the wedding feast is higher owing apparently to the necessity of supplying food for more people.)

As I have stressed elsewhere (Alexander 1979), evolution is a simple process, not particularly difficult to understand, which means that it will be extremely difficult to apply broadly to problems as complex as understanding human social behavior. Anyone who finds it easy to assume that the first Darwinian hypothesis he thinks of is good enough should review the torturous efforts of biologists to use Darwinian theory to understand some comparatively simple attributes of life, such as sex ratios, sexuality, or outbreeding.

To digress a moment, the most serious scientific questions about behavioral studies involve when and how predictions from hypotheses are made and data purporting to test the predictions are gathered. Data can be divided into two classes, those involving more or less unequivocal decisions of a yes–no nature (e.g. did the subject pull his ear or not) and those involving highly subjective decisions (e.g. distinguishing different levels of agonism, especially when the grades of agonism cannot be separated by absolute breaks).

Data can be gathered before or after a hypothesis is generated and its predictions established; each sequence has advantages and disadvantages. Anyone who locates data already gathered to test a hypothesis generated later, *and independently*, is lucky indeed, especially if (1) he can prove that the data were unavailable to him, or unanalyzed, so that the hypothesis was indeed generated independently of them and (2) the data really are appropriate to test the particular hypothesis involved. If these two conditions can be satisfied, whether the data are subjective or objective (involve unequivocal decisions) is not important.

If, on the other hand, data are gathered explicitly to test a hypothesis already generated, then if the data involve subjective decisions they must be gathered by observers who are 'blind' to the hypothesis. Otherwise there is no obligation to accept the study as valid and no excuse for publishing it. This is particularly true when one outcome will further the career of the investigator substantially more than the alternative. Deliberate distortion need not be involved, for evidently investigators may deceive themselves without knowing it. If the data involve unequivocal yes–no observations we tend to be less concerned about 'blind' observations because deliberate distortion is necessary and the costs of this activity, if it is detected, typically involve termination of a career.

On this basis we are presented, then, with three kinds of 'scientific' investigations' as set out in Table 20.1.

This volume presents us with all three kinds of studies, and a few problems in respect to some of them. Crook and Crook, Brown and Hotra, Boone, Voland, Gaulin and Hoffman, and Low utilize data gathered prior to their studies. Low (Chapter 6), for example, uses data from the existing ethnographic literature to test a hypothesis generated orally by William D. Hamilton in 1981: that degree of polygyny in humans may correlate with variations in the severity of certain kinds of parasites. Low's data are sometimes subjective, but there can be no doubt that the data and the hypothesis are independent; and the tests are easily repeated. Low also deals with the problem of human uniqueness, here with respect to the amount of female choice that is likely involved in mate selection in polygynous societies, as compared to other organisms. Her conclusions, as we might expect, are not entirely unequivocal; but they point the way to further studies.

Chagnon, Betzig, Borgerhoff Mulder, Berté, Turke, Flinn, Essock-Vitale and McGuire, Hewlett, and Hill and Kaplan all gathered their own data. At least in some cases, the data were gathered with an evolutionary hypothesis in mind, or under the general assumption that evolution by natural selection has molded human behavior. All of the authors in this volume seem favorably inclined to this hypothesis (as am I), and when they seem to be performing tests of it they appear to be attempting to convince an audience that has not yet accepted it. What these authors are really interested in, and taking up, is the *next* level of investigation – namely, how knowing about evolution and assuming that selection has operated on human behavior can lead to predictions and findings that are unlikely to have been uncovered using any other general approach. This 'next level' of investigation includes not only what people do in particular circumstances, and how such things relate to the eventualities of culture, but, as well, what are their conscious motivations and reflections about what they are doing and why do the two realms connect as they do. As Symons (1987, pers. comm.) emphasizes (see also Ghiselin 1969, Trivers 1971, 1985, Alexander 1979, 1987), a Darwinian psychology lies ahead of us, and it will unfold as multiple levels of proximateness in (1) life function, (2) the structure of human effort and design of lifetimes, and (3) the makeup and activities of the human psyche.

The distinction between testing general evolutionary theory and seeking the next level of hypothesis is not trivial. *Ad hoc* hypothesizing is one of the most prominent complaints registered against evolutionary biologists examining human behavior. It consists of generating a new hypothesis when the old one has failed, *while continuing to adhere to the original general paradigm* (i.e. the sequence, 6, 8, 9, 10, Figure 20.1). The people who accuse evolutionary biologists of this supposed scientific sin are saying that if one hypothesis derived from considerations of natural selection is wrong, then the investigator is only being scientific if he discards the entire evolutionary paradigm. As Williams (1985) notes, however, if an automobile fails to run, 'Any sane engineer would first look for trivial rather than profound causes of failure, and test them in the expectation of confirming at least one.' The reason is that motors *usually run*; and

in biology the motors of explaining organisms by natural selection have been running very well indeed, for a very long time.

The papers in this volume are, of course, not all methodologically flawless, and one of the problems comes from comparing the sequence of arguments or findings as given in the published articles with the actual sequence of discoveries in the investigations themselves. This is not an isolated problem in science. I remember reading Karl von Frisch's (1954) book and marvelling at the logical sequence of his thoughts and his experiments – until it dawned on me that he was telling a story. No long-term investigation works so flawlessly. No investigator plans so perfectly. All scientists reorder the parts of their investigations and findings so that the narrative of their publications will be briefer and more understandable to readers (and editors!). But reordering can also needlessly obscure what really happened, in ways that make results look more convincing than they would if the details were known to the reader. This is how all of the old falsehoods arose about the singularity of 'scientific method' that used to be taught in American high schools.

Suppose, for example, that it was found that the best Ache hunters (cf. Hill and Kaplan) hunt for longer periods than less successful hunters, not shorter ones, and that originally this puzzled the investigators, who knew that meat is divided evenly back at the camp. Subsequently the idea arose that hunting prowess might be important in sexual competition. From this hypothesis the investigators predict that men who hunt more successfully are also more successfully sexually. This hypothesis is confirmed. So it amounts to a test – not necessarily definitive – of the earlier hypothesis that hunting prowess is important in sexual selection. But the investigators could not legitimately turn the sequence around and say that they had originally predicted that hunting prowess is important in sexual competition and then argue that they had secured *two* results supporting the prediction – namely, not only that better hunters are sexually more successful but, as well, that better hunters hunt longer even though their catches are going to be divided evenly among the entire group later. There is an irony in the fact that if the investigators in this case reported the findings and hypotheses in the precise sequence in which they occurred, the original (and puzzling) finding that Ache hunters hunt longer would provide *some* additional support for the hypothesis that prowess in hunting is important in sexual selection because the discovery was independent of any such hypothesis, and made in the absence of any apparent explanation. In my opinion such a sequence should be reported, and the reader has a right to expect that he has not been confused by shifts in sequences of actual events during an investigation.

This particular reporting sequence is probably common in science, and it is probably the most serious methodological criticism I can level at any of the papers in this volume. Unless my biases are causing me to be a poor critic, that speaks well for the level of effort exhibited here.

Considering the procedural problems that I have discussed so far, it may not be surprising that those who attempt to study human behavior find it exceptionally difficult to be scientific (i.e. to do repeatable, quantitative studies) and simultaneously to avoid being trivial. Unfortunately, as I have stressed, most people also would agree that errors in studies of human behavior are more important than errors in analyses of the behavior of other organisms. These two problems are simply crosses that all students of humans have to bear.

How do these papers compare with those presented in earlier volumes – say, Chagnon and Irons (1979) or Alexander and Tinkle (1981)? I think the big difference is that a higher proportion of the papers is empirical as opposed to theoretical, and a higher proportion use data gathered by the investigators themselves. It would be nice if we could say that there are now many times as many investigators active in this general arena, but in truth we cannot. The number of people involved is still disappointingly small. It would be wonderful if we could say that new quantitative field studies are being generated on every hand, but we cannot. There are probably more new studies represented here, and more quantitative data, than in any previous anthropological symposium volume. Some of the data, however, derive from information gathered years ago, and either unpublished until now or else used one or more times already. Why is this true? It is true in part because the distinguished social anthropologist I quoted at the outset was right: The anthropology panels of the US Natio-

nal Science Foundation have not funded much work of the sort reported here, and most of these authors have extensively used their own personal funds to complete their research. Nevertheless, of the studies reported in this volume, six acknowledge support from US federal grant sources, three were supported by US private foundations, and one by a non-US foundation.

But that same distinguished social anthropologist could not have been more wrong than to apply the word 'fad' to the use of an evolutionary approach to examine human behavior. Perhaps the current hiatus with respect to acceptance of use of evolution in studies of human behavior will last many more years. Perhaps not. But it will be passed through. And as that process takes place it will become increasingly advantageous for young social scientists, competing for positions in the tight academic job market by producing notable research results, to know how to employ evolutionary arguments and hypotheses when they are useful and how to bypass or discard them when they are not. The people contributing to this volume have demonstrated that they know how to do these things.

Conclusion

There is probably no area of investigation in which it is more difficult to be scientific than that involving human behavior. Pitfalls and hostilities lurk at every turn. The expense and effort required to secure significant data on important questions is, to say the least, daunting. But if we evolutionists persevere, our academic descendants will probably prevail. My own view of the optimal outcome would be for the significance of evolution to become so widely known and so thoroughly imbedded in the understanding of all those working in human-oriented disciplines, that its tenets can be employed, without fanfare, when they are useful, and ignored or discarded when they are not. This is in fact the situation that prevails throughout most of the biological sciences, even if there are also flurries of dismay and controversy there when significant shortcomings are discovered in theory or its application.

References

Alexander, R. D. (1974) The evolution of social behavior. *Annual Review of Ecology and Systematics*, 5, 325–83.

Alexander, R. D. (1977) Natural selection and the analysis of human sociality. In *Changing Scenes in the Natural Sciences: 1776–1976*, ed. C. E. Goulden, pp. 283–337. Bicentennial Symposium Monograph, Philosophical Academy of Natural Science Special Publication 12.

Alexander, R. D. (1978) Natural selection and societal laws. In *The Foundations of Ethics, Vol. 3, Morals, Science, and Society*, ed. T. Engelhardt and D. Callahan. pp. 138–82. Hastings-on-Hudson, NY: Hastings Institute.

Alexander, R. D. (1979) *Darwinism and Human Affairs*. Seattle: University of Washington Press.

Alexander, R. D. (1985) Genes, consciousness, and behavior theory. In *A Century of Psychology as Science*, eds. S. Koch and D. E. Leary, pp. 783–802. New York: McGraw-Hill.

Alexander, R. D. (1987) *The Biology of Moral Systems*. Hawthorne, NY: Aldine-deGruyter.

Alexander, R. D. and Tinkle, D. W. (eds.) (1981) *Natural Selection and Social Behavior: Recent Research and New Theory*. New York: Chiron Press.

Barash, D. (1977) *Sociobiology and Behavior*. New York: Elsevier.

Betzig, L. L. (1986) *Despotism and Differential Reproduction: A Darwinian View of History*. Hawthorne, NY: Aldine-deGruyter.

Betzig, L. L. and Turke, P. (1986) Parental investment by sex on Ifaluk. *Ethology and Sociobiology*, 7, 29–37.

Brues, A. (1964) The cost of evolving vs. The cost of not evolving. *Evolution*, 18, 379.

Brues, A. (1969) Genetic load and its varieties. *Science*, 164, 1130.

Buss, D. M. (1985) Human mate selection. *American Scientist*, 73, 47–51.

Buss, D. M. (1987) Sex differences in human mate selection criteria. An evolutionary perspective. In *Sociobiology and Psychology: Ideas, Issues, and Applications*, eds. C. Crawford, M. Smith, and D. Krebs. Hillsdale, NJ: Erlbaum (in press).

Chagnon, N. A. and Irons, W. (eds.) (1979) *Evolutionary Biology and Human Social Behavior: An Anthropological Perspective*. North Scituate, MA: Duxbury Press.

Conant, J. R. (1951) *On Understanding Science*. New York: The New American Library (Mentor).

Daly, M. and Wilson, M. (1981) Abuse and neglect of children in evolutionary perspective. In *Natural Selection and Social Behavior: Recent Research and New Theory*, eds. R. D. Alexander and D. W. Tinkle, pp. 405–16. New York: Chiron Press.

Daly, M. and Wilson, M. (1983) *Sex, Evolution, and Behavior*, 2nd edition. Boston: Willard Grant Press.

Darwin, C. (1859) *On the Origin of Species*. A facsimile of the first edition with an introduction by Ernst Mayr, published in 1967. Cambridge, MA: Harvard University Press.

Dawkins, R. (1976) *The Selfish Gene*. New York: Oxford University Press.

Dickemann, M. (1979) The reproductive structure of stratified human societies: a preliminary model. In *Evolutionary Biology and Human Social Organization: An Anthropological Perspective*, eds. N. A. Chagnon and W. G. Irons, pp. 321–67. North Scituate, MA: Duxbury Press.

Ember, C. R. (1974) An evaluation of alternative theories of matrilocal versus patrilocal residence. *Behavior Science Research*, 9, 135–49.

Ember, M. and Ember, C. R. (1971) The conditions favoring matrilocal versus patrilocal residence. *American Anthropologist*, 73, 571–94.

Fisher, R. A. (1930 [1958]) *The Genetical Theory of Natural Selection*. 2nd edition, 1958. New York: Dover.

Flinn, M. V. (1981) Uterine versus agnatic kinship and associated cousin marriage preferences: an evolutionary biological analysis. In *Natural Selection and Social Behavior: New Research and Theory*, eds. R. D. Alexander and D. W. Tinkle. New York: Chiron Press.

Flinn, M. V. and Alexander, R. D. (1982) Culture theory: The developing synthesis from biology. *Human Ecology*, 10, 383–400.

Frisch, K. von (1954) *The Dancing Bees: An Account of the Life and Senses of the Honey Bee* (trans. Dora Ilse). London: Methuen and Co.

Gaulin, J. C. and Schlegel, A. (1980) Paternal confidence and paternal investment: a cross-cultural test of a sociobiological hypothesis. *Ethnology and Sociobiology*, 1, 301–9.

Ghiselin, M. T. (1969) *The Triumph of the Darwinian Method*. Berkeley: University of California Press.

Gould, S. J. and Lewontin, R. C. (1979) The spandrels of San Marco and the panglossian paradigm: A critique of the adaptationist program. *Proceedings of the Royal Society, London, B*, 205, 581–98.

Haldane, J. B. S. (1957) The cost of natural selection. *Journal of Genetics*, 55, 511.

Hamilton, W. D. (1964) The genetical evolution of social behavior. I, II, *Journal of Theoretical Biology*, 7, 1–52.

Harris, M. (1979) *Cultural Materialism: The Struggle for a Science of Culture*. New York: Random House.

Hartung, J. (1976) On natural selection and the inheritance of wealth. *Current Anthropology*, 17, 607–22.

Hoogland, J. L. (1977) The evolution of coloniality in white-tailed and black-tailed prairie dogs (Sciuridae: *Cynomys leucurus* and *C. ludovicianus*). Ph.D. Dissertation, University of Michigan.

Hoogland, J. L. and Sherman, P. W. (1976) Advantages and Disadvantages of bank swallow (*Tiparia riparia*) coloniality. *Evolutionary Monographs*, 46, 33–58.

Kamin, L. (1985) Genes and behavior: The missing link. *Psychology Today*, 19, 76–8.

Kitcher, P. (1985) *Vaulting Ambition*. MIT Press.

Konner, M. and Worthman, C. (1980) Nursing frequency, gonadal function, and birth spacing among !Kung hunter–gatherers. *Science*, 207, 788–91.

Kurland, J. A. (1979) Paternity, mother's brother, and human sociality. In *Evolutionary Biology and Human Social Behavior: An Anthropological Perspective*, ed. N. A. Chagnon and W. G. Irons, pp. 145–80. North Scituate, MA: Duxbury Press.

Lack, D. (1965) Natural selection and human nature. In *Biology and Personality: Frontier Problems in Science, Philosophy, and Religion*, ed. I. T. Ramsey, pp. 40–8. New York: Barnes and Noble Inc.

Lewontin, R. C. (1979) Sociobiology as an adaptationist program. *Behavioural Sciences*, **24**, 5–14.

Lewontin, R. C., Rose, S. and Kamin, L. J. (1985) *Not in Our Genes: Biology, Ideology, and Human Nature*. New York: Pantheon Books.

Maynard Smith, J. (1983) Current controversies in evolutionary biology. In *Dimensions of Darwinism*, ed. M. Grene, pp. 273–86. Cambridge: Cambridge University Press.

Maynard Smith, J. (1984) Science and myth. *Natural History*, **93**, 10–25.

Maynard Smith, J. (1985) Biology and the behaviour of man. *Nature*, **318**, 121–2.

Muller, H. J. (1950) Our load of mutations. *American Journal of Human Genetics*, **2**, 111–76.

Popper, K. (1963) Science: conjectures and refutations. In *The Growth of Scientific Knowledge*, pp. 33–7. New York: Harper Torch Books.

Raymond, J. C. (1982) Rhetoric: The methodology of the humanities. *College English*, **44** (8), 777–83.

Sahlins, M. D. (1976) *The Use and Abuse of Biology: An Anthropological Critique of Sociobiology*. Ann Arbor: University of Michigan Press.

Schneider, D. (1961) Introduction. In *Matrilineal Kinship*, eds. D. M. Schneider and K. Gough, pp. 1–29. Berkeley: University of California Press.

Schneirla, T. C. (1950) The relationship between observation and experimentation in the field study of behavior. *Annals of the New York Academy of Science*, **51**, 1032–44.

Segerstrale, U. (1986) Colleagues in conflict: An 'in vivo' analysis of the sociobiology controversy. *Biology and Philosophy*, **1**, 53–87.

Sherman, P. W. (1977) Nepotism and the evaluation of alarm cells. *Science*, **197**, 1246–53.

Smith, P. (1984) *Dissenting Opinions: Selected Essays*. San Francisco: North Point Press.

Symons, D. (1987) If we're all Darwinians, what's the fuss about? In *Sociobiology and Psychology: Ideas, Issues, and Applications*, eds. C. B. Crawford, M. F. Smith and D. L. Krebs. Hillsdale, NJ: Erlbaum (in press).

Trivers, R. L. (1971) The evolution of reciprocal altruism. *Quarterly Review of Biology*, **46**, 35–57.

Trivers, R. L. (1985) *Social Evolution*. Menlo Park, CA: Benjamin/Cummings.

Trivers, R. L. and Willard, D. E. (1973) Natural selection of parental ability to vary the sex ratio of offspring. *Science*, **179**, 90–8.

Vining, D. R. (1986) Social versus reproductive success: the central theoretical problem of human sociobiology. *Behavioral and Brain Sciences*, **9**, 167–87.

Wallace, B. (1968) *Topics in Population Biology*. New York: W. W. Norton.

White, L. (1947) The expansion of the scope of science. *Journal Washington Academy of Sciences*, **37**, 181–210.

Williams, G. C. (1966) *Adaptation and Natural Selection: A Critique of Some Current Evolutionary Thought*. Princeton: Princeton University Press.

Williiams, G. C. (1985) *A Defense of Reductionism in Biology*. Oxford Surveys in Evolutionary Biology, **2**, 1–27.

Wilson, E. O. (1975) *Sociology: The New Synthesis*. Cambridge, MA: Harvard University Press.

Index

The discussion of the subject of this volume, 'Human reproductive behaviour', necessarily involves the frequent use of some very common words, which occur either in pairs (e.g. brother–sister, father–mother, husband–wife, male–female, man–woman) or singly (e.g. child, family, kin, marriage, offspring). In order to avoid printing long strings of useless page numbers after these headings (keywords), they have, wherever possible, been lumped together, in two ways. Thus, 'mothers, 41–6' means that the word 'mother' occurs *at least once* on each of the pages mentioned, and 'mother, 144–228 *passim*' means that the word 'mother' occurs sporadically in these pages but not on every one of them.

An extra indentation in the run-on sub-headings indicates the beginning of a particularly important sub-heading and (subsequently) the resumption of the ordinary sub-headings.

Index

benefit (*see also* fitness), 10–11, 52–192 *passim*, 238–9, 244–5, 280, 283–8, 302–3, 309, 313, 336; benefit of care, 238; benefits to investment in offspring, 239; benefit-to-cost ratio, 182; benefits to courtship, 239; fitness, 299, 302; future, 73; 'managerial', 336; material, 54–5, 197; monetary cost-benefit, 85; nutritional, 284; of labor invested in farming, 94; of peasant productive activities, 84; productive and reproductive, 60; ratio of reproductive, to cost, 9; reproductive, 13, 184; resource, 296; social and economic, 73; vicarious, 73

biologist, vii, 164, 166, 173–4, 317–18, 321, 323, 327, 329, 333, 335, 337; American, 52; behavioral, 277; evolutionary, 237, 273, 317, 321–3, 325; modern, 327

biology, 40, 145, 161, 238, 279, 318, 321–4, 334, 338; 'biology', 332; evolutionary, vii, viii, 5, 223, 253, 263–4, 317, 322–3; molecular, 162; of human species, 97; proximate, of spatial ability, 133; theoretical, 29; biological advantage, 222; factors, 165; 'needs', 168; science, 331, 339; systems, 164; theory, 322

birds, 99, 176, 297; larger, full-adult, 286; monogamous, 280; territorial-nesting, 286; young, 286; young male, 286

birth, 59, 75, 156, 158, 180, 204, 227, 232, 242, 294–5, 297, 310, 328, 333; birth histories, 266; birth of the first child, 287; date of, 69, 180, 204–5, 207, 282; frequencies and sex ratios of all reported, 203; first birth, 180; husband's year of, 58; intervals (*see also* interbirth intervals), 58, 178–80, 182, 184, 243, 309, 312; optimal birth interval, 295; physiological constraints on, 184; live births, 156–8, 180, 227, 231–2, 267, 296; spacing, 10, 294–5, 302, 328; still births, 227; surviving birth, 312; year of, 57–8, 182

birth control, 231, 310; ills, 228; usage, 231

birth order, 5, 110, 202, 210–12, 217, 254, 258, 271, 287; effect of, 211; place in, 311

birth rank, 254, 257–9

birth rates, 28, 111–12, 329; high, for Catholics, 310; random variations in the, 164

boys, 33, 53, 67, 130, 136–7, 139, 142–4, 174, 254, 257; older, 87

brain, 133–4; brain damage, left-hemisphere, 135–6; right-hemisphere, 135; unilateral, 135; brain function, 145; cognitive abilities of right and left hemispheres, 134; female, 135; male, 135; lateralization (laterality), 133, 139, 145–6; cerebral-speech, 135; hemispheric, 140; linguistic, 134; of cognitive processes, 134; sex differences in, 135–6; left hemisphere in the human brain, 133–5; right hemisphere, 133–6; mammalian brain, 137

Brazil: Catrimani River Basin in, 47; Shavante headmen in, 49

breadfruit, 52, 54; season, 56

breeding: pattern, 153; population, 213; ranges, 133; season, 132; structure, patrilineal-polygynous-hypergynous, 205; system, polygynous, 4; breeding-system ratio (BSR), 153–4, 156, 158

brides, 66–79, 90–1, 123, 164, 216, 288, 336–7; 'accompanied', 71–2, 75; age of potential, 74; bride's age, 78; at circumcision (*see also* circumcision), 68, 74; at menarche, 71, 73, 78; bride's family, 66, 90, 122, 216; bride's father (BF), 67–73, 75–7, 208, 336; wealth of the, 69; bride's labor, 72; parents, 67; price, 76;

village, 91; early-maturing, 79; ideal, 230; local, 73; non-local, 72; nulliparous, non-pregnant, 70, 73; physically handicapped, 70; of high reproductive value, 78; plump, 79; pregnant, 71; pregnant, low bride-wealth of, 70; pregnant, reduced intrinsic value of, 70; reproductive value of the, 79; 'skin' or 'body' of the, 78; 'suboptimal', 164; 'unaccompanied', 71–2, 75

bride price, 7, 91, 111, 121–2, 163–4; bride-price conventions, nature of, 167

bride-service, 90, 121, 265–6, 270

bride-wealth, 65–79; amounts of, 68, 70; index, 68; Kipsigis bride-wealth payments, 15, 65, 79; amount of variance in, 74; negotiations, 77; negotiated bride-wealth payments, variation in, 79; negotiated bride-wealth settlements, 79; paid for non-pregnant brides, 71; paid for pregnant brides, 71; payments, 65, 67–71, 74–5, 78–9; variance in, 74; inflation of, in Kenya, 79; intracultural variability in, 76; settlement, 78; token, 75; transaction, 77; units, 69; valuables, availability and fluidity of, 79; values, 68, 73; variability, 79; variability, cross-cultural and intracultural studies of, 79; variability in, among the Kipsigis, 74; variations in, 336

brother, 9, 28, 33, 38, 50, 52, 89, 99, 101, 104, 106, 108, 110–12, 175, 179, 207, 215, 248, 253, 266, 270–2, 274, 336; 'brothers', 24; brother-in-law, 34, 36; 'brother–sister' exchange, 24, 26; co-husbanding, 112; deceased, 29; eldest, 101, 112; full, 33, 108, 110, 271; junior brother's strategy, 112; marrying, 107, 112; 'my little', 37; older (elder), 52, 108, 110–11, 210, 335; reproductively active older, 31; teenage, 110; unmarrying, 108; younger, 99, 108, 110, 166, 215, 335–6

bureaucracy: local-government, 167; royal, 203, 207, 209, 213

canoe: houses, 55, 177; sailing, 177

capital, 86; assets, 78; inherited, vii

care (*see also* child-care *and* infants, care), 176, 180, 184, 237–9, 241–8, 265, 293; active, 243; age/sex dimensions of, 242, 246; alloparental, 237, 249; care behavior, 241; care-giver, 237–8, 241, 243–5; age, 238; male as, to offspring, 222, 229; potential, 246; sex, 238; care-giving, 237, 265; recipients of care-giving behavior, 242; care-receiver, 237; care-taker, 7, 239, 241–3, 245–7, 265, 293, 300; identification of, 247; identity of, 245; non-parental, 245; secondary, 273; adult secondary, 274; care-taking, 244–5, 273–4, 301; ability, 238; assistance in, 247; male, 246; tasks, 269; direct care, 183, 237–8, 242–3, 246, 248–9, 266, 268, 271, 273–4, 293, 295; low paternal participation in, 238; general care, 241, 244–5; indirect care, 183, 238, 246, 248; intensive, 247; male, 249; night-time, 241; unrecorded night-time, 241; non-nursing, 244, 246; normalized, 246; of children, 240; outside the village, 243; parental, 237, 280; passive, 243; physical, 249; sources of, 244; total, 241–2

carnivores, social, 176, 286

carrier, 243–4 (child)-carrying, 241–4, 248; carrying/holding, 243–5

cash, 67–8, 91, 174; cash cropping, 85, 239; cash crops, 190; earnings, 67; economy, 86; employment, 68

344

Index

Index

psyche: female, 154; human, make-up and activities of the, 338; male, 154

pyschiatry: psychiatric inpatients, 226; treatment, 226; inpatient, 226

psychologists, vii, 318, 324

psychology, 318; 'folk psychology', 325; sex differences in, 15; psychological differentiation, 142; mechanisms, evolved, 313; mechanisms, proximate, 260

puberty, 137–9, 145, 293–4, 300

range, 132–3, 143–4, 267; annual, 133; breeding, 133; exploration, 266–7; hearing, 270; home, 132, 143, 265; male, 132, 139; mating, 266; normal female, 139; parentally defined spatial-range restriction, 143; ranges of boys, 144; of girls, 144; range sizes, home, 132, 144, 265; sex differences in, 143–4; sexually dimorphic, 133; spatial, 143; visual, 270

ranging, 141–3; activity, 145; behavior of children, 143; behavior of men and women, 144; experiences, 141–2, 145–6; sex differences in, 141–3, 145; patterns, 133, 141, 143; sex differences in, 133

rank, 5, 52, 59, 183, 325, 327–9, 333; élite, 211; high, 50, 232; high-ranking men, 57; matrilineally inherited chiefly, 52; men of, 53, 57; of higher social, 204; people without, 54; top-ranking, 333

reciprocity ('reciprocity'), 49–50, 247–9

redistribution, 49, 51, 53, 55, 59–60, 100, 104; ritual, of furs, 50; social function of, 50

redistributor, 49–50

relatedness, 11–13, 15, 34–5, 67, 91–3, 145, 238–9, 242, 245–9, 301, 332–3; average, 54; coefficients of, 12; genealogical, 87, 93, 95, 190; coefficient of, 11; of plot 'owners', 92–3; genetic, 313; patterns of, 297; variations in, 335; local, 92; asymmetry, 194; status, 91; to potential laborers, 93; to the local pool of potential laborers, 93

relationship (relation), 69, 70, 91, 98, 155, 222, 247, 299, 334; adaptive, 98; biological, 298; close spatial psychosocial, between mother and infant, 256; closeness of, 12; coefficient of, to the infant, 247; cousin, 175; exchange, 249; illicit sexual, 155, 230; male, to female kin, 41; mating and marriage, 190; network of, within the village community, 167; parent–child, 260; parent–offspring, 191, 193; productive, 91; between affines, 68; between age of mother and risk of parental violence towards step-children, 257; between individual strategies and conventional moral and jural rules, 312; between individual strategies, and social rules and cultural traditions, 313; between social rules and individual strategies, 311; to perpetrator of sexual assault, 228; within a community, 161; polyandrous, 158; recurring pattern of dominant–subordinate, 214; simultaneous and sequential, 156; social, 222, 230; unconscious relationship-calculator, 324

relatives, 30, 34–5, 39, 43–5, 87, 90, 101, 163–4, 174, 180, 191, 270, 310, 327–8, 335–6; a child's, 246; ascending-generation, 12; assistance to, other than offspring, 89; blood, 228; classified, 37; closest, 332; collateral, 328–9, 335; collateral male, 89; co-resident, 44; descendant, 335; descending-generation, 37; distant, 98; (older) female, 41–2, 123, 193; genetic, 89, 167, 174; kinship categories of, 167; male, 121–3,

332; (close) matrilineal, 12, 175; 'my darling [younger] female', 37; 'my darling [younger] male', 37; own-generation, 12, 37; size of the family of older, 110; unmarried male, 177; very young, 38

religion, 222, 225, 232, 308, 310, 319; childhood, 231–2; current, 231–2; effect of, on reproduction, 310; religious activities, 233; beliefs, 165; career, 202; classification, 225, community, membership of, 310; houses (see monasteries and Tibet); organizations, 226; preference, 225, 232; services, 226

remarriage, 154, 157, 159, 254–5, 258–60, 309; date of the, 259; mother's, 258; of males, 157; of the (surviving) investor, 258; rate of, 122

repeatability, 319–20

reproduction, 13, 25, 40, 51, 59–60, 83, 98, 110–11, 119, 132, 165–6, 174, 179–81, 184, 186, 211, 223, 227, 230, 238, 249, 264, 277, 294, 297, 300–3, 307–9, 325–7, 329; a mother's rate of, 244; age at first, 5, 287; age differences at first, 26; age of, 26, 30; biological, 167; biology of mammalian, 238; completed, 180; continued, 301; costs of, male–female differences in the, 238; differential, 6, 60–1, 205–6, 254, 260; direct, 56, 89, 173, 176–7, 181–2, 186, 308–9; each adult's lifetime, 333; effect of religion on, 310; family, 102; élite family, 206; (direct) female, 25, 182, 207, 239, 308; first, 294; indirect, 309; investment in current, 253; late age of female, 294; male, 25, 207, 211, 213, 301; means to, 5; modes of, 61; offspring, 238; parents', 288; personal, 163; probability of successful, 301; psychology and physiology of, 184; rapid, 112; rates of, high, 184, 210; per generation, 103; potential, 238; reduced future, 174; reproduction, 50, 60; scheduling of, 293; sexual, 15; spouse's age at first, 5; strategies of, 78; successful, 294, 300; suppression of, 202; variance in, 158; balanced, 159

reproductive (reproductive) advantage, 5, 23, 47, 51, 58–9, 74, 78, 93, 110, 311, 313; the female's, 274

reproductive benefit (see also benefit), 60, 74, 174, 196, 333; additional, 288; net, 9

reproductive career, 67, 173, 177, 186, 206, 211, 228, 233, 287–8, 300, 304, 311; differences in the duration of male and female, 239

reproductive cost-benefit: analyzers, 325; assessment, 325

reproductive cycle (cycling), 295, 302

reproductive decisions, 184, 277–8, 291, 302; female, 280; male, 280, 302; reproductive decision-making, 302; women's, 299

reproductive effort, 3–4, 7, 9, 11, 15, 83, 89, 121, 129, 133, 174, 176, 280, 309, 327; expenditures of, 12; human, 3

reproductive fitness (see fitness)

reproductive history, 93, 226–7, 234, 281; Ache, 296; of adults, 90

reproductive interests, 29, 55, 76; individual, 102; mutual, 87; woman's, 121

reproductive maturity, 87, 90

reproductive opportunities, 68, 176

reproductive performance, 75–6, 204–14; differences in, 207; differential, 207; female, 202, 204–5, 207; human, 257; male, 205–7, 213; measurement of, 204; of newly married males, 206; range of variation in, 207

Index